KU-013-120

Diabetic Retinopathy

CONTEMPORARY DIABETES

ARISTIDIS VEVES, MD

SERIES EDITOR

The Diabetic Foot: *Second Edition,* edited by *Aristidis Veves, MD, John M. Giurini, DPM, and Frank W. LoGerfo, MD, 2006*

The Diabetic Kidney, edited by *Pedro Cortes, MD and Carl Erik Mogensen, MD, 2006*

Obesity and Diabetes, edited by *Christos S. Mantzoros, MD, 2006*

Diabetic Retinopathy, edited by *Elia J. Duh, MD, 2008*

Diabetic Retinopathy

Edited by

Elia J. Duh, MD
The Wilmer Ophthalmological Institute
Johns Hopkins University
School of Medicine
Baltimore, MD, USA

Humana Press

Editor
Elia J. Duh, MD
The Wilmer Ophthalmological Institute
Johns Hopkins University School of Medicine
Baltimore, MD
USA

Series Editor
Aristides Veves
Beth-Israel Deaconess Medical Center
Boston, MA
USA

ISBN: 978-1-934115-83-1 e-ISBN: 978-1-59745-563-3
DOI: 10.1007/978-1-59745-563-3

Library of Congress Control Number: 2008936769

© 2008 Humana Press, a part of Springer Science+Business Media, LLC
All rights reserved. This work may not be translated or copied in whole or in part without the written permission of the publisher (Humana Press, 999 Riverview Drive, Suite 208, Totowa, NJ 07512 USA), except for brief excerpts in connection with reviews or scholarly analysis. Use in connection with any form of information storage and retrieval, electronic adaptation, computer software, or by similar or dissimilar methodology now known or hereafter developed is forbidden.
The use in this publication of trade names, trademarks, service marks, and similar terms, even if they are not identified as such, is not to be taken as an expression of opinion as to whether or not they are subject to proprietary rights.
While the advice and information in this book are believed to be true and accurate at the date of going to press, neither the authors nor the editors nor the publisher can accept any legal responsibility for any errors or omissions that may be made. The publisher makes no warranty, express or implied, with respect to the material contained herein.

Printed on acid-free paper

9 8 7 6 5 4 3 2 1

springer.com

Preface

Diabetic retinopathy is the most common microvascular complication of diabetes and remains a major cause of new-onset visual loss in the United States and other industrialized nations. In addition to the morbidity and suffering caused by visual loss, the economic impact from diabetic retinopathy is tremendous. Despite significant advances in scientific understanding of diabetic retinopathy, the major treatments for this condition have largely remained the same for many years. Indeed, laser photocoagulation for proliferative diabetic retinopathy emerged in the late 1960's, and the Early Treatment Diabetic Retinopathy Study (ETDRS) guidelines for laser treatment of macular edema were formulated around the mid-1980's. Guidelines for vitrectomy for vitreous hemorrhage and retinal detachment were also formulated in the 1980's.

However, new therapeutic strategies are being advanced, which raise the prospect that the years ahead will see very significant additions to the options for treatment of diabetic retinopathy. Both corticosteroids and anti-VEGF treatments are serving as additional options in the clinical management of DR. The emergence of anti-VEGF treatments strongly highlights the advent of rational drug therapy based on the identification of causative mechanisms and molecular targets. There is ample reason to anticipate additional significant therapeutic advances in the not too distant future, made possible by the great progress that has been made in identifying new molecules, pathways, and processes that promote diabetic retinopathy, all of which serve as potential therapeutic targets.

For these reasons, this is a very appropriate time to assess the current state of knowledge regarding the clinical management of DR as well as its underlying mechanisms. This book is intended to depict the current clinical understanding of DR as well as the many scientific advances in understanding this condition. The first section encompasses the current understanding of diabetic retinopathy from a clinical standpoint, including current clinical practice. The second section serves as a description of the current understanding of the pathophysiology of DR from the standpoint of biomedical research. Many of these advances may serve as the basis for the development of additional therapeutic strategies. The pathogenesis of DR is certainly multi-factorial, and there is clearly interplay between many of these factors. Although a wide array of topics is covered, this section certainly does not encompass the entire gamut of pathogenic mechanisms of this complex disease, and it is anticipated that further important molecules and processes will emerge in the years ahead. The third and final section discusses new and more recent concepts relating to management and treatment of DR.

I am grateful to the many authors who contributed the chapters in this text. These individuals are internationally recognized leaders in diabetic retinopathy, and their prominence and expertise in their respective fields are invaluable to this discussion. Indeed, I have every expectation that they will continue to be among the leaders in advancing the understanding and treatment of diabetic retinopathy in the years to come. This is an exciting time in the research and management of DR, and it is my hope that this text will help in stimulating further advances in this field.

Elia J. Duh, MD

Contents

Contributors

ANTHONY P. ADAMIS • *Jerini Ophthalmic, Inc., New York, NY, USA*
LLOYD P. AIELLO • *Joslin Diabetes Center, Harvard Medical School, Boston, MA, USA*

DAVID A. ANTONETTI • *Department of Cellular and Molecular Physiology and Ophthalmology, Penn State College of Medicine, Hershey, PA, USA*

ALISTAIR J. BARBER • *The Penn State Retina Research Group, Penn State University College of Medicine, Hershey, PA, USA*

MICHAEL BOULTON • *Department of Ophthalmology and Visual Sciences, The University of Texas Medical Branch, Galveston, TX, USA*

SERGIO CABALLERO • *Dept. of Pharmacology and Therapeutics, University of Florida, Gainesville, Florida*

RUTH B. CALDWELL • *Vascular Biology Center, Medical College of Georgia Augusta, GA*

ROBERT W. CALDWELL • *Department of Pharmacology & Toxicology, Medical College of Georgia, Augusta, GA*

POOI-SEE CHAN • *Kresge Eye Institute, Wayne State University, Detroit, MI*

NING CHEUNG • *Centre for Eye Research Australia, the University of Melbourne, Royal Victorian Eye and Ear Hospital, Melbourne*

EMILY Y. CHEW • *National Eye Institute, National Institutes of Health, Bethesda, Maryland*

RONALD P. DANIS • *Department of Ophthalmology and Visual Sciences, University of Wisconsin-Madison, Madison, WI*

ARUP DAS • *Department of Surgery, and Cell Biology & Physiology, University of New Mexico School of Medicine, Albuquerque, NM; New Mexico VA Health Care System, Albuquerque, NM*

MATTHEW D. DAVIS • *Department of Ophthalmology and Visual Sciences, University of Wisconsin-Madison, Madison, WI*

DIANA V. DO • *The Wilmer Eye Institute, The Johns Hopkins University School of Medicine, Baltimore, Maryland*

Elia J. Duh • *The Wilmer Eye Institute, The Johns Hopkins University School of Medicine, Baltimore, MD*

Azza E.B. El-Remessy • *College of Pharmacy, University of Georgia, Augusta, GA*

Yuxi Feng • *5th Medical Department, University Hospital Mannheim, University of Heidelberg, Mannheim, Germany*

Frederick L. Ferris III • *National Eye Institute, National Institutes of Health, Bethesda, Maryland*

Thomas W. Gardner • *The Penn State Retina Research Group, Penn State University College of Medicine, Hershey, PA*

Mark C. Gillies • *Department of Clinical Ophthalmology, Save Sight Institute, University of Sydney, Australia*

Maria B. Grant • *Dept. of Pharmacology and Therapeutics, University of Florida, Gainesville, Florida*

Julia A. Haller • *The Wilmer Eye Institute, The Johns Hopkins University School of Medicine, Baltimore, Maryland*

Rola Hamam • *Joslin Diabetes Center, Harvard Medical School, Boston, MA*

Hans-Peter Hammes • *5th Medical Department, University Hospital Mannheim, University of Heidelberg, Mannheim, Germany*

Antonia M. Joussen • *Department of Ophthalmology, University of Düsseldorf, Düsseldorf, Germany*

Peter K. Kaiser • *Cole Eye Institute, Cleveland Clinic Foundation, Cleveland, OH*

Timothy S. Kern • *Department of Medicine, Case Western Reserve University, Cleveland, OH*

George L. King • *Joslin Diabetes Center, Harvard Medical School, Boston, MA*

Ronald Klein • *Department of Ophthalmology and Visual Sciences, University of Wisconsin School of Medicine and Public Health, Madison, WI*

Renu A. Kowluru • *Kresge Eye Institute, Wayne State University, Detroit, MI*

Alexander V. Ljubimov • *Ophthalmology Research Laboratories, Cedars-Sinai Medical Center and Department of Medicine, David Geffen School of Medicine at UCLA, Los Angeles, CA*

Mara Lorenzi • *Schepens Eye Research Institute, Harvard Medical School, Boston, MA*

Cheng Mao-Lin • *Department of Cellular and Molecular Physiology and Ophthalmology, Penn State College of Medicine, Hershey, PA*

RON MARGOLIS • *Cole Eye Institute, Cleveland Clinic Foundation, Cleveland, OH*

PAUL G. MCGUIRE • *Department of Surgery, and Cell Biology & Physiology, University of New Mexico School of Medicine, Albuquerque, NM*

CATHERINE B. MEYERLE • *National Eye Institute, National Institutes of Health, Bethesda, Maryland*

DEEPTI NAVARATNA • *Department of Cell Biology & Physiology, University of New Mexico School of Medicine, Albuquerque, NM*

QUAN DONG NGUYEN • *The Wilmer Eye Institute, The Johns Hopkins University School of Medicine, Baltimore, Maryland*

PETER J. OATES • *Pfizer Global Research and Development, CVMED Department, Groton, CT*

FREDERICK PFISTER • *5th Medical Department, University Hospital Mannheim, University of Heidelberg, Mannheim, Germany*

MANVI PRAKASH • *Joslin Diabetes Center, Harvard Medical School, Boston, MA*

SYED MAHMOOD SHAH • *The Wilmer Eye Institute, The Johns Hopkins University School of Medicine, Baltimore, Maryland*

ALAN W. STITT • *Centre for Vision Science, Queens University of Belfast, Northern Ireland, UK*

CARLA STRIATA • *Ophthalmology Europe, Pfizer Ltd UK*

JENNIFER K. SUN • Joslin Diabetes Center, Harvard Medical School, Boston, MA

LAUREN E. SWENARCHUK • *Zola Associates, Englewood Cliffs, New Jersey*

HEATHER D. VANGUILDER • *The Penn State Retina Research Group, Penn State University College of Medicine, Hershey, PA*

LINDA E. WHETTER, DVM • *Zola Associates, Englewood Cliffs, New Jersey*

TIEN Y. WONG, FRANZCO • *Centre for Eye Research Australia, the University of Melbourne, Royal Victorian Eye and Ear Hospital, Melbourne*

I

Clinical Aspects of Diabetic Retinopathy

1 Nonproliferative Diabetic Retinopathy

Catherine B. Meyerle, Emily Y. Chew, and Frederick L. Ferris III

CONTENTS

ABSTRACT

Nonproliferative diabetic retinopathy (NPDR) is a microvascular complication of diabetes mellitus that can lead to irreversible visual loss. Intraretinal microvascular changes, such as altered retinal vascular permeability and eventual retinal vessel and capillary closure, characterize NPDR. Macular edema, the most frequent cause of visual loss in NPDR, may result from increased vascular leakage. Retinal hypoxia, secondary to chronic hyperglycemia, triggers the pathologic processes of NPDR. Additionally, there is increasing evidence that inflammatory mechanisms may play a role in the pathogenesis. Systemic factors such as glycemic control, hypertension, and serum lipid level also contribute to the development and progression of NPDR. Prompt and appropriate initiation of laser photocoagulation for macular edema or severe retinal nonperfusion, along with optimal control of systemic factors, can prevent visual loss.

Key Words: Diabetes mellitus; Diabetic retinopathy; Macular edema; Laser photocoagulation.

From: *Contemporary Diabetes*: *Diabetic Retinopathy*
Edited by: E. Duh © Humana Press, Totowa, NJ

NONPROLIFERATIVE DIABETIC RETINOPATHY

Diabetes is an epidemic affecting more than 18 million people in the United States *(1)*. Chronic hyperglycemia triggers a cascade of molecular events that leads to microvascular damage. Diabetic retinopathy is the most prevalent microvascular complication and can lead to irreversible visual loss. Epidemiologic studies show that diabetic retinopathy is a leading cause of acquired blindness in people aged 20–74 years in the United States, with 12,000–24,000 new cases of legal blindness each year *(1–3)*. The retinal manifestations of diabetes mellitus are broadly classified as either nonproliferative diabetic retinopathy (NPDR) or proliferative diabetic retinopathy (PDR).

Nonproliferative diabetic retinopathy occurs when there are only intraretinal microvascular changes, such as altered retinal vascular permeability and eventual retinal vessel closure. Clinically, the hallmark of the nonproliferative phase is microaneurysms and intraretinal abnormalities. Neovascularization is not a component of the nonproliferative phase. However, in advanced NPDR, nonperfusion of the retina may develop and lead to the proliferative phase. Proliferative diabetic retinopathy is characterized by new vessels and sometimes fibrous bands proliferating on the retinal surface. In both nonproliferative and proliferative diabetic retinopathy, macular edema can occur as increased retinal vascular permeability leads to accumulation of fluid in the retinal area serving central vision. This chapter focuses on the clinical aspects of NPDR.

PATHOPHYSIOLOGY OF NONPROLIFERATIVE DIABETIC RETINOPATHY

Effective and appropriate management of NPDR is dependent on a clear understanding of the disease course. Chronic hyperglycemia in poorly controlled diabetes results in biochemical alterations and altered hemodynamics of the retinal vasculature, which lead to chronic hypoxia *(4, 5)*. Since the retina is a highly metabolic tissue dependent on optimal oxygenation, compensatory pathways, such as upregulation of vascular endothelial growth factor (VEGF) protein, are targeted against this retinal hypoxia. These efforts are futile, however, and ultimately result in the pathologic processes of NPDR: retinal capillary microaneurysms, vascular permeability, and eventual vascular occlusion, or capillary closure.

Inflammatory Mechanisms

Increasing evidence suggests that inflammation may play a role in the pathogenesis of diabetic retinopathy. Multiple animal and human tissue studies have indicated that chronic inflammation contributes to diabetic vascular damage.

Intercellular adhesion molecule 1 (ICAM-1), a member of the immunoglobulin superfamily involved in immune activation and inflammation, and its counter-receptor CD18 are thought to play a pivotal role *(6, 7)*. ICAM-1 mediates leukocyte migration into inflammatory sites via its interaction with different cytokines. Increased leukocyte adhesion to the diabetic vascular endothelium can promote endothelial apoptosis, resulting in vascular permeability and capillary nonperfusion *(7, 8)*. In the rat model of streptozotocin-induced diabetes *(9)*, retinal leukostasis increased within days of developing diabetes and correlated with the increased expression of retinal ICAM-1. Additionally,

ICAM-1 blockade in this rat model prevented diabetic retinal leukostasis and vascular leakage by 48.5 and 85.6%, respectively. Other rat models have shown that antibody-based inhibition of ICAM-1 and CD18 may prevent acellular capillary formation via the suppression of endothelial cell injury and death *(10)*.

Studies of human tissue have also suggested an inflammatory role in the pathogenesis of diabetic retinopathy. Immunoassays for the quantitative determination of soluble ICAM-1 in the vitreous of PDR patients undergoing vitrectomy showed elevated ICAM-1 levels when compared with that in the control group *(6)*. In another study *(11)*, frozen sections of a donor eye obtained at autopsy from a patient with documented severe NPDR and diabetic macular edema were compared with a normal nondiabetic eye. Immunoperoxidase staining was positive for inflammatory chemokines such as monocyte chemoattractant protein, RANTES (Regulated on Activation Normal T Cell Expressed and Secreted), and ICAM-1 in the retina of the diabetic eye, while the non-diabetic eye showed little reactivity. Serum levels of inflammatory mediators also appear to correlate with increasing diabetic retinopathy severity. In one study of 93 participants, the serum levels of proinflammatory RANTES and stromal cell-derived factor were significantly elevated in patients with at least severe NPDR, compared with those in patients with less severe diabetic retinopathy *(11)*. Similar to the animal studies, these human studies suggest that inflammation may play a central role in the development of diabetic retinopathy.

While the precise components of the inflammatory pathways in the pathogenesis of diabetic retinopathy are still being investigated, the recognition of the role of inflammation in this retinal disease suggests the potential utility of using anti-inflammatory therapies. Further research is required to translate these scientific findings into clinical care.

Microaneurysms

The retinal capillary microaneurysm usually is the first visible sign of diabetic retinopathy. Microaneurysms, identified clinically by ophthalmoscopy as deep-red dots varying from 15 to 60 μm in diameter, are most common in the posterior pole. Although microaneurysms can be associated with other retinal vascular diseases, particularly those associated with vascular occlusion such as branch and central vein occlusions, they are the hallmark of NPDR.

Histologically, microaneurysms are hypercellular saccular outpouchings of the capillary wall, as demonstrated by trypsin digest retinal mounts *(12)*. Experimental models of diabetic retinopathy in dogs and rats and studies of human autopsy eyes indicate that the initial step in the pathogenesis of diabetic retinopathy is the loss of intramural capillary pericytes. Subsequently, microaneurysms form and capillary closure ensues, leading to the development of acellular capillaries. Another early morphologic finding in diabetic retinopathy is the thickening of the basement membrane of the retinal capillaries. The importance of this thickening in the pathogenesis of diabetic retinopathy is unknown *(13–15)*.

The mechanism for the formation of microaneurysms is also unknown. Possible mechanisms include release of a vasoproliferative factor with endothelial cell proliferation, weakness of the capillary wall (from loss of pericytes), abnormalities of the adjacent retina, and increased intraluminal pressure *(16–18)*.

Microaneurysms may be difficult to differentiate from punctate hemorrhages seen in diabetic retinopathy. However, on the early frames of a fluorescein angiogram, microaneurysms are easily distinguished from intraretinal hemorrhages because they exhibit bright hyperfluorescence against the darker choroidal background, whereas retinal hemorrhages block fluorescence (Figs. 1 and 2). Microaneurysms may show little change over many years, but the lumens can occlude, as demonstrated by hyperfluorescence on fluorescein angiography, and after recanalization the microaneurysms can disappear *(19)*. It is typical for individual microaneurysms to appear and disappear with time. Without the other components of diabetic retinopathy, microaneurysms alone have no apparent clinical significance. However, an increase in the number of microaneurysms in the retina is associated with progression of retinopathy *(20–22)*. When the number of microaneurysms increases, there is an increased likelihood that the other microvascular changes of diabetic retinopathy may also be present.

Vascular Permeability

As microvascular damage increases in the presence of excessive blood glucose, increased vascular permeability occurs through multiple pathways. Vascular endothelial growth factor (VEGF) protein is thought to play a pivotal role. A healthy human retina contains little VEGF, but its level is increased in response to hypoxia that can occur in states such as diabetic retinopathy. Originally described as vascular permeability factor, VEGF is not only a mediator of new blood vessel formation seen in PDR, but also an inducer of vascular permeability, which can lead to retinal edema seen in both nonproliferative and proliferative diabetic retinopathy *(23–25)*. The molecular pathway for this

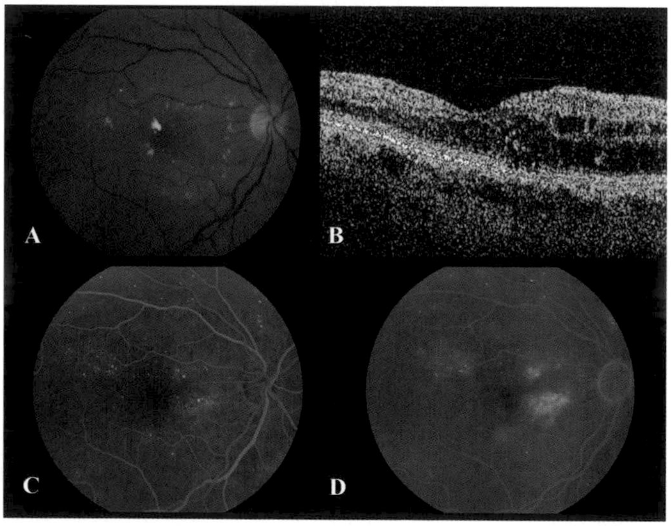

Fig. 1. The right eye of a 55-year-old woman with mild macular edema. (**A**) Color photograph shows circinate ring of lipid and microaneurysms. Best-corrected vision is 20/25. (**B**) Optical coherence tomography shows mild macular edema with preservation of the foveal contour. (**C**) Early phase of fluorescein angiogram highlights the multiple microaneurysms. (**D**) Late phase of fluorescein angiogram shows patchy areas of leakage.

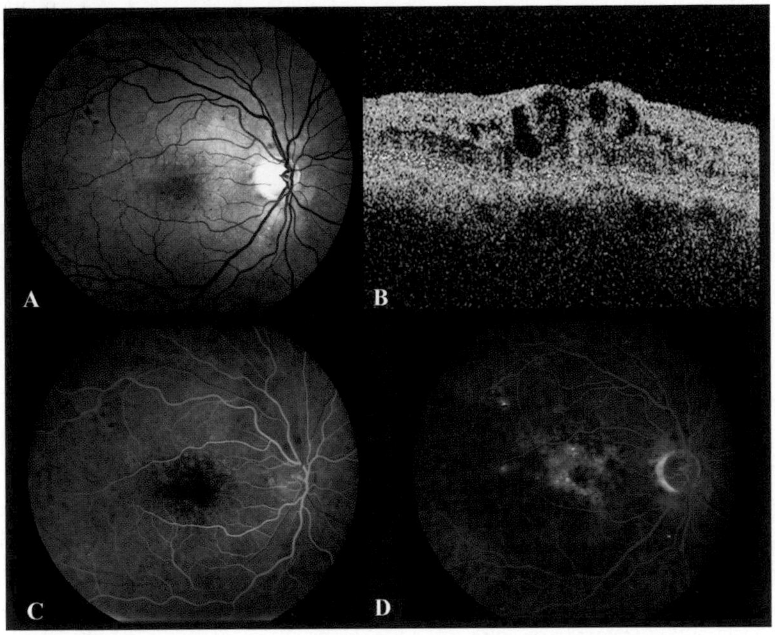

Fig. 2. The right eye of a 68-year-old man with chronic macular edema. (**A**) Red-free photograph shows multiple microaneurysms in this patient with type 2 diabetes for 45 years. Best-corrected visual acuity was 20/63 despite multiple treatments over many years, including focal laser, subtenon triamcinolone, and intravitreal bevacizumab. (**B**) Optical coherence tomography shows large intraretinal cysts and foveal distortion. (**C**) Early fluorescein angiogram highlights the multiple microaneurysms. (**D**) Late fluorescein angiogram shows petalloid edema.

pro-angiogenic factor involves VEGF tyrosine kinase receptors located on endothelial cells. This homodimeric protein promotes endothelial cell proliferation, migration, apoptosis, and vascular tube formation. On a molecular level, VEGF induces vessel permeability by causing conformational changes in the tight junctions of the retinal vascular endothelial cells *(26)*. Additionally, some animal studies suggest that VEGF contributes to the inflammatory component of diabetic retinopathy by upregulating ICAM-1 *(7)*. Other molecules suspected to be involved in vascular permeability include protein kinase C-beta (PKC-beta) *(27, 28)*. In addition to vessel permeability changes, PKC-beta is associated with other classic pathological changes seen in diabetes, such as basement membrane thickening and prolonged retinal circulation time *(29–32)*.

Retinal edema resulting from increased vascular permeability is particularly significant if it occurs in the macula. Macular edema is defined clinically as retinal thickening from accumulation of fluid within 1 disc diameter of the macula *(24, 33, 34)*. As the fluid disrupts the architecture of the macular region serving central visual acuity, macular edema can cause significant visual loss. Fluorescein angiography can be used to identify excessive permeability and may demonstrate the classic petalloid leakage pattern that occurs as fluid accumulates in the radially oriented layer of Henle (Fig. 2). While fluorescein angiography may be useful to guide focal laser treatment of macular edema and to identify macular nonperfusion contributing to visual loss, it is not required to make the diagnosis of macular edema. Macular edema is best detected with a combination of techniques, including slit-lamp biomicroscopy, stereoscopic fundus photography, and optical coherence tomography. On clinical examination, a contact lens is particularly helpful for detecting subtle fluid changes in the macula. Stereoscopic fundus photography is useful, but requires a skilled photographer. Optical coherence tomography is an imaging modality that uses near-infrared light beams to create high-resolution cross-sections of the vitreoretinal interface, retina, and subretinal space. Essentially, it provides an in vivo histological section that can demonstrate the cystic spaces that occur in macular edema (Figs. 1–3). Optical coherence tomography can also detect any traction contributing to the macular edema and provide quantitative measurements of the macular fluid.

Clinically, hard exudates often accompany macular edema and appear as well-defined, yellowish white intraretinal deposits. They generally occur in the posterior pole at the border of edematous and nonedematous retinas. These hard exudates are lipid deposits that presumably accumulate in association with lipoprotein leakage caused by breakdown of endothelial tight junctions in microaneurysms or retinal capillaries.

Edema fluid may wax and wane within the retina without visual consequence in some cases, but can result in permanent visual loss if the fluid chronically disrupts the delicate macular architecture. Lipid deposits, especially when under the center of the macula, are a poor prognostic sign as they are often associated with permanent visual loss *(35, 36)*. Increased serum lipid is significant because it correlates with the degree of retinal lipid deposits *(37, 38)*.

Capillary Closure

One of the most serious consequences of diabetic retinopathy is the obliteration of the retinal capillaries. When patches of acellular capillaries, seen early in the course of diabetic retinopathy, increase and become confluent, the terminal arterioles that supply these capillaries often become occluded. Adjacent to these areas of nonperfused retina, clusters of microaneurysms and tortuous, hypercellular vessels often develop. It is difficult to determine whether these vessels are dilated preexisting capillaries or

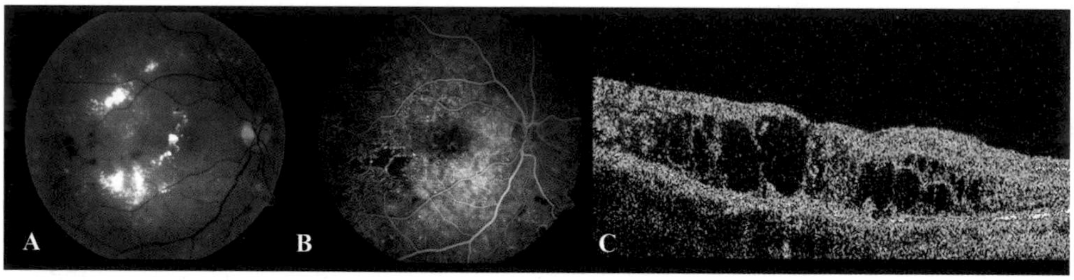

Fig. 3. The right eye of a 65-year-old woman with a history of nonperfusion and severe macular edema. (**A**) Red-free photograph shows a ring of hard exudates with marked retinal thickening and edema involving the center of the macula, although not visible in this nonstereoscopic photograph. Several microaneurysms are also visible within the thickened areas. Best-corrected visual acuity was 20/200. Panretinal photocoagulation scars initiated for severe nonperfusion are also evident in this photograph. (**B**) Fluorescein angiogram at 28 s shows patches of nonperfusion temporal to the fovea and some perifoveal leakage. (**C**) Optical coherence tomography illustrates the loss of foveal contour in the setting of extensive cystic edema.

neovascularization within the retina. These vessels have been referred to as *intraretinal microvascular abnormalities* (IRMA) clinically to include both possibilities (Fig. b).

As capillary closure becomes extensive, it is common to see many intraretinal hemorrhages or dilated segments of retinal veins (venous beading), or both. The severity of IRMA, intraretinal hemorrhages, and venous beading is directly associated with increasing nonperfusion and resulting ischemia. This ischemia has a major pathogenic role in the development of retinal neovascularization. Endothelial proliferation occurs following ischemia with the subsequent preretinal new vessel proliferation and progression to the proliferative phase of diabetic retinopathy.

CLASSIFICATION OF NONPROLIFERATIVE RETINOPATHY

Diabetic retinopathy is broadly categorized as nonproliferative (NPDR) or proliferative. In the nonproliferative stage, retinopathy is categorized further into four levels of severity: mild, moderate, severe, and very severe (Table 1). Accurate diagnosis of the stage of NPDR is essential as it determines the risk for progression to PDR and the appropriate timing for clinical examinations. The extent of IRMA, venous abnormalities, and the retinal hemorrhages are the factors that determine the level of severity of nonproliferative disease. In the mild-to-moderate nonproliferative categories (formerly termed *background retinopathy*), there are relatively few intraretinal hemorrhages and microaneurysms. The severe nonproliferative stage (formerly termed *preproliferative retinopathy*) represents increasing ischemia and is clinically detected by evaluating the four midperipheral retinal quadrants using the so-called 4–2–1 rule *(39)*. Patients with any one of the following features are considered to have severe nonproliferative retinopathy: (1) severe intraretinal hemorrhages and microaneurysms in all *four* quadrants (Fig. 4a), (2) venous beading in *two* or more quadrants (Fig. 4b), or (3) moderate IRMA in at least *one* quadrant (Fig. 4b). If any two of these features are present, the retinopathy level is considered to be very severe nonproliferative.

Table 1
Classification of Severity of Nonproliferative Diabetic Retinopathy

Level of severity	*Lesions present*
No retinopathy	No retinal lesions
Mild	Mild levels of microaneurysms and intraretinal hemorrhage
Moderate	Moderate levels of microaneurysms and intraretinal hemorrhage
Severe	Presence of one of the following features (4:2:1 rule) *(39)*: 1. Severe intraretinal hemorrhage in all 4 quadrants 2. Venous beading in 2 or more quadrants 3. Moderate IRMA in at least 1 quadrant
Very severe	Presence of two or more of the above-mentioned features described in severe nonproliferative diabetic retinopathy

IRMA intraretinal microvascular abnormalities

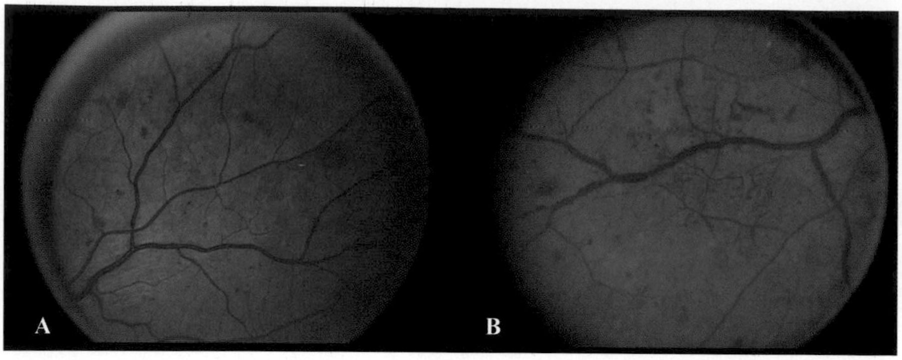

Fig. 4. "4–2–1" Rule. (**A**) Using the 4–2–1 rule, the presence of hemorrhages and microaneurysms in at least four midperipheral fields, equaling or exceeding this standard photograph, would qualify as severe nonproliferative diabetic retinopathy. (**B**) This standard photograph shows both venous beading and intraretinal microvascular abnormalities (IRMA). If there is venous beading in at least two quadrants or if there is IRMA in at least one quadrant, the patient has severe nonproliferative diabetic retinopathy according to the 4–2–1 rule.

MACULAR EDEMA

Macular edema is the most frequent cause of visual impairment in patients with NPDR. The breakdown of endothelial tight junctions and loss of the "blood–retinal" barrier seen in diabetic macular edema can occur in either nonproliferative or proliferative diabetic retinopathy at any stage. The prevalence of macular edema after 15 years of known diabetes, according to the Wisconsin Epidemiologic Study of Diabetic Retinopathy, is ~20% in patients with type 1 diabetes, 25% in patients with insulin-dependent type 2 diabetes, and 14% in patients with non-insulin dependent type 2 diabetes *(40)*. In macular edema, as VEGF is upregulated, excessive vascular permeability occurs because of increasing endothelial cell fenestrations *(26)*. This vascular permeability results in the leakage of fluid and plasma constituents, such as lipoproteins, into the retina and eventually leads to thickening of the retina. Macular edema is best detected by stereoscopic examination techniques and optical coherence tomography (Fig. 1–3). One study comparing the detection of diabetic foveal edema with contact lens biomicroscopy and OCT suggested that mild diabetic macular edema may be more readily detected by OCT *(41)*.

When thickening involves or threatens the center of the fovea, there is a higher risk of visual loss. In the Early Treatment Diabetic Retinopathy Study (ETDRS), the 3-year risk of moderate visual loss (a doubling of the initial visual angle, e.g., 20/30 to 20/60, or a decrease of 3 lines or more on a logarithmic visual acuity chart) was 32%. The ETDRS investigators classified macular edema by its severity. It was defined as *clinically significant macular edema* if any of the following features were present: (1) thickening of the retina at or within 500 μm of the center of the macula, (2) hard exudates at or within 500 μm of the center of the macula, if associated with thickening of the adjacent retina (not residual hard exudates remaining after the disappearance of retinal thickening), or (3) a zone or zones of retinal thickening 1 disc area or larger, any part of which is within 1 disc diameter of the center of the macula (Table 2) *(42)*.

Table 2
Definition of Clinically Significant Macular Edema

Clinically significant macular edema
Thickening of the retina at or within 500 μm of the center of the macula
Or
Hard exudates at or within 500 μm of the center of the macula, if associated with thickening of the adjacent retina (not residual hard exudates remaining after the disappearance of retinal thickening)
Or
Zone of retinal thickening 1 disc area or larger, any part of which is within 1 disc diameter of the center of the macula

RISK FACTORS FOR PROGRESSION OF RETINOPATHY

Severity of Retinopathy

As NPDR progresses, the risk of developing PDR or visual loss also increases. In the ETDRS Study, eyes with very severe NPDR or mild-to-moderate PDR, or both, had a 60-fold increased risk of developing high-risk PDR after 1 year of follow-up, compared with eyes with mild NPDR (48.5% vs. 0.8%). After 5 years of follow-up, there was still a fivefold increased risk (74.4% vs. 14.3%) *(43)*.

The importance of retinopathy severity in predicting progression of retinopathy also was evaluated in the population-based Wisconsin Epidemiological Study of Diabetic Retinopathy *(44)*. In 708 insulin-dependent patients younger than 30 years at time of diagnosis of diabetes, the odds ratio for 4-year progression to PDR was 2.1 for each step increase in baseline retinopathy severity on an 11-step scale. For patients with bilateral moderate NPDR, the 4-year risk of progression to PDR increased by 40-fold when compared with patients who had microaneurysms in only one eye.

Glycemic Control

Hyperglycemia is the instigator of a cascade of events leading to microvascular complications in diabetes. The landmark studies investigating glycemic control and its effects on diabetic complications include the Diabetes Control and Complications Trial (DCCT), Epidemiology of Diabetes Interventions and Complications Trial (EDIC), and the United Kingdom Prospective Diabetes Study (UKPDS). These studies all demonstrated that tight blood glucose control decreases, but does not eliminate, the risk of diabetic retinopathy development and progression (Table 3).

The Diabetes Control and Complications Trial

The DCCT was a randomized, multicenter, prospective trial designed to determine whether intensive insulin treatment, with the goal of near-normal glucose levels, would affect the development and progression of diabetic complications. The 1,441 participant patients with type 1 diabetes were randomly assigned to either conventional or intensive

Table 3
Glycemic control studies

Diabetes Control and Complications Trial (DCCT)	*Epidemiology of Diabetes Interventions and Complications Trial (EDIC)*	*United Kingdom Prospective Diabetes Study (UKPDS)*
Summary		
• Type 1 diabetes mellitus • Intensive vs. conventional glucose control	• Follow-up to DCCT cohort (type 1 diabetes mellitus) • Both the DCCT conventional-therapy and intensive-therapy groups were treated with the same intensive glucose control therapy	• Type 2 diabetes mellitus • Intensive vs. conventional glucose control
Results		
• For participants with no retinopathy at baseline – 75% reduction in 3-year risk of developing retinopathy for intensive group when compared with conventional controls • For participants with preexisting retinopathy – 50% reduction in rate of progression, as compared with conventional controls • 35–40% reduction of risk of retinopathy progression for every 10% decrease in HbA_1C (e.g. 8% – 7.2%)	• After 4 years, proportion of patients who had worsening retinopathy was lower in the DCCT intensive-therapy group than in the DCCT conventional-therapy group despite both having the same HbA_1C level on intensive treatment in EDIC • Suggestive of metabolic memory	• 25% reduction in risk of any diabetic microvascular endpoint (e.g., need for retinal photocoagulation) for intensive group, compared with conventional controls • 35% reduction in risk of microvascular complications for every point decrease in HbA_1C (e.g., 8% – 7%)

insulin treatment and followed up for a period of 4–9 years *(45–49)*. Of the participants, 726 had no retinopathy at baseline (the primary-prevention cohort) and 715 had mild nonproliferative retinopathy (the secondary-intervention cohort). Intensive therapy consisted of an external insulin pump or three or more daily insulin injections guided by frequent blood glucose monitoring, while conventional therapy consisted of one or two daily insulin injections.

Intensive insulin treatment in the DCCT study was associated with a decreased risk of either the development or progression of diabetic retinopathy in patients with type 1 diabetes. In patients without any visible retinopathy when enrolled in the DCCT, the 3-year risk of developing retinopathy was reduced by 75% in the intensive insulin treatment group when compared with the standard treatment group. However, even in the intensively treated group, retinopathy could not be completely prevented over the 9-year course of the study.

The benefit of the strict control was also evident in patients with existing retinopathy. There was a 50% reduction in the rate of progression of retinopathy when compared with controls. At 6- and 12-month visits, a small adverse effect of intensive treatment on retinopathy progression was seen, similar to that described in other trials of glucose control. However, in eyes with little or no retinopathy at the time of initiating intensive glucose control, this early worsening of retinopathy is unlikely to threaten vision. When the DCCT results were stratified by glycosylated hemoglobin (HbA_1C) levels, there was a 35–40% reduction in the risk of retinopathy progression for every 10% decrease in HbA_1C (e.g., from 8% to 7.2%). This represented a fivefold increase in the risk for patients with HbA_1C of about 10% vs. those with a HbA_1C of 7%. Furthermore, there was a statistically significant reduction in both diabetic neuropathy and nephropathy with intensive blood glucose control in the DCCT. The current recommendation for glycemic control is to achieve a HbA_1C level below 7% for patients in general and a level as close to normal (<6%) as possible without significant hypoglycemia for individual patients *(50)*.

Epidemiology of Diabetes Interventions and Complications Trial

EDIC is the long-term follow-up to the DCCT *(51)*. At the conclusion of the DCCT, intensive glucose control was recommended for all participants and the conventional group started intensive diabetic management. Care of all participants was transferred to personal physicians during the EDIC study. Four years after the end of DCCT, the difference in HbA_1C levels between the DCCT conventional-therapy and intensive-therapy groups had narrowed and both groups had a HbA_1C level of ~8%. This likely occurred in EDIC because the original intensive group was not monitored as frequently and the conventional group started intensive therapy. Retinopathy during the fourth year after the conclusion of DCCT was evaluated on the basis of centrally graded fundus photographs. Interestingly, despite the same HbA_1C level in EDIC, the proportion of patients who had worsening retinopathy, including proliferative retinopathy, macular edema, and the need for laser therapy, was lower in the original intensive-therapy group than in the original conventional-therapy group (odds reduction, 72–87%; $P < 0.001$). These data suggest that the original intensive-therapy group had a prolonged benefit in delaying progression of retinopathy. This phenomenon of cells "remembering" tight control for extended periods is known as *metabolic memory*. Clinically, as per the concept of metabolic memory and EDIC results, early intervention with intensive glucose management is critical for preventing long-term complications of retinopathy.

The United Kingdom Prospective Diabetes Study

The effect of glycemic control on the incidence and progression of diabetic retinopathy is similar in patients with type 2 diabetes. UKPDS *(52)*, the largest and longest study of patients with type 2 diabetes, evaluated the effect of conventional vs. intensive glucose management on diabetic complications in 3,867 newly diagnosed patients. Intensive management involved either sulphonylureas or insulin, while conventional treatment relied on diet alone, with drugs added only if there were hyperglycemic symptoms or fasting plasma glucose greater than 15 mmol L^{-1}. The UKPDS showed a 25% reduction in the risk of the "any diabetes-related microvascular end point," including the need for retinal photocoagulation, in the intensive treatment group, compared with the conventional treatment group. After 6 years of follow-up, a smaller proportion of patients in the intensive treatment group, compared with the conventional group, had a two-step progression (worsening) in diabetic retinopathy. Epidemiologic analysis of the UKPDS data showed a continuous relationship between the risk of microvascular complications and glycemia; for every percentage point decrease in HbA_1C (e.g., 9% to 8%), there was a 35% reduction in the risk of microvascular complications.

Hypertension

Hypertension is theorized to exacerbate diabetic retinopathy through mechanical stretching of endothelial cells, resulting in increased VEGF release *(53)*. The findings of multiple studies assessing the importance of blood pressure in the progression of NPDR, however, are inconsistent *(54)*. Large studies correlating tight blood pressure control with reduced risk of retinopathy progression include the UKPDS and Appropriate Blood Pressure Control in Diabetes (ABCD) trials.

The United Kingdom Prospective Diabetes Study

In UKPDS, a randomized comparison of more intensive blood pressure control and less intensive blood pressure control in persons with type 2 diabetes demonstrated that intensive blood pressure control was associated with a decreased risk of retinopathy progression. Of the 1,148 hypertensive patients in the UKPDS, 758 were allocated to tight blood pressure control arm and 390 to less tight control arm, with a median follow-up of 8.4 years *(55)*. Tight blood pressure control resulted in a 37% reduction in microvascular diseases, predominantly reduced risk of retinal photocoagulation, when compared to less tight control. A previously published study of blood pressure medication in diabetic retinopathy suggested that there might be a specific benefit of angiotensin-converting enzyme (ACE) inhibition and blood pressure reduction, even in "normotensive" persons, on the progression of diabetic retinopathy *(56)*. The UKPDS included a randomized comparison of beta-blockers and ACE inhibitors in the tight blood pressure control arm of that study. Benefits from tight blood pressure control were present in both the beta-blocker and ACE inhibitor treatment groups, with no statistically significant difference between them. This suggests that the treatment effect is more likely to be secondary to blood pressure reduction than to a specific effect of ACE inhibitors.

Appropriate Blood Pressure Control in Diabetes Trials

The ABCD trials also showed a correlation between tight blood pressure control and decreased risk of retinopathy *(54, 57)*. This prospective, controlled, randomized study evaluated the effect of intensive vs. moderate diastolic blood pressure control on diabetic vascular complications in 480 normotensive type 2 diabetic patients. Over a 5-year follow-up period, there was less progression of diabetic retinopathy 35% for the intensive therapy group vs. 46% for the moderate control group).

Elevated Serum Lipid Levels

The Wisconsin Epidemiological Study of Diabetic Retinopathy, a population-based study, and the ETDRS found that elevated levels of serum cholesterol were associated with increased severity of retinal hard exudate *(37, 38)*. Independent of the accompanying macular edema, the severity of retinal hard exudate at baseline was associated with decreased visual acuity in the ETDRS. The severity of retinal hard exudate also was a significant risk factor for moderate visual loss (15-letter or more loss) during the course of the study. In addition, the strongest risk factor for the development of subretinal fibrosis in ETDRS patients with diabetic macular edema was the presence of severe hard exudate *(58)*.

The DCCT investigators also evaluated the association of severity of retinopathy and retinal hard exudates with serum lipids *(59)*. The lipoproteins in the total cholesterol were further characterized by nuclear magnetic resonance lipoprotein subclass profile (NMR-LSP), apoA1, apoB, lipoprotein (a), and susceptibility of LDL to oxidation. They found that the severity of retinopathy was associated with increasing triglycerides and inversely associated with HDL cholesterol. The NMR-LSP results showed an increasing severity of retinopathy with small and medium VLDL and an inverse relationship with VLDL size. These data support the potential role of dyslipoproteinemia in the pathogenesis of diabetic retinopathy. More recently, a small controlled prospective study showed reduction in retinal hard exudates after treatment with atorvastatin, although visual acuity was not affected *(60)*. Another small controlled prospective study found that simvastatin lowered the risk of retinopathy progression but did not cause any statistically significant change in visual acuity *(61)*.

Given the well-known systemic benefits of serum lipid control and the current data regarding lipid levels and retinopathy, it is reasonable to recommend optimal control of hyperlipidemia in all diabetic patients. Further studies are required, however, to elucidate the specific benefits of various lipid-lowering therapies on diabetic retinopathy.

Pregnancy and Diabetic Retinopathy

Pregnancy is a risk factor for progression of diabetic retinopathy. The mechanism for disease acceleration may be a result of the pregnancy itself or the changes in metabolic control *(62–65)*. Risk factors for The Diabetes in Early Pregnancy Study *(62)*, a prospective cohort study of 155 diabetic women followed up from the periconceptional period to 1 month postpartum, demonstrate that the stage of retinopathy prior to conception is a predictor of disease progression. 10.3% of patients with no retinopathy, 21.1% of patients with only microaneurysms, and 18.8% with mild nonproliferative retinopathy progressed during this study. However, 54.8% of patients with moderate-to-severe nonproliferative retinopathy at baseline worsened during the study period. Additional risk factors for retinopathy progression in the pregnant population include pregnancy-associated hypertension and poor glycemic control prior to conception *(66)*.

Ideally, patients who are planning to become pregnant should have their eyes examined before they attempt to conceive and should make every attempt to lower their blood glucose levels to as near normal as possible for the health of the fetus, as well as their own health. Panretinal photocoagulation for severe NPDR should be considered. During the first trimester, another eye examination should be performed; subsequent follow-up will depend on the findings at the time of this examination. Pregnant women with less than severe NPDR should be examined every 3 months, whereas those with more severe stages should be seen every 1–3 months according to current guidelines.

Other Systemic Risk Factors

Diabetic nephropathy, as measured by albuminuria, proteinuria, or renal failure, is found to be a risk factor associated with progression of retinopathy in some, but not all, studies *(43, 67, 68)*. Anemia has also been reported to be associated with progression of diabetic retinopathy in two small case series and two epidemiologic studies *(43, 69–71)*. There was a progressive increase in the risk of development of high-risk PDR with decreasing hematocrit in an adjusted multivariate model in the ETDRS. This may add substantially to the evidence supporting the importance of anemia as a risk factor for diabetic retinopathy. History of diabetic neuropathy and cardiovascular autonomic neuropathy have also been suggested to be associated with increased risk of progression of retinopathy *(43, 72, 73)*.

MANAGEMENT OF NONPROLIFERATIVE DIABETIC RETINOPATHY

The treatment recommendations of diabetic retinopathy are based on the results of two major randomized clinical trials of laser photocoagulation, the Diabetic Retinopathy Study (DRS), and the Early Treatment Diabetic Retinopathy Study (ETDRS). The treatment of NPDR depends on the severity of retinopathy and the presence or absence of clinically significant macular edema, which may be present at any stage of NPDR.

Photocoagulation

The DRS enrolled patients with severe nonproliferative or proliferative diabetic retinopathy and visual acuity of 20/100 or better. The DRS results demonstrated a 50% reduction in severe visual loss (visual acuity of 5/200 or worse at two or more consecutively completed follow-up visits scheduled at 4-month intervals) in eyes that had received photocoagulation (scatter and focal photocoagulation), compared with eyes that did not. DRS reports also identify retinopathy features associated with a particularly high risk of severe visual loss *(74–77)*. These "high-risk" characteristics seen in the proliferative phase, which can be summarized as either neovascularization accompanied by vitreous hemorrhage or obvious neovascularization on or near the optic disc, even in the absence of vitreous hemorrhage, are described in further detail in Chap. 2.

Patients in the DRS had severe nonproliferative or proliferative retinopathy and were randomly assigned to either immediate photocoagulation or no photocoagulation, regardless of retinopathy progression. Although that study identified a group of patients at high risk for visual loss, it could not assess the appropriate timing of scatter photocoagulation. However, the ETDRS was designed to address this clinical question, as well as to evaluate the effects of laser photocoagulation for diabetic macular edema *(78)*. To be eligible for the ETDRS, patients had to have diabetic retinopathy in both eyes with less than high-risk proliferative retinopathy (allowing for mild, moderate, and severe nonproliferative and early proliferative retinopathy) with or without macular edema. One eye of each patient was randomly assigned to early photocoagulation using one of several strategies, and the fellow eye was assigned to deferral of photocoagulation *(79)*.

Scatter Photocoagulation for Nonproliferative Diabetic Retinopathy

The comparison of early photocoagulation vs. deferral in the ETDRS revealed a small reduction in the incidence of severe visual loss in the early-treated eyes, but 5-year rates were low in both the early treatment and deferral groups (2.6% and 3.7%, respectively) *(80)*. For eyes with only mild-to-moderate NPDR, rates of severe visual loss were even lower, and any reductions in visual loss from early photocoagulation did not seem sufficient to compensate for the unwanted side effects of scatter photocoagulation. As the retinopathy advances to the severe or very severe nonproliferative or early proliferative stage, the risk–benefit ratio becomes more favorable, and it is reasonable to consider initiating scatter photocoagulation before the development of high-risk PDR. Recent analyses of ETDRS data suggested that early scatter treatment is particularly effective in reducing severe visual loss in patients with type 2 diabetes *(81)*. While no studies have been performed evaluating intraocular VEGF levels after scatter photocoagulation for NPDR, successful panretinal photocoagulation for ocular neovascularization was found to reduce intraocular VEGF by 75% in one study *(82)*. These data provide an additional reason to recommend early scatter photocoagulation in older patients with very severe nonproliferative or early proliferative diabetic retinopathy.

If patients with either type 1 or 2 diabetes present with both clinically significant macular edema and very severe nonproliferative or early proliferative diabetic retinopathy, the treatment of the macular edema should be considered first, if possible. Data from the ETDRS demonstrated that initial scatter photocoagulation in such patients can actually worsen the macular edema.

Scatter Photocoagulation for Proliferative Retinopathy

The technique of scatter photocoagulation for PDR is discussed in Chap. 2. This technique is used for some eyes that are approaching high-risk PDR, for example, eyes with severe nonproliferative or early proliferative retinopathy. A standard "full" scatter panretinal photocoagulation should be applied (1,200–1,600 moderate intensity burns of ~500 µm in diameter).

Focal Photocoagulation for Diabetic Macular Edema

The ETDRS results also provide clinically important information to guide the treatment of diabetic macular edema *(42, 79, 83, 84)*. In the ETDRS, eyes with mild or moderate NPDR and macular edema were randomly assigned to early focal/grid photocoagulation or no photocoagulation unless high-risk PDR developed. The main outcome variable was a decrease of 3 lines on a logarithmic visual acuity chart. This 3-line decrease represents a doubling of the initial visual angle, for example, a change from 20/20 to 20/40 or from 20/100 to 20/200. After 3 years of follow-up, 24% of the control group experienced such a visual loss when compared with 12% of the treated eyes. Focal/grid photocoagulation reduced the risk of moderate visual acuity loss for all eyes with diabetic macular edema and mild-to-moderate NPDR by about 50%. The group of untreated eyes with macular edema at highest risk for visual loss was the group with edema involving the center of the macula. Prompt photocoagulation is indicated for these eyes, but treatment should be deferred for eyes with edema that is more remote from the macular center. Also, if a large plaque of hard exudate is threatening the center, prompt treatment may be advised.

The effect of focal laser photocoagulation on diabetic macular edema was evaluated in eyes with a broad range of baseline edema severity, visual acuity levels, and various baseline fluorescein angiographic characteristics in the ETDRS *(85)*. Although these analyses were performed in eyes with mild-to-moderate NPDR only, the most important factor to consider in deciding whether to treat macular edema remains involvement of the center of the fovea.

Patients can sometimes notice scotomata related to the focal laser burns, although there was limited documentation of this using the visual fields as measured in the ETDRS. For eyes with leakage arising close to the center of the macula, it may be preferable to observe closely or consider alternative treatment other than laser because of increased risk of damage from direct laser treatment and possible subsequent migration of laser treatment scars. Careful follow-up with intervention when retinal thickening or lipid deposits threaten or involve the center of the macula can reduce the risk of visual loss and limit the number of patients needing treatment.

The ETDRS used two types of treatment for diabetic macular edema, focal and grid. Focal refers to the direct treatment of all leaking microaneurysms in the edematous retina between 500 and 3,000 μm from the center of the macula. Individual microaneurysms are treated with a spot size of 50–100 μm and an exposure time of 0.1 s. The power in ETDRS was set initially low and slowly increased to obtain either whitening or darkening of the microaneurysm with minimal power. The grid treatment in ETDRS was used primarily for areas of diffuse leakage with no identifiable focal areas of leakage. The grid was composed of light intensity burns, 50 to rarely 200 μm in diameter, producing a grid of equally spaced burns more than one burn width apart. One of the reported adverse effects of focal laser photocoagulation is the development of choroidal neovascularization and subsequent subretinal fibrosis *(86, 87)*. However, in the ETDRS, only 9 of 109 eyes with subretinal fibrosis associated with diabetic macular edema could be directly attributed to focal photocoagulation. The strongest risk factor for the development of subretinal fibrosis was the presence of severe hard exudate deposition in the retina, which is associated with elevated serum lipid levels *(58)*. With further clinical experience, we have learned that photocoagulation scars can expand with time, resulting in increased retinal and retinal pigment epithelial atrophy. Therefore, most ophthalmologists today treat with lighter and less intense burns than originally described in ETDRS, aiming for a grey burn as opposed to a white burn, in order to avoid central visual acuity loss or central scotomata that can be associated with expanding laser scars.

Other Treatment of Diabetic Macular Edema

Although focal photocoagulation based on ETDRS guidelines is effective in most cases, there are limitations to laser therapy. First, laser scars can expand with time and encroach upon the fovea. Second, some cases of diabetic macular edema are refractory to focal laser photocoagulation. One alternative treatment is pars plana vitrectomy. The rationale for surgical intervention is that removal of any vitreoretinal traction can result in amelioration of macular edema and improved visual acuity *(88, 89)*. The major drawbacks to this therapy are the invasive nature of vitrectomy and that it may be appropriate only for a subset of macular edema patients with vitreoretinal tractional.

Other treatment possibilities involve pharmacological intervention. Multiple case series and some small controlled trials have suggested that intravitreal injection of the slow-release steroid triamcinolone acetonide is an effective therapy*(90–94)*. However, intravitreal triamcinolone acetonide has been associated with multiple complications such as steroid-induced intraocular pressure elevation and cataract, in addition to the typical risks from intravitreal injections such as retinal detachment and endophthalmitis. A study of rabbit eyes found that intravitreal triamcinolone can be toxic to the outer retina *(95)*. Given the complications associated with steroids and our recent understanding of upregulation of VEGF, molecules targeting VEGF such as intravitreal ranibizumab or bevacizumab are sometimes used to treat refractory macular edema *(96)*. Other therapies targeting VEGF that are under investigation include PKC-beta inhibitors. These emerging treatment concepts are discussed further in Sect. 3.

Medical Therapy

Aspirin and Antiplatelet Treatments

Three randomized controlled clinical trials of antiplatelet treatments have been performed in patients with diabetic retinopathy. None has demonstrated a clinically beneficial effect of treatment. The Dipyridamole Aspirin Microangiopathy of Diabetes (DAMAD) Study *(97)* and the Ticlopidine Microangiopathy of Diabetes Study *(98)* enrolled 475 and 435 patients, respectively. These two studies found similar results with little difference in change in retinopathy severity as judged by visual acuity measurements or ophthalmoscopy. Antiplatelet therapy had been a focus of research in the past because some earlier studies suggested that platelet aggregation may be increased early in diabetes mellitus and may be involved in the genesis of diabetic microangiopathy *(99–103)*.

In the ETDRS, all patients were randomly assigned to 650 mg aspirin per day or a placebo, and one eye of each patient was randomly assigned to immediate photocoagulation, whereas the fellow eye was assigned to deferral of photocoagulation, that is, careful follow-up and prompt scatter photocoagulation if high-risk retinopathy developed. The eyes assigned to deferral of laser photocoagulation were assessed for the effects of aspirin on the progression of diabetic retinopathy. Aspirin use did not affect the progression of retinopathy, nor did it affect the risk of visual loss *(84)*. Additionally, aspirin did not increase the risk of vitreous hemorrhage in patients with proliferative retinopathy *(104, 105)*. Aspirin use was associated with a 17% reduction in morbidity and mortality from cardiovascular disease *(106)*. Therefore aspirin should be considered for persons with diabetes, not because of any effect on their diabetic retinopathy, but because of the benefits of aspirin that have been demonstrated for persons at increased risk of cardiovascular disease. The presence of PDR should not be considered a contraindication to aspirin use.

While the DAMAD and ETDRS showed little benefit of salicylates to inhibit diabetic retinopathy, there is currently renewed interest in this therapy, given the new emphasis on the inflammatory component of diabetic retinopathy. A recent animal study *(107)* showed that salicylate-based anti-inflammatory drugs were able to significantly inhibit the degeneration of retinal capillaries in diabetic rats. Interestingly, this study used a higher dosage of salicylates per kilogram body weight than was given in the DAMAD and ETDRS studies. Also, this animal study began salicylate therapy as soon as diabetes was induced in the rats, compared with the human studies where intervention was not begun until the patients already had retinal manifestations of diabetes. As we learn more about the inflammatory cascade involved in diabetic retinopathy, further studies may investigate the role of salicylate therapy begun earlier in the course of diabetes at a different dose.

Aldose Reductase Inhibitors

A medical approach for preventing the development of retinopathy that has been hypothesized for decades involves blocking the effects of the enzyme aldose reductase *(108)*. In hyperglycemic states, this enzyme facilitates the conversion of glucose to sorbitol. Build-up of sorbitol is thought to disrupt retinal cellular function via induction of apoptosis and osmotic changes *(109)*. Animal experiments suggest that an aldose reductase inhibitor could slow the development of diabetic retinopathy *(110–114)*. Clinical trials of aldose reductase inhibitors have resulted in a decrease in capillary cell death, microaneurysm count, fluorescein leakage, nonperfusion status, and VEGF expression *(5, 115–119)*. However, none of these observations have resulted in any slowing of the progression of retinopathy. One of the largest human trials, the Sorbinil Retinopathy Trial, enrolled 497 diabetic patients with little or no retinopathy. After 3–4 years of follow-up, progression of diabetic retinopathy and neuropathy were apparently unaffected by the administration of the aldose reductase inhibitor *(115, 120)*.

Other Medical Treatments

A variety of other medical approaches for reducing the secondary complications of diabetes are currently under evaluation. Current clinical studies are evaluating protein kinase C inhibitors, such as oral ruboxistaurin, as potential modulators of diabetes-induced retinal hemodynamic abnormalities *(29)*. This therapy was found to reduce the rate of sustained moderate visual loss in a randomized controlled clinical trial by 40% (P 0.034 with 9.1% in placebo-treated patients vs. 5.5% of ruboxistaurin-treated patients) *(121)*. Ultimately, prevention is more effective than treatment, and so a healthy lifestyle, including weight control and regular exercise, is essential as illustrated by the Diabetes Prevention Program *(122)*.

This clinical trial *(122)* evaluated diabetes prevention in 3,234 nondiabetic, overweight persons with elevated fasting and postload plasma glucose concentrations. The mean body-mass index, weight in kilograms divided by the square of the height in meters, was 34. The participants were randomized to placebo, metformin (850 mg twice daily), or a lifestyle-modification program with the goals of at least a 7% weight loss and at least 150 min of physical activity per week. The results indicated success for the lifestyle modification group. Specifically, the incidence of diabetes was 11.0, 7.8, and 4.8 cases per 100 person-years in the placebo, metformin, and lifestyle groups, respectively,

Table 4
Recommended Scheduling of Examinations Based on the Timing of Diabetes Mellitus Onset

Time of onset	*Recommended time for first examination*	*Routine minimum follow-up*
Age less than 30 years	5 years after onset	Yearly
Age 30 and older	At time of diagnosis	Yearly
Before pregnancy	Before or soon after conception	At least every 3 months

Table 5
Recommended Follow-up Based on the Status of the Retinopathy

Status	*Follow-up (months)*
No retinopathy or microaneurysms only	12
Mild/moderate NPDR without macular edema	6–12
Mild/moderate NPDR with macular edema that is not clinically significant	4–6
Mild/moderate NPDR with clinically significant macular edema	3–4
Severe/very severe NPDR	3–4

NPDR nonproliferative diabetic retinopathy

The lifestyle intervention reduced the incidence by 58% (95% confidence interval, 48–66%) and metformin by 31% (95% confidence interval, 17–43%), compared with placebo. Therefore, a healthy lifestyle is a cost-saving, effective method to prevent the development of diabetic complications.

SUMMARY

On the basis of the results of controlled clinical trials that have accumulated over the past several decades, we now have beneficial methods for the treatment of diabetic retinopathy. However, diabetic retinopathy remains a leading cause of visual loss in the United States among working-age Americans. This is unfortunate, because when properly treated, the 5-year risk of blindness for patients with PDR is reduced by 90% and the risk of visual loss from macular edema is reduced by 50%. (80) Appropriate follow-up (Tables 4 and 5) and timely intervention are essential and may help prevent blinding complications of diabetic retinopathy. With the advent of emerging therapies, prevention strategies, and heightened awareness of the extensive microvascular complications in diabetes, the future for effective clinical management of diabetic retinopathy is optimistic.

ACKNOWLEDGMENT

This chapter was based on, and reprinted from, *Retina*, 4th Edition, Vol. 2 (eds Ryan SJ, Schachat AP), Drs. E.Y. Chew and F.L. Ferris III, "Nonproliferative Diabetic Retinopathy", pp. 1271–1284, 2006, with permission from Elsevier.

REFERENCES

1. Wild S, Roglic G, Green A, Sicree R, King H. Global prevalence of diabetes: estimates for the year 2000 and projections for 2030. Diabetes Care 2004;27:1047–1053.
2. D'Amico D. Diseases of the retina. N Engl J Med 1994;331(2):95–106.
3. National Society to Prevent Blindness. Vision problems in the US: data analysis, definitions, data sources, detailed data table, analyses, interpretation. New York, USA, 1980.
4. Ciulla T, Harris A, Latknay P, Piper HC, Arend O, Garzozi H, Martin B. Ocular perfusion abnormalities in diabetes. Acta Ophthalmol Scand 2002;80(5):468–477.
5. Comer GM, Ciulla TA. Current and future pharmacological intervention for diabetic retinopathy. Expert Opin Emerg Drugs 2005;10(2):441–455.
6. Esser P, Bresgen M, Fischbach R, Heimann K, Wiedemann P. Intercellular adhesion molecule-1 levels in plasma and vitreous from patients with vitreoretinal disorders. Ger J Ophthalmol 1995;4(5):269–274.
7. Joussen AM, Poulaki V, Qin W, Kirchhof B, Mitsiades N, Wiegand SJ, Rudge J, Yancopoulos GD, Adamis AP. Retinal vascular endothelial growth factor induces intercellular adhesion molecule-1 and endothelial nitric oxide synthase expression and initiates early diabetic retinal leukocyte adhesion in vivo. Am J Pathol 2002;160(2):501–509.
8. Joussen AM, Poulaki V, Le ML, Koizumi K, Esser C, Janicki H, Schraermeyer U, Kociok N, Fauser S, Kirchhof B, Kern TS, Adamis AP. A central role for inflammation in the pathogenesis of diabetic retinopathy. FASEB J 2004;18(12):1450–1452.
9. Miyamoto K, Khosrof S, Bursell SE, Rohan R, Murata T, Clermont AC, Aiello LP, Ogura Y, Adamis AP. Prevention of leukostasis and vascular leakage in streptozotocin-induced diabetic retinopathy via intercellular adhesion molecule-1 inhibition. Proc Natl Acad Sci USA 1999;96:10836–10841.
10. Joussen AM, Murata T, Tsujikawa A, Kirchhof B, Bursell SE, Adamis AP. Leukocyte-mediated endothelial cell injury and death in the diabetic retina. Am J Pathol 2001;158:147–152.
11. Meleth AD, Agron E, Chan CC, Reed GF, Arora K, Byrnes G, Csaky KG, Ferris FL III, Chew EY.Serum inflammatory markers in diabetic retinopathy. Invest Ophthalmol Vis Sci 2005;46(11):4295–4301.
12. Kuwabara T, Cogan DG. Retinal vascular patterns. I. Normal architecture. Arch Ophthalmol 1960;64:904–911.
13. Bloodworth JMB. Fine structure of retina in human and canine diabetes mellitus. In Kimuara, SJ, Caygill, WM, eds, Vascular complications of diabetes mellitus. St Louis: Mosby, 1967.
14. Engerman RL. Pathogenesis of diabetic retinopathy. Diabetes 1989;38:1203–1206.
15. Frank RN. On the pathogenesis of diabetic retinopathy – a 1990 update. Ophthalmology 1991;98:586–593.
16. Cogan DG, Toussaint D, Kuwabara T. Retinal vascular patterns. IV. Diabetic retinopathy. Arch Ophthalmol 1961;66:366–378.
17. Frank RN. Etiologic mechanisms in diabetic retinopathy. In Ryan SJ, Schachat AP, Murphy RP, Patz A, eds, Retina, vol 2, Medical retina, 1st ed., St Louis: Mosby, 1989.
18. Wise GN. Retinal neovascularization. Trans Am Ophthalmol Soc 1956;54:729–826.
19. De Venecia G, Davis M, Engerman R. Clinicopathologic correlations in diabetic retinopathy. I. Histology and fluorescein angiography of microaneurysms. Arch Ophthalmol 1976;94:1766–1773.
20. Klein R, Meuer SM, Moss SE, Klein BEK. The relationship of retinal microaneurysm counts to the 4-year progression of diabetic retinopathy. Arch Ophthalmol 1989;107:1780–1785.
21. Klein R, Meuer SM, Moss SE, Klein BEK. Retinal micro-aneurysm counts and 10-year progression of diabetic retinopathy. Arch Ophthalmol 1995;113:1386–1391.
22. Kohner EM, Sleightholm M, and The Kroc Collaborative Study Group. Does microaneurysm count reflect severity of early diabetic retinopathy? Ophthalmology 1986;93:586–589.
23. Funatsu H, Yamashita H, Ikeda T, Mimura T, Eguchi S, Hori S. Vitreous levels of interleukin-6 and vascular endothelial growth factor are related to diabetic macular edema. Ophthalmology 2003; 110(9):1690–1696.
24. Funatsu H, Yamashita H, Nakamura S, Mimura T, Eguchi S, Noma H, Hori S. Vitreous levels of pigment epithelium-derived factor and vascular endothelial growth factor are related to diabetic macular edema. Ophthalmology 2006;113(2):294–301.

25. Aiello LP, Avery RL, Arrigg PG, Keyt BA, Jampel HD, Shah ST, Pasquale LR, Thieme H, Iwamoto MA, Park JE, et al. Vascular endothelial growth factor in ocular fluid of patients with diabetic retinopathy and other retinal disorders. N Engl J Med 1994;331(22):1480–1487.
26. Gardner TW, Antonetti DA, Barber AJ, LaNoue KF, Levision SW. Diabetic retinopathy: more than meets the eye. Surv Ophthalmol 2002;47 (Suppl 2):S253–S262.
27. Koya D, King GL. Protein kinase C activation and the development of diabetic complications. Diabetes 1998;47(6):859–866.
28. Ishii H, Koya D, King GL. Protein kinase C activation and its role in the development of vascular complications in diabetes mellitus. J Mol Med 1998;76(1):21–31.
29. Aiello LP, Clermont A, Arora V, Davis MD, Sheetz MJ, Bursell SE. Inhibition of PKC beta by oral administration of ruboxistaurin is well tolerated and ameliorates diabetes-induced retinal hemodynamic abnormalities in patients. Invest Ophthalmol Vis Sci 2006;47(1):86–92.
30. Shiba T, Inoguchi T, Sportsman JR, Heath WF, Bursell S, King GL. Correlation of diacylglycerol level and protein kinase C activity in rat retina to retinal circulation. Am J Physiol 1993;265(5 Pt 1):E783–E793.
31. Yan SF, Lu J, Zou YS, Kisiel W, Mackman N, Leitges M, Steinberg S, Pinsky D, Stern D. Protein kinase C-beta and oxygen deprivation. A novel Egr-1-dependent pathway for fibrin deposition in hypoxemic vasculature. J Biol Chem 2000;275(16):11921–11928.
32. Wolf BA, Williamson JR, Easom RA, Chang K, Sherman WR, Turk J. Diacylglycerol accumulation and microvascular abnormalities induced by elevated glucose levels. J Clin Invest 1991;87(1):31–38.
33. Ferris FL III, Patz A. Macular edema: a complication of diabetic retinopathy. Surv Ophthalmol 1984;28 (suppl):452–461.
34. Patz A, Schatz H, Berkow JW, Gittelsohn AM, Ticho U. Macular edema – an overlooked complication of diabetic retinopathy. Trans Am Acad Ophthalmol Otolaryngol 1973;77:34–42.
35. King RC. Exudative diabetic retinopathy. Br J Ophthalmol 1963;47:666–672.
36. Sigurdsson R, Begg I. Organized macular plaques in exudative diabetic maculopathy. Br J Ophthalmol 1980;64:392–397.
37. Chew EY, Klein ML, Ferris FL III, Remaley NA, Murphy RP, Chantry K, Hoogwerf BJ, Miller D, for the Early Treatment Diabetic Retinopathy Study Research Group. Association of elevated serum lipid levels with retinal hard exudate in diabetic retinopathy. Arch Ophthalmol 1996;114:1079–1084.
38. Klein BEK, Moss SE, Klein R, Surawicz TS. The Wisconsin Epidemiologic Study of Diabetic Retinopathy. XIII. Relationship of serum cholesterol to retinopathy and hard exudates. Ophthalmology 1991;98:1261–1265.
39. Wilkinson CP. Achieving consensus on an international clinical classification for diabetic retinopathy. Program and abstracts of the American Academy of Ophthalmology 2002 Annual Meeting, Orlando, FL, October 20–23, 2002.
40. Klein R, Klein B, Moss S, Davis M, DeMets D. The Wisconsin Epidemiologic Study of Diabetic Retinopathy. IV. Diabetic macular edema. Ophthalmology 1984;91:1464–1474.
41. Brown JC, Soloman S, Bressler SB, Schachat AP, DiBernardo C, Bressler NM. Detection of diabetic foveal edema. Contact lens biomicroscopy compared with optical coherence tomography. Arch Ophthalmol 2004;122:330–335.
42. Early Treatment Diabetic Retinopathy Study Research Group. Photocoagulation for diabetic macular edema, ETDRS report no 1. Arch Ophthalmol 1985;103:1796–1806.
43. Davis MD, Fisher MR, Gangnon RE, Barton F, Aiello LM, Chew EY, Ferris FL III, Knatterud GL. Risk factors for high-risk proliferative diabetic retinopathy and severe visual loss, ETDRS report no 18. Invest Ophthalmol Vis Sci 1998;39:233–252.
44. Klein R, Klein BEK, Moss SE, Davis MD, DeMets DL. Is blood pressure a predictor of the incidence or progression of diabetic retinopathy? Arch Intern Med 1989;149:2427–2432.
45. Diabetes Control and Complications Trial Research Group. The effect of intensive treatment of diabetes on the development and progression of long-term complications in insulin-dependent diabetes mellitus. N Engl J Med 1993;329:977–986.
46. Diabetes Control and Complications Trial Research Group. The effect of intensive diabetes treatment on the progression of diabetic retinopathy in insulin-dependent diabetes mellitus. Arch Ophthalmol 1995;113:36–51.

47. Diabetes Control and Complications Trial Research Group. The relationship of glycemic exposures (HbA_1C) to the risk of development and progression of retinopathy in the Diabetes Control and Complications Trial. Diabetes 1995;44:968–983.
48. Diabetes Control and Complications Trial Research Group. Perspectives in diabetes: the absence of a glycemic threshold for the development of long-term complications. The perspective of the Diabetes Control and Complications Trial. Diabetes 1996;45:1289–1298.
49. Reichard P, Nilsson BY, and Rosenqvist U. The effect of long-term intensified insulin treatment on the development of microvascular complications of diabetes mellitus, N Engl J Med 1993;329:304–309.
50. American Diabetes Association. Standards of medical care in diabetes – 2007. Diabetes Care 2007;30:S4–S41.
51. The Diabetes Control and Complications Trial/Epidemiology of Diabetes Interventions and Complications Research Group. Retinopathy and nephropathy in patients with type 1 diabetes four years after a trial of intensive therapy. N Engl J Med 2000;342:381–389.
52. UK Prospective Diabetes Study Group. Intensive blood-glucose control with sulphonylureas or insulin compared with conventional treatment and risk of complications in patients with type 2 diabetes (UKPDS 33). Lancet 1988;352:837–853.
53. Suzuma I, Hata Y, Clermont A, Pokras F, Rook SL, Suzuma K, Feener EP, Aiello LP. Cyclic stretch and hypertension induce retinal expression of vascular endothelial growth factor and vascular endothelial growth factor receptor-2: potential mechanisms for exacerbation of diabetic retinopathy by hypertension. Diabetes 2001;50(2):444–454.
54. Yam JC, Kwok AK. Update on the treatment of diabetic retinopathy. Hong Kong Med J 2007;13(1): 46–60.
55. UK Prospective Diabetes Study Group. Tight blood pressure control and risk of macrovascular and microvascular complications in type 2 diabetes (UKPDS 38). Br Med J 1998;317:703–713.
56. Chaturvedi N, Sjolie AK, Stephen JM, Heidemarie A, Deipes M, Castellarin A, Rogulja-Pepeonik X, Fuller JH. and the EUCLID Study Group. Effect of lisinopril on progression of retinopathy in normotensive people with type 1 diabetes. Lancet 1998;351:28–31.
57. Schrier RW, Estacio RP, Esler A, Mehler P. Appropriate blood pressure control in hypertensive and normotensive type 2 diabetes mellitus: a summary of the ABCD trial. Nat Clin Pract Nephrol. 2007 Aug;3(8):428–438.
58. Fong DS, Segal PP, Myers F, Ferris FL, Hubbard LD, Davis MD. Subretinal fibrosis in diabetic macular edema, ETDRS report no 23. Arch Ophthalmol 1997;115:873–877.
59. Lyons TJ, Jenkins AJ, Zhen D, Lackland DT, McGee D, Garvey WT, Klein RL, the DCCT/EDIC Research Group. Diabetic retinopathy and serum lipoprotein subclasses in the DCCT/EDIC cohort. Invest Ophthalmol Vis Sci 2004;45:910–918.
60. Gupta A, Gupta V, Thapar S, Bhansali A. Lipid-lowering drug atorvastatin as an adjunct in the management of diabetic macular edema. Am J Ophthalmol 2004;137(4):675–682.
61. Sen K, Misra A, Kumar A, Pandey RM.Simvastatin retards progression of retinopathy in diabetic patients with hypercholesterolemia. Diabetes Res Clin Pract 2002;56(1):1–11.
62. Chew EY, Mills JL, Metzger BE, Remaley NA, Jovanovic-Peterson L, Knopp RH, Conley M, Rand L, Simpson JL, Holmes JB, Aarons J. Metabolic control and progression of retinopathy. The Diabetes in Early Pregnancy Study. National Institute of Child Health and Human Development Diabetes in Early Pregnancy Study. Diabetes Care 1995;18:631–637.
63. Klein BEK, Moss SE, Klein R. Effect of pregnancy on progression of diabetic retinopathy. Diabetes Care 1990;13:34–40.
64. Phelps RL, Sakol P, Metzger BE, Jampol LM, Freinkel N. Changes in diabetic retinopathy during pregnancy: correlations with regulation of hyperglycemia. Arch Ophthalmol 1986;104: 1806–1810.
65. The Diabetes Control and Complications Trial Research Group. Effect of pregnancy on the microvascular complications. Diabetes Care 2000;23:1084–1091.
66. Schultz KL, Birnbaum AD, Goldstein DA. Ocular disease in pregnancy. Curr Opin Ophthalmol 2005;16(5):308–314.
67. Janka HU, Warram JH, Rand LI, Krolewski AS. Risk factors for progression of background retinopathy in long-standing IDDM. Diabetes 1989;38:460–464.

68. Rand LI, Prud'homme GJ, Ederer F, Canner PL, and the Diabetic Retinopathy Study Research Group. Factors influencing the development of visual loss in advanced diabetic retinopathy, DRS report no 10. Invest Ophthalmol Vis Sci 1985;26:983–991.
69. Berman DH, Friedman EA. Partial absorption of hard exudates in patients with diabetic end-stage renal disease and severe anemia after treatment with erythropoietin. Retina 1994;14:1–5.
70. Qiao Q, Keinanen-Kiukaanniemi S, Laara E. The relationship between hemoglobin levels and diabetic retinopathy. J Clin Epidemiol 1997;50:153–158.
71. Shorb SR. Anemia and diabetic retinopathy. Am J Ophthalmol 1985;100:434–436.
72. Krolewski AS, Barzilay J, Warram JH, Martin BC, Pfeifer M, Rand LI. Risk of early-onset proliferative diabetic retinopathy in IDDM is closely related to cardiovascular autonomic neuropathy. Diabetes 1992;41:430–437.
73. Tesfaye S, Stevens LK, Stephenson JM, et al. Prevalence of diabetic peripheral neuropathy and its relation to glycaemic control and potential risk factors: The EURODIAB IDDM Complications Study. Diabetologia 1996;39:1377–1384.
74. Diabetic Retinopathy Study Research Group. Photocoagulation treatment of proliferative diabetic retinopathy, DRS report no 2. Ophthalmology 1978;85:82–105.
75. Diabetic Retinopathy Study Research Group. Four risk factors for severe visual loss in diabetic retinopathy, DRS report no 3. Arch Ophthalmol 1979;97:654–655.
76. Diabetic Retinopathy Study Research Group. Clinical application of Diabetic Retinopathy Study (DRS) findings, DRS report no 8. Ophthalmology 1981;88:583–600.
77. Diabetic Retinopathy Study Research Group. Photocoagulation treatment of proliferative diabetic retinopathy: relationship of adverse treatment effects to retinopathy severity. Dev Ophthalmol 1981;2:248–261.
78. Early Treatment Diabetic Retinopathy Study Research Group. Early Treatment Diabetic Retinopathy Study design and baseline patient characteristics, ETDRS report no 7. Ophthalmology 1991; 98:741–756.
79. Early Treatment Diabetic Retinopathy Study Research Group. Techniques for scatter and local photocoagulation treatment of diabetic retinopathy, ETDRS report no 3. Int Ophthalmol Clin 1987;27:254–264.
80. Early Treatment Diabetic Retinopathy Study Research Group. Early photocoagulation for diabetic retinopathy, ETDRS report no 9. Ophthalmology 1991;98 (suppl):767–785.
81. Ferris F. Early photocoagulation in patients with either type I or type II diabetes. Trans Am Ophthalmol Soc 1996;94:505–537.
82. Aiello LP, Avery RL, Arrigg PG, Keyt BA, Jampel HD, Shah ST, Pasquale LR, Thieme H, Iwamoto MA, Park JE, Nguyen HV, Aiello LM, Ferrara N, King GL. Vascular endothelial growth factor in ocular fluid of patients with diabetic retinopathy and other retinal disorders. N Engl J Med 1994;331(22):1480–1487.
83. Early Treatment Diabetic Retinopathy Study Research Group. Photocoagulation for diabetic macular edema, ETDRS report no 4. Int Ophthalmol Clin 1987;27:265–272.
84. Early Treatment Diabetic Retinopathy Study Research Group. Treatment techniques and clinical guidelines for photocoagulation of diabetic macular edema, ETDRS report no 2. Ophthalmology 1987;94:761–774.
85. Early Treatment Diabetic Retinopathy Study Research Group. Photocoagulation for diabetic macular edema: relationship of treatment effect to fluorescein angiographic and other retinal characteristics at baseline, ETDRS report no 19. Arch Ophthalmol 1995;113:1144–1155.
86. Han DP, Miller WF, Burton TC. Submacular fibrosis after photocoagulation for diabetic macular edema. Am J Ophthalmol 1992;113:513–521.
87. Lewis H, Schachat AP, Haimann MH, et al. Choroidal neovascularization after laser photocoagulation for diabetic macular edema. Ophthalmology 1990;97:503–511.
88. Yamamoto T, Akabane N, Takeuchi S. Vitrectomy for diabetic macular edema: the role of posterior vitreous detachment and epimacular membrane. Am J Ophthalmol 2001;132:369–377.
89. Lewis H, Abrams G, Blumenkranz M, Campo R. Vitrectomy for diabetic macular traction and edema associated with posterior hyaloidal traction. Ophthalmology 1992;99:753–759.
90. Martidis A, Duker JS, Greenberg PB, Rogers AH, Puliafito CA, Reichel E, Baumal C. Intravitreal triamcinolone for refractory diabetic macular edema. Ophthalmology 2002;109:920–927.

91. Jonas JB, Kreissing I, Sofker A, Degenring RF. Intravitreal injection of triamcinolone for diffuse macular edema. Arch Ophthalmol 2003;121:57–61.
92. Massin P, Audren F, Haouchine B, Erginay A, Bergmann JF, Benosman R, Caulin C, Gaudric A. Intravitreal triamcinolone acetonide for diabetic diffuse macular edema. Ophthalmology 2004; 111:218–225.
93. Gillies MC, Sutter FK, Simpson JM, Larsson J, Ali H, Zhu M. Intravitreal triamcinolone for refractory diabetic macular edema: two-year results of a double-masked, placebo-controlled, randomized clinical trial. Ophthalmology 2006;113(9):1533–1538.
94. Jonas JB, Kamppeter BA, Harder B, Vossmerbaeumer U, Sauder G, Spandau UH. Intravitreal triamcinolone acetonide for diabetic macular edema: a prospective, randomized study. J Ocul Pharmacol Ther 2006;22(3):200–207.
95. Yu SY, Damico FM, Viola F, D'Amico DJ, Young LH. Retinal toxicity of intravitreal triamcinolone acetonide: a morphological study. Retina 2006;26(5):531–536.
96. Massin P, Audren F, Haouchine B, Erginay A, Bergmann JF, Benosman R, Caulin C, Gaudric A. Intravitreal triamcinolone acetonide for diabetic diffuse macular edema: preliminary results of a prospective controlled trial. Ophthalmology 2004;111(2):218–225.
97. Dipyridamole Aspirin Microangiopathy of Diabetes Study Group. Effect of aspirin alone and aspirin plus dipyridamole in early diabetic retinopathy: a multicenter, randomized, controlled clinical trial. Diabetes 1989;38:491–498.
98. Ticlopidine Microangiography of Diabetes Study Group. Ticlopidine treatment reduces the progression of nonproliferative diabetic retinopathy. Arch Ophthalmol 1990;108:1577–1583.
99. Carroll WW, Geeraets WJ. Diabetic retinopathy and salicylates. Ann Ophthalmol 1972;4:1019–1046.
100. Dobbie JG, Kwaan HC, Colwell JA, et al. The role of platelets in pathogenesis of diabetic retinopathy. Trans Am Acad Ophthalmol Otolaryngol 1973;77:43–46.
101. Powell EDU, Field RA. Diabetic retinopathy and rheumatoid arthritis. Lancet 1964;2:17–18.
102. Regnault F. Role des plaguettes dans la pathogenie de la retinopathie diabetique. Sem Hop Paris 1972;48:893–902.
103. Sagel J, Colwell JA, Crook L, et al. Increased platelet aggregation in early diabetes mellitus. Ann Intern Med 1975;82:733–738.
104. Chew EY, Klein ML, Murphy RP, Remalely NA, Ferris FL. Effects of aspirin on vitreous/preretinal hemorrhage in patients with diabetes mellitus, ETDRS report no 20. Arch Ophthalmol 1995; 113:52–55.
105. Early Treatment Diabetic Retinopathy Study Research Group. Effects of aspirin treatment on diabetic retinopathy, ETDRS report no 8. Ophthalmology 1991;98:757–765.
106. Early Treatment Diabetic Retinopathy Study Research Group. Aspirin effects on mortality and morbidity in patients with diabetes mellitus, ETDRS report no 14. JAMA 1992;268:1292–1300.
107. Zheng L, Howell SJ, Hatala DA, Huang K, Kern TS. Salicylate-based anti-inflammatory drugs inhibit the early lesion of diabetic retinopathy. Diabetes 2007;56(2):337–345.
108. Frank RN. Perspectives in diabetes: the aldose reductase controversy. Diabetes 1994;43:169–172.
109. Asnaghi V, Gerhardinger C, Hoehn T, Adeboje A, Lorenzi M. A role for the polyol pathway in the early neuroretinal apoptosis and glial changes induced by diabetes in the rat. Diabetes 2003; 52(2):506–511.
110. Engerman RL, Kern TS. Experimental galactosemia produces diabetic-like retinopathy. Diabetes 1984;33:97–100.
111. Kador PF, Akagi Y, Takahashi Y, Ikebe H, Wyman M, Kinoshita JH. Prevention of retinal vessel changes associated with diabetic retinopathy in galactose-fed dogs by aldose reductase inhibitors. Arch Ophthalmol 1990;108:1301–1309.
112. Kador PF, Akagi Y, Takahashi Y, Wyman M, Kinoshita JH. Prevention of pericyte ghost formation in retinal capillaries of galactose-fed dogs by aldose reductase inhibitors. Arch Ophthalmol 1988;106:1099–1102.
113. Robison WG Jr, Laver NM, Jacot JL, et al. Diabetic-like retinopathy ameliorated with the aldose reductase inhibitor WAY-121,509. Invest Ophthalmol Vis Sci 1996;37:1149–1156.
114. Robison WG Jr, Nagata M, Laver N, Hohman TC, Kinoshita JH. Diabetic-like retinopathy in rats prevented with an aldose reductase inhibitor. Invest Ophthalmol Vis Sci 1989;30:2285–2292.

115. Sorbinil Retinopathy Trial Research Group. A randomized trial of sorbinil, an aldose reductase inhibitor, in diabetic retinopathy. Arch Ophthalmol 1990;108:1234–1244.
116. Van Gerven Boot JP, Lemkes HH, van Best JA. Effects of aldose reductase inhibition with tolrestat on diabetic retinopathy in a six months double blind trial. Doc Ophthalmol 1994;87(4):355–365.
117. Stevens MJ, Henry DN, Thomas TP, Killen PD, Greene DA. Aldose reductase gene expression and osmotic dysregulation in cultured human retinal pigment epithelial cells. Am J Physiol 1993;265(3 Pt 1): E428–E438.
118. Obrosova IG, Minchenko AG, Vasupuram R, White L, Abatan OI, Kumagai AK, Frank RN, Stevens MJ. Aldose reductase inhibitor fidarestat prevents retinal oxidative stress and vascular endothelial growth factor overexpression in streptozotocin-diabetic rats. Diabetes 2003;52(3):864–871.
119. Cusick M, Chew E, Ferris F, Cox TA, Chan CC, Kador PF. Effects of aldose reductase inhibitors and galactose withdrawal on fluorescein angiographic lesions in galactose-fed dogs. Arch Ophthalmol 2003;121(12):1745–1751.
120. Sorbinil Retinopathy Trial Research Group. The sorbinil retinopathy trial: neuropathy results. Neurology 1993;43:1141–1149.
121. PKC-DRS2 Group, Aiello LP, Davis MD, Girach A, Kles KA, Milton RC, Sheetz MJ, Vignati L, Zhi XE. Effect of ruboxistaurin on visual loss in patients with diabetic retinopathy. Ophthalmology 2006;113(12):2221–2230.
122. Diabetes Prevention Program Research Group. Reduction in the incidence of type 2 diabetes with lifestyle intervention or metformin. N Engl J Med 2002;346:393–403.

2 Proliferative Diabetic Retinopathy

Ronald P. Danis and Matthew D. Davis

CONTENTS

ABSTRACT

Proliferative diabetic retinopathy continues to be a major cause of blindness throughout the world. The natural history demonstrates that its development is primarily related to progressive retinal ischemia from diabetic retinopathy. The primary complications leading to vision loss, tractional retinal detachment and vitreous hemorrhage, are dependent upon the relationship between the neovascular tissue and the vitreous. The major risk factors are duration of diabetes and the level of glycemic control of the patient, with glycemic control being the modifiable risk factor as demonstrated in the DCCT/EDIC and UKPDS trials. Timely treatment with laser photocoagulation has been demonstrated to be of immense value for the preservation of vision, as reported by the DRS, ETDRS, and other studies. Pars plana vitrectomy is indicated for some patients with vitreous hemorrhage, retinal detachment, and other complications. With growing understanding of the cell biology of diabetes complications, pharmacologic therapies are emerging as promising treatment options.

Key Words: Diabetes mellitus; Diabetic retinopathy; Neovascularization; Laser photocoagulation Vitrectomy.

DEVELOPMENT AND NATURAL HISTORY

Histopathology and Early Development

Endothelial proliferation and new vessel formation in the retina are stimulated by ischemia of its inner layers secondary to regional closure of the retinal capillary bed

From: *Contemporary Diabetes: Diabetic Retinopathy*
Edited by: E. Duh © Humana Press, Totowa, NJ

(1–4). Retinal hypoxia induces upregulation of genes such as hypoxia inducible factor that in turn stimulate the production of a variety of endothelial mitogens, most notably vascular endothelial growth factor (VEGF). Chronic ischemia also produces a localized low-grade inflammatory response within the vessels, with the subsequent migration and stimulation of immunogenic cells in the tissue, which also produce a variety of mitogenic cytokines. These growth factors promote a neovascular (NV) response locally and by diffusing through the vitreous to other areas of the retina, to the optic disc, and into the anterior chamber *(5–7)*.

The background of intraretinal lesions against which preretinal new vessels arise is variable. The risk of proliferative diabetic retinopathy (PDR) is greatest in eyes with severe NPDR (nonproliferative diabetic retinopathy, also called preproliferative retinopathy), characterized by the presence of soft exudates (cotton-wool patches), intraretinal microvascular abnormalities (IRMAs, a term chosen so as to be neutral about whether these abnormal vessels represent intraretinal new vessels or dilated preexisting vessels), venous beading, and extensive retinal hemorrhage or microaneurysms (Fig. 1). In the Diabetic Retinopathy Study (DRS) severe NPDR was basically defined as the presence of at least three of the four above-mentioned characteristics, each generally involving at least two quadrants of the fundus. About 50% of such eyes assigned to the untreated control group had developed PDR within 15 months *(8)*. The presence and extent of retinal and optic nerve head NV in the diabetic retina are roughly correlated with the extent of capillary loss on fluorescein angiography *(1)*.

Although there is little doubt that the presence of severe NPDR is predictive of subsequent NV, the characteristic intraretinal lesions are not always present when preretinal

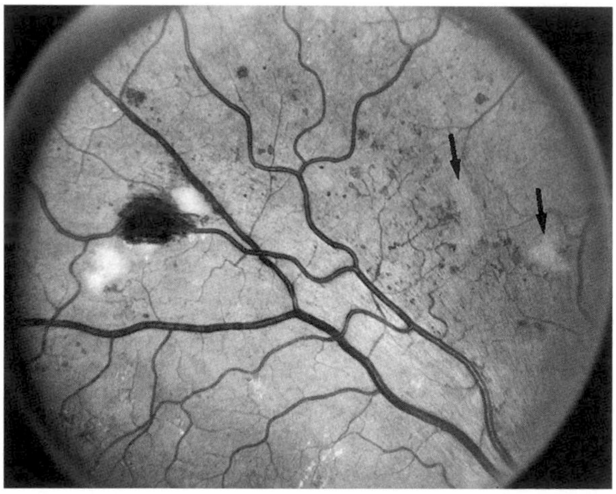

Fig. 1. Severe nonproliferative diabetic retinopathy. Two prominent cotton-wool spots (soft exudates) are noted on the left side with a large blot hemorrhage between them. Venous beading is present where the superior branch of the superotemporal vein passes by the upper exudate. On the right are two faint soft exudates (*arrows*) and many intraretinal microvascular abnormalities. (Courtesy Early Treatment Diabetic Retinopathy Study Research Group.)

new vessels are first recognized. A possible explanation for this is the relatively transient nature of some of these lesions. Soft exudates usually disappear within 6–12 months. Blot hemorrhages and IRMA tend to disappear after extensive capillary closure, when the number of small vascular branches decreases and some small arterioles become white threads, producing a picture aptly described as featureless retina (Fig. 2).

Some, but probably a minority, of the IRMAs eventually develop into neovascular tissue *(9)*. IRMAs feature endothelial proliferation and vascular caliber larger than retinal capillaries with loose adventitia, similar to NV lesions. A critical distinction is that IRMAs lie exclusively below the level of the internal limiting membrane (ILM) of the retina, whereas NV lies above the ILM, growing along the interface between the retina and posterior vitreous face, where they can become elevated as vitreous detachment occurs.

Although new vessels may arise anywhere in the retina, they are most frequently seen within 10–15 mm of the optic disc, and on the disc itself (Davis *(10)*: 69% of 155 eyes with PDR; Taylor and Dobree *(11)*: 73% of 86 eyes). In the DRS, among 1,377 control group eyes with new vessels present in baseline photographs, 15% had new vessels only on or within 1 disc diameter (DD) of the disc, 40% had new vessels only outside this zone, and 45% had new vessels in both zones *(12)*.

Neovascularization of the optic disc (NVD) begins as fine loops or networks of vessels lying on the surface of the disc or bridging across the physiologic cup. The most satisfactory examining methods are those that provide a magnified stereoscopic view, either biomicroscopy with contact or precorneal lens or stereoscopic 30-deg photography. If any doubt remains, it can usually be resolved by fluorescein angiography, which demonstrates the profuse leakiness characteristic of preretinal new vessels. Wide-angle angiography can be helpful in identifying ischemia and NV, particularly when NV

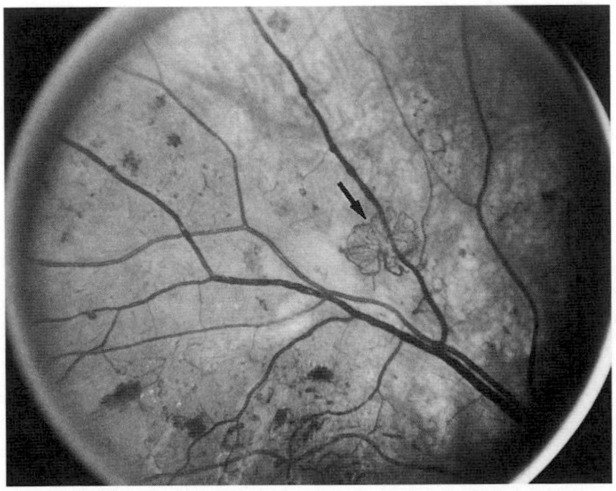

Fig. 2. Early proliferative diabetic retinopathy. New vessels form a small wheel-like network (*arrow*) in the superotemporal quadrant of an eye with venous beading, cotton-wool spots (soft exudates), intraretinal microvascular abnormalities, and blot hemorrhages. (Courtesy Early Treatment Diabetic Retinopathy Study Research Group.)

lesions are suspected (e.g., due to recent vitreous hemorrhage) but are not found on clinical examination. The possibility that the vitreous hemorrhage may come from a peripheral retinal tear, unrelated to diabetic retinopathy, should be kept in mind, and a careful examination of the peripheral fundus with scleral depression should be performed.

Early new vessels elsewhere (NVE) may be difficult to distinguish from IRMA, particularly if the IRMA are extensive and NVE do not yet show any of their unique features, such as formation of wheel-like networks, extension across both arterial and venous branches of the underlying retinal vascular network, accompanying fibrous proliferations, or elevation. The true nature of such borderline lesions soon becomes clear with careful follow-up.

NV requires a scaffold or matrix in which to grow *(13)*; therefore, NV does not typically occur in areas where the vitreous has detached or has been surgically removed *(14)*. In fact, in an eye with complete posterior vitreous detachment with severe NPDR, the clinical concern should be more for the possibility of the development of rubeosis iridis, NV of the iris, than of PDR. In some instances, small buds or "popcorn kernels" of NV may appear in eyes with vitreous separation, but such lesions rarely progress or lead to complication. Some investigators have suggested that iatrogenic induction of posterior vitreous detachment in eyes with NPDR, or drug treatment to prevent vitreous senescence and detachment, would be beneficial, since it would prevent the development and complications of PDR *(15)*.

Proliferation and Regression of New Vessels

Initially, new vessels may be very subtle on clinical examination. Their caliber may eventually range up to that of a major retinal vein at the disc margin (Fig. 3). New vessels frequently form wheel-like networks (see Fig. 2). NV networks also may be irregular in

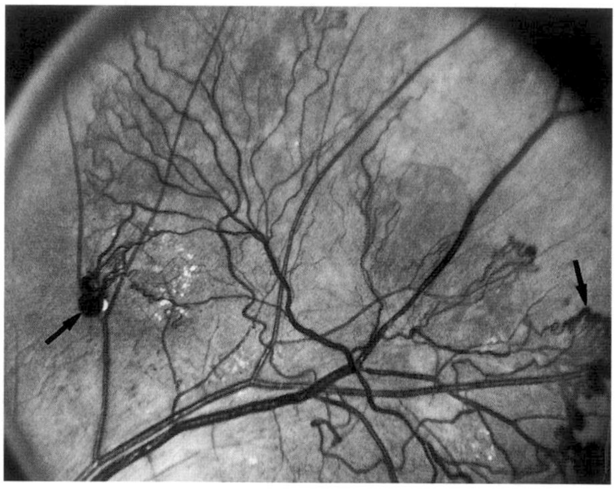

Fig. 3. New vessels elsewhere without prominent network formation. Over much of their course, these new vessels did not form networks. Large aneurysmal dilations were present at the end of a long new vessel loop (*left arrow*) and at the circumference of a partial wheel-like network (*right arrow*). (Courtesy Diabetic Retinopathy Study Research Group.)

shape, without a distinct radial pattern. New vessel patches often lie over retinal veins and appear to drain into them. The superotemporal vein is involved somewhat more frequently than others *(10, 11)*. At times new vessels grow for several disc diameters across the retina without forming prominent networks (Fig. 3).

The rate of growth of NV is variable. In some patients a patch of vessels may show little change over years, whereas in others a definite increase may be seen in 1 or 2 weeks. Early in their evolution, new vessels appear bare, but later delicate white fibrous tissue usually becomes visible within the complex. Histopathologically, NV always has a variety of cell types, including pericytes, fibrocytes, macrophages, and glial cells, in addition to the endothelial cells of the vessels themselves. Hence, even when the vessels have the clinical appearance of bare, naked vessels, the common clinical convention of referring to such tissue as "fibrous" or "fibrovascular" is technically correct *(16, 17)*. In many cases, as the NV complex matures or involutes, the nonvascular whitish component becomes more prominent (Fig. 4a–d). In such cases, the extravascular cellular proliferation has become prominent relative to the vascular component. Vascular lumina containing blood cells are nearly always present in involuted fibrous-appearing tissue on microscopy, even if blood-filled vessels are not visible on clinical examination.

NV lesions characteristically follow a cycle of enlargement, followed by partial or complete regression *(10, 18)*. Regression of a wheel-shaped net of new vessels typically begins with a decrease in the number and caliber of the vessels at the center of the patch, followed by their partial replacement with fibrous tissue. Simultaneously, the peripheral vessels tend to become more narrow, although they may still be growing in length and the patch may still be enlarging (Fig. 4a). At times, regressing new vessels appear to become sheathed. The width of the sheath, which presumably represents opacification and thickening of the vessel wall, increases until only a network of white lines without visible blood columns remains (see Fig. 4d). At times certain new vessels seem to become preferential channels, enlarging while adjacent vessels regress and disappear. Fresh, active new vessels are commonly seen emerging from the edges of partially regressed patches, and new vessels are frequently seen at different stages of development in different areas of the same eye. Early in their evolution, the fibrous components of fibrovascular proliferations tend to be translucent and are easily underestimated. Subsequently, with increasing growth, contraction, or separation from the retina, they become more prominent.

A feature of fibrocytic proliferation is eventual contraction, a complication responsible for most of the complications of PDR. If contraction of the vitreous and fibrovascular proliferations does not occur, new vessels may pass through all the stages described here without causing any visual symptoms. Concurrently, a decrease in intraretinal lesions and in the caliber of major retinal vessels may occur as retinopathy enters the burned-out stage. Occasionally, new vessels appear to regress completely, leaving no trace of their previous presence *(19)*.

Contraction of the Vitreous and Fibrovascular Proliferations

Before the onset of posterior vitreous detachment, NV networks appear to be on or slightly anterior to the retina, both by biomicroscopy and in stereophotographs. At this stage, slit-lamp examination of new vessel patches that appear to be slightly elevated

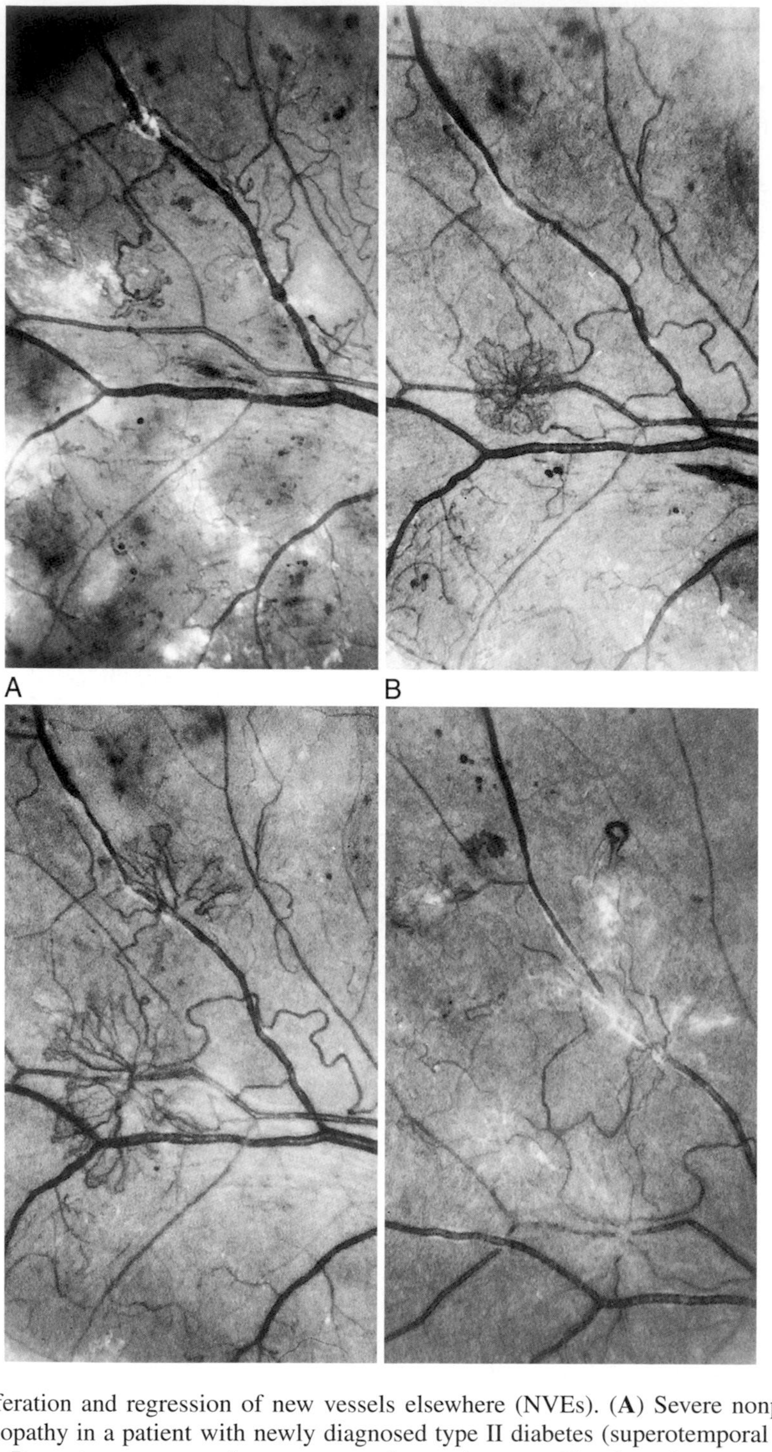

Fig. 4. Proliferation and regression of new vessels elsewhere (NVEs). (**A**) Severe nonproliferative diabetic retinopathy in a patient with newly diagnosed type II diabetes (superotemporal quadrant of the right eye). Present were many microaneurysms, hemorrhages, and hard exudates, as well as extensive retinal edema and venous beading. Most of the tortuous small vessels appeared to be within the retina (large intraretinal microvascular abnormalities), but some may have been on its surface (NVEs). (**B**) Eight months later, marked improvement in the intraretinal abnormalities was noted, but a wheel-like network of new vessels had appeared on the surface of the retina. Venous beading had decreased,

shows no change in the vitreous adjacent to them nor any separation between them and the retina. Nearly all NV is adherent to the posterior vitreous surface. This adhesion becomes apparent when posterior vitreous detachment occurs adjacent to the patch, pulling its edge forward. If vitreous detachment surrounds the patch, all its edges become more elevated than its center, giving its anterior surface a concave appearance.

Before the beginning of posterior vitreous detachment, new vessels usually are asymptomatic *(10, 18)*. Small hemorrhages in the posterior vitreous are occasionally seen near the growing ends of the new vessels, but they usually remain subhyaloid or hang suspended in the most posterior portion of the vitreous without becoming apparent to the patient. When symptomatic vitreous hemorrhages do occur, some evidence of localized posterior vitreous detachment usually can be found. When only a small area of the posterior vitreous surface is detached, it appears flat and very close to the retina; but as detachment becomes more extensive, this surface moves forward and assumes a curved contour more or less parallel to the retina and slightly anterior to it. This otherwise smoothly curved surface is held posteriorly by vitreoretinal adhesions at the sites of new vessels. The new vessels in turn tend to be pulled forward in these same areas. Vitreous strands and opacities usually can be seen anterior to the posterior vitreous surface, whereas posteriorly the vitreous cavity is optically empty or contains red blood cells *(10, 20)*. The principal force pulling the posterior vitreous surface forward usually appears to be the forward vector resulting from contraction of this surface and the fibrovascular proliferations growing along it.

Posterior vitreous detachment usually begins near the posterior pole. Detachment often spreads fairly rapidly (within hours, days, or weeks) to the periphery of the quadrant in which it begins, unless such spread is halted by vitreoretinal adhesions associated with patches of new vessels. Circumferential extension into other quadrants of the fundus tends to be slower, sometimes requiring months or years to reach completion. Detachment of the vitreous from the disc usually is prevented by adhesions between the vitreous and fibrovascular proliferations arising there. Vitreous detachment is not a smoothly progressive process. It occurs in abrupt steps, usually halting whenever its advancing edge meets a patch of active or regressed new vessels. Traction on such patches may lead to recurrent vitreous hemorrhages. If contraction continues, the patch is pulled forward, with or without the underlying retina, and vitreous detachment spreads beyond it. At times the peripheral spread of posterior vitreous detachment is temporarily stopped by invisible adhesions to the retina in areas where no new vessels are present *(21)*.

Traction exerted on the new vessels appears to be the primary factor contributing to the recurrent vitreous hemorrhages and these coincide with extension of vitreous

Fig. 4. *(continued)* and venous sheathing had increased. (**C**) Three months later, the new vessel patch had enlarged, and a second patch had developed above it. During the next 2 years, the new vessels continued to grow slowly at the edges of the patches, while regressing at their centers. (**D**) Three years after they had appeared, most of the new vessels had regressed, although there was still one dilated loop at the upper edge of the upper patch. No contraction of fibrous proliferation or vitreous had occurred, no vitreous hemorrhage was present, and vision remained good.

detachment. Hemorrhages also occur independently, sometimes apparently in relation to bouts of severe coughing or vomiting and occasionally at the time of insulin reactions. In such cases, the increased venous backpressure from a Valsalva maneuver may be etiologically related to the rupture of fragile NV vessels. More often vitreous hemorrhages occur during sleep and are unrelated to any obvious factor *(22, 23)*.

Blood in the fluid vitreous posterior to the detached vitreous framework is usually absorbed within weeks or several months, retaining its red color until absorbed. Hemorrhage in the formed vitreous tends to lose its red color and become white or ochre-colored before absorption is complete. Absorption of a large hemorrhage from the formed vitreous usually is slow, requiring many months and sometimes not reaching completion before fresh hemorrhage occurs. As PDR enters the burned-out stage or if a vitreous detachment is complete so that there is no longer any vitreous traction, the hemorrhaging may cease. Particularly in eyes that have had involuted or partially involuted NV, a vitreous hemorrhage may be accompanied by the appearance of a fibrous membrane on the posterior hyaloid face where the fibrous complex has been completely avulsed from the surface of the retina. As noted, if there is a complete vitreous separation at this point, the patient's eye may have a very low risk of subsequent vitreous bleeding *(21)*.

The arrangement and movement of blood in the posterior fluid vitreous often make it possible to define the limits of posterior vitreous detachment ophthalmoscopically *(10, 20)*. In areas of vitreous detachment, the presence of fresh blood in the posterior fluid vitreous obscures fundus details, distinguishing these areas from adjacent ones in which the vitreous remains attached and details of the retina are clear. In the upper quadrants of the fundus, blood tends to become deposited in thin meridional streaks on the detached posterior vitreous surface, identifying its position. Blood may pool between the detached vitreous and attached retina, outlining the inferior extent of vitreous detachment and often forming a fluid-level or boat-shaped hemorrhage. At times, even when posterior vitreous detachment cannot definitely be identified with slit lamp and contact lens, a thin, curving line of subhyaloid hemorrhage parallel to and behind the inferior equator can be seen, presumably marking the lower edge of an area of vitreous detachment. When posterior vitreous detachment is complete, blood in the posterior fluid vitreous can be made to flow into the periphery of any quadrant by positioning the patient's head to make that quadrant dependent. Because of the tendency of vitreous hemorrhage to accumulate in dependent portions of the globe, many clinicians advise patients with dense vitreous hemorrhage to sleep with the head elevated so that blood does not accumulate in the macula, but rather in the inferior periphery. Some patients will remark that this maneuver makes their vision clearer upon arising in the morning. Often, with motion as the patient ambulates, the vitreous hemorrhage will redistribute and the vision clouds once more.

Retinal Distortion and Detachment

With contraction of an extensive sheet of fibrovascular proliferations, distortion or displacement ("dragging") of the macula may occur *(24)*. Since the most common site of extensive fibrovascular proliferations is on and near the disc, the macula usually is dragged nasally and often also somewhat vertically (Fig. 5). Occasionally, a displaced

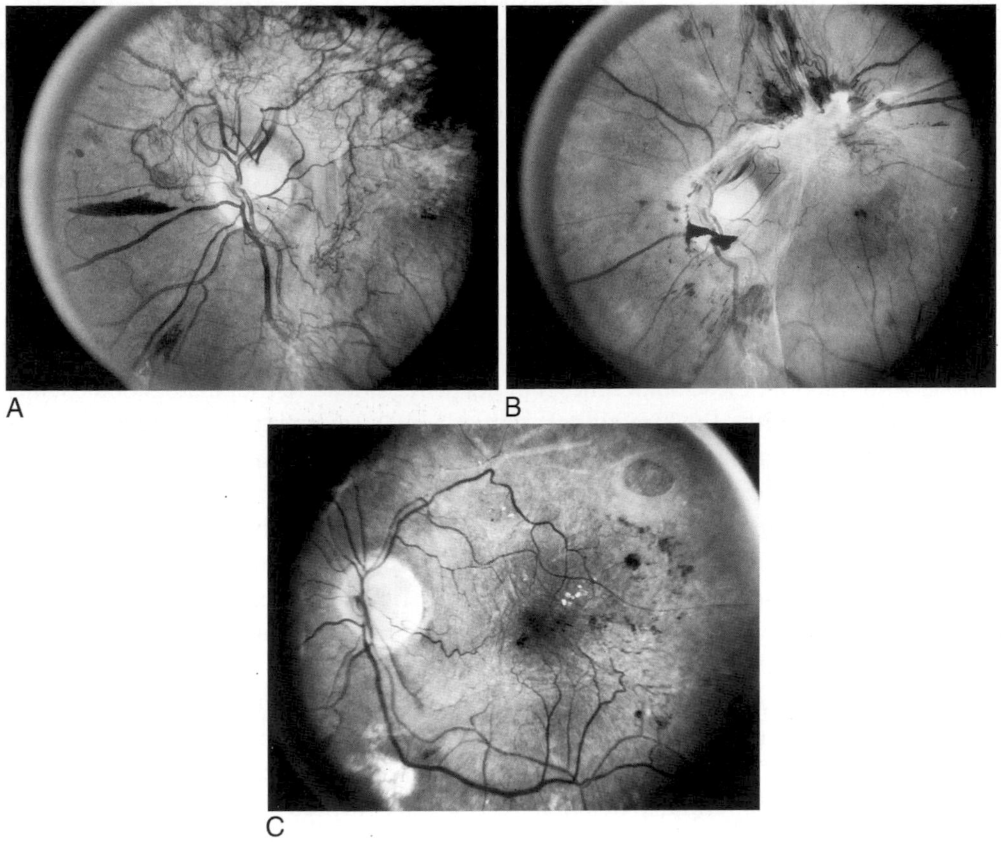

Fig. 5. Dragging of the macula. (**A**) In the left eye of this 39-year-old white woman, whose age at diagnosis of diabetes was 10 years, extensive fibrovascular proliferations were present on and adjacent to the disc, centered superotemporally. The temporal edge of the patch of proliferations was tightly apposed to the retina, and the nasal edge was elevated about one third of a disc diameter by localized posterior vitreous detachment, the lower edge of which was marked by a preretinal hemorrhage. Visual acuity was 20/60. Scatter photocoagulation was initiated. (**B**) Three weeks after photocoagulation, the patient noted a marked decrease in visual acuity and returned for examination. There had been marked regression of the new vessels. Contraction of the proliferations had pulled the neurosensory macula (but not the corresponding, more deeply pigmented retinal pigment epithelium) up and nasally. Vitrectomy was carried out. (**C**) Two months later (postvitrectomy), visual acuity had improved to 20/30, and the neurosensory macula had returned to near-normal position. There appeared to be a rather large, full-thickness retinal break (near upper right corner), but this did not lead to retinal detachment during the remaining 3 years of follow-up. At 4-year follow-up, vision had improved to 20/20. (Courtesy Diabetic Retinopathy Vitrectomy Study Research Group.)

macula will retain good acuity potential, but more often there is a decline in acuity proportionate to the extent of distortion and striae. An eye with a displaced macula may retain good visual acuity for a time, but tractional membranes also cause macular edema. Chronic edema and secondary pigmentary changes will lead to a gradual decline in acuity. Diplopia and metamorphopsia are also common symptoms.

Contraction of the vitreous or fibrovascular proliferations also may lead to retinal detachment. This may be limited to avulsion of a retinal vessel, sometimes accompanied by vitreous hemorrhage. Alternatively, a relatively thin fold of retina may become elevated, with only a narrow zone of retinal detachment adjacent to its base. In other cases retinal detachment may be more extensive, but the concave shape that is typical of traction detachment generally is maintained. If subretinal fluid from a tractional retinal detachment involves the macula, the prognosis for retention of acuity is grave *(25)*. At times, what may appear clinically to be a shallow retinal detachment may be a schisis-like splitting of the retina upon optical coherence tomography *(26)*. Tractional retinoschisis of the retina results in severe retinal dysfunction of the involved region.

At times, small, apparently full-thickness retinal holes may be seen near the proliferations with traction; these sometimes, but not always, lead to rhegmatogenous detachment combined with the tractional components (a tractional–rhegmatogenous detachment). When such A detachment occurs, it tends to have a flat or convex anterior surface and be more extensive, even to the ora serrata. The occurrence and severity of retinal detachment are influenced by the timing and degree of shrinkage of the vitreous and fibrovascular proliferations and by the type, extent, and location of the vitreoretinal adhesions. New vessels with little accompanying fibrous tissue tend to produce less extensive vitreoretinal adhesions and less risk of retinal detachment, particularly when posterior vitreous detachment begins soon after the onset of neovascularization. At times, new vessels that extend for a considerable distance along the surface of the retina appear to be adherent to the retina only at their sites of origin and to the vitreous only near their distal ends. In this case the posterior vitreous surface can pull away before exerting traction on the retina. When new vessels are confined to the surface of the disc, vitreous detachment can reach completion without producing traction on the retina, since there are no vitreoretinal adhesions, but the vitreous remains tethered at the disc. Retinal detachment does not occur in such eyes, but recurrent vitreous hemorrhage from the new vessels is a risk.

Burned-Out Proliferative Diabetic Retinopathy

PDR may be considered to no longer be active when vitreous contraction has reached completion (i.e., when the vitreous has detached from all areas of the retina except those where vitreoretinal adhesions associated with new vessels prevent such detachment) *(10, 18, 27, 28)*. Vitreous hemorrhages decrease in frequency and severity and may stop entirely, although many months may elapse before substantial vitreous clearing occurs. If retinal detachment is absent or only localized and the macula remains intact, visual acuity may be good. Frequently, however, dragging or distortion of the macula or long-standing macular edema leads to substantial reduction in vision. In many cases retinal detachment involves the entire posterior pole, with resultant severe loss of vision. Although spontaneous partial reattachment occasionally occurs, if the macula has been detached for months or years, usually no significant return of vision occurs. A marked reduction in the caliber of retinal vessels is characteristic of this stage. Previously dilated or beaded veins return to normal caliber or become narrower and often appear sheathed; fewer small venous branches are visible. Changes in the arterioles are often even more striking, with decreased caliber and marked reduction of the number of visible branches. Some small arterioles now appear to be white threads without visible blood columns. Characteristically, only occasional retinal hemorrhages and microaneurysms are present. New vessels usually are reduced in caliber and number and are quiescent; at times no patent new vessels can be seen. Marked loss of vision at this stage often seems best explained by severe retinal ischemia *(21)*.

SYSTEMIC ASSOCIATIONS

Relationship of Proliferative Diabetic Retinopathy to Type and Duration of Diabetes

The factor most closely related to prevalence of PDR is duration of diabetes, particularly in those with type 1 (T1DM) *(29)*. In type 2 diabetes (T2DM, adult-onset diabetes) typically discovered in older patients who are often overweight, patients with retinopathy may be asymptomatic at the time of diagnosis, and may even present with significant retinopathy. Such cases occur because of a lengthy period of unrecognized hyperglycemia. It is rare, however, for T2DM patients to present with PDR.

Comparisons of retinopathy features in T1DM and T2DM have been hampered by the difficulty in classifying diabetes type, by the scarcity of studies that have evaluated patients of both types with the same methods, and by the even greater rarity of population-based studies. A population-based stereophotographic study (the Wisconsin Epidemiologic Study of Diabetes, WESDR) was carried out by Klein *(30)*, beginning in the early 1980s. The prevalence of PDR in insulin-taking patients younger than 30 years at diagnosis (mainly T1DM) was near zero when duration of diabetes was less than 10 years and then rose rapidly to about 50% in persons with 20 or more years of diabetes. In an older-onset (30 years or more) insulin-taking group, which included both diabetes types, prevalence of PDR rose from 2% in persons with less than 5 years of diabetes to about 25% in those with 20 years or more. In the older-onset, non-insulin-using T2DM group, prevalence of PDR increased only slightly with duration, from less than 5% before 20 years to about 5% thereafter (Fig. 6). Among patients with PDR, its severity did not appear to differ between the younger-onset and the combined older-onset groups; in each case in the worse eye about 25% of patients had DRS high-risk characteristics and 15% had ungradable retinopathy severity because of extensive vitreous hemorrhage, phthisis bulbi, or enucleation secondary to complications of diabetic retinopathy. In patients with PDR, macular edema was more common in the combined older-onset group; retinal thickening or scars of previous focal photocoagulation were present in at least one eye in about 45% (vs. 30% in the younger-onset group). Given the overall better glycemic control of diabetic patients in developed countries in the current decade, it is likely that the incidence of complications of DM is decreasing, but the greater incidence of disease may offset the overall prevalence data *(31)*.

The Diabetic Retinopathy Vitrectomy Study (DRVS) found a substantial variation in severity of PDR by diabetes type among persons with vitreous hemorrhage severe enough to reduce visual acuity to 5/200 or less for a period of at least 1 month *(25)*. In this study the severity of new vessels, fibrous proliferations, and vitreoretinal adhesions was greater in T1DM than in T2DM. T2DM has a four- or fivefold greater prevalence

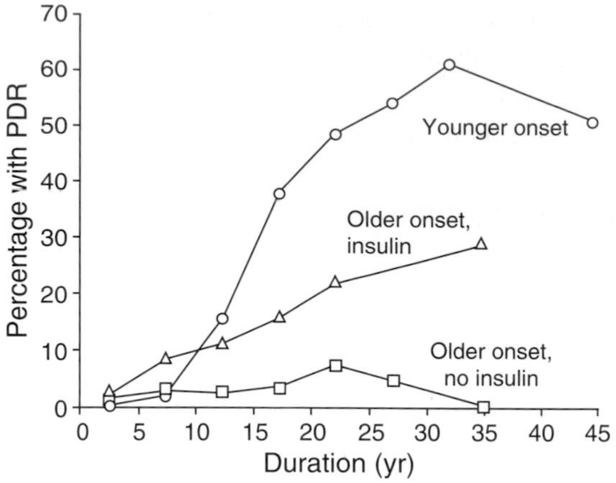

Fig. 6. Percentage of people with PDR by duration of diabetes in each of the three groups. (Reprinted from *(141)*, with permission from Springer Science and Business Media.)

than T1DM, and in clinical practice, PDR is seen with about equal frequency in the younger- and older-onset groups. Klein *(30)* estimated that, in the population they surveyed, 43% of patients with PDR were in the younger-onset group, 42% were in the older-onset insulin-taking group, and 15% were in the non-insulin-taking group. In the DRS, in which more than 90% of the 1,742 patients examined had PDR in at least one eye, 44% were classified as juvenile-onset (younger than 20 years at diagnosis and taking insulin at entry into the study); 28% as adult-onset, possibly insulin-dependent (age 20 years or older at diagnosis, not overweight, and taking insulin); and 26% as classic adult-onset (mild symptomatic or asymptomatic onset at 20 years or older and either overweight or not taking insulin at study entry). The remaining 2% were not classifiable. Aiello et al. *(32)* found the age at diagnosis of diabetes among 244 consecutive patients with PDR to be less than 20 years, 53%; 20–39 years, 25%; and 40 years or older, 22%.

Proliferative Diabetic Retinopathy and Glycemic Control

The Diabetes Control and Complications Trial (DCCT), a large multicenter trial in which patients with type I diabetes were followed up for as long as 9 years, demonstrated conclusively that the long-term risks both for the development of diabetic retinopathy and for its progression from very early to later stages can be reduced markedly by improving blood glucose control with intensive insulin treatment *(33, 34)*. A total of 1,441 patients with no or minimal complications were randomly assigned to either conventional or intensive insulin treatment *(35)*. Conventional treatment was characterized by one or two daily insulin injections, daily self-monitoring of urine or blood glucose, and diet and exercise education. Intensive treatment consisted of insulin administered three or more times daily by injection or an external pump, with doses adjusted according to self-monitored blood glucose results obtained at least four times per day, as well as anticipated dietary intake and exercise, and with the goal of lowering HbA_{1c} (measured monthly) to within the nondiabetic range (6.05%). Seven-field stereoscopic color fundus photographs were taken at baseline and every 6 months thereafter, and they were graded (masked to treatment) centrally using the Early Treatment of Diabetic Retinopathy Study (ETDRS) protocol *(36)*.

Mean HbA_{1c} at baseline was 8.9% in each treatment group (nondiabetic mean, 5.1; SD, 0.5). Over the entire study period, means were 9.1% and 7.2%, respectively, in the conventional and intensive treatment groups. One of the principal outcome measures analyzed was the prevalence of progression by three or more steps on the ETDRS retinopathy severity scale at each visit *(37)*. After 4 years, there was about a fivefold reduction in the risk of progression in the intensive treatment group, compared with that in the conventional. There were similar large risk reductions for progression from NPDR to PDR, which became evident after 3 years of follow-up and exceeded 80% (crude relative risk, 0.17) in the 5.5- to 9-year interval (Table 1).

The Epidemiology of Diabetes Intervention and Complications (EDIC) study was initiated at the close of the DCCT to provide longer-term observations of these patients *(38)*. Patients in the conventional-therapy group were offered intensive therapy and instructed in its use, and the care of all patients was transferred back to their own physicians. In EDIC, patients were evaluated at annual intervals. The most important finding was the continuation of the strong beneficial effect in the group originally randomized to intensive treatment in spite of marked narrowing of the difference in glycemic control between the two treatment groups (HbA_{1c} 8.2% and 7.9%, respectively, in the conventional and intensive treatment groups, vs. 9.1% and 7.2% during the DCCT). In addition, the increasing duration of diabetes in the cohort during the DCCT provided more patients with moderate NPDR or worse than had been available at the beginning of the DCCT (Table 1). At the EDIC 4-year visit 42% of 110 such patients in the original conventional treatment group vs. 22% of 58 patients in the intensive treatment group had progressed (by at least 3 steps on the ETDRS severity scale and in most cases to PDR), representing an odds reduction of 60% (95% CI, 18, 80; $P = 0.012$) *(39)*.

Evidence that better glycemic control in patients with severe NPDR or early PDR reduces their risk of further progression is provided by ETDRS multivariable analyses of risk factors for progression to high-risk PDR in such patients, in which HbA_{1c} at

Table 1
DCCT: Rates of Progression from Nonproliferative Diabetic Retinopathy to Proliferative Diabetic Retinopathy and Crude Relative Risks (RRs), by Follow-Up Time Period

Time period (years)t	*Conventional (C) rate (cases/person-years)*[a]	*Intensive (I) rate (cases/person-years)*[a]	*Crude RR, I:C*
0–1	0.86 (3/351)	0.55 (2/362)	0.65
1.5–3	1.60 (11/688)	1.41 (10/711)	0.88
3.5–5	1.86 (12/646)	0.88 (6/681)	0.47
5.5–9	3.97 (20/504)	0.69 (4/580)	0.17

Modified from *(33)*, Copyright American Medical Association
[a]Rates in cases per 100 person-years at risk

baseline was a strong factor, with odds ratios ranging from 1.6 to 1.9 for patients in the highest vs. the lowest categories, 12% and 8.3%, respectively ($P = 0.0001$) *(39)*. Even in the lowest category the 5-year rate of high-risk PDR was high (50%), and so large odds ratios were not to be expected. These analyses suggest that the benefits of better control continue to be manifest even after severe NPDR or PDR has developed.

The United Kingdom Prospective Diabetes Study (UKPDS) reported results consistent with those of the DCCT in patients with type II diabetes. This randomized trial enrolled 3,867 patients with newly diagnosed type II diabetes and assigned them to intensive treatment with a sulfonyl-urea or insulin, or to conventional treatment beginning with diet only. The HbA_{1c} levels of the intensively and conventionally treated cohorts (medians, 7.0% and 7.9%, respectively, over 10 years of follow-up) were separated by about one half the amount observed in the DCCT. Retinopathy progression over a 9-year period was observed in 31% of 1,171 patients assigned to intensive treatment vs. 38% of 459 patients assigned to conventional treatment ($P = 0.012$) *(40, 41)*. However, this trial did not report rates of progression to PDR.

Caution and close observation are appropriate when a patient with severe NPDR or early untreated PDR is abruptly transitioned from poor to excellent glycemic control because of a phenomenon called "early worsening." As described in the DCCT *(42)*, a greater proportion of subjects in the intensive control groups had worsening of DR at the 6th or 12th month visits, compared with that in the conventional treatment group (13.1% vs. 7.6%, $P < 0.001$). Three eyes of 2 patients in the DCCT progressed from moderate NPDR to HR-PDR within 12 months, all in the intensive control group. Other reports have also noted that severe NPDR or PDR does not respond or even worsens after short-term strict glycemic control intervention, and progression to severe vision loss has been reported *(43–48)*.

Other Risk Factors for Proliferative Diabetic Retinopathy

Results of the ETDRS multivariable analyses of risk factors for progression to high-risk PDR mentioned earlier demonstrate that the strongest factor was retinopathy severity; however, decreased visual acuity was also a strong factor, as was HbA_{1c}. Additional significant factors were the presence of diabetic neuropathy, decreased hematocrit, increased serum triglyceride, and decreased plasma albumin (odds ratios for highest vs. lowest categories of each factor ranged from 1.2 to 1.6) *(49)*.

Severe anemia is an infrequent problem in diabetic patients, but its association with increased risk of severe retinopathy may be important to these patients, as suggested by these ETDRS analyses and other reports. In a multivariable cross-sectional analysis of 1,386 patients in Finland, the relative risk of severe retinopathy (among all patients with retinopathy) was 5 for those with hemoglobin <12 g dL^{-1}, compared with the relative risks of those with higher levels *(50)*. One small case series reported improvement in hard exudates and visual acuity in 3 patients after successful treatment of severe anemia with erythropoietin *(51)*.

Hypertension was not a risk factor for development of high-risk PDR in the ETDRS, and findings in previous studies have been variable *(28, 49)*. In the UKPDS, patients with hypertension were randomized between more and less intensive regimens of blood pressure control, and retinopathy progression was significantly less common in the former, as was the incidence of photocoagulation and of a three or more line decrease in visual acuity, with risk reductions after 7.5 years ranging from 35 to 45% for these outcomes. Progression to PDR was too infrequent for analysis *(41, 52)*. These findings provide strong support for inclusion of intensive blood pressure control in the management of diabetes and diabetic retinopathy.

OTHER TYPES OF INTRAOCULAR NEOVASCULAR PROLIFERATION IN DIABETES

Rubeosis Iridis

The retinal ischemia causing PDR may also lead to new vessels in locations in the eye not on the retina or optic nerve head. Rubeosis iridis, neovascularization of the iris, may occur with or without concurrent PDR in patients with diabetes. In some diabetic patients with PDR, subtle new vessels on the pupil margin may be seen. These vessels may remain relatively stable, particularly after panretinal laser photocoagulation *(53)*. However, the risk of neovascular glaucoma is substantial in the setting of iris neovascularization, as the new vessels tend to invade the angle and root of the iris, causing peripheral synechiae with secondary neovascular glaucoma. As noted previously, in patients who develop spontaneous posterior vitreous detachment, or in vitrectomized eyes, there is no extracellular scaffold upon which neovascular tissue can proliferate out of the retina. Therefore, rubeosis iridis may occur in the absence of PDR. T2DM patients with severe NPDR and PVD should be observed for the potential development of rubeosis iridis. Panretinal laser photocoagulation is generally helpful in preventing the progression of the iris neovascularization after it has been detected.

Anterior Hyaloidal Fibrovascular Proliferation

In eyes with PDR that have had vitrectomy surgery, particularly those with recurrent hemorrhage and retinal detachment, severe fibrovascular proliferation from the sclerotomy sites in the pars plana can occur, called anterior hyaloidal fibrovascular proliferation *(54)*. This ominous complication can sometimes be treated with aggressive laser and repeated surgery *(55)*. If progressive, the eyes are often lost, as the fibrovascular proliferation leads to development of a cyclitic membrane, which in turn, presages the development of hypotony and eventual phthisis.

MANAGEMENT OF PROLIFERATIVE DIABETIC RETINOPATHY

Pituitary Ablation

Although no longer performed, pituitary ablation was an interesting historical footnote in the treatment of PDR; it reached its most widespread use in the 1950s and 1960s. Building on the fundamental discovery of Houssay *(56)* that hypophysectomy reduced the severity of diabetes in pancreatectomized dogs, Luft et al. *(57)* carried out hypophysectomy in the hope of ameliorating the vascular complications of diabetes. Further impetus was provided by Poulsen's *(58)* report of remission of diabetic retinopathy in a woman with postpartum anterior pituitary insufficiency (Sheehan's syndrome). Over the next 25 years, various types of pituitary suppression were used, ranging from external irradiation to transfrontal hypophysectomy, and consensus developed among advocates of these procedures that complete or nearly complete suppression of anterior pituitary function (pituitary ablation) produced rapid improvement in eyes with the intraretinal lesions characteristic of severe NPDR and in those eyes with actively growing new vessels not yet accompanied by extensive fibrous proliferations. Although only two randomized trials have been reported *(59, 60)*, both small and neither in itself compelling, the weight of evidence supports the strongly held opinion of those most experienced with this procedure that it is beneficial. Particularly persuasive are comparisons between patients in whom transsphenoidal implantation of radioactive yttrium was followed by complete or nearly complete anterior pituitary suppression and similar patients in whom little or no suppression was achieved; substantially better outcome was observed in the former group *(61)*. Additional support is provided by a nonrandomized comparison of eyes with very extensive new vessels and IRMAs, in which outcome was better in the eyes of patients undergoing pituitary ablation than in similar eyes receiving photocoagulation or no treatment *(62)*.

The obvious risks of the procedures and difficulty in managing the side effects of pan-hypopituitarism in diabetic patients made this treatment obsolete once the efficacy of panretinal laser photocoagulation was demonstrated. However, the favorable effect of pituitary ablation on retinopathy, which is thought to be mediated by suppression of growth hormone activity, provides rationale for medical interventions designed to achieve this effect. In one such study, daily subcutaneous injections of a genetically engineered growth hormone receptor antagonist, pegvisomant, were given for 3 months in 25 patients with non-high-risk PDR. Regression of new vessels did not occur in any patient, although the serum level of insulin-like growth factor 1, a growth factor whose secretion is stimulated by growth hormone, did decrease, on an average, by 55% compared to baseline levels *(63)*. Several small randomized trials have suggested benefit of octreotide, an inhibitor of insulin-like growth factor 1, for prevention and treatment of PDR *(64–66)*. Paired placebo-controlled phase 3 trials of a long-acting octreotide given subcutaneously every 4 weeks have been conducted but not yet reported in the peer-reviewed literature (Grant M. Treating diabetic retinopathy with insulin-like growth factor 1 antagonists. Diabetic retinopathy – diagnostic and treatment novelties. Symposium. Program and abstracts of the American Diabetes Association 66th scientific sessions, Washington, DC, 9–13 June 2006.). One of these trials demonstrated a reduction in the rate of retinopathy progression with the highest dose of study drug ($P < 0.043$), but the companion trial with identical endpoints did not.

Photocoagulation

The first use of a device to cause intentional burns to the retina utilized solar radiation, but a later device utilizing a xenon arc source was developed by Meyer-Schwickerath of Munich *(67)*. The treatment of PDR involved direct treatment of new vessels on the surface of the retina, particularly those that appeared to be the source of vitreous hemorrhage. Large, slow, moderately intense burns were used, the result of heat generated when light was absorbed by the RPE or by hemorrhage within the retina or on its surface *(68)*. These intense burns usually involved the full thickness of the retina and often led to nerve fiber bundle field defects, particularly if hemorrhages were present in or on the retina. When new vessels were located some distance from the RPE, either in the vitreous or on the optic disc, they could not be treated directly with the xenon arc photocoagulator because it was not possible to concentrate enough energy in a short enough time to coagulate the rapidly flowing blood within them. The possibility of a much more exciting effect of extensive photocoagulation began to emerge with the observation that regression of new vessels and diminution of retinal edema and vascular congestion at some distance from the areas of retina directly treated could occur *(67, 69, 70)*. Beetham et al. *(69)* and Aiello et al. *(71)* began a study in which ruby laser burns were scattered across the retina from the posterior pole to the midperiphery. The long wavelength and very brief exposure time of the ruby laser limited burns mainly to the outer layers of the retina, without immediately visible effects in new vessels on its surface. The rationale initially proposed for regression of new vessels after this indirect treatment was that ischemic retina, which was postulated to be producing a vasoformative factor, was destroyed; hence the term retinal ablation, paralleling pituitary ablation. Indeed this mechanism has been proven by the discovery that the powerful angiogenic protein VEGF is found in high levels in the vitreous of patients with active, but not inactive, PDR *(72)*. Hypoxia upregulates the production of VEGF *(73)*, VEGF levels are associated with intraocular neovascularization in animal models *(74)*, and its inhibition causes the regression of neovascularization in animal models *(75)*. VEGF appears to be a major mediator of the hypoxic neovascular response in PDR.

Photocoagulation may improve oxygenation of the ischemic inner retinal layers by destroying some of the metabolically highly active photoreceptor cells and allowing the oxygen normally diffusing from the choriocapillaris to supply these cells to continue into the inner layers of the retina, relieving hypoxia and removing the stimulus for expression of angiogenic factors such as VEGF *(76–79)*. This theory fails to explain why stronger burns sometimes seem more effective clinically. Retinal blood flow decreases and the autoregulatory response to breathing pure oxygen improves following scatter photocoagulation, as might be expected if more oxygen were reaching the inner retina from the choroid *(80, 81)*. However, the choriocapillaris, which presumably is an important source of the oxygen postulated to be relieving inner retinal ischemia, has been found to be destroyed beneath at least some scatter burns *(82)*. The cells of the RPE produce growth-stimulating and growth-inhibiting factors and the response of these cells to photocoagulation injury may change the balance of these factors *(7, 83, 84)*.

Randomized Clinical Trials of Laser Photocoagulation

The Diabetic Retinopathy Study

The early reports concerning treatment of PDR with photocoagulation suffered from small numbers of patients, brief periods of follow-up, or lack of a randomly selected control group *(85)*. Two collaborative randomized trials were initiated in the early 1970s: the British multicenter trial using xenon arc photocoagulation *(86)* and the National Eye Institute's DRS, which compared xenon arc and argon laser photocoagulation *(8)*. Patients entering the DRS had PDR in at least one eye or severe NPDR in both eyes and visual acuity of 20/100 or better. Each patient was randomized to either the argon or xenon treatment group; one eye was randomly assigned to treatment and the other to indefinite deferral of treatment (i.e., no treatment ever) *(8)*.

The DRS treatment techniques were either xenon arc photocoagulation or argon laser photocoagulation. The argon treatment technique specified 800–1,600, 500-μm scatter burns of 0.1-s duration and direct treatment of new vessels on the disc and elsewhere, whether flat or elevated. Direct treatment was also applied to microaneurysms or other lesions thought to be causing macular edema. Follow-up treatment was applied as needed at 4-month intervals. The xenon technique was similar, but burns were fewer, of longer duration, and stronger, and direct treatment was not applied to elevated new vessels or those on the surface of the disc.

As its principal outcome variable, the DRS chose visual acuity of <5/200 at each of two consecutively completed follow-up visits, scheduled at 4-month intervals, using for this the term severe visual loss. Visual acuity of <5/200 was chosen as the level at which vision becomes too poor to be useful for walking about or for other self-care activities; the requirement of two consecutive visits was included because of the variability in visual acuity assessment: the rate of recovery to better visual acuity after a single visit at the <5/200 level was 29% in the control group and 49% in the treated group; after two visits, it was 12 and 29%, respectively *(8)*.

For all eyes in the untreated control group, the risk of severe visual loss within 2 years was 15.9%, and this was reduced to 6.4% by treatment. The risk was greatest (36.9% in the control group) in eyes that had preretinal or vitreous hemorrhage and NVD exceeding those in standard photograph 10A of the Modified Airlie House

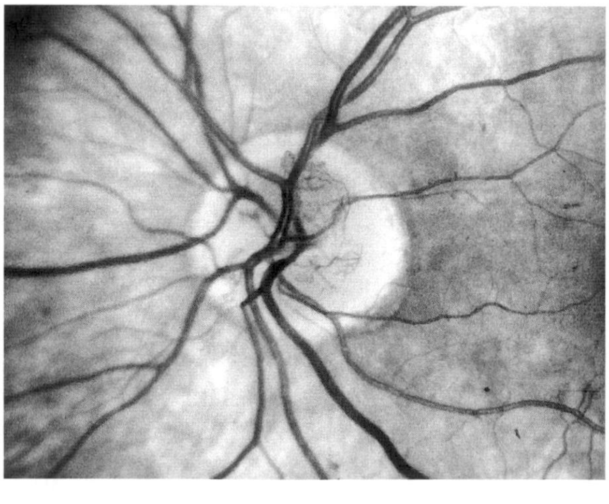

Fig. 7. Standard photograph 10A of the Modified Airlie House classification, defining the lower limit of moderate new vessels on or within 1 disc diameter of the disc. (From *(90)*, with permission from the Association of Research in Vision and Ophthalmology.)

classification (Fig. 7). The risk appeared somewhat lower for eyes with NVD of this severity without hemorrhage (26.2% in the control group). Similar risks (25.6 and 29.7%, respectively) were observed for untreated eyes with vitreous or preretinal hemorrhage and less severe new vessels (Figs. 8 and 9) *(8)*. Treatment reduced the risk of severe visual loss by 50–65% at both 2 and 4 years, except for those eyes with NPDR at 2 years (Fig. 9).

The DRS identified features in eyes with particularly high risk for severe vision loss. Such eyes had three or four new vessel-vitreous hemorrhage risk factors, these factors being (1) new vessels present, (2) new vessels located on or within 1 DD of the disc (NVD), (3) new vessels moderate to severe (NVD equaling or exceeding those in standard photograph 10A (Fig. 7) or, for eyes without NVD, NVE equaling or exceeding one-half disc area in at least one photographic field), and (4) vitreous or preretinal

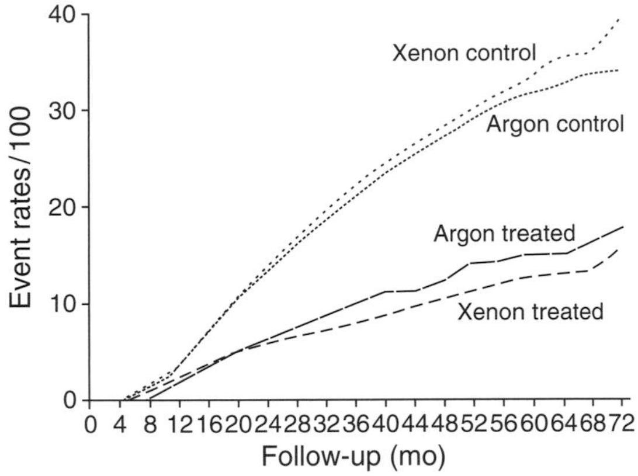

Fig. 8. Cumulative rates of severe visual loss by treatment group. (From *(142)*, copyright Elsevier).

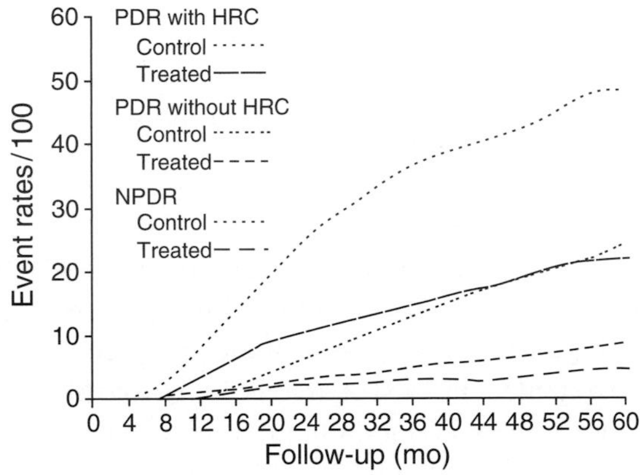

Fig. 9. Cumulative rates of severe visual loss for eyes classified by the presence of proliferative retinopathy (PDR) and high-risk characteristics (HRC) in baseline fundus photographs, argon and xenon groups combined. *NPDR* nonproliferative diabetic retinopathy. (From *(143)*, copyright Elsevier).

Table 2
Diabetic Retinopathy Study Risk Characteristics

- Any new vessels
- New vessels on or within 1,500 μm (1 standard disc diameter) from the disc
- New vessels on the disc ≥ standard photograph 10A (Fig. 7)
- If no disc new vessels, a patch of new vessels on the retina ≥ ½ disc area
- Vitreous or preretinal hemorrhage

3 or more is high-risk PDR

hemorrhage (or both) present (Table 2). In counting the risk factors, the presence and severity of NVE were considered only in eyes without NVD because a subgroup analysis indicated that in eyes with NVD the presence of moderate or severe NVE did not further increase the risk of severe visual loss.

The DRS investigators concluded in 1976 that prompt photocoagulation treatment usually was desirable for eyes with high-risk characteristics. The protocol was therefore modified to allow treatment of eyes originally assigned to the untreated control group, if they had high-risk characteristics then or developed them in the future *(8)*.

Some smaller reports support the results of the DRS. The British multicenter trial, a small randomized study of xenon photocoagulation, reported that of 77 patients observed at the 5-year follow-up visit, 27 untreated eyes (35%) were blind (visual acuity, 6/60 or less), compared with 8 treated eyes (10%) *(86, 87)*. About 2,700 eyes treated for PDR with xenon arc photocoagulation were reported by Okun et al. *(68)*, with about 1,200 eyes observed at the 4-year follow-up visit. Cumulative rates of severe visual loss were almost identical to those observed in DRS-treated eyes, both in eyes with high-risk characteristics and in those with less severe PDR. Decreases in visual acuity of one to four lines were similar to those observed with DRS xenon treatment. Little *(88)* reported results in 457 eyes with NVD exceeding one-fourth disc area treated with 2,000–4,000, 500-μm argon laser burns. New vessels regressed completely in 50% of eyes and showed some decrease in nearly all the remainder. Last recorded visual acuity was <20/200 in about 18% of 241 eyes followed for 5 or more years, an outcome similar to that observed in the DRS.

Risks and Benefits Photocoagulation in the DRS

A temporary decrease in visual acuity is frequently noted after extensive scatter photocoagulation, with recovery to the pretreatment level in most cases within several weeks. In the DRS, visual acuity decreases of one or more lines from which recovery did not occur were attributed to treatment in 14% of argon-treated and 30% of xenon-treated eyes. Visual field losses also were more common in the xenon group (Table 3) *(89)*. In a small subgroup of eyes with severe fibrous proliferations or localized traction retinal detachment, or both, visual acuity decreases of five lines or more were attributed to xenon treatment in 18% of eyes but were not significantly more frequent in argon-treated than in control eyes *(89)*. Because the harmful effects of the DRS argon treatment were less than

Table 3
Estimated Percentages of Wyes with Harmful Effects Attributable to Diabetic Retinopathy Study Treatment

	Argon (%)	*Xenon (%)*
Constriction of visual field (Goldmann IVe4 test object) to an average of ≤45 deg, >30 deg per meridian ≤30 deg per meridian	5	25
Decrease in visual acuity	0	25
1 line	11	19
≥2 lines	3	11

From *(143)*, copyright Elsevier

those observed with the xenon treatment used in the DRS, argon was given preference, and in the hope of further reducing harmful side effects, scatter treatment was more often divided between two or more episodes several days apart.

For eyes with severe NPDR or PDR without high-risk characteristics, the DRS concluded that either prompt treatment or careful follow-up with prompt treatment if high-risk characteristics developed was satisfactory and that DRS results were not helpful in choosing between these strategies. In univariate analyses of DRS control group eyes that had PDR without high-risk characteristics, the severity of each of three retinopathy characteristics was associated with risk of visual loss: retinal hemorrhages or microaneurysms, arteriolar abnormalities, and venous caliber abnormalities. These lesions – and soft exudates and IRMAs – also were risk factors for visual loss in control group eyes with NPDR *(90)*. A multivariable analysis that included all DRS control group eyes found baseline visual acuity; extent of NVD; elevation of NVD (a measure of contraction of vitreous and fibrous proliferations); and severity of hemorrhages or microaneurysms, arteriolar abnormalities, venous caliber abnormalities, and vitreous or preretinal hemorrhage all to be risk factors for visual loss. Neither in this analysis nor in a similar one confined to DRS control group eyes that were free of NVD was the extent of NVE found to be a risk factor *(91)*. These findings support clinical impressions that NVE on the surface of the retina often proliferate and regress over a period of years, remaining asymptomatic unless contraction of vitreous and fibrous proliferations begins, and that the severity of intraretinal lesions may be of greater prognostic importance than the extent of NVE.

The Early Treatment Diabetic Retinopathy Study

For eyes with severe NPDR or early (not high-risk) PDR, DRS results were not helpful in determining which of two treatment strategies would be attended by a more favorable visual outcome: (1) immediate photocoagulation or (2) frequent follow-up and prompt initiation of photocoagulation only if high-risk PDR developed. One of the goals of the ETDRS, a randomized clinical trial sponsored by the National Eye Institute, was to compare these alternatives (designated "early photocoagulation" and "deferral of photocoagulation," respectively) in patients with mild-to-severe NPDR or early PDR, with or without macular edema *(92)*. Other goals were to evaluate photocoagulation for diabetic macular edema and to determine the possible effects of aspirin on diabetic retinopathy. Between 1980 and 1985, 3,711 patients were enrolled. One eye of each patient was randomly assigned to early photocoagulation and the other to deferral. Follow-up ranged from 3 to 8 years. Eyes assigned to early photocoagulation were randomly assigned to either of two scatter treatment protocols, full or mild. The full scatter protocol called for 500-μm, 0.1-s argon blue-green or green laser burns of moderate intensity, placed one-half burn apart, extending from the posterior pole to the equator. Between 1,200 and 1,600 burns were applied, divided between two or more episodes. The mild scatter protocol was the same, except that 400–650 more widely spaced burns were applied to the same area in a single episode. Direct (local) treatment was specified for patches of surface NVE that were two disc areas or less in extent using confluent, moderately intense burns that extended 500 μm beyond the edges of the patch *(93)*.

One important outcome measure used in the ETDRS was the first occurrence of either severe visual loss, as defined in the DRS, or vitrectomy *(92)*. These events were combined because progression to a stage requiring vitrectomy may rightly be considered a bad outcome for ETDRS-eligible eyes and because presumably most eyes selected for vitrectomy before the occurrence of severe visual loss (68% of the 243 ETDRS eyes undergoing vitrectomy) would have developed severe visual loss within several months if vitrectomy had not been done.

The outcome was more frequent in eyes with more severe retinopathy (in the deferral group, 10% in eyes with severe NPDR or early PDR vs. 4% in eyes with mild-to-moderate NPDR). In both of these retinopathy subgroups, early treatment reduced the event rate to about one half that of the deferral group, but the percentage of eyes treated that benefited was only 2–4% (Table 4). Some harmful effects of scatter photocoagulation also were

Table 4
Cumulative 5-year Rates of Severe Visual Loss or Vitrectomy, and Relative Risks For the Entire Period of Follow-Up, by Baseline rRetinopathy Status and Treatment Group

Baseline retinopathy	*Treatment group*				*Relative risk*
	Early photocoagulation		*Deferral*		
	No. at baseline	*5-year rate (%)*	*No. at baseline*	*5-year rate (%)*	
Mild-to-moderate NPDR with macular edema	1,448	2	1,429	4	0.55 (0.33–0.94)[a]
Severe NPDR or early PDR with macular edema	1,090	6	1,103	10	0.68 (0.47–0.99)
Moderate-to-severe NPDR or early PDR without macular edema	1,173	4	1,179	5	0.78 (0.47–1.29)

From *(93)*, copyright Elsevier
NPDR nonproliferative diabetic retinopathy, *PDR* proliferative diabetic retinopathy
[a]Values in parentheses are 99% confidence interval

observed in the ETDRS: an early decrease in visual acuity (a doubling or more of the visual angle at the 4-month visit in about 10% of eyes assigned to early full scatter, compared with about 5% of eyes assigned to deferral) and some decrease in visual field. Both beneficial and harmful effects were somewhat greater with full than with mild scatter.

The ETDRS recommended that scatter treatment not be used in eyes with mild-to-moderate NPDR, but that it be considered for eyes approaching the high-risk stage (i.e., eyes with very severe NPDR or moderate PDR) and that it usually should not be delayed when the high-risk stage is present. The recommendation to consider photocoagulation for eyes approaching the high-risk stage was made because, although both the benefits and risks of treatment were small and roughly in balance, the risk/benefit ratio was approaching a clearly favorable range. A policy of continued observation would be expected to spare only a minority of eyes from the risks of treatment, while increasing the risk that rapid progression might occur between follow-up visits and that entry into the high-risk stage might be marked by occurrence of a large vitreous hemorrhage, making satisfactory treatment difficult. In choosing between prompt treatment and deferral, the commitment of the patient to careful follow-up and the state of the fellow eye are important factors. Eyes with moderate PDR have a nearly 50% risk of severe vision loss at 1 year. A particular subgroup of eyes with very severe NPDR had about the same risk (Fig. 10 and Table 5).

These initial ETDRS recommendations were made without regard to patient age or type of diabetes. Subsequent analyses of ETDRS data suggest that, among patients whose retinopathy is in the severe NPDR to non-high-risk PDR range, the benefit of prompt treatment is greater in those who have type II diabetes (or are older than 40 years; these characteristics are highly correlated, and analyses using either gave almost identical results) *(94)*. In the type II group, the 5-year rate of severe visual loss or vitrectomy was about 5% in eyes assigned to early photocoagulation vs. 13% in eyes

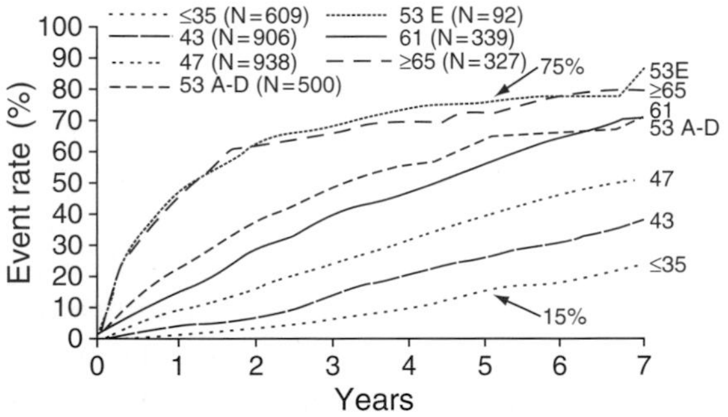

Fig. 10. Cumulative incidence of high-risk PDR in the eyes of Early Treatment Diabetic Retinopathy Study (ETDRS) patients assigned to deferral of photocoagulation. The 5-year rate for eyes with mild NPDR (level 35) was 15%. For eyes with very severe NPDR (level 53E) or moderate PDR (level 65), the 5-year rate was about 75% and the 1-year rate was almost 50%. Levels 43 and 47 represent moderate NPDR; level 53A–D, severe NPDR; and level 61, mild PDR (NVE less than half disc area or fibrous proliferation only). *NPDR* nonproliferative diabetic retinopathy, PDR proliferative diabetic retinopathy, *NVE* new vessels elsewhere. (From *(93)*, copyright Elsevier).

Table 5
Characteristics of severe and very severe NPDR (4–2–1 rule)

Severe NPDR (any one of the following)
• H/MA ≥ Fig. 68–21 in four quadrants
• VB definitely present in ≥ two quadrants
• IRMA ≥ Fig. 68–22 in ≥ one quadrant
Very severe NPDR (two or more of the above characteristics)

NPDR nonproliferative diabetic retinopathy, *H/MA* hemorrhage/microaneurysms, *VB* venous bleeding, *IRMA* intraretinal microvascular abnormalities

assigned to deferral, whereas in the type I group the rates were about 8% in both treatment groups. In eyes assigned to deferral, severe visual loss or vitrectomy developed over the first 3 years at about the same rate in both diabetes types; apparently, the greater treatment effect in type II diabetes resulted mainly from greater responsiveness to early treatment. The DRS also found greater photocoagulation treatment benefit in patients with type II diabetes *(94)*. These studies are consistent with the clinical impression that in patients with type II diabetes high-risk PDR is often first detected on the basis of a symptomatic vitreous hemorrhage in an eye in which new vessels had not been observed on previous visits, whereas in patients with type I diabetes, NVD is more often the first sign of high-risk PDR, an occurrence more easily managed with photocoagulation.

Indications for Photocoagulation of PDR

Treatment should be carried out promptly in most eyes with PDR that have well-established NVD or vitreous or preretinal hemorrhage. Treatment is particularly urgent when localized fresh vitreous or preretinal hemorrhage is present because of the risk that dispersion of the hemorrhage throughout the vitreous or recurrent bleeding may soon make laser treatment more difficult or impossible. In the great majority of such eyes, new vessels of sufficient extent to fulfill the definition of DRS high-risk characteristics can either be seen ophthalmoscopically or be presumed to be present behind the hemorrhage. When visible or suspected new vessels seem insufficient to explain the hemorrhage, special consideration should be given to other possible causes, such as fresh retinal tears, partially avulsed retinal veins, or small patches of new vessels that have been completely avulsed from the disc or retina. Complete avulsion of a small new vessel patch from its connections to the disc or retina should be considered as a possible explanation of a recent vitreous hemorrhage when the detached posterior vitreous surface can be seen anterior to the disc or retina and contains a subtle opacity, suggesting a small patch of empty new vessels *(95)*.

Progressive contraction of fibrous proliferations leading to displacement or detachment of the macula sometimes follows scatter photocoagulation for high-risk characteristics in eyes with extensive fibrous proliferations (Fig. 11). Experience with such cases has led to some reluctance to advise photocoagulation in this situation and to proceed with vitrectomy as a first line management option or to schedule surgery soon after PRP.

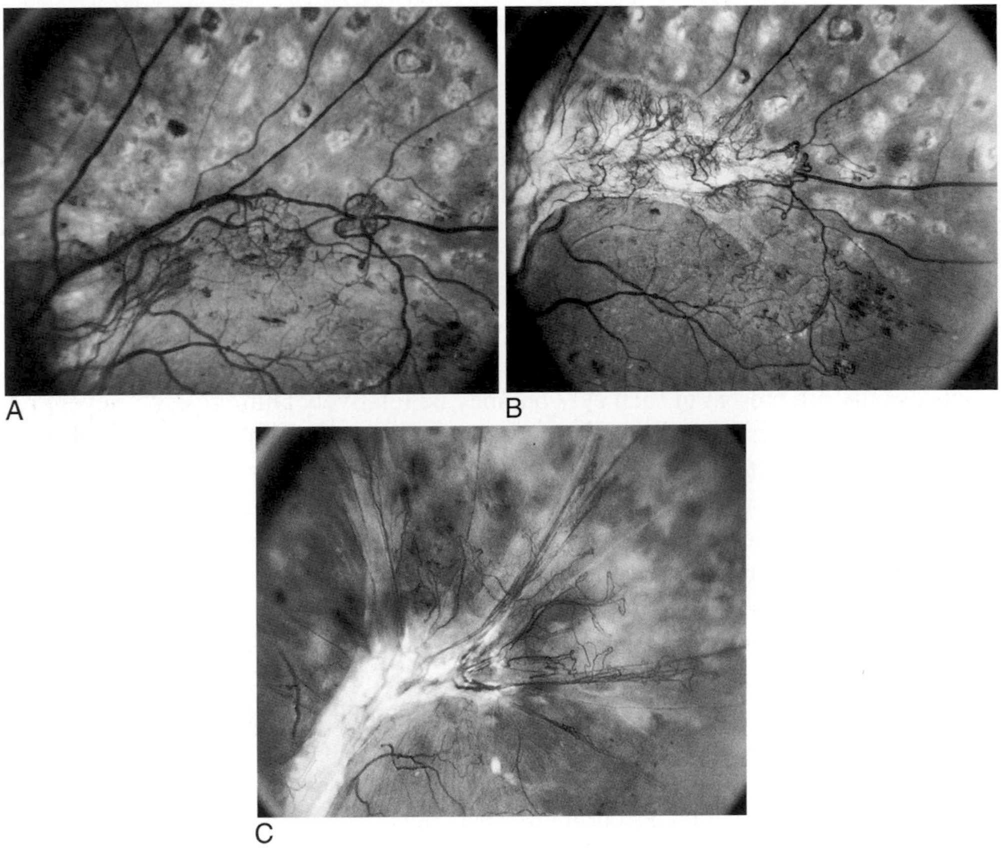

Fig. 11. Contraction of fibrovascular proliferations leading to extensive retinal detachment. (**a**) In the left eye of this 35-year-old man, whose age at diagnosis of diabetes was 14 years, networks of new vessels extended over the surface of the retina along the superotemporal vein. Scars were typical of initial scatter photocoagulation, with space between scars available for additional treatment. (**b**) Four months later, new vessels had increased, and dense fibrous tissue had appeared. (**c**) Seven months later, fibrous proliferations had contracted. Broad adhesions prevented them from pulling away from the retina. Instead, the retina was pulled forward (detached) throughout the area shown in the figure. The photocoagulation scars were blurred by the overlying detached retina (and are out of focus). (Courtesy Diabetic Retinopathy Vitrectomy Study Research Group).

Few such eyes were included in the DRS, but analyses of them indicated that outcome was better with photocoagulation than without it; however, vitrectomy instrumentation and procedures in the current era carry a lower risk of intraoperative and postoperative complications, and the risk/benefit ratio may favor surgery in some situations. When high-risk characteristics are definitely present, scatter photocoagulation usually should be carried out, despite the presence of fibrous proliferations or localized traction retinal detachment. Areas of fibrous proliferations and retinal detachment should be avoided, and treatment strength should be mild to moderate. It may be desirable to divide treatment between several episodes. Of course, photocoagulation is not indicated when PDR is entering the stage of regression, with few or no new vessels and extensive fibrous proliferations.

Extensive neovascularization in the anterior chamber angle is a strong indication for scatter photocoagulation, if it is feasible, regardless of the presence of high-risk characteristics. If this treatment is carried out before extensive closure of the angle has occurred, full-blown neovascular glaucoma can be prevented. When opacities of the media preclude retinal photocoagulation, cryoapplications or vitrectomy with endophotocoagulation may be used.

The presence of extensive retinal hemorrhages, IRMAs, venous beading, and opaque small arteriolar branches, often accompanied by prominent soft exudates, suggests rapidly progressive closure of the retinal capillary bed and severe retinal ischemia. New vessels usually are present in such eyes but may be relatively unimpressive. Severe retinal ischemia increases the urgency to initiate scatter photocoagulation, whether or not DRS high-risk characteristics are present, since eyes so affected appear to be at greater risk of anterior segment neovascularization *(4)*. Patients should be aware of this risk and the risk of a sudden decrease in central vision, which may occur with occlusion of the remaining arterioles supplying the macula.

Systemic factors also should be considered in deciding whether to initiate treatment in patients with very severe NPDR or moderate PDR. Clinical impression suggests that progression of retinopathy may accelerate during pregnancy *(96–100)* or with the development of renal failure *(101–105)*. If photocoagulation is deferred until high-risk characteristics develop, and this occurs in the later stages of pregnancy or when renal transplantation or dialysis is required, these more pressing problems may make it difficult to complete photocoagulation according to a schedule considered optimal from the ophthalmologic point of view. If measures to improve long-standing poor glycemic control are planned when retinopathy is already at this stage, photocoagulation of at least one eye should be considered because of the phenomenon of early worsening, described earlier.

PRP and Macular Edema

Macular edema sometimes increases, at least temporarily, after scatter photocoagulation, and this may be followed by transient or persistent reduction of visual acuity *(106, 107)*. The ETDRS documented small early harmful effects of scatter photocoagulation, particularly full scatter, in eyes with macular edema, as well as in those without. The DRS also found early harmful effects, which were greater in the xenon group. At the 6-week posttreatment visit, 21% of argon-treated and 46% of xenon-treated eyes that had macular edema and were free of high-risk characteristics at baseline had a decrease in visual acuity of two or more lines, compared with 9% of untreated eyes. Comparable percentages for eyes with neither macular edema nor high-risk characteristics were 9%, 18%, and 3%, respectively. After 1 year of follow-up, the greater progression of retinopathy in untreated eyes had led them to catch up with treated eyes; in the group having macular edema without high-risk characteristics at baseline, the percentages with a decrease in visual acuity of two or more lines were 32, 33, and 34%, respectively, in the argon-treated, xenon-treated, and control groups *(108)*. A multivariable analysis confirmed the independent effects of macular edema and treatment and provided no evidence of any interaction *(109)*. Both the

ETDRS and the DRS support the clinical impression that eyes with macular edema requiring scatter treatment are at less risk of visual acuity loss when focal or grid treatment to reduce the macular edema precedes scatter photocoagulation. If a delay of scatter treatment seems undesirable, the ETDRS protocol can be used, combining focal/grid treatment for macular edema with scatter treatment in the nasal quadrants at the first episode of photocoagulation and adding scatter in the temporal quadrants at one or more subsequent episodes *(110)*. Certainly, scatter treatment should not be delayed when the risks of vitreous hemorrhage or neovascular glaucoma seem high, regardless of the status of the macula.

PRP Treatment Techniques

It is important to realize that the size of the burn produced depends not only on the spot-size setting used, but also on power and duration; so it is difficult to compare techniques, even those using the same wavelength and spot-size setting, on the basis of number and theoretical size of burns. It is also difficult to describe burn strength; power level is not very helpful, since the required power for a burn of given strength depends on the clarity of the media and the pigmentation of the fundus, even if spot-size setting and duration are kept constant. One useful measure of burn strength is the need for retrobulbar anesthesia. What we consider to be optimal burn strength with the argon laser is just below the level at which treatment under topical anesthesia with 300–500-μm, 0.1-s burns becomes painful for most patients. With topical anesthesia only, it usually is difficult or impossible to obtain burns of adequate strength when their duration is longer than 0.1 or 0.15 s or their size is >500 μm. The ETDRS protocol for full scatter treatment provides useful guidelines for initial treatment, calling for a total of 1,200–1,600, 500-μm, 0.1-s argon laser burns of moderate intensity placed one-half to one burn apart and divided between two or more episodes (at least 2 weeks apart, if two episodes; at least 4 days apart, if three or more episodes). Burns usually appear to enlarge slightly within several minutes after their application, resulting in the closer spacing of the scatter burns.

Blankenship *(111)* suggested that keeping the posterior limit of scatter treatment farther from the posterior pole may reduce harmful treatment effects. More peripheral treatment protocol may provide a useful alternative for initial treatment of eyes with macular edema in which the urgency of treatment for severe PDR is thought to preclude division of scatter treatment between two or more episodes.

Among the techniques currently in use, the number of episodes in which initial scatter treatment is carried out varies from one to four or more. Those techniques using a smaller number of larger burns tend toward a single episode with retrobulbar anesthesia, whereas those using a larger number of smaller burns nearly always divide treatment into two or more episodes. Multiple episodes make it easier to avoid retrobulbar anesthesia and its occasional complications, but they may cause delays and inconvenience for patients who must travel long distances for treatment. Angle-closure glaucoma secondary to serous detachment of the peripheral choroid and ciliary body is less common when scatter treatment is carried out in two or more sessions over a period of 1 or 2 weeks *(112, 113)*, and some observers believe that small losses in visual acuity also may be less common.

Substantial regression of new vessels usually occurs within days or weeks after the initial application of scatter photocoagulation, and eyes in which new vessels continue to grow despite initial treatment, or recur after partial or complete regression, usually respond well to additional treatment *(114–117)*. Because techniques, assessments, and inclusion criteria between studies vary, it is difficult to directly compare them to report the response rate to an initial course of full PRP. It appears that, on average, about two thirds of eyes have a satisfactory response to initial scatter treatment. As mentioned earlier, this ratio tends to be more favorable in patients with type II diabetes. Patients with severe intraretinal lesions and actively growing new vessels, who typically have type I diabetes, often need multiple treatments. In most cases re-treatment gives positive results *(36, 117)*.

The ETDRS protocol contains guidelines for follow-up treatment that seem suitable for general use. Six factors are considered: (1) change in new vessels since the last visit or last photocoagulation treatment, (2) appearance of the new vessels (caliber, degree of network formation, extent of accompanying fibrous tissue), (3) frequency and extent of vitreous hemorrhage since the last visit or last photocoagulation treatment, (4) status of vitreous detachment, (5) extent of photocoagulation scars, and (6) extent of traction retinal detachment and fibrous proliferations *(118)*. If new vessels appear to be active, as suggested by formation of tight networks, paucity of accompanying fibrous tissue, and increase in extent in comparison to the previous visit, additional photocoagulation is considered. A single episode of vitreous hemorrhage coincident with the occurrence of extensive posterior vitreous detachment, particularly if the only vitreoretinal adhesion remaining is at the disc, argues less for additional photocoagulation than do recurrent hemorrhages unrelated to such an occurrence. The extent and location of photocoagulation scars also may influence the decision regarding additional photocoagulation treatment. If the previous scatter burns appear widely spaced, or if there are areas where scatter was omitted, additional photocoagulation is considered more seriously.

Vitrectomy for PDR

When vitrectomy was initially introduced in 1970 by Machemer et al. *(119)*, the major indications in eyes with PDR were severe vitreous hemorrhage that had failed to clear spontaneously after a year and traction retinal detachment involving the center of the macula. As this procedure came into widespread use, it was recognized that it might be of value earlier in the course of very severe PDR *(120)*. A clinical trial, the Diabetic Retinopathy Vitrectomy Study (DRVS), was established by the National Eye Institute to explore this possibility. In one part of the DRVS, eyes with recent severe vitreous hemorrhage (hemorrhage sufficient to completely obscure the posterior pole and to reduce visual acuity to 5/200 or less for at least 1 month) were randomly assigned to either early vitrectomy or conventional management (i.e., follow-up without vitrectomy unless retinal detachment involving the center of the macula occurred or the hemorrhage failed to clear during a 1-year waiting period) *(25)*. After 2 years of follow-up, recovery of good vision (visual acuity of 10/20 or better) was observed more frequently in the early vitrectomy group, but loss of light perception tended also to occur more frequently in the early vitrectomy group (Table 6). Early vitrectomy appeared to be clearly advantageous only in patients with T1DM. These results suggest that early vitrectomy

Table 6
Percentages of eyes with visual acuities of 10/20 or better and no light perception (NLP) at the 2-year follow-up visit, by type and duration of diabetes and treatment group

	Visual acuity (%)							
	No. of eyes		*≥10/20*			*NLP*		
Baseline factor	*E*	*D*	*E*	*D*	*Difference (E – D)*	*E*	*D*	*Difference (D – E)*[a]
Diabetes type								
Type 1	101	103	35.6	11.7	23.9	27.7	26.2	−1.5
Mixed	70	69	18.6	17.4	1.2	24.3	15.9	−8.4
Type 2	82	72	15.9	18.1	−2.2 (*P* = 0.007)	22.0	12.5	−9.5 (*P* = 0.48)
Duration of diabetes (years)								
All diabetes types								
<20	131	129	21.4	10.1	11.3	28.2	24.8	−3.4
≥20	122	115	27.9	20.9	7.0 (*P* = 0.29)	21.3	13.0	−8.3 (*P* = 0.36)
Type 1 only								
<20	50	53	34.0	1.9	32.1	34.0	35.8	1.8
≥20	51	50	37.3	22.0	15.3 (*P* = 0.007)	21.6	16.0	−5.6 (*P* = 0.50)

E early vitrectomy group, *D* deferral group
From *(25)*, copyright American Medical Association
[a]D minus E rather than E minus D (as for visual acuity ≥10/20), so that a positive value is a difference in favor of early vitrectomy, as is the case for visual acuity ≥10/20

should be considered in eyes with recent severe diabetic vitreous hemorrhage when it is known from prior examination that fibrovascular proliferations are severe, particularly if it appears that macular potential is good. Older patients with severe vitreous hemorrhage sometimes have surprisingly mild PDR, and in such patients it usually is preferable to allow more time for spontaneous clearing of vitreous hemorrhage before considering vitrectomy, particularly if vision in the fellow eye is good.

As vitrectomy techniques have evolved and improved and the frequency of serious complications decreased, additional indications have been suggested. These included traction on the disc, peripapillary retina, or macula that distorts these structures and leads to substantial reduction in visual acuity; opaque fibrous proliferations in front of the macula; and extensive preretinal hemorrhage *(120–122)* (Fig. 5b, c).

In a second study the DRVS compared early vitrectomy vs. conventional management in eyes that had extensive active neovascular or fibrovascular proliferations and useful vision, 65% of which had had previous photocoagulation (Table 7) *(14, 123)*. In eyes with the most severe new vessels (the *severe* and *very severe* categories), early vitrectomy appeared to provide a greater chance of good vision with no increase in risk

Table 7
Percentage of Eyes with Specified Visual Acuity at the 4-year Follow-up Visit for Early Vitrectomy and Conventional Management Groups, and Differences between Groups, by Severity of New Vessels in Baseline Stereoscopic Color Fundus Photographs

	Visual Activity							
	No. of eyes		*≥10/20*			*NLP*		
Baseline factor	*E*	*D*	*E*	*D*	*Difference (E – D)*	*E*	*D*	*Difference (D – E)*[a]
New vessels combined								
Least severe	35	34	42.9	41.2	1.7	20.0	5.9	−14.1
Moderately severe	46	36	50.0	36.1	13.9	23.9	13.9	−10.0
Severe[a]	39	49	43.6	20.4	23.2	17.9	22.4	4.5
Very severe[a]	25	19	36.0	10.5	25.5	32.0	42.1	10.1
P (for interaction)					0.0784			0.0419

NLP no light perception, *E* early vitrectomy, *C* conventional management, *NVD* new vessels on or within 1 DD of the disc, *NVE* new vessels elsewhere

From *(124)*, copyright Elsevier

[a]Eyes with either NVD 1.5 disc areas or more in extent or NVE 2.5 disc areas or more in extent in at least one of the seven standard photographic fields were classified as *severe*; eyes with both NVD and NVE of this extent were classified as *very severe*

of NLP. These results are consistent with those of the earlier DRVS study and support the use of vitrectomy in cases with very severe PDR that do not respond promptly to scatter photocoagulation or in which it cannot be applied because of vitreous hemorrhage.

Pharmacologic Treatment of PDR

Owing to the lack of effective alternative treatments in age-related macular degeneration, pharmacologic management of neovascularization with intravitreal injection of drugs was first introduced for this disease. With greater familiarity with intravitreal injection procedures in the office setting and the tolerability of the procedure among patients, use of these agents has gradually expanded to include treatment of select cases of PDR, but published reports are sparse and most exist as uncontrolled case series.

Steroids are potent antiangiogenic agents and were the first class of such drugs discovered by Folkman *(13)*. Intravitreal triamcinolone acetonide, a potent steroid with a long drug half-life in the eye after intravitreal injection, has been extensively used for treatment of DME. Some literature demonstrates potential efficacy in the treatment of PDR. Although demonstrating good efficacy in pilot reports for neovascularization due to uveitis *(124)*, and intriguing positive reports of its utility in the management of neovascular glaucoma *(125)*, its side effect profile of cataractogenesis *(126)* and secondary steroid-induced glaucoma *(127)* prohibit its widespread use for a condition that already has an effective and tolerable treatment such as PRP. Nevertheless, cases of regression of PDR following intraocular triamcinolone establish that this treatment can be effective in select cases *(128–130)*, and may be used adjunctively with PRP.

The relationship between intraocular NV and intraocular VEGF has been well demonstrated *(74, 75, 131)*. By specifically blocking VEGF activity, therapies with bevacizumab, ranibizumab, and pegaptanib have been reported to temporarily ameliorate neovascular lesions in PDR *(132–134)*, and have been considered as adjunctive therapies for eyes requiring vitrectomy *(135)* and also as adjunctive for PRP. Owing to the invasiveness of intravitreal injection and apparent temporary effects of the above-mentioned drugs, it appears that the use of current agents in the management of PDR is reserved for occasional difficult cases, where there is considerable potential for benefit.

Protein Kinase C beta (PKCβ) is a regulatory intracellular protein that is activated by hyperglycemia and angiogenic growth factors such as VEGF *(136, 137)*. A phase 3 trial demonstrated a modest effect of a specific inhibitor on preservation of vision and reduction in progression of DME, but no effect on the progression of moderate-to-severe NPDR to more severe levels or to PDR *(138)*.

Although eyes with severe vitreous hemorrhage from PDR often proceed to vitrectomy surgery if there is delayed clearing, particularly if there has been no preceding PRP treatment, there has been interest in treatments to promote clearing of vitreous hemorrhage to avoid the risks of surgery and to allow PRP in those cases requiring more laser. Intravitreal hyaluronidase injection has been demonstrated to have modest efficacy with a good safety profile *(139, 140)*. However, the clinical trials failed to achieve their primary endpoint, and hyaluronidase has not been approved by the FDA for this indication.

Pharmacologic management of PDR, either as primary therapy or as adjunctive therapy, has not yet become commonplace. With the intense level of interest in ocular antiangiogenic therapy for treatment of macular degeneration, undoubtedly new treatments will be introduced and tested in the near future. While laser photocoagulation treatment is well tolerated, with relatively rare serious adverse effects, and has excellent efficacy when applied appropriately, there is still opportunity to improve upon this great success.

ACKNOWLEDGMENT

Supported in part by an unrestricted grant from Research to Prevent Blindness, Inc., and by a Research to Prevent Blindness Senior Scientific Investigator Award (M.D.D.).

This chapter was based on and reprinted from *Retina*, 4th edition, Vol. 2 (eds Ryan SJ, Schachat AP), Davis MD, Blodi BA, "Proliferative Diabetic Retinopathy", pp 1285–1322, 2006, with permission from Elsevier.

REFERENCES

1. Shimizu K, Kobayashi Y, Muraoka K. Midperipheral fundus involvement in diabetic retinopathy. *Ophthalmology* 1981;88:601–12.
2. Wise GN. Retinal neovascularization. *Trans Am Ophthalmol Soc* 1956;54:729–826.

3. Kuwabara T, Cogan DG. Retinal vascular patterns. VII. Acellular change. *Invest Ophthalmol* 1965;4:1049–64.
4. Bresnick GH, De Venecia G, Myers FL, Harris JA, Davis MD. Retinal ischemia in diabetic retinopathy. *Arch Ophthalmol* 1975;93:1300–10.
5. Patz A. Clinical and experimental studies on retinal neovascularization. XXXIX Edward Jackson memorial lecture. *Am J Ophthalmol* 1982;94:715–43.
6. Miller JW, Adamis AP, Aiello LP. Vascular endothelial growth factor in ocular neovascularization and proliferative diabetic retinopathy. *Diabetes Metab Rev* 1997;13:37–50.
7. Patel JI, Tombran-Tink J, Hykin PG, Gregor ZJ, Cree IA. Vitreous and aqueous concentrations of proangiogenic, antiangiogenic factors and other cytokines in diabetic retinopathy patients with macular edema: implications for structural differences in macular profiles. *Exp Eye Res* 2006;82:798–806.
8. The Diabetic Retinopathy Study Research Group. Photocoagulation treatment of proliferative diabetic retinopathy: the second report of diabetic retinopathy study findings. *Ophthalmology* 1978;85:82–106.
9. Imesch PD, Bindley CD, Wallow IH. Clinicopathologic correlation of intraretinal microvascular abnormalities. *Retina* 1997;17:321–9.
10. Davis MD. Vitreous contraction in proliferative diabetic retinopathy. *Arch Ophthalmol* 1965;74:741–51.
11. Taylor E, Dobree JH. Proliferative diabetic retinopathy. Site and size of initial lesions. *Br J Ophthalmol* 1970;54:11–18.
12. Report 6. Design, methods, and baseline results. *Invest Ophthalmol Vis Sci* 1981;21:149–209.
13. Folkman J, Ingber DE. Angiostatic steroids. Method of discovery and mechanism of action. *Ann Surg* 1987;206:374–83.
14. Early vitrectomy for severe proliferative diabetic retinopathy in eyes with useful vision. Clinical application of results of a randomized trial – Diabetic Retinopathy Vitrectomy Study report 4. *Ophthalmology* 1988;95:1321–34.
15. Sebag J. Abnormalities of human vitreous structure in diabetes. *Graefes Arch Clin Exp Ophthalmol* 1993;231:257–60.
16. Kampik A, Kenyon KR, Michels RG, Green WR, de la Cruz ZC. Epiretinal and vitreous membranes. Comparative study of 56 cases. *Arch Ophthalmol* 1981;99:1445–54.
17. Nork TM, Wallow IH, Sramek SJ, Anderson G. Muller's cell involvement in proliferative diabetic retinopathy. *Arch Ophthalmol* 1987;105:1424–9.
18. Dobree JH. Proliferative diabetic retinopathy: Evolution of the retinal lesions. *Br J Ophthalmol* 1964;48:637–49.
19. Bandello F, Gass JD, Lattanzio R, Brancato R. Spontaneous regression of neovascularization at the disk and elsewhere in diabetic retinopathy. *Am J Ophthalmol* 1996;122:494–501.
20. Tolentino FI, Lee PF, Schepens CL. Biomicroscopic study of vitreous cavity in diabetic retinopathy. *Arch Ophthalmol* 1966;75:238–46.
21. Davis MD, Myers F, Engerman RL, deVenicia G, Magli YL. Clinical observations regarding the pathogenesis of diabetic retinopathy. In: Goldberg MF, Fine SL, eds. *Symposium on the treatment of diabetic retinopathy* (pub. no. 1890). Washington, DC: US Public Heath Service; 1969.
22. Tasman W. Diabetic vitreous hemorrhage and its relationship to hypoglycemia. *Mod Probl Ophthalmol* 1979;20:413–14.
23. Anderson B, Jr. Activity and diabetic vitreous hemorrhages. *Ophthalmology* 1980;87:173–5.
24. Bresnick GH, Haight B, de Venecia G. Retinal wrinkling and macular heterotopia in diabetic retinopathy. *Arch Ophthalmol* 1979;97:1890–5.
25. The Diabetic Retinopathy Vitrectomy Study Research Group. Early vitrectomy for severe vitreous hemorrhage in diabetic retinopathy. Two-year results of a randomized trial. Diabetic Retinopathy Vitrectomy Study report 2. *Arch Ophthalmol* 1985;103:1644–52.
26. Panozzo G, Parolini B, Gusson E et al. Diabetic macular edema: an OCT-based classification. *Semin Ophthalmol* 2004;19:13–20.
27. Beetham WP. Visual prognosis of proliferating diabetic retinopathy. *Br J Ophthalmol* 1963;47:611–19.
28. Ramsay WJ, Ramsay RC, Purple RL, Knobloch WH. Involutional diabetic retinopathy. *Am J Ophthalmol* 1977;84:851–8.
29. Klein R, Klein BE, Moss SE. Epidemiology of proliferative diabetic retinopathy. *Diabetes Care* 1992;15:1875–91.

30. Klein R. The epidemiology of diabetic retinopathy: findings from the Wisconsin Epidemiologic Study of Diabetic Retinopathy. *Int Ophthalmol Clin* 1987;27:230–8.
31. Wong TY, Loon SC, Saw SM. The epidemiology of age related eye diseases in Asia. *Br J Ophthalmol* 2006;90:506–11.
32. Aiello LM, Rand LI, Briones JC, Wafai MZ, Sebestyen JG. Diabetic retinopathy in Joslin Clinic patients with adult-onset diabetes. *Ophthalmology* 1981;88:619–23.
33. The Diabetes Control and Complications Trial Research Group. The effect of intensive diabetes treatment on the progression of diabetic retinopathy in insulin-dependent diabetes mellitus. The Diabetes Control and Complications Trial. *Arch Ophthalmol* 1995;113:36–51.
34. The effect of intensive treatment of diabetes on the development and progression of long-term complications in insulin-dependent diabetes mellitus. *N Engl J Med* 1993;329:977–86.
35. The Diabetes Control and Complications Trial (DCCT): Results of the Feasibility Study and Design of the Full-Scale Clinical Trial. *Pediatr Adolesc Endocrinol* 1989;18:15–21.
36. Early Treatment Diabetic Retinopathy Study design and baseline patient characteristics. ETDRS report no 7. *Ophthalmology* 1991;98:741–56.
37. Diabetes Control and Complications Trial Research Group. Progression of retinopathy with intensive versus conventional treatment in the Diabetes Control and Complications Trial. *Ophthalmology* 1995;102:647–61.
38. Epidemiology of Diabetes Interventions and Complications (EDIC) Research Group. Epidemiology of Diabetes Interventions and Complications (EDIC). Design, implementation, and preliminary results of a long-term follow-up of the Diabetes Control and Complications Trial cohort. *Diabetes Care* 1999;22:99–111.
39. The Diabetes Control and Complications Trial/Epidemiology of Diabetes Interventions and Complications Research Group. Retinopathy and nephropathy in patients with type 1 diabetes four years after a trial of intensive therapy. *N Engl J Med* 2000;342:381–9.
40. UK Prospective Diabetes Study (UKPDS) Group. Effect of intensive blood-glucose control with metformin on complications in overweight patients with type 2 diabetes (UKPDS 34). *Lancet* 1998;352:854–65.
41. UK Prospective Diabetes Study (UKPDS) Group. Tight blood pressure control and risk of macrovascular and microvascular complications in type 2 diabetes: UKPDS 38. *BMJ* 1998;317:703–13.
42. Early worsening of diabetic retinopathy in the Diabetes Control and Complications Trial. *Arch Ophthalmol* 1998;116:874–86.
43. Lawson PM, Champion MC, Canny C et al. Continuous subcutaneous insulin infusion (CSII) does not prevent progression of proliferative and preproliferative retinopathy. *Br J Ophthalmol* 1982;66:762–6.
44. Puklin JE, Tamborlane WV, Felig P, Genel M, Sherwin RS. Influence of long-term insulin infusion pump treatment of type I diabetes on diabetic retinopathy. *Ophthalmology* 1982;89:735–47.
45. Agardh CD, Eckert B, Agardh E. Irreversible progression of severe retinopathy in young type I insulin-dependent diabetes mellitus patients after improved metabolic control. *J Diabetes Complications* 1992;6:96–100.
46. Moskalets E, Galstyan G, Starostina E, Antsiferov M, Chantelau E. Association of blindness to intensification of glycemic control in insulin-dependent diabetes mellitus. *J Diabetes Complications* 1994;8:45–50.
47. Roysarkar TK, Gupta A, Dash RJ, Dogra MR. Effect of insulin therapy on progression of retinopathy in noninsulin-dependent diabetes mellitus. *Am J Ophthalmol* 1993;115:569–74.
48. Henricsson M, Nilsson A, Janzon L, Groop L. The effect of glycaemic control and the introduction of insulin therapy on retinopathy in non-insulin-dependent diabetes mellitus. *Diabet Med* 1997;14:123–31.
49. Davis MD, Fisher MR, Gangnon RE et al. Risk factors for high-risk proliferative diabetic retinopathy and severe visual loss: Early Treatment Diabetic Retinopathy Study report no 18. *Invest Ophthalmol Vis Sci* 1998;39:233–52.
50. Qiao Q, Keinanen-Kiukaanniemi S, Laara E. The relationship between hemoglobin levels and diabetic retinopathy. *J Clin Epidemiol* 1997;50:153–8.
51. Berman DH, Friedman EA. Partial absorption of hard exudates in patients with diabetic end-stage renal disease and severe anemia after treatment with erythropoietin. *Retina* 1994;14:1–5.

52. Matthews DR, Stratton IM, Aldington SJ, Holman RR, Kohner EM. Risks of progression of retinopathy and vision loss related to tight blood pressure control in type 2 diabetes mellitus: UKPDS 69. *Arch Ophthalmol* 2004;122:1631–40.
53. Kaufman SC, Ferris FLR, Swartz M. Intraocular pressure following panretinal photocoagulation for diabetic retinopathy. Diabetic retinopathy report no 11. *Arch Ophthalmol* 1987;105:807–9.
54. Bhende M, Agraharam SG, Gopal L et al. Ultrasound biomicroscopy of sclerotomy sites after pars plana vitrectomy for diabetic vitreous hemorrhage. *Ophthalmology* 2000;107:1729–36.
55. Ho T, Smiddy WE, Flynn HW, Jr. Vitrectomy in the management of diabetic eye disease. *Surv Ophthalmol* 1992;37:190–202.
56. Houssay B, Biasotti A. La diabetes pancreatica de los perros hipofisoprivos. *Soc Argent Biol* 1930;6:251–96.
57. Luft R, Olivecrona H, Sjogren B. [Hypophysectomy in man.]. *Nord Med* 1952;47:351–4.
58. Poulsen JE. Diabetes and anterior pituitary insufficiency. Final course and postmortem study of a diabetic patient with Sheehan's syndrome. *Diabetes* 1966;15:73–7.
59. Kohner EM, Joplin GF, Blach RK, Cheng H, Fraser TR. Pituitary ablation in the treatment of diabetic retinopathy (a randomized trial). *Trans Ophthalmol Soc UK* 1972;92:79–90.
60. Lundbaek K, Malmros R, Andersen R et al. Hypophysectomy for diabetic retinopathy: a controlled clinical trial. In: Goldberg MF, Fine SL, eds. *Diabetic retinopathy*. New York: Thieme-Stratton; 1969.
61. Panisset A, Kohner EM, Cheng H, Fraser TR. Diabetic retinopathy: new vessels arising from the optic disc. II. Response to pituitary ablation by yttrium 90 implant. *Diabetes* 1971;20:824–33.
62. Kohner EM, Hamilton AM, Joplin GF, Fraser TR. Florid diabetic retinopathy and its response to treatment by photocoagulation or pituitary ablation. *Diabetes* 1976;25:104–10.
63. The effect of a growth hormone receptor antagonist drug on proliferative diabetic retinopathy. *Ophthalmology* 2001;108:2266–72.
64. Croxen R, Baarsma GS, Kuijpers RW, van Hagen PM. Somatostatin in diabetic retinopathy. *Pediatr Endocrinol Rev* 2004;1 (Suppl 3):518–24.
65. Grant MB, Caballero S, Jr. The potential role of octreotide in the treatment of diabetic retinopathy. *Treat Endocrinol* 2005;4:199–203.
66. Grant MB, Mames RN, Fitzgerald C et al. The efficacy of octreotide in the therapy of severe nonproliferative and early proliferative diabetic retinopathy: a randomized controlled study. *Diabetes Care* 2000;23:504–9.
67. Meyer-Schwickerath RE, Schott K. Diabetic retinopathy and photocoagulation. *Am J Ophthalmol* 1968;66:597–603.
68. Okun E, Johnston GP, Boniuk I, Arribas NP, Escoffery RF, Grand MG. Xenon arc photocoagulation of proliferative diabetic retinopathy. A review of 2688 consecutive eyes in the format of the Diabetic Retinopathy Study. *Ophthalmology* 1984;91:1458–63.
69. Beetham WP, Aiello LM, Balodimos MC, Koncz L. Ruby-laser photocoagulation of early diabetic neovascular retinopathy: preliminary report of a long-term controlled study. *Trans Am Ophthalmol Soc* 1969;67:39–67.
70. Okun E. The effectiveness of photocoagulation in the therapy of proliferative diabetic retinopathy (PDR) (a controlled study in 50 patients). *Trans Am Acad Ophthalmol Otolaryngol* 1968;72:246–52.
71. Aiello L, Beetham WP, Balodimos MC, Chazan B, Bradley R. Ruby laser photocoagulation in treatment of diabetic proliferating retinopathy: preliminary report. In: Goldberg MF, Fine SL, eds. *Symposium on the treatment of diabetic retinopathy* (pub. no. 1890). Washington, DC: US Public Health Service; 1969.
72. Aiello LM, Cavallerano J. Diabetic retinopathy. *Curr Ther Endocrinol Metab* 1994;5:436–46.
73. Aiello LP, Pierce EA, Foley ED et al. Suppression of retinal neovascularization in vivo by inhibition of vascular endothelial growth factor (VEGF) using soluble VEGF-receptor chimeric proteins. *Proc Natl Acad Sci USA* 1995;92:10457–61.
74. Miller JW, Adamis AP, Shima DT et al. Vascular endothelial growth factor/vascular permeability factor is temporally and spatially correlated with ocular angiogenesis in a primate model. *Am J Pathol* 1994;145:574–84.
75. Adamis AP, Shima DT, Tolentino MJ et al. Inhibition of vascular endothelial growth factor prevents retinal ischemia-associated iris neovascularization in a nonhuman primate. *Arch Ophthalmol* 1996;114:66–71.

76. Molnar I, Poitry S, Tsacopoulos M, Gilodi N, Leuenberger PM. Effect of laser photocoagulation on oxygenation of the retina in miniature pigs. *Invest Ophthalmol Vis Sci* 1985;26:1410–14.
77. Pournaras CJ. Retinal oxygen distribution. Its role in the physiopathology of vasoproliferative microangiopathies. *Retina* 1995;15:332–47.
78. Pournaras CJ, Tsacopoulos M, Strommer K, Gilodi N, Leuenberger PM. Experimental retinal branch vein occlusion in miniature pigs induces local tissue hypoxia and vasoproliferative microangiopathy. *Ophthalmology* 1990;97:1321–8.
79. Stefansson E, Hatchell DL, Fisher BL, Sutherland FS, Machemer R. Panretinal photocoagulation and retinal oxygenation in normal and diabetic cats. *Am J Ophthalmol* 1986;101:657–64.
80. Patel V, Rassam S, Newsom R, Wiek J, Kohner E. Retinal blood flow in diabetic retinopathy. *BMJ* 1992;305:678–83.
81. Grunwald JE, Riva CE, Brucker AJ, Sinclair SH, Petrig BL. Altered retinal vascular response to 100% oxygen breathing in diabetes mellitus. *Ophthalmology* 1984;91:1447–52.
82. Wilson DJ, Green WR. Argon laser panretinal photocoagulation for diabetic retinopathy. Scanning electron microscopy of human choroidal vascular casts. *Arch Ophthalmol* 1987;105:239–42.
83. Adamis AP, Shima DT, Yeo KT et al. Synthesis and secretion of vascular permeability factor/vascular endothelial growth factor by human retinal pigment epithelial cells. *Biochem Biophys Res Commun* 1993;193:631–8.
84. Gao G, Li Y, Zhang D, Gee S, Crosson C, Ma J. Unbalanced expression of VEGF and PEDF in ischemia-induced retinal neovascularization. *FEBS Lett* 2001;489:270–6.
85. Ederer F, Hiller R. Clinical trials, diabetic retinopathy and photocoagulation. A reanalysis of five studies. *Surv Ophthalmol* 1975;19:267–86.
86. Cheng H. Multicentre trial of xenon-arc photocoagulation in the treatment of diabetic retinopathy. A Randomized controlled study. Interim report. *Trans Ophthalmol Soc UK* 1975;95:351–7.
87. Photocoagulation for proliferative diabetic retinopathy: a randomised controlled clinical trial using the xenon-arc. *Diabetologia* 1984;26:109–15.
88. Little H. Proliferative diabetic retinopathy: pathogenesis and treatment. In: Little H, Patz A, Forsham P, eds. *Diabetic retinopathy*. New York: Thieme-Stratton; 1983.
89. The Diabetic Retinopathy Study Research Group. Photocoagulation treatment of proliferative diabetic retinopathy: relationship of adverse treatment effects to retinopathy severity. Diabetic Retinopathy Study report no 5. *Dev Ophthalmol* 1981;2:248–61.
90. Diabetic Retinopathy Research Group. Diabetic Retinopathy Study, Report 7. A modification of the Airlie House classification of diabetic retinopathy. *Invest Ophthalmol Vis Sci* 1981;21:210–26.
91. Rand LI, Prud'homme GJ, Ederer F, Canner PL. Factors influencing the development of visual loss in advanced diabetic retinopathy. Diabetic Retinopathy Study (DRS) report no 10. *Invest Ophthalmol Vis Sci* 1985;26:983–91.
92. Early Treatment Diabetic Retinopathy Study Research Group. Early photocoagulation for diabetic retinopathy. ETDRS report no 9. *Ophthalmology* 1991;98:766–85.
93. The Early Treatment Diabetic Retinopathy Study Research Group. Techniques for scatter and local photocoagulation treatment of diabetic retinopathy: Early Treatment Diabetic Retinopathy Study report no 3. *Int Ophthalmol Clin* 1987;27:254–64.
94. Ferris F. Early photocoagulation in patients with either type I or type II diabetes. *Trans Am Ophthalmol Soc* 1996;94:505–37.
95. The Early Treatment Diabetic Retinopathy Study Research Group. Case reports to accompany Early Treatment Diabetic Retinopathy Study reports 3 and 4. *Int Ophthalmol Clin* 1987;27:273–333.
96. Phelps RL, Sakol P, Metzger BE, Jampol LM, Freinkel N. Changes in diabetic retinopathy during pregnancy. Correlations with regulation of hyperglycemia. *Arch Ophthalmol* 1986;104:1806–10.
97. Klein BE, Moss SE, Klein R. Effect of pregnancy on progression of diabetic retinopathy. *Diabetes Care* 1990;13:34–40.
98. Chew EY, Mills JL, Metzger BE et al. Metabolic control and progression of retinopathy. The Diabetes in Early Pregnancy Study. National Institute of Child Health and Human Development Diabetes in Early Pregnancy Study. *Diabetes Care* 1995;18:631–7.
99. Lovestam-Adrian M, Agardh CD, Aberg A, Agardh E. Pre-eclampsia is a potent risk factor for deterioration of retinopathy during pregnancy in type 1 diabetic patients. *Diabet Med* 1997;14:1059–65.

100. Temple RC, Aldridge VA, Sampson MJ, Greenwood RH, Heyburn PJ, Glenn A. Impact of pregnancy on the progression of diabetic retinopathy in type 1 diabetes. *Diabet Med* 2001;18:573–7.
101. Jensen T. Albuminuria – a marker of renal and generalized vascular disease in insulin-dependent diabetes mellitus. *Dan Med Bull* 1991;38:134–44.
102. Kostraba JN, Klein R, Dorman JS et al. The epidemiology of diabetes complications study. IV. Correlates of diabetic background and proliferative retinopathy. *Am J Epidemiol* 1991;133:381–91.
103. Cruickshanks KJ, Ritter LL, Klein R, Moss SE. The association of microalbuminuria with diabetic retinopathy. The Wisconsin Epidemiologic Study of Diabetic Retinopathy. *Ophthalmology* 1993;100:862–7.
104. Agardh CD, Agardh E, Torffvit O. The association between retinopathy, nephropathy, cardiovascular disease and long-term metabolic control in type 1 diabetes mellitus: a 5 year follow-up study of 442 adult patients in routine care. *Diabetes Res Clin Pract* 1997;35:113–21.
105. Klein R, Zinman B, Gardiner R et al. The relationship of diabetic retinopathy to preclinical diabetic glomerulopathy lesions in type 1 diabetic patients: the Renin-Angiotensin System Study. *Diabetes* 2005;54:527–33.
106. McDonald HR, Schatz H. Visual loss following panretinal photocoagulation for proliferative diabetic retinopathy. *Ophthalmology* 1985;92:388–93.
107. Meyers SM. Macular edema after scatter laser photocoagulation for proliferative diabetic retinopathy. *Am J Ophthalmol* 1980;90:210–6.
108. Indications for photocoagulation treatment of diabetic retinopathy: Diabetic Retinopathy Study report no 14. *Int Ophthalmol Clin* 1987;27:239–53.
109. Ferris FLR, Podgor MJ, Davis MD. Macular edema in Diabetic Retinopathy Study patients. Diabetic Retinopathy Study report no 12. *Ophthalmology* 1987;94:754–60.
110. Techniques for scatter and local photocoagulation treatment of diabetic retinopathy: Early Treatment Diabetic Retinopathy Study report no 3. *Int Ophthalmol Clin* 1987;27:254–64.
111. Blankenship GW. A clinical comparison of central and peripheral argon laser panretinal photocoagulation for proliferative diabetic retinopathy. *Ophthalmology* 1988;95:170–7.
112. Doft BH, Blankenship GW. Single versus multiple treatment sessions of argon laser panretinal photocoagulation for proliferative diabetic retinopathy. *Ophthalmology* 1982;89:772–9.
113. Liang JC, Huamonte FU. Reduction of immediate complications after panretinal photocoagulation. *Retina* 1984;4:166–70.
114. Doft BH, Blankenship G. Retinopathy risk factor regression after laser panretinal photocoagulation for proliferative diabetic retinopathy. *Ophthalmology* 1984;91:1453–7.
115. Reddy VM, Zamora RL, Olk RJ. Quantitation of retinal ablation in proliferative diabetic retinopathy. *Am J Ophthalmol* 1995;119:760–6.
116. Rogell GD. Incremental panretinal photocoagulation. Results in treating proliferative diabetic retinopathy. *Retina* 1983;3:308–11.
117. Vander JF, Duker JS, Benson WE, Brown GC, McNamara JA, Rosenstein RB. Long-term stability and visual outcome after favorable initial response of proliferative diabetic retinopathy to panretinal photocoagulation. *Ophthalmology* 1991;98:1575–9.
118. Treatment techniques and clinical guidelines for photocoagulation of diabetic macular edema. Early Treatment Diabetic Retinopathy Study report no 2. *Ophthalmology* 1987;94:761–74.
119. Machemer R, Buettner H, Norton EW, Parel JM. Vitrectomy: a pars plana approach. *Trans Am Acad Ophthalmol Otolaryngol* 1971;75:813–20.
120. Shea M. Early vitrectomy in proliferative diabetic retinopathy. *Arch Ophthalmol* 1983;101:1204–5.
121. O'Hanley GP, Canny CL. Diabetic dense premacular hemorrhage. A possible indication for prompt vitrectomy. *Ophthalmology* 1985;92:507–11.
122. Ramsay RC, Knobloch WH, Cantrill HL. Timing of vitrectomy for active proliferative diabetic retinopathy. *Ophthalmology* 1986;93:283–9.
123. Early vitrectomy for severe proliferative diabetic retinopathy in eyes with useful vision. Results of a randomized trial – Diabetic Retinopathy Vitrectomy Study report 3. *Ophthalmology* 1988;95:1307–20.
124. Young S, Larkin G, Branley M, Lightman S. Safety and efficacy of intravitreal triamcinolone for cystoid macular oedema in uveitis. *Clin Exp Ophthalmol* 2001;29:2–6.

125. Jonas JB, Hayler JK, Sofker A, Panda-Jonas S. Regression of neovascular iris vessels by intravitreal injection of crystalline cortisone. *J Glaucoma* 2001;10:284–7.
126. Thompson JT. Cataract formation and other complications of intravitreal triamcinolone for macular edema. *Am J Ophthalmol* 2006;141:629–37.
127. Bakri SJ, Beer PM. The effect of intravitreal triamcinolone acetonide on intraocular pressure. *Ophthalmic Surg Lasers Imaging* 2003;34:386–90.
128. Jonas JB, Hayler JK, Sofker A, Panda-Jonas S. Intravitreal injection of crystalline cortisone as adjunctive treatment of proliferative diabetic retinopathy. *Am J Ophthalmol* 2001;131:468–71.
129. Zein WM, Noureddin BN, Jurdi FA, Schakal A, Bashshur ZF. Panretinal photocoagulation and intravitreal triamcinolone acetonide for the management of proliferative diabetic retinopathy with macular edema. *Retina* 2006;26:137–42.
130. Bandello F, Polito A, Pognuz DR, Monaco P, Dimastrogiovanni A, Paissios J. Triamcinolone as adjunctive treatment to laser panretinal photocoagulation for proliferative diabetic retinopathy. *Arch Ophthalmol* 2006;124:643–50.
131. Miller JW, Stinson WG, Folkman J. Regression of experimental iris neovascularization with systemic alpha-interferon. *Ophthalmology* 1993;100:9–14.
132. Adamis AP, Altaweel M, Bressler NM et al. Changes in retinal neovascularization after pegaptanib (Macugen) therapy in diabetic individuals. *Ophthalmology* 2006;113:23–8.
133. Spaide RF, Fisher YL. Intravitreal bevacizumab (Avastin) treatment of proliferative diabetic retinopathy complicated by vitreous hemorrhage. *Retina* 2006;26:275–8.
134. Avery RL. Regression of retinal and iris neovascularization after intravitreal bevacizumab (Avastin) treatment. *Retina* 2006;26:352–4.
135. Krzystolik MG, Filippopoulos T, Ducharme JF, Loewenstein JI. Pegaptanib as an adjunctive treatment for complicated neovascular diabetic retinopathy. *Arch Ophthalmol* 2006;124:920–1.
136. Aiello LP, Bursell SE, Clermont A et al. Vascular endothelial growth factor-induced retinal permeability is mediated by protein kinase C in vivo and suppressed by an orally effective beta-isoform-selective inhibitor. *Diabetes* 1997;46:1473–80.
137. Aiello LP. The potential role of PKC beta in diabetic retinopathy and macular edema. *Surv Ophthalmol* 2002;47 (Suppl 2):S263–9.
138. Aiello LP, Davis MD, Girach A et al. Effect of ruboxistaurin on visual loss in patients with diabetic retinopathy. *Ophthalmology* 2006;113:2221–30.
139. Kuppermann BD, Thomas EL, de Smet MD, Grillone LR. Pooled efficacy results from two multinational randomized controlled clinical trials of a single intravitreous injection of highly purified ovine hyaluronidase (Vitrase) for the management of vitreous hemorrhage. *Am J Ophthalmol* 2005;140: 573–84.
140. Kuppermann BD, Thomas EL, de Smet MD, Grillone LR. Safety results of two phase III trials of an intravitreous injection of highly purified ovine hyaluronidase (Vitrase) for the management of vitreous hemorrhage. *Am J Ophthalmol* 2005;140:585–97.
141. Klein R et al. The Wisconsin Epidemiologic Study of Diabetic Retinopathy: a comparison of retinopathy in younger and older onset diabetic persons. In: Vranic M, Hollenberg C, Steiner G, eds. *Comparison of type I and II diabetes*. New York: Plenum; 1985.
142. Photocoagulation treatment of proliferative diabetic retinopathy. Clinical application of Diabetic Retinopathy Study (DRS) findings, DRS Report Number 8. *Ophthalmology* 1981;88:583.

3 The Epidemiology of Diabetic Retinopathy

Ronald Klein, MD, MPH

Contents

Abstract

Over the past 25 years, there have been dramatic changes in the management of diabetes and its complications resulting from the application of evidence from randomized controlled clinical trials showing the efficacy of photocoagulation treatment (e.g., Diabetic Retinopathy Study [DRS], Early Treatment Diabetic Retinopathy Study [ETDRS]), and glycemic and blood pressure control (e.g., Diabetes Control and Complications Trial [DCCT], United Kingdom Prospective Diabetes Study [UKPDS]) *(1–6)*. Translation of these findings to clinical care have resulted in changes in the incidence and progression of retinopathy and resultant visual loss in persons with diabetes. The purpose of this chapter is to review the epidemiology of diabetic retinopathy over this period of change.

Key Words: Diabetic retinopathy; epidemiology; incidence; risk factors.

From: *Contemporary Diabetes: Diabetic Retinopathy*
Edited by: E. Duh © Humana Press, Totowa, NJ

BRIEF HISTORICAL BACKGROUND

Shortly after the invention of the ophthalmoscope by Helmholtz in 1851, the first descriptions of lesions defining diabetic retinopathy appeared. Classification systems for diabetic retinopathy were first developed at the end of the nineteenth century by Hirschberg *(7)*.

Prior to 1921, signs of diabetic retinopathy were limited primarily to persons with older-onset noninsulin-dependent diabetes because younger-onset persons with insulin-dependent diabetes rarely survived long enough to develop signs of retinopathy. The discovery and use of insulin by Banting and Best led to longer survival of persons with younger-onset insulin-dependent type 1 diabetes. With longer survival, the presence and severity of retinopathy increased as did visual loss due to retinopathy.

The role of glycemia in the pathogenesis of diabetic retinopathy remained uncertain for many years after the discovery of insulin. Retinopathy was thought by some to be related to high blood sugar while others thought it to be associated with arteriosclerosis, high blood pressure, and serum high cholesterol levels and not hyperglycemia *(8)*. This latter belief was based on the observation that retinopathy was present in some diabetic patients despite seemingly good glycemic control while it was absent in others despite relatively poor glycemic control. The University Group Diabetes Program (UGDP), initiated in 1960, was a long-term prospective randomized controlled clinical trial that evaluated the effects of four methods of treatment (oral hypoglycemic agents, insulin in fixed or variable doses, and diet only) on mortality and vascular complications in persons with type 2 diabetes *(9)*. Data from this trial showed no statistically significant differences in the incidence or progression of retinopathy in the groups studied for 5 and 12 years (for the insulin and diet groups) despite differences in levels of glycemic control as measured by fasting blood glucose values. These findings provided further evidence supporting those who believed that poor glycemic control was not causally related to the incidence and progression of diabetic retinopathy.

The lack of certainty regarding the efficacy of glycemia in preventing the development of diabetic vascular complications and the high frequency of complications, such as severe hypoglycemia associated with intensive insulin treatment, resulted in a long period beginning in the 1940s through the 1990s where blood sugar in persons with diabetes was relatively poorly controlled by today's standards. By the 1970s, diabetic retinopathy was considered the leading cause of legal blindness in persons 25–74 years of age in the United States *(10)*. In 1978, Kelly West in his seminal book "Epidemiology of Diabetes and its Vascular Lesions" wrote: "The extent to which the level of hyperglycemia determines the risk of retinopathy is not at all clear. This is the most important issue at hand and deserves high priority in epidemiologic research" *(11)*.

The Wisconsin Epidemiologic Study of Diabetic Retinopathy (WESDR) was funded by the National Eye Institute in 1979 with its primary aims to: *(1)* describe the prevalence and severity of retinopathy and visual loss in persons with diabetes and their relationship to other systemic complications and mortality; *(2)* quantitate the association of risk factors with retinopathy; and *(3)* provide information on health care delivery and quality of life in persons with diabetes. Over the next 25 years, it provided estimates of the prevalence, incidence, and progression of diabetic retinopathy, its risk factors, and information on the management of retinopathy and other diabetic complications. This ongoing study has taken place in a period of profound change which included: *(1)* the development of new approaches to the management and treatment of diabetes including the self-monitoring of blood glucose, implementation of insulin infusion systems, development of new insulins, insulin sensitizers, and oral hypoglycemic agents; *(2)* the development of new antihypertensive drugs and the use of them earlier in the course of diabetes; *(3)* the promulgation of guidelines, standards, and ophthalmologic care including normalization of glycemia, blood pressure, and lipid levels; *(4)* the development of new education programs promoting dilated eye examinations for earlier detection and treatment of diabetic retinopathy; and *(5)* the initiation of telemedicine screening approaches using digital photographic technology and centralized grading of images for earlier detection of vision-threatening retinopathy. The purpose of this chapter is to review the epidemiology of diabetic retinopathy using data from the WESDR, other population-based studies, and clinical trials to examine how these data have been used to develop public health approaches to reduce visual loss due to retinopathy.

THE WESDR

The study design and methods have been described in detail in previous reports *(12–14)*. In brief, 452 of the 457 physicians who provided primary care to diabetic patients in an 11 county area in southern Wisconsin participated in the study. The 452 physicians kept lists of all their diabetic patients for whom they provided primary care from July 1, 1979 to June 30, 1980. During this 1-year period, 10,135 diabetic patients were identified. A sample of 2,990 persons was selected for the baseline examination. This sample was composed of two groups. The first consisted of all patients diagnosed as having diabetes before 30 years of age who took insulin (1,210 patients); this group is referred to as "younger-onset" and is made up of those with type 1 diabetes. The second group consisted of a probability sample of 1,780 persons of the 5,431 patients who met the eligibility criteria of being diagnosed as having diabetes at 30 years of age or older and who had their diagnosis confirmed by a casual or a postprandial serum glucose level of at least 11.1 mmol/L or a fasting serum glucose level of at least 7.8 mmol/L on at least two occasions; this group is referred to as "older-onset." The latter group was stratified by duration of disease (<5 years, 576 persons; 5–14 years, 579 persons; and ≥ 15 years, 625 persons). Of these, 824 were taking insulin and 956 were not.

Of the 2,990 eligible patients, 2,366 (79.1%) participated in the baseline examination from 1980 through 1982. The younger-onset WESDR cohort was re-examined in 1984–1986, 1990–1992, 1994–1996, 2000–2002, and in 2005–2007, while the older-onset cohort was re-examined in 1984–86 and 1990–92 and interviewed only in 1994–1996. The main reason for nonparticipation in the study for both groups was death. In the WESDR, stereoscopic color fundus photographs of the DRS seven standard fields were taken of each eye *(15)*. Objective masked grading of retinopathy using standard protocols assured reproducible assessment and classification of the severity of retinopathy *(16, 17)*.

PREVALENCE OF DIABETIC RETINOPATHY

At the time of the WESDR baseline examination (1980–1982), 71% of younger-onset persons had retinopathy, and 23% of these had PDR of whom 10% had Diabetic Retinopathy Study High Risk Characteristics (DRS-HRC) for severe visual loss (Table 1) *(13)*. Retinopathy was found in 70% and 39% of the older onset persons taking and not taking insulin, respectively, of whom 5% and 1% had signs of PDR

Table 1
Prevalence and Severity of Retinopathy and Macular Edema at the Baseline Examination in the Wisconsin Epidemiologic Study of Diabetic Retinopathy

Retinopathy status	*Younger-onset, taking insulin (n=996)*	*Older-onset, taking insulin (n=673)*	*Older-onset, not taking insulin (n=673)*
None	29.3	29.9	61.3
Early nonproliferative	30.4	30.6	27.3
Moderate to severe nonproliferative	17.6	25.7	8.5
Proliferative without DRS high-risk characteristics	13.2	9.1	1.4
Proliferative with DRS high-risk characteristics or worse	9.5	4.8	1.4
Clinically significant macular edema	5.9	11.6	3.7

DRS Diabetic Retinopathy Study
Modified from Ref. 206. Copyright © Elsevier 1995

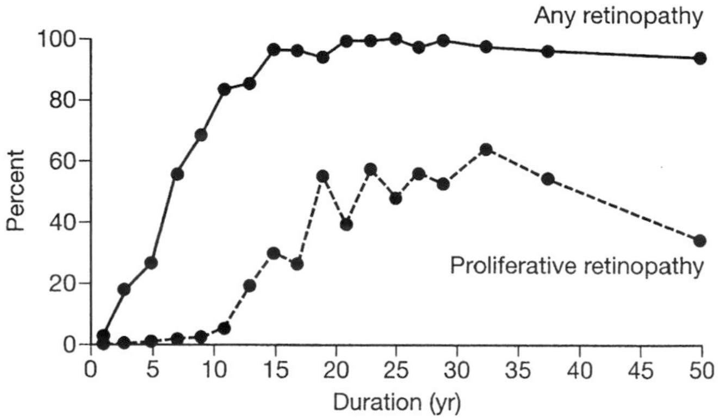

Fig. 1. Prevalence of any retinopathy and of proliferative diabetic retinopathy in insulin-taking patients diagnosed with diabetes at age < 30 years, by duration of diabetes. Data are from Wisconsin Epidemiologic Study of Diabetic Retinopathy (WESDR) 1980–1982.
Source: Reproduced with permission from Ref. *205*.

with DRS-HRC, respectively (Table 1) *(14)*. Six percent of the younger, 12% of the older-onset taking insulin, and 4% of the older-onset not taking insulin subjects had clinically significant macular edema (CSME) *(18)* Based on these data, it was estimated that the burden of PDR with HRC and/or CSME in the 5.8 million persons with known diabetes at the time of the 1980–1982 examination in the United States was approximately 400,000.

For younger- and older-onset persons, both the frequency and severity of retinopathy (Figs. 1 and 2) and CSME (Fig. 3) increased with increasing duration of diabetes

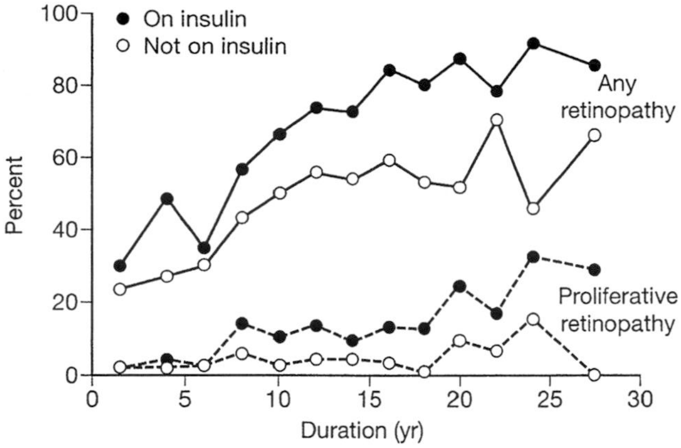

Fig. 2. Prevalence of any retinopathy and of proliferative diabetic retinopathy in patients diagnosed with diabetes at age 30 years or older, by duration of diabetes. Data are from WESDR 1980–1982. **Source:** Reproduced with permission from Klein R, Klein BEK, Moss SE. Risk factors for retinopathy. In: Feman SS (ed). Ocular problems in diabetes mellitus. Boston: Blackwell Publishing; 1992:39.

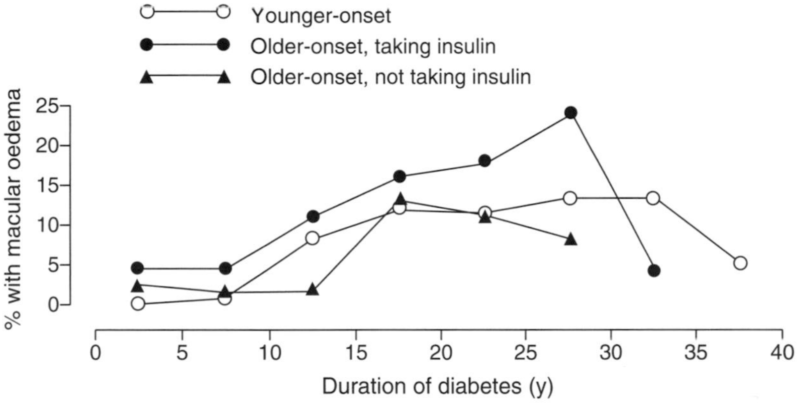

Fig. 3. Frequency of clinically significant macular edema (CSME, as defined in the Early Treatment Diabetic Retinopathy Study) by duration of diabetes in younger-onset persons taking insulin ($n = 996$) and older-onset persons taking insulin ($n = 674$) or not taking insulin ($n = 696$) who participated in the WESDR, 1980–1982.
Source: Reproduced with permission from Reproduced with permission from Klein R, Klein BEK, Moss SE. Risk factors for retinopathy. In: Feman SS (ed). Ocular problems in diabetes mellitus. Boston: Blackwell Publishing; 1992:39.

(13, 14, 18). In the younger-onset group, the prevalence of retinopathy during the first 5 years after the diagnosis of diabetes was 14%, and in all cases it was mild. On the other hand, in younger-onset persons with diabetes for 20 or more years, 53% had signs of PDR, and 11% had signs of CSME. After diagnosis of diabetes, retinopathy was more frequent in the older-onset group compared with the younger-onset group (Figs. 1, 2). In the first 5 years after diagnosis of diabetes, 33% of the older-onset group had retinopathy, 2% had PDR (Fig. 2), and 3% had CSME (Fig. 3). However, after 20 years or

Table 2
Studies Included in Estimates of the Prevalence of Diabetic Retinopathy

Variable	*Barbados Eye Study, Barbados, West Indies*	*BDES Beaver Dam, Wis*	*BMES, Blue Mountain, Australia*	*Melbourne VIP, Melbourne Australia*	*Proyecto VER, Nogales and Tucson, Ariz*	*SAHS, San Antonio, Tex*[a]	*SLVDS, San Luis Valley, Colo*	*WESDR, Southern Wis*
Year study conducted	1988–1992	1988–1990	1992–1994	1991–1998	1999–2000	1985–1987	1984–1988	1980–1982
No. of participants with diabetes mellitus[b]	615	410	252	233	899	351	360	1,313
Photographic fields taken[c]	1 and 2	1–7	1–5	1 and 2	1, 2, and 4	1–7	1, 2, and 4	1–7
Age, years								
40–49	19.2	6.6	0.0	9.9	17.8	31.2	22.9	7.4
50–64	47.2	36.3	38.9	40.8	44.6	66.7	55.8	35.9
65–74	26.3	34.9	36.5	31.7	25.4	12.5	31.4	33.8
≥ 75	7.3	22.2	24.6	17.6	12.2	NA	NA	22.8
Gender								
Women	63.4	56.8	47.2	43.8	63.0	58.7	56.4	53.2
Men	36.6	43.2	52.8	56.2	37.0	41.3	33.6	46.8
Race/ethnicity								
Black	100.0	NA	NA	NA	NA	NA	NA	NA
Hispanic	NA	NA	NA	NA	100.0	80.6	64.7	NA
White	NA	100	100.0	100	NA	19.4	35.3	100.0
Crude prevalence								
Mild NPDR	19.8	22.9	21.0	16.3	36.6	18.2	20.6	36.6

Moderate NPDR	8.0	10.0	4.4	6.9	1.7	13.7	10.3	6.8
Severe NPDR and/or PDR	1.0	2.2	3.6	4.3	6.0	4.3	4.4	6.9
Macular edema	8.6	1.2	4.8	2.2	8.9	2.6	3.3	5.1
DR of any type	28.8	35.1	29.0	27.5	44.3	36.2	35.3	50.3
VTDR	9.1	3.2	6.4	4.3	8.9	5.3	6.4	10.0

Abbreviations: BDES Beaver Dam Eye Study; BMES Blue Mountains Eye Study; DR diabetic retinopathy; NA not applicable; NPDR nonproliferative diabetic retinopathy; PDR proliferative diabetic retinopathy; SAHS San Antonio Heart Study; SLVDS San Luis Valley Diabetes Study; VER Vision Evaluation Research; VIP Visual Impairment Project; VTDR Vision-Threatening Diabetic Research; WESDR Wisconsin Epidemiologic Study of Diabetic Retinopathy

Dates are given as percentage of persons unless otherwise indicated

Source: Reprinted with permission from The American Diabetes Association. The Eye Diseases Prevalence Research Group. Ref. 28. Copyright © 2004 American Medical Association. All rights reserved

[a]Persons with adult-onset diabetes mellitus only

[b]The number of persons reported for each study in this table reflects the number contributing to our estimates in the current article and not necessarily the total number of participants in the original study as published

[c]The photographic fields are described in reference *15*

more of diabetes, fewer people with older-onset diabetes had signs of PDR (22% vs. 53%) than younger-onset people. These findings, in part, provided the rationale for the development of guidelines for need for dilated eye examination by eye doctors experienced in detection and treatment of diabetic retinopathy: at the time of diagnosis in older-onset persons and yearly thereafter; after age 12 years and/or 5 years duration of diabetes in younger-onset persons; and yearly or more frequently thereafter based on retinopathy severity *(19)*.

Prevalence data from more recently conducted population-based studies show lower frequencies than that found in the WESDR *(20–27)*. To provide more up-to-date estimates of prevalence of diabetic retinopathy in the United States population, data were pooled from eight population-based studies, including the WESDR, most of which used the ETDRS classification scheme to evaluate the severity of diabetic retinopathy *(28)*. These pooled analyses included 1,415 diabetic persons who were Hispanic and 615 individuals who were black. The prevalence estimates were limited to persons 40 years of age and older. The estimates of retinopathy were higher in the WESDR group compared to the seven other studies, all of which were performed at least 10 years after the WESDR baseline examination (Table 2). Based on these analyses, it was estimated that among persons with diabetes, the crude prevalence of diabetic retinopathy was 40% and the crude prevalence of severe retinopathy (preproliferative and PDR or macular edema) was 8% in persons 40 years of age or older. Projection of these rates to the diabetic population 40 years of age or older in the United States resulted in an estimate of 4 million persons with retinopathy of whom 900,000 have signs of vision-threatening retinopathy in 2004.

The above pooled data were largely limited to those with type 2 diabetes. There are recent data from two population-based epidemiological studies also suggesting a possible decrease in the prevalence of retinopathy in persons with type 1 diabetes *(29, 30)*. The Wisconsin Diabetes Registry Study (WDRS) cohort was established in 1987–1992 to examine persons at the time of their diagnosis with type 1 diabetes *(29)*. The cohort was reexamined over the next 10 years. The WDRS data showed lower than expected prevalence of retinopathy compared to previous age- and duration-specific estimates from WESDR persons with type 1 diabetes (Fig. 4), suggesting a decrease in prevalence of this complication in those who were more recently diagnosed. In another study, data from the Epidemiology of Diabetes Complications study in Pittsburgh showed a nonstatistically significant decline in the prevalence of PDR in those with 20 or more years of type 1 diabetes diagnosed at later times *(30)*. These data suggest similar lowering of the prevalence of diabetic retinopathy in type 1 diabetic persons as found in those with type 2 diabetes.

Comparisons among studies must be made cautiously because prevalence of retinopathy is influenced by possible differences in age, sociodemographic, and genetic factors, how diabetes and its component complications are defined, and in the methods used to detect and classify retinopathy among groups under study. Furthermore, without adjusting for duration of diabetes, glycemia, blood pressure levels, and other factors associated with the prevalence of retinopathy, comparisons among populations are limited. However, some of these (e.g., glycemia, blood pressure) probably explain why recent prevalence of diabetic retinopathy is lower.

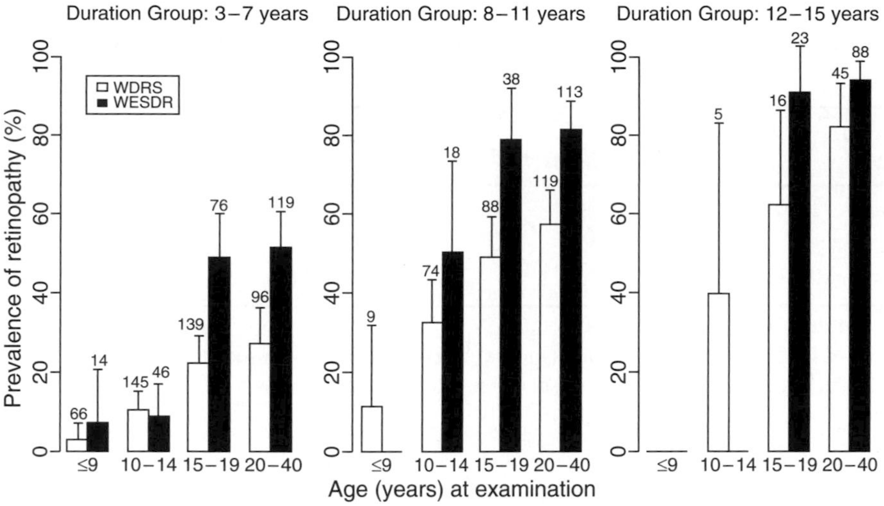

Fig. 4. Prevalence of diabetic retinopathy by duration of type 1 diabetes and age at examination in the Wisconsin Diabetes Registry Study (WDRS) (1990–2002) and the WESDR (1979–1980). Duration groups: 3–7 years (7- or 4-year examination), 8–11 years (9-year examination), and 12–15 years (14-year examination). T-shaped bars show 95% confidence intervals. The number of persons in each age-and-duration group is noted above the bar.

Source: From Ref. 29. Copyright © 2006. Reprinted with permission from Oxford University Press.

INCIDENCE OF DIABETIC RETINOPATHY

Less information is available regarding the incidence and progression of retinopathy in population-based studies *(31–44)*. In the WESDR, the overall incidence of retinopathy in a 10-year interval from 1980–1982 to 1990–1992 was 74%, rate of progression was 64%, and progression to PDR 17% *(36)*. The 10-year incidence and rates of progression of diabetic retinopathy in the WESDR by type of diabetes are presented in Table 3. The younger-onset group using insulin had the highest 10-year incidence, rate of progression, and progression to PDR, while the older-onset group not using insulin had the lowest rates. The older-onset group taking insulin had the highest 10-year incidence of macular edema (data not shown) *(45)*. While the incidence of PDR was higher in the younger-onset group, the estimates of the number of incident cases in the 10-year period were higher in the older- than in the younger-onset group (387 vs. 226 persons) due to the higher frequency of people with older-onset diabetes *(36)*. Based on the WESDR data, it is estimated that each year, of the 10 million Americans estimated to have known diabetes mellitus in 1990–1992, 96,000 will develop PDR, 48,000 will develop PDR with DRS-HRC for severe loss of vision, and 121,000 people will develop macular edema. Due to lower glycemia and blood pressure levels, new definitions of diabetes and greater numbers of persons diagnosed to have diabetes since 1980–1982, these numbers may no longer correctly estimate the annual numbers of diabetic persons developing these complications in 2007.

Is the incidence of late complications (e.g., PDR) declining? In the WESDR, the estimated annual rates of progression to PDR were compared for the first four years of the study with the next six or 10 years of the study *(36, 41)*. The estimated annual

Table 3
10-Year Incidence of Progression of Diabetic Retinopathy in the Wisconsin Epidemiologic Study of Diabetic Retinopathy, 1980–1982 to 1990–1992

Retinopathy	*Younger-onset (%)*	*Older-onset taking insulin (%)*	*Older-onset not taking insulin (%)*
Incidence	89	79	67
Progression	76	69	53
Progression to PDR	30	24	10

PDR proliferative diabetic retinopathy
Source: Reprinted with permission from The American Diabetes Association. Modified from Ref. 36.
Copyright © 1994 American Medical Association. All rights reserved

incidence of PDR was found to be similar in 1994–1996 compared to the first four years of the study (1980–1984). While adjusting for the severity of retinopathy or duration of diabetes at baseline and the 4-year follow-up, the estimated annual incidence of PDR was higher in the next 6-year period than in the first 4-year period in the older-onset groups. These data suggest that the incidence of PDR worsened or remained the same despite improvements in glycemic control over the course of the study.

There are few other population-based studies in which incidence data have been collected over a long period of time using objective measures to detect retinopathy. Data from a clinic-based study in Denmark showed that the incidence of PDR for a specific duration of diabetes was declining for each subsequent 5 years at year of diagnosis from 1965–1969 through 1979–1980 (Fig. 5) *(46)*. This was associated with statistically significant trends of decreasing glycosylated hemoglobin, mean arterial blood pressure levels, and earlier treatment of hypertension in each subsequent period. Long-term follow-up of existing population-based cohorts of diabetic patients are needed to examine whether the incidence of severe diabetic retinopathy is continuing to fall as new treatments are introduced.

RACIAL ETHNIC DIFFERENCE IN PREVALENCE OF DIABETIC RETINOPATHY

Prior to 1980, there were only anecdotal clinical observations that the rates of severe diabetic retinopathy were higher among African Americans and Hispanic Americans than among non-Hispanic European Americans *(47)*. Since that time there has been one population-based study in African American persons with type 1 diabetes, the New Jersey 725, and two studies, the Los Angeles Latino Eye Study (LALES) and the Proyecto VER, providing estimates of diabetic retinopathy in Mexican Americans *(22, 48–52)*. Furthermore, population-based studies such as the Atherosclerosis Risk in Communities (ARIC) Study *(53)* and the Cardiovascular Health Study (CHS) *(54)* have compared diabetic retinopathy prevalence among non-Hispanic European Americans and African Americans. The National Health and Nutrition Survey (NHANES) III *(55)* compared prevalence of diabetic retinopathy among three racial/ethnic groups: non-Hispanic European Americans, African Americans, and Mexican Americans. Another

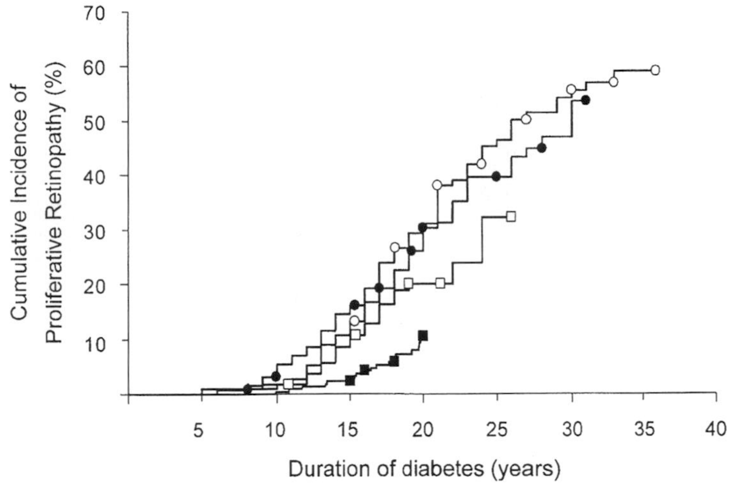

Fig. 5. Cumulative incidence of proliferative retinopathy in 600 type 1 diabetic patients with onset of diabetes from 1965 to 1979 (*n* = 113, group A [*circle*]), 1970–1974 (*n* = 130, group B [*filled circle*]), 1975–1979 (*n* = 113, group C [*square*]), and 1979–1984 (*n* = 244, group D [*filled square*]). *P* < 0.001, log-rank test, pooled over strata. Not all patients in group D have yet been followed for 20 years. For pairwise log-rank test over strata after 20 years of diabetes.
Source: Copyright © 2003 American Diabetes Association. From Ref. 46. Reprinted with permission from *The American Diabetes Association*.

study, the Multi-Ethnic Study of Atherosclerosis (MESA) *(56)*, compared prevalence of diabetic retinopathy among four racial ethnic groups: non-Hispanic European Americans, African Americans, Hispanics, and Chinese Americans.

Diabetic Retinopathy in African American and Hispanic Whites

In the New Jersey 725 study of African Americans conducted from 1993–1997 and using similar methodology for detecting retinopathy as in the WESDR, for persons with type 1 diabetes, the prevalences for any diabetic retinopathy and for PDR are fairly comparable to those of persons with type 1 diabetes in the WESDR (predominantly white European Americans) *(49–51)*. The prevalence of 71% for any retinopathy in WESDR is comparable to 64% in the New Jersey 725 study; similarly, the prevalence of PDR of 23% in WESDR is similar to that prevalence of 19% in the New Jersey 725 study. Because of the infrequency of type 1 diabetes among Hispanics, there are no population-based estimates of differences with white Europeans.

There are more data available regarding retinopathy in African Americans and Hispanics with type 2 diabetes. Data from two population-based studies using the same methodology, the NHANES III (Fig. 6) and the MESA (Fig. 7), showed that diabetic retinopathy prevalence and severity was higher in African Americans and Hispanics than in whites *(55, 56)*. In the NHANES III, the crude prevalence and severity of diabetic retinopathy among African Americans was about twice that of non-Hispanic European Americans *(55)*. However, after controlling for glycosylated hemoglobin, systolic blood pressure, duration of diabetes, and severity of diabetes (measured by need

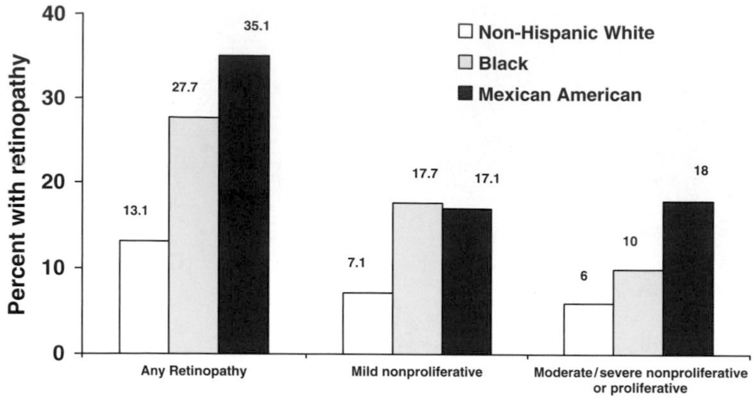

Fig. 6. Severity of retinopathy in whites, blacks, and Mexican Americans with diagnosed non insulin-dependent diabetes mellitus in the National Health and Nutrition Examination III, 1988–1991. **Source**: Copyright © 1998. American Diabetes Association. From Ref. 55. Reprinted and modified with permission from *The American Diabetes Association.*

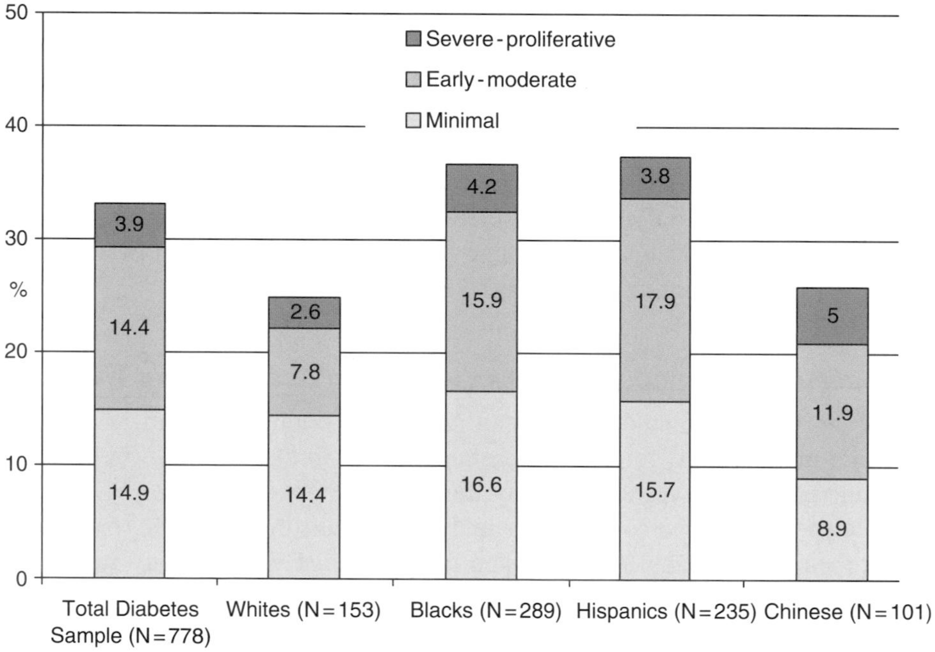

Fig. 7. Prevalence of diabetic retinopathy in the Multi-Ethnic Study of Atherosclerosis subdivided into minimal, mild-moderate, and severe-proliferative grades, in the total diabetes sample and in different racial/ethnic groups.
Source: This article was published in American Journal of Ophthalmology, Ref. 56. Copyright Elsevier © 2006.

for insulin therapy), there were no significant differences between non-Hispanic African Americans and non-Hispanic European Americans in the prevalence and severity of retinopathy in this study. Furthermore, the effect of these known risk factors appeared to be similar in the two groups. The NHANES III investigators concluded that the higher prevalence of retinopathy in African Americans with type 2 diabetes appears due, in part, to poorer glycemic and blood pressure control than in non-Hispanic whites. These are both factors that can be influenced by treatment and patient involvement. In the NHANES III, Mexican Americans diagnosed with type 2 diabetes were three times more likely than non-Hispanic European Americans with type 2 diabetes to have any retinopathy and to have moderate/severe nonproliferative retinopathy or PDR. Although the Mexican Americans were more likely to have poor glycemic control and high systolic blood pressure than non-Hispanic European Americans, these differences were not sufficient to account for the higher prevalence of retinopathy in Mexican Americans than in whites. The odds ratio (OR) for Mexican Americans, after controlling for other factors, was 2.15, with 95% confidence interval (CI) of 1.95–4.04. A similar twofold increase in risk for Mexican Americans has been reported from an analysis of pooled data from the Proyecto VER study, the LALES, and the Beaver Dam Eye Study *(22, 27, 48)*. It is not clear what factors account for differences between Mexican Americans and non-Hispanic European Americans. It is possible that these findings reflect subpopulation differences associated with medical care or perhaps sample design, rather than a general genetic predisposition to more severe complications of diabetes.

Native Americans and Asian Americans

A higher prevalence and incidence of diabetic retinopathy has been reported in Native Americans than in whites and Asians *(57, 58)*. However, the duration-adjusted 4-year cumulative incidence rate of retinopathy in one Native American group, the Pima, was lower than that in whites in the WESDR *(59)*.

Based on grading of fundus photographs, Chinese Americans (25%) were found to have a similar frequency of retinopathy as non-Hispanic European Americans (26%) in the MESA (Fig. 7) *(56)*. Based on self-report in the 2001 Behavioral Risk Factor Surveillance System, Asian Americans had a similar prevalence of retinopathy as non-Hispanic whites *(60)*.

Age and Puberty

For a similar duration of diabetes, the prevalence and incidence of diabetic retinopathy is less frequent prior to than after puberty *(61)*. In the WESDR, duration of diabetes after menarche, a marker of puberty, was associated with an approximate 30% increase in the risk of having any retinopathy compared with duration before menarche *(62)*. The reason for this is not known. Changes in insulin resistance, hormonal levels, and compliance after puberty have been suggested as accounting for this finding. Based on these observations, when type 1 diabetes is diagnosed prior to puberty, guidelines suggest that the first dilated eye examination should begin after puberty and if no retinopathy is present, yearly thereafter.

Genetic and Familial Factors

The reader is referred to recent reviews which describe the genetics of diabetic retinopathy *(63, 64)*.

MODIFIABLE RISK FACTORS

Hyperglycemia

Because of the difficulty in achieving good glycemic control and the lack of certainty of the efficacy of such control in preventing microvascular and macrovascular complications, patients with diabetes, on average, were poorly controlled in the 1970s (see above). For example, at the baseline WESDR eye examination in 1980–1982, the mean glycosylated hemoglobin A1c in younger-onset type 1 participants was 10.1% while in older-onset type 2 participants it was 9.0% compared to 6.0% in nondiabetic persons in the same study. The WESDR provided an excellent opportunity to examine the relationship of retinopathy in a diabetic cohort with a wide range of glycosylated hemoglobin levels (from 6 to 20%) at baseline.

Data from the WESDR (Fig. 8) showed a strong association of glycosylated hemoglobin levels with the 10-year incidence and progression of retinopathy and the incidence of PDR and macular edema (data not shown) *(65)*. On close inspection of Fig. 8, it is apparent that the 10-year progression of diabetic retinopathy in the younger-onset type 1 cohort and older-onset type 2 cohort is similar for persons whose glycosylated hemoglobin levels fell within the 2nd and 3rd quartile ranges at baseline. This observation contradicted the widespread impression at the time that persons with type 2 diabetes had a "milder" form of diabetes and were at a lower risk of progression of retinopathy than persons with type 1 diabetes. These data showed that it is the level of glycemic control and not the type of diabetes that is important in determining progression of retinopathy.

Data from the WESDR also showed that the risk of incidence or progression of retinopathy was similar for a given glycosylated hemoglobin level at any duration of diabetes or at any stage of retinopathy prior to the onset of PDR in persons with both type 1 and 2 diabetes (Figs. 9 and 10) *(65)*. Analyses of the epidemiological data in the DCCT showed less progression of retinopathy when reduction of glycosylated hemoglobin was achieved earlier than later in the course of type 1 diabetes or when milder compared to more moderate nonproliferative retinopathy was present *(66)*. Similarly, epidemiological data from the UKPDS showed that people presenting with type 2 diabetes with lower fasting blood sugars at the start of the study had a lower incidence of retinopathy despite similar glycemic progression *(67)*. Taken together, these data suggest a lower risk of incidence and progression of diabetic retinopathy with earlier intervention to achieve better glycemic control that is maintained throughout the course of the disease.

A 1% change in glycosylated hemoglobin level in the WESDR between the baseline and 4-year follow-up was associated with lower odds of 6-year incidence and progression of retinopathy, incidence of visual loss, nephropathy, lower extremity amputation, and ischemic heart disease mortality in both type 1 and 2 diabetic participants in the WESDR *(68)*. While data from the WESDR and other observational cohort studies have shown a strong and consistent association of reduction in risk of incidence and progression of retinopathy, these observational epidemiological data were not able to demonstrate a cause and effect relationship, that is, they could not demonstrate that a reduction in glycosylated hemoglobin would lead to reduction in incidence and progression of diabetic retinopathy. Two randomized controlled clinical trials, the DCCT and UKPDS were needed to show this *(3, 4)*.

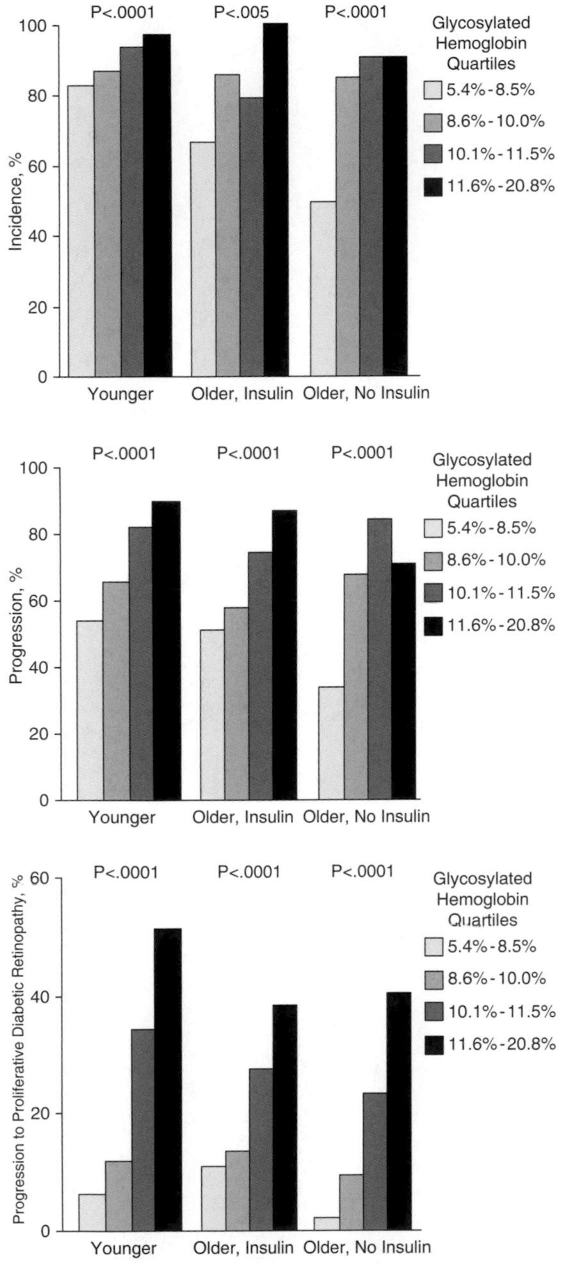

Fig. 8. The relationship of incidence, in persons with younger-onset diabetes, persons with older-onset diabetes taking insulin, and persons with older-onset diabetes not taking insulin over a 10-year period to glycosylated hemoglobin levels by quartiles for the whole population at baseline. *P*-values are based on the Mantel–Haenszel test of trend.
Source: Reprinted with permission from Ref. *65*, The American Diabetes Association. Copyright © 1994 American Medical Association. All rights reserved.

Derby Hospitals NHS Foundation Trust
Library and Knowledge Service

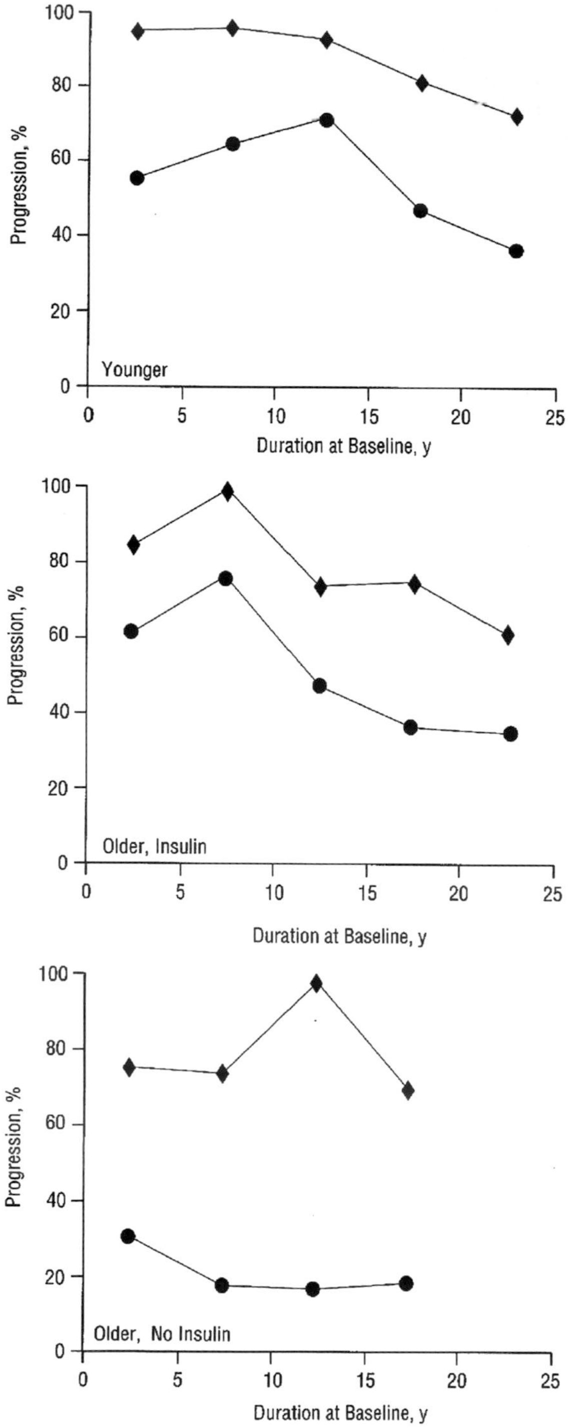

Fig. 9. Ten-year progression of retinopathy by first (*circles*) and fourth (*diamonds*) quartiles of glycosylated hemoglobin levels and by duration of diabetes at the baseline examination in persons with younger-onset diabetes (*top*), in persons with older-onset diabetes taking insulin (*center*), and in persons with older-onset diabetes not taking insulin (*bottom*).

Source*:* Reprinted with permission from Ref. 65, The American Diabetes Association. Copyright © 1994 American Medical Association. All rights reserved.

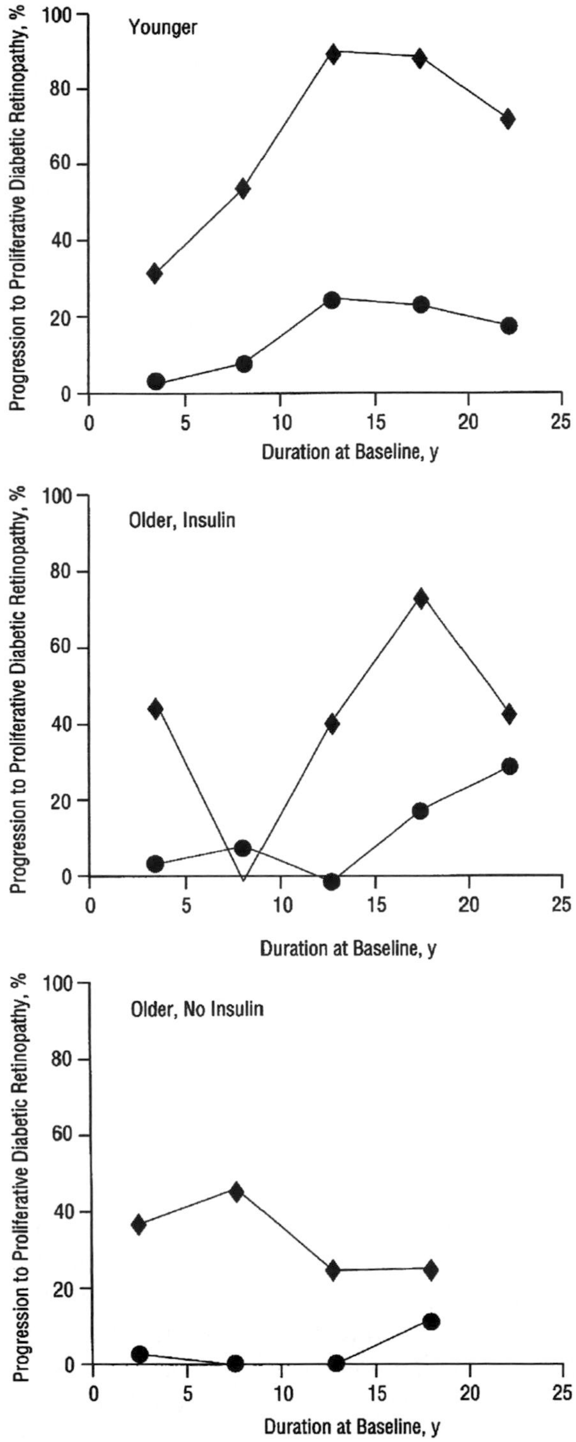

Fig. 10. Ten-year progression to proliferative diabetic retinopathy by first (*circles*) and fourth (*diamonds*) quartiles of glycosylated hemoglobin levels and by duration of diabetes at the baseline examination in persons with younger-onset diabetes (*top*), in persons with older-onset diabetes taking insulin (*center*), and in persons with older-onset diabetes not taking insulin (*bottom*).
Source: Reprinted with permission from Ref. 65, The American Diabetes Association. Copyright © 1994 American Medical Association. All rights reserved.

CLINICAL TRIALS OF INTENSIVE TREATMENT OF GLYCEMIA

Diabetes Control and Complications Trial

The DCCT was designed to compare intensive with conventional diabetes therapy with regard to their effects on the development and progression of retinopathy in persons with type 1 diabetes *(3)*. The study was designed to make recommendations regarding the benefits and risks associated with intensive therapy. Two of the main questions asked in the study were *(1)* Will intensive therapy prevent the development of diabetic retinopathy in patients with no retinopathy (primary prevention)? and *(2)* Will intensive therapy affect the progression of early retinopathy (secondary intervention)? Other issues investigated in the DCCT involved the magnitude of the effect of intensive insulin treatment on progression and regression of retinopathy, the degree to which this effect changes over time, and the relation of the effect to the level of severity of the retinopathy at baseline *(3, 66, 69)*. Persons included in the DCCT at baseline were 13–39 years of age and did not have hypertension, hypercholesterolemia, or severe complications associated with diabetes. From 1983 to 1989, 1,441 persons were randomized to either conventional or intensive insulin therapy *(3)*. Conventional therapy consisted of one or two daily injections of insulin per day, daily self-monitoring of urine or blood glucose, and education about exercise and diet. No attempts were made to do daily adjustments of the insulin dosage. The most important primary outcome measure was a sustained (at two consecutive 6-month visits) three-step progression of diabetic retinopathy along an ordinal ETDRS severity scale based on retinopathy scores in both eyes.

An important finding of the trial was the significant reduction in risk of sustained incidence of retinopathy of approximately 50% in the intensive therapy group compared to the conventional therapy group in the primary-prevention cohort after 5 years of follow-up (Fig. 11) *(3)*. Intensive treatment was found to reduce the adjusted mean risk of retinopathy progression by three or more steps by 76%. In the secondary-intervention cohort, patients assigned to the intensive-therapy group had a reduction of average risk of progression by 54% during the entire study period compared to patients assigned to the conventional-therapy group. In addition, when both cohorts were combined, the intensive-therapy group also had a reduction in risk for development of severe nonproliferative retinopathy or PDR by 47% and of treatment with photocoagulation by 51%. These findings were statistically significant. There was a decrease in the incidence of CSME in the group assigned to intensive therapy compared to those assigned to conventional therapy. However, this difference did not reach statistical significance.

On average, it took about 3 years to demonstrate the beneficial effect of intensive treatment. After 3 years, the beneficial effect of intensive insulin treatment increased over time. An early worsening of retinopathy in the first year of treatment of the intensive therapy group in the secondary-intervention cohort was observed. This was similar to what previously had been reported by earlier feasibility clinical trials of intensive treatment in patients with insulin-dependent diabetes mellitus (IDDM) *(70–74)*.

The DCCT investigators also examined whether there was an association of glycosylated hemoglobin values < 8% vs. those > 8% for progression of retinopathy and found no support to the concept of a glycemic threshold regarding progression of retinopathy *(69)*. These finding are consistent with the lack of a glycemic threshold found in the WESDR.

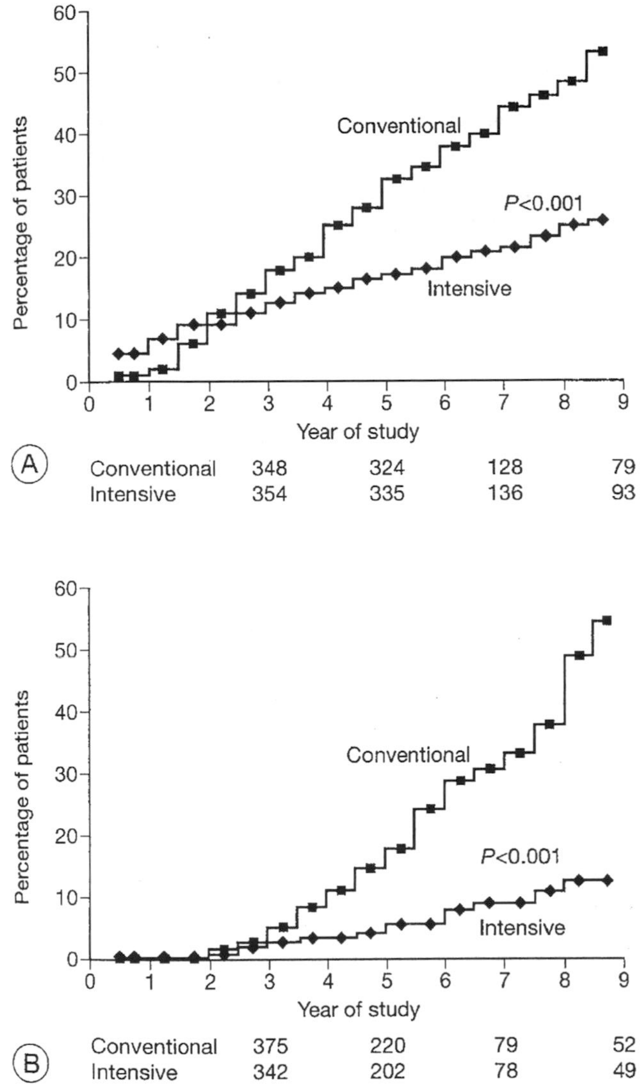

Fig. 11. Cumulative incidence of a sustained change in retinopathy in patients with type 1 diabetes mellitus receiving intensive or conventional therapy in A, the primary-prevention and B, the secondary-intervention arms of the Diabetes Control and Complications Trial.
Source*:* From Ref. 3. Copyright © 1993 Massachusetts Medical Society. All rights reserved.

The most important adverse event found in the DCCT was a two-to-threefold increase in severe hypoglycemia in the intensive insulin treatment group compared to the conventional group *(3)* There was a 33% increase in the mean adjusted risk of becoming overweight (body weight more than 120% above the ideal) in persons in the intensive compared to the conventional insulin treatment group.

The DCCT investigators concluded that intensive therapy should form the backbone of any health care strategy aimed at reducing the risk of visual loss from diabetic retinopathy in persons with IDDM *(75)*. Their analyses showed that intensive therapy, as practiced in the DCCT, would result in a gain of 920,000 years of sight, 691,000 years free from end-stage renal disease, 678,000 years free from lower extremity amputation, and 611,000 years of life at an additional cost of 4 billion dollars over the lifetime of the 120,000 persons with type 1 diabetes in the United States who meet DCCT eligibility criteria. The incremental cost per year of life gained was $28,661, and when adjusted for quality of life, intensive therapy costs $19,987 per quality of life year gained. These findings were similar to cost-effectiveness ratios for other medical interventions in the United States.

After the trial phase of the DCCT was finished, long-term follow-up of the cohort showed a long-term advantage in terms of reduction in incidence and progression of retinopathy by intensive glycemic control that remained more than four years later despite comparability of glycosylated hemoglobin levels between conventionally and intensively treated subjects (Fig. 12) *(76)*. Thus, while there is a suggestion of reduction of risk at any point in time after diagnosis of diabetes, more benefit appears to result if lowering of blood sugar occurs earlier in the course of the type 1 diabetes. The reason for this is not fully understood.

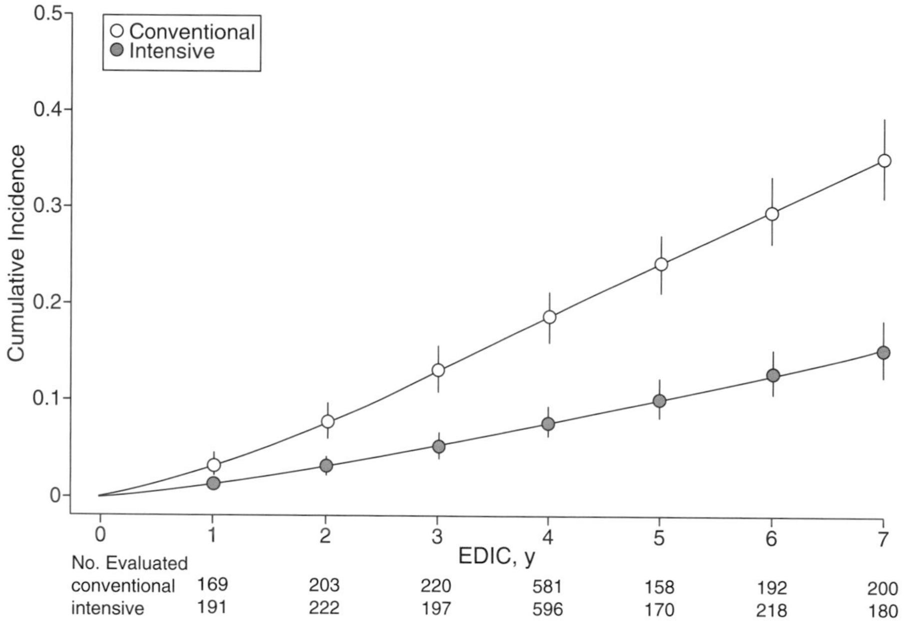

Fig. 12. Estimated cumulative incidence of progression of retinopathy 3 steps on the Early Treatment Diabetic Retinopathy Scale from the level at Diabetes Control and Complications Trial closeout over 7 years of Epidemiology of Diabetes Interventions and Complications. At each EDIC year, approximately one-fourth of the treatment groups were examined by fundus photography, except for year 4 when approximately 85% were examined. Risk reduction with intensive therapy is 62% (95% confidence interval, 51–70%; *P*<.001). The *curves* show the cumulative incidences estimated by a proportional hazards regression model for interval-censored event times that are assumed to follow an underlying Weibull distribution. Error bars represent 95% confidence intervals.

Source: Reprinted from Ref. 76. Copyright © 2002 American Medical Association. All rights reserved.

The United Kingdom Diabetes Prospective Study (UKPDS)

The UKPDS was a randomized controlled clinical trial involving 3,867 newly diagnosed patients with type 2 diabetes (4,77,78). Patients with a mean of two fasting plasma glucose concentrations of 6.1–15.0 mmol/L were randomly assigned to intensive glycemic control with either insulin, a sulfonylurea, or conventional glycemic control. The latter group was further divided into those who were overweight or not. Metformin was included as one of the treatment arms for 1,704 overweight patients and analyses included comparison of the effect of metformin against conventional therapy in overweight patients.

There was a reduction in the 12-year rate of progression of diabetic retinopathy of 21% and reduction in need for laser photocoagulation of 29% in the intensive vs. the conventional treatment group *(4)*. In addition, there were no differences in reduction in the incidence of the retinopathy endpoints among the three agents used in the intensive treatment group (glibenclamide, chlorpropamide, and insulin), but the chlorpropamide treatment group failed to show a reduced rate of retinopathy requiring photocoagulation. Furthermore, there was no difference in vision outcomes between conventional and intensive treatments. The study concluded that metformin was preferred as the first-line pharmacological therapy in newly diagnosed type 2 diabetic patients who were overweight based on their finding of a significant (39%) reduction in myocardial infarction compared to the conventional treatment group.

The intensive treatment group suffered significantly more major hypoglycemic episodes and weight gain than patients in the conventional group. Economic analyses of the clinical trial data suggested that intensive glucose control increased treatment costs but substantially reduced complication costs and increased the time free of such complications *(78)*.

Two new clinical trials which permit evaluation of near normalization of glycemic level on the incidence of cardiovascular disease and retinopathy are underway. The first, the Glycemic Control and Complications in Diabetes Mellitus Type 2, is an ongoing 7-year randomized controlled parallel-treatment trial, and its secondary objective is the evaluation of glycemic control on the incidence and progression of diabetic retinopathy in American war veterans, 41 years of age or older whose glycemia is inadequately controlled on maximal therapy *(79)*. The approach used in this trial is an intensification of combination therapy and frequent blood glucose monitoring to achieve glycosylated hemoglobin A1c levels within normal limits (at or below 6.0%). Another new large randomized controlled clinical trial that began in February 2003, the Action to Control Cardiovascular Risk in Diabetes (ACCORD), is studying the effect of near normalization of blood glucose (defined as keeping glycosylated hemoglobin A1c levels close to 6%) on the incidence and progression of retinopathy in persons with type 2 diabetes. Both studies should provide additional information regarding the risks and benefits of intensive treatment resulting in near normalization of glycemic level in persons with type 2 diabetes, a level of control not achieved in the UKPDS.

In summary, based on the results of the DCCT and the UKPDS, in the absence of preventing diabetes itself, intensive therapy is the primary public health care strategy for reducing the risk of visual loss from diabetic retinopathy in persons with both type 1 and 2 diabetes. Data from the DCCT and UKPDS have provided further support for the American Diabetes Association guidelines of a target goal of glycosylated hemoglobin of 7% for persons with diabetes *(80)*. However, data from the WESDR *(81)* and the NHANES III *(82)* suggest that few persons with diabetes achieve this targeted level of glycemic control.

HYPERTENSION

In 1934, Wagener et al., in a case-series of 1,052 diabetic persons seen at the Joslin clinic, reported that retinopathy was more likely to be manifest when patients had hypertension in addition to diabetes than just diabetes alone *(83)*. Damage to small retinal blood vessels has been shown to result from higher blood flow in eyes of hypertensive diabetic patients and thought to result in increased risk of retinopathy *(84)*. In a small randomized clinical trial, Patel et al. showed that the use of angiotensin converting enzyme (ACE) inhibitors in patients with diabetes reduced retinal blood flow as measured by laser Doppler velocimetry compared to an increase in retinal blood flow in controls *(85)*. They concluded that such treatment might protect against the progression of diabetic retinopathy.

However, blood pressure has inconsistently been shown to be associated with diabetic retinopathy, due, in part, to selective drop-out of patients and small sample sizes in some of these epidemiological studies *(13, 14, 18, 32, 41, 86–98)*. In a recent study of normotensive normoalbuminuria type 1 diabetic patients, while controlling for age, duration of diabetes, and glycosylated hemoglobin, persons whose nighttime systolic ambulatory blood pressure was in the upper three quartiles (>103 mmHg) had a higher risk of having diabetic retinopathy than those whose nighttime systolic ambulatory blood pressure was in the first quartile (OR 3.71, 95% CI 1.50–9.16, $P = 0.004$) *(99)*. There was no relation of clinical blood pressure with the severity of diabetic retinopathy in this study. These data suggest that ambulatory blood pressure may have an advantage over clinical blood pressure measurements as a marker of risk of diabetic retinopathy prior to the onset of hypertension.

In the WESDR, blood pressure was associated with the 14-year incidence of diabetic retinopathy in people with type 1 diabetes *(41)*. In the epidemiological data from the UKPDS, for each 10 mmHg decrease in mean systolic blood pressure, there was a 13% reduction in microvascular complications, including retinopathy in persons with newly diagnosed type 2 diabetes *(100)*. Stratton et al. assessed the interactive effects of glycemia and systolic blood pressure exposures on the risk of diabetic complications over a median of 10.4 years *(101)*. They reported risk reductions of microvascular complications, including retinopathy of 21% per 1% glycosylated hemoglobin A1c decrement and 11% per 10 mmHg systolic blood pressure decrement and concluded that intensive treatment of both of these risk factors is needed to substantially reduce the incidence of these complications. In the WESDR, independent of glycosylated hemoglobin levels, a 10 mmHg rise in diastolic blood pressure was associated with a 230% increase in the 4-year risk of developing macular edema in those with type 1 diabetes and a 110% increase in the risk in those with type 2 diabetes *(45)*.

While epidemiological data suggested a relationship of blood pressure to diabetic retinopathy, randomized controlled clinical trial data are necessary to show that reductions in blood pressure result in reductions in the incidence and progression of retinopathy.

The results of such trials have not been consistent. The EURODIAB Controlled Trial of Lisinopril in Insulin-Dependent Diabetes Mellitus (EUCLID) study examined the role of the ACE inhibitor lisinopril in reducing the incidence and progression of retinopathy in a group of largely normoalbuminuric normotensive type 1 diabetic patients *(102)*. Those taking lisinopril had a 50% reduction in the progression of retinopathy over a 2-year period. However, while controlling for other factors, the relationship was not statistically significant ($P = 0.06$). Progression to PDR was also reduced, although the relation was also not statistically significant.

The UKPDS also included a randomized controlled clinical trial to determine whether lowering blood pressure was beneficial in reducing macrovascular and microvascular complications associated with type 2 diabetes (5, 103). One thousand forty-eight patients with hypertension (mean blood pressure 160/94 mmHg) were randomized to a regimen of tight control with either captopril (an ACE-inhibitor) or atenolol (a beta blocker) and another 390 patients to less tight control of their blood pressure. The aim in the group randomized to the tight control treatment group (by the standards at the beginning of the clinical trial) was to achieve blood pressure values <150/<85 mmHg, while the aim in the group randomized to less tight control was to achieve blood pressure values <180/<105 mmHg. By 4.5 years after randomization, there was a highly significant difference in number of retinal microaneurysms with 23% in the tight blood pressure control group and 33.5% in the less tight blood pressure control group having five or more microaneurysms (relative risk (RR) 0.70; $P = 0.003$). The effect continued to 7.5 years (RR, 0.66; $P < 0.001$). Similarly, there was a 47% reduction in hard exudates and cotton wool spots in the tight blood pressure control group (RR, 0.53; $P < 0.001$) compared to the less tight blood pressure control group. There was a 25% reduction in progression of retinopathy and a 42% reduction in photocoagulation for diabetic macular edema in the tightly controlled group compared to the less tightly controlled group. The cumulative incidence of the end point of legal blindness (Snellen visual acuity, ≤ 20/200) in 1 eye was 2.4% (18/758) for the tightly controlled blood pressure group compared with 3.1% (12/390) for less tightly controlled blood pressure equating to a 24% reduction in risk. They found no detectable differences in outcome between the two randomized therapies of ACE-inhibition and beta-blockade suggesting that blood pressure reduction itself was more important than the type of medication used to reduce it. The effects of blood pressure control were independent of those of glycemic control. These findings support the recommendations for blood pressure control in patients with type 2 diabetes as a means of preventing visual loss from diabetic retinopathy.

The Appropriate Blood Pressure Control in Diabetes (ABCD) Trial consisted of two randomized masked clinical trials comparing the effects of intensive and moderate blood pressure control in persons with type 2 diabetes. The first trial included a diastolic blood pressure goal of 75 mmHg in the intensive group and a diastolic blood pressure of 80–89 mmHg in the moderate group in 470 hypertensive subjects (baseline diastolic blood pressure of > 90 mmHg) with type 2 diabetes (6,104). The mean blood pressure achieved was 132/78 mmHg in the intensive group and 138/86 mmHg in the moderate control group. Over a 5-year follow-up period, there was no difference between the intensive and moderate groups with regard to progression of diabetic retinopathy. There was no difference in nisoldipine vs. enalapril in progression of retinopathy. The authors concluded that the lack of efficacy in their study compared to the UKPDS might have resulted from the lower average blood pressure control in the ABCD Trial (144/82 mmHg vs. 154/87 mmHg in the UKPDS), the shorter time period of the ABCD Trial (5 years vs. 9 years on average for the UKPDS), and poorer glycemic control in the ABCD Trial than the UKPDS (5, 104). These data may also be interpreted as showing a threshold effect below which there is minimal reduction in the risk of progression of retinopathy by further reduction of blood pressure.

However, results from a second clinical trial from the same ABCD group suggested otherwise *(6)*. In the second ABCD Trial, the question was whether lowering blood pressure in normotensive (BP < 140/90 mmHg) patients with type 2 diabetes offered any beneficial results on vascular complications. The effect of intensive vs. moderate diastolic blood pressure control on diabetic vascular complications in 480 normotensive type 2 diabetic patients was examined in a prospective, randomized controlled trial. Over the 5-year period, the intensive blood pressure control group showed less progression of diabetic retinopathy (34% vs. 46%, $P = 0.019$) than the moderate therapy group with no difference whether enalapril or nisoldipine was used as the initial antihypertensive agent. There was no difference in the incidence of retinopathy between the moderate and the intensive groups (39% vs. 42%, respectively). The authors concluded that "over a five-year follow-up period, intensive (approximately 128/75 mmHg) control of blood pressure in normotensive type 2 diabetic patients decreased the progression of diabetic retinopathy." They concluded that the specific initial agent used (calcium channel blocker vs. ACE inhibitor) appears to be less important than the achievement of the lower blood pressure values in normotensive type 2 diabetic patients.

In an open parallel trial, patients with diabetes at the Steno clinic in Denmark were allocated to standard treatment (Danish guidelines, $n = 80$) or intensive treatment (stepwise implementation of behavior modification, pharmacological therapy targeting hyperglycemia, hypertension, dyslipidemia, and microalbuminuria, $n = 80$) *(105)*. After 3 years of follow-up, patients in the intensive group had significant (55%) reduction in odds of progression of retinopathy compared to those in the standard group.

The ACCORD trial is also examining whether in the context of good glycemic control, a "therapeutic strategy that targets a systolic blood pressure of < 120 mmHg will reduce the rate of cardiovascular disease events compared to a strategy that targets a systolic blood pressure of < 140 mmHg" in persons with type 2 diabetes. In that trial, the effect of blood pressure control on the incidence and progression of retinopathy will be examined. The aim of another clinical trial that is underway, the Diabetic Retinopathy Candesartan Trials (DIRECT), consisting of three randomized double-masked, parallel, placebo-controlled studies, is to determine the impact of treatment with candesartan, an angiotensin II type 1 receptor blockade, on the incidence and progression of diabetic retinopathy *(106)*.

American Diabetes Association guidelines recommend blood pressure level targets of less then 130/85 mmHg based on the above clinical trial data *(107)*. However, a study at an academically affiliated institution found only 15% of diabetic patients in that study achieved the ADA goals *(108)*. Similarly, in the NHANES, among U.S. adults with diabetes in 1999–2002, 49.8% had A1c < 7%; and nearly 40% met ADA blood pressure recommendations *(109)*. Reduction of weight, increased physical activity, and other behaviors that might help reduce blood pressure beyond use of antihypertensive agents are often not achieved in people with diabetes *(110)*. These data show the difficulty of achieving recommendations based on findings from clinical trials in clinical practice and the need for new approaches for meeting these goals.

LIPIDS

Retinal hard exudates result from the deposition of lipoproteins in the outer layers of the retina that have leaked from retinal capillaries and microaneurysms in persons with diabetes. So, it is not surprising that epidemiological data have shown that higher levels of serum lipids are associated with a higher frequency and incidence of retinal hard exudates in persons with diabetes *(53, 111–114)*. In the WESDR, while controlling for duration of diabetes, blood pressure, glycosylated hemoglobin, and diabetic nephropathy, higher serum total cholesterol was associated with the presence of hard exudates in both younger-onset persons (OR per 50 mg/dL 1.65, 95% CI, 1.24–2.18) and older-onset persons (OR 1.50, 95% CI, 1.01–2.22) taking insulin *(111)*. In the ETDRS, diabetic persons with higher serum triglycerides, low-density lipoproteins (LDL), and very-low-density lipoproteins at baseline were about twice as likely to have retinal hard exudates at baseline as persons with normal levels and were more likely to develop hard exudates and visual loss during the course of the study *(112)*. In the Hoorn study, higher serum total cholesterol (OR per 1.19 mmol/L, 1.59, 95% CI, 1.13–2.23) and LDL cholesterol (OR per 1.05 mmol/L, 1.63, 95% CI, 1.12–2.37) but not HDL cholesterol (OR per 0.36 mmol/L 1.03, 95% CI, 0.69–1.53) or triglyceride level (OR per 50 mmol/L 1.23, 95% CI, 0.93–1.63) were related to hard exudates in persons with type 2 diabetes *(113)*. In the Atherosclerosis Risk in Communities study, while controlling for age, gender, duration of diabetes, serum glucose, and type of diabetes medications taken, the presence of retinal hard exudates was associated with plasma LDL cholesterol (OR/10 mg/dL 1.18, 95% CI, 1.09–1.29) and plasma Lp(a) (OR/10 mg/dl 1.02, 95% CI, 1.00–1.05) *(53)*. In the DCCT, both the serum total-to-high density lipoprotein (HDL) cholesterol ratio and LDL cholesterol level predicted the incidence of CSME (RR for extreme quintiles 3.84, *p*-test for trend = 0.03 for serum total-to-HDL cholesterol ratio, and RR 1.95, *p*-test for trend = 0.03 for serum LDL cholesterol) and hard exudate (RR 2.44, *p* for trend = 0.0004 for total-to-HDL cholesterol ratio, and RR 2.77, *p* for trend = 0.002 for LDL cholesterol) in patients with type 1 diabetes *(114)*. Lipid levels at baseline were not associated with progression of diabetic retinopathy in this study. In Mexican patients with type 2 diabetes, Santos et al. showed the frequency of severe retinal hard exudates was higher in those with 4 allele polymorphism of the apolipoprotein E gene *(115)*.

While higher serum lipids appear associated with hard exudates in observational studies, it is not certain that intensive control of dyslipidemia with cholesterol lowering agents reduce the incidence of hard exudate, macular edema, and visual loss in persons with diabetic retinopathy. Earlier clinical trials of clofibrate showed that treatment with this medication reduced lipid levels and the incidence of hard exudate but did not restore vision to eyes when macular edema was present at the onset of the trial *(116)*. Due to the association of clofibrate with liver toxicity, it is no longer used. Few clinical trial data are available regarding the efficacy of statins in preventing the incidence of hard exudates and macular edema. Data from small short-term pilot studies suggested that statin therapy may have a possible benefit in preventing or reducing the severity of macular edema *(117–119)*. However, there have been no completed large clinical trials showing the efficacy of lipid lowering agents in reducing the progression of retinopathy, the incidence of macular edema or the loss of vision. In persons with type 2 diabetes, the ACCORD study will permit examination of whether raising the serum HDL cholesterol and lowering triglyceride levels in the context of good glycemic control reduces the incidence of macular edema and progression of retinopathy compared to a strategy that only achieves desirable levels of LDL cholesterol and glycemic control.

SUBCLINICAL AND CLINICAL DIABETIC NEPHROPATHY

Both retinopathy and nephropathy have been linked together as sharing a common "microvascular" origin and similar risk factors. This notion has been supported by data from most studies showing associations between diabetic nephropathy, as manifest by microalbuminuria or gross proteinuria, and retinopathy *(13, 14, 39, 87, 89, 91, 94, 120–122)*. Independent of levels of blood sugar and blood pressure, it has been hypothesized that inflammatory, lipid, rheological, and platelet abnormalities associated with nephropathy may be involved in the pathogenesis of retinopathy.

Microalbuminuria and Diabetic Retinopathy

In the WESDR, in cross-sectional analyses while controlling for duration of diabetes, glycosylated hemoglobin, and diastolic blood pressure, persons with microalbuminuria were more likely to have retinopathy present (for those with type 1 diabetes, OR 1.90, 95% CI, 0.95–3.78 and for those with type 2 diabetes, OR 1.80, 95% CI, 1.22–2.65) than those with normoalbuminuria *(123)*. In multivariable analyses, microalbuminuria remained statistically significantly associated with PDR in those with type 1 (OR 2.14, 95% CI, 1.27–3.61) but not type 2 diabetes (OR 1.05, 95% CI, 0.56–1.96). While controlling for other risk factors, the relationship of microalbuminuria to CSME was not statistically significant in either persons with type 1 diabetes (OR 2.05, 95% CI, 0.81, 5.17, $P = 0.13$) or those with type 2 diabetes (OR 1.26, 95% CI, 0.52–3.06, $P = 0.62$). In a cross-sectional analysis of 982 Danish patients with type 1 diabetes, the prevalence of proliferative retinopathy and vision loss increased with increasing levels of albuminuria, being 12% and 1%, respectively, in persons with normoalbuminuria, 28% and 6% in those with microalbuminuria, and 58% and 11% in those with gross proteinuria *(124)*.

While data from cross-sectional studies suggest early nephropathy, as manifest by microalbuminuria, is associated with more severe retinopathy, data regarding the longitudinal relationship of microalbuminuria to incident and progressed retinopathy are less consistent. In a clinic-based study, persons with type 1 diabetes and microalbuminuria had a higher annual incidence of PDR (10–15%) compared to only 1% in patients without signs of nephropathy *(125)*. In another study of 82 patients with type 1 diabetes, of the 13 who developed a progressive increase in their albumin excretion rate and persistent microalbuminuria during the study period, 62% (8/13) developed macular edema or PDR compared with 7% (5/69) who remained normoalbuminuric *(126)*. In the population-based Epidemiology of Diabetes Complications (EDC) Study, persons with type 1 diabetes and higher albumin excretion rates were more likely to develop incident PDR *(127, 128)*. In the WESDR, while controlling for other factors at baseline, microalbuminuria status was not associated with the incidence of retinopathy, its progression to CSME, or the incidence of proliferative disease *(123)*.

Gross Proteinuria and Retinopathy

In cross-sectional analyses in the WESDR, those with gross proteinuria were more likely to have signs of any retinopathy, PDR, or CSME at baseline than those without gross proteinuria *(123)*. While controlling for other factors, the odds of having PDR present when gross proteinuria was present varied from 4.58 (95% CI, 3.10–6.77) in those with type 1 diabetes to 2.27 (95% CI, 1.65–3.11) in those with type 2 diabetes compared to those without gross proteinuria; for CSME, the odds were 2.42 (95% CI, 1.20–4.88) and 1.47 (95% CI, 0.83–2.61) in type 1 and type 2 diabetes, respectively. These findings are also consistent with other epidemiological and clinical studies. In Hispanics, gross proteinuria was cross-sectionally related to diabetic retinopathy (OR 11.14, 95% CI, 1.2–103), but there was no relationship in whites *(129)*.

In a clinical study in Denmark, the cumulative 5-year incidence of nonproliferative retinopathy and PDR in persons with type 1 diabetes with gross proteinuria was 93% and 74%, respectively, and it was 37% and 14%, respectively, in those without *(130)*. In Oklahoma Indians with type 2 diabetes, gross proteinuria was associated with retinopathy at baseline but was not found to be a risk factor for the development of retinopathy *(95, 96)*. In Pima Indians with type 2 diabetes, while controlling for other risk factors, the presence of proteinuria or renal insufficiency at baseline predicted the development of PDR *(131)*. The incidence–rate ratio was 4.8. However, in people with type 2 diabetes in Rochester, Minnesota, persistent proteinuria was not an independent predictor of subsequent incidence of retinopathy *(88)*. In the WESDR, the presence of gross proteinuria was associated with the 10-year incidence of PDR in type 1 diabetes; otherwise, gross proteinuria was not associated with the progression of retinopathy or incidence of CSME *(123)*. The lack of an association in the WESDR may have been due, in part, to the high risk of persons with gross proteinuria who develop severe retinopathy dying and not being seen at follow-up.

There are no clinical trial data to show that interventions that prevent or slow diabetic nephropathy reduce the incidence and progression of retinopathy.

In summary, while both retinopathy and nephropathy are linked together as "microvascular" in origin and share similar risk factors, the fact that after long duration of disease most individuals develop retinopathy but only about two-thirds develop clinical signs of nephropathy suggests possible genetic differences making susceptibility to damage of each system different for a given level of exposure of blood pressure, glycemia, and other risk factors. Epidemiological data support nephropathy as a risk indicator and risk factor for retinopathy and suggest that nephrotic patients might benefit from having regular ophthalmologic evaluation.

Diabetic Retinopathy as a Risk Indicator of Subclinical Nephropathy

Diabetic retinopathy severity has been shown to be related to preclinical glomerulopathy lesions in the baseline biopsies in normotensive normoalbuminuric persons with type 1 diabetes and normal or increased glomerular filtration rate *(132)*. The severity of diabetic retinopathy was significantly associated with renal structural endpoints such as glomerular basement membrane mesangial fractional volume while controlling for other risk factors such as age, diabetes duration, sex, glycosylated hemoglobin A1c, mean arterial blood pressure, and body mass index (BMI), suggesting that retinopathy may be a marker of subclinical renal disease.

OTHER RISK FACTORS FOR RETINOPATHY

Smoking and Drinking

Smoking, through its hypoxic effects on tissue and its effects on increasing platelet adhesiveness and aggregability, both hypothesized mechanisms involved in the pathogenesis of diabetic retinopathy, would be expected to be associated with retinopathy *(133–135)*. However, most epidemiologic data do not show a relationship between cigarette smoking and a higher incidence or rate of progression of diabetic retinopathy *(87, 88, 94, 96, 135–137)*. It is not known whether there are substances in cigarette smoke, such as nicotine, that neutralize the presumed detrimental effect of hypoxia and platelet dysfunction on retinopathy pathogenesis. Regardless, smoking should be discouraged in diabetic persons because of an increased risk of cardiovascular and respiratory disease and cancer. In the WESDR, while controlling for other risk factors, persons who smoked with type 1 diabetes or type 2 diabetes were 2.4 times and 1.6 times, respectively, as likely to die as those who did not smoke *(138)*.

Alcohol through decreased platelet aggregation and adhesiveness might be thought of as having a possible protective effect in reducing the incidence and progression of retinopathy *(139)*. However, no consistent relation between a history of alcohol consumption and retinopathy has been found. Data from some studies have shown alcohol to be beneficial, while others have shown no or a detrimental effect on risk of retinopathy *(23, 140, 141)*. In the UKPDS, a relation of increased alcohol consumption to increased severity of retinopathy was found only in newly diagnosed men with type 2 diabetes *(142)*. In the WESDR, there was no relationship between alcohol consumption at the 4-year examination and the incidence and progression of retinopathy in either persons with type 1 or 2 diabetes at the 10-year follow-up *(143)*. With lack of a harmful effect of moderate alcohol consumption on retinopathy, the finding in the WESDR of a protective effect on cardiovascular disease mortality in persons with type 2 diabetes suggests that such behavior might be of benefit *(144)*.

Inflammation and Endothelial Dysfunction and Cellular Adhesion Molecules

Inflammatory processes have been hypothesized to be involved in the pathogenesis of diabetic retinopathy *(145, 146)*. Elevations in the level of markers of inflammation attributed to hyperglycemia, advanced glycation end-products, and increased BMI *(147, 148)* have been found in persons with type 1 diabetes *(146–148)*. While inflammatory biomarkers such as serum fibrinogen, tumor necrosis factor alpha (TNF-α), and C-reactive protein (CRP) may be elevated, there are few data regarding the role of inflammation in the progression of diabetic retinopathy *(148–152)*. In two case–control studies, diabetic subjects with macular edema *(151)* or PDR *(150)* had higher levels of vascular endothelial growth factors and cytokines in their vitreous than those without macular edema or PDR. In a cross-sectional study of normotensive persons with type 1 diabetes, CRP and fibrinogen levels were positively associated with diabetic retinopathy severity *(148)*. In a case series of 93 diabetic patients, serum chemokines were significantly elevated in patients with at least severe nonproliferative diabetic retinopathy compared with those who had less severe retinopathy *(153)*. Data from the Hoorn study in persons with type 2 diabetes also showed retinopathy to be associated with serum CRP and soluble intercellular adhesion molecule-1 (sICAM-1) levels, a marker of endothelial dysfunction *(154)*. While some treatments for chronic macular edema have been focused on use of intravitreal anti-inflammatory agents, e.g., steroids, there are few data showing that decreasing inflammatory activity stops the development or progression of diabetic retinopathy or restores visual acuity.

Endothelial dysfunction may result in increased vascular permeability, alteration of blood flow, oxidative stress, and angiogenesis and has been postulated to play a role in the pathogenesis of diabetic retinopathy *(155–162)*. Endothelial dysfunction is characterized by elevated levels of several systemic markers (e.g., von Willebrand factor, Factor VIII, soluble E-selectin). In addition, homocysteine levels, which have been found to be elevated in persons with type 1 diabetes, have been shown to damage endothelial cells via generation of hydrogen peroxide *(162, 163)*. Homocysteine, von Willebrand factor, and other markers of endothelial dysfunction have been inconsistently associated with the prevalence, severity, and incidence of diabetic retinopathy *(148, 164–172)*. Fewer data are available about potentially protective factors such as folate and vitamins B12 and B6 levels for progression of retinopathy and incidence of proliferative retinopathy in persons with diabetes *(166, 170)*.

Leucocyte adherence to retinal endothelium has been postulated as a cause of capillary occlusion, a factor in the pathogenesis of diabetic retinopathy *(173)*. Adherence of leucocytes to capillary and arteriolar endothelium occurs as a result of a process involving expression of adhesion molecules (e.g., selectins, intercellular adhesion molecules [ICAM-1], and vascular cell adhesion molecules [VCAM]-1) *(174–179)*. Levels of two adhesion molecules, soluble E-selectin and soluble VCAM-1, have been shown to be elevated in patients with type 1 diabetes with more severe retinopathy *(153, 180)*. However, there are neither prospective nor population-based data showing that elevation in concentrations of these molecules precedes the progression of retinopathy nor whether these associations remain while controlling for glycosylated hemoglobin, blood pressure levels, and signs of diabetic nephropathy.

Body Mass Index and Physical Activity

Data from epidemiological studies show that when other risk factors, e.g., hyperglycemia and hypertension, are controlled for, neither BMI, a measure of obesity, nor physical activity are associated with a higher risk of diabetic retinopathy *(13, 87, 88, 131, 181–187)*.

Hormone and Reproductive Exposures in Women

The evidence to date suggests that estrogen exposure is not associated with risk of retinopathy. Use of oral contraceptives, which contain estrogens as well as progestins, or hormone replacement therapy after menopause does not appear to increase the risk of retinopathy *(188, 189)*.

Progression of retinopathy in pregnancy is related to glycemia, blood pressure level, and prior duration of diabetes *(190, 191)*. However, pregnancy has been shown to be associated with more rapid progression of retinopathy independent of the level of glycemia and blood pressure *(192–194)*. Despite the apparent adverse effect of pregnancy on retinopathy, the number of past pregnancies has been reported to be unrelated to the severity of diabetic retinopathy in women with type 1 diabetes *(189, 195)*. Close observation of women with type 1 diabetes, especially those with retinopathy, is indicated during pregnancy and after delivery.

PREVALENCE AND INCIDENCE OF VISUAL IMPAIRMENT

Data from the WESDR showed the relatively high prevalence and incidence of visual impairment in persons with both type 1 and 2 diabetes first studied in 1980 (Table 4) *(196, 197)*. In 1980–1982, the results of the ETDRS, DCCT, and UKPDS had not been reported, control of glycemia and blood pressure was poorer, and people at risk of visual impairment from diabetic retinopathy were not getting dilated retinal examinations by experienced ophthalmoscopists. Much has changed since. However, few data are available

Table 4
Prevalence of Any and Severe Visual Impairment by Age and Sex in the Wisconsin Epidemiologic Study of Diabetic Retinopathy, 1980–1982

	Females		*Males*	
Age, years	% Any	% Severe	% Any	% Severe
Type 1, Younger Onset				
0–17	2.3	0	3.6	0
18–24	4.9	1	3.5	0.9
25–34	5.8	0.7	8.6	2.0
35–44	10.6	3.0	12.7	4.2
45–54	17.5	0	23.1	2.6
55+	26.7	3.3	21.4	0
Total	7.9	1.2	8.8	1.6
Type 2, Older Onset				
30–44	0	0	0	0
45–54	7.3	0.4	1.2	0.4
55–64	4.2	0.5	4.0	0.2
65–74	11.3	2.0	8.1	0.6
75–84	27.6	2.0	26.6	6.2
85+	48.7	10.7	58.7	3.2
Total	13.3	1.7	10.4	1.4

Any visual impairment defined as best corrected 20/40 or worse in better eye; severe visual impairment as 20/200 or worse in better eye

Modified from Ref. 207. Copyright © Elsevier 1984

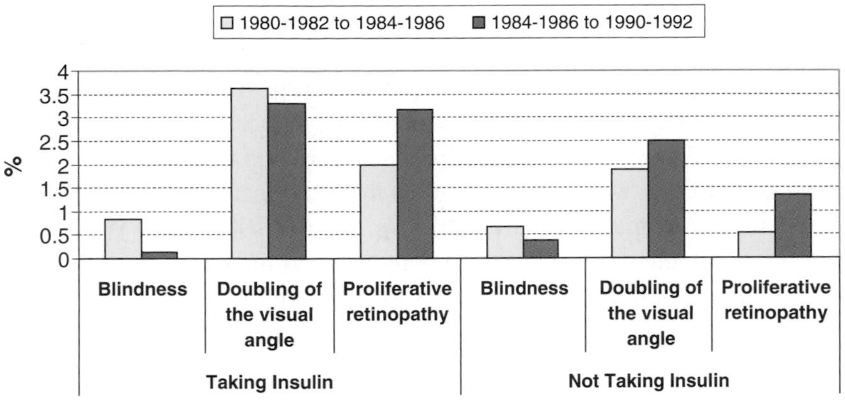

Fig. 13. Annual incidence rates of legal blindness, doubling of the visual angle, and proliferative retinopathy by examination period in persons with older-onset diabetes in the (WESDR).

that have examined changes in the prevalence and incidence of visual loss associated with diabetic retinopathy over the past 25 years. Estimated visual impairment in 2004 attributed to diabetic retinopathy was lower in persons 40 years of age or older than that reported approximately 25 years earlier *(198, 199)*. In the WESDR, in persons with type 1 disease, estimated annual incidence of severe visual impairment due to diabetic retinopathy was lower in follow-up examination periods than at baseline (Fig. 13) *(197)*. Furthermore, in the WESDR, at any given duration of diabetes in persons with type 1 diabetes, those whose year of diagnosis was earlier were more likely to have visual impairment than in those whose diagnosis was at a later date (Klein R. unpublished data). For example, in those with type 1 diabetes for 25–29 years, visual impairment was 25% in those who were diagnosed in 1953–1957, 18% in those diagnosed in 1958–1962, 7% in those diagnosed 1963–1967, and 2% in those diagnosed in 1968–1972. In another study in Denmark in 2004, the prevalence of visual impairment was lower than anticipated from the existing literature *(200)*. Causes other than diabetic retinopathy, such as age-related macular degeneration, contributed significantly to the occurrence of visual loss in this study. This was also found in the Beaver Dam Eye Study, where diabetic retinopathy accounted for only 3% of the 15-year cumulative incidence of blindness in people 43–86 years of age *(201)*. There is the need for ongoing surveillance for providing estimates of diabetic retinopathy and visual loss in the U.S. population.

CONCLUSIONS

Data from the WESDR and other population-based studies have shown associations of glycosylated hemoglobin, blood pressure, and serum total cholesterol with the incidence and progression of retinopathy and other microvascular and macrovascular complications *(19, 41, 198, 202, 203)*. However, these factors only explain a small proportion of the progression of retinopathy (R^2 = 9%) and incidence of PDR (R^2 = 10%). For example, of persons with the poorest glycemic control over the first four WESDR examinations (glycosylated hemoglobin A1c ≥ 10.2%), 17% had no or minimal retinopathy despite a mean duration of 27 years of type 1 diabetes, while 68% of those in the best glycemic control (glycosylated hemoglobin A1c ≤ 8.4%) had no or minimal retinopathy (Klein R, unpublished data). Thus, while glycemic control is associated with less severe retinopathy, there are people with type 1 diabetes who appear to be relatively protected despite poor control. This was corroborated in the experience of the DCCT *(3)*. Moreover, while intensive glycemic control is beneficial in reducing complications, in the DCCT it was associated with a threefold increase in severe hypoglycemic reactions resulting in coma or seizures (16.3 vs. 5.4 per 100/patient years of follow-up comparing those on intensive to those on conventional insulin therapy), making it difficult for many persons with type 1 diabetes to adhere to an intensive insulin treatment regimen *(204)*. Thus, because intensive insulin treatment is associated with significant morbidity (e.g., hypoglycemia), because glycemia control is difficult, and because glycemia appears to account for only a small proportion of those who experience progression of complications, it is important to search for other factors that would prevent or delay the progression of diabetic retinopathy. Similarly, it is difficult for persons with type 2 diabetes to normalize their blood sugar and pressure. Identification of novel risk factors and genetic factors for diabetic retinopathy will be important in the future.

Tertiary prevention through early detection and treatment by photocoagulation can prevent visual loss due to severe diabetic retinopathy. However, many barriers still need to be overcome. Secondary prevention may play a more important role than tertiary prevention in reducing visual loss due to diabetic retinopathy. Ongoing monitoring of vision in populations is needed to assess efficacy of early detection programs and new interventions.

ACKNOWLEDGMENTS

This chapter was supported by National Institutes of Health grant # EY016379 (R Klein and BEK Klein).

REFERENCES

1. The Diabetic Retinopathy Study Research Group. Photocoagulation treatment of proliferative diabetic retinopathy. Clinical application of Diabetic Retinopathy Study (DRS) findings, DRS Report Number 8. Ophthalmology. 1981;88:583–600.
2. Early Treatment Diabetic Retinopathy Study Research Group. Effects of aspirin treatment on diabetic retinopathy. ETDRS report number 8. Ophthalmology. 1991;98:757–65.
3. The Diabetes Control and Complications Trial Research Group. The effect of intensive treatment of diabetes on the development and progression of long-term complications in insulin-dependent diabetes mellitus. N Engl J Med. 1993;329:977–86.
4. UK Prospective Diabetes Study (UKPDS) Group. Intensive blood-glucose control with sulphonylureas or insulin compared with conventional treatment and risk of complications in patients with type 2 diabetes (UKPDS 33). Lancet. 1998;352:837–53.
5. UK Prospective Diabetes Study (UKPDS) Group. Tight blood pressure control and risk of macrovascular and microvascular complications in type 2 diabetes: UKPDS 38. BMJ. 1998;317:703–13.
6. Schrier RW, Estacio RO, Esler A, Mehler P. Effects of aggressive blood pressure control in normotensive type 2 diabetic patients on albuminuria, retinopathy and strokes. Kidney Int. 2002;61:1086–97.
7. Hirschberg J. Ueber Diabetische Netzhautentzundung. Deutsche Medicinische Wochenschrift. 1893;16:1181–5, 1236–9.
8. Friedenwald H. The Doyne memorial lecture: pathological changes in the retinal blood-vessels in arterio-sclerosis and hypertension. Trans Ophthal Soc UK. 1930;50:531.

9. University Group Diabetes Program. Effects of hypoglycemic agents on vascular complications in patients with adult-onset diabetes. VIII. Evaluation of insulin therapy: final report. Diabetes. 1982;31 Suppl 5:1–81.
10. Vision problems in the U.S. Data analysis. Definitions, data sources, detailed data tables, analysis, interpetation. In: New York: National Society to Prevent Blindness; 1980:1–46.
11. West KM. Epidemiology of diabetes and its vascular lesions. New York: Elsevier; 1978.
12. Klein R, Klein BE, Moss SE, DeMets DL, Kaufman I, Voss PS. Prevalence of diabetes mellitus in southern Wisconsin. Am J Epidemiol. 1984;119:54–61.
13. Klein R, Klein BE, Moss SE, Davis MD, DeMets DL. The Wisconsin Epidemiologic Study of Diabetic Retinopathy. II. Prevalence and risk of diabetic retinopathy when age at diagnosis is less than 30 years. Arch Ophthalmol. 1984;102:520–6.
14. Klein R, Klein BE, Moss SE, Davis MD, DeMets DL. The Wisconsin Epidemiologic Study of Diabetic Retinopathy. III. Prevalence and risk of diabetic retinopathy when age at diagnosis is 30 or more years. Arch Ophthalmol. 1984;102:527–32.
15. Early Treatment Diabetic Retinopathy Study Research Group. Grading diabetic retinopathy from stereoscopic color fundus photographs–an extension of the modified Airlie House classification. ETDRS report number 10. Ophthalmology. 1991;98:786–806.
16. Klein BE, Davis MD, Segal P, et al. Diabetic retinopathy. Assessment of severity and progression. Ophthalmology. 1984;91:10–7.
17. Early Treatment Diabetic Retinopathy Study Research Group. Fundus photographic risk factors for progression of diabetic retinopathy. ETDRS report number 12. Ophthalmology. 1991;98:823–33.
18. Klein R, Klein BE, Moss SE, Davis MD, DeMets DL. The Wisconsin Epidemiologic Study of Diabetic Retinopathy. IV. Diabetic macular edema. Ophthalmology. 1984;91:1464–74.
19. Aiello LP, Gardner TW, King GL, et al. Diabetic retinopathy. Diabetes Care. 1998;21:143–56.
20. Lopez IM, Diez A, Velilla S, Rueda A, Alvarez A, Pastor CJ. Prevalence of diabetic retinopathy and eye care in a rural area of Spain. Ophthalmic Epidemiol. 2002;9:205–14.
21. Broadbent DM, Scott JA, Vora JP, Harding SP. Prevalence of diabetic eye disease in an inner city population: the Liverpool Diabetic Eye Study. Eye. 1999;13 (Pt 2):160–5.
22. West SK, Klein R, Rodriguez J, et al. Diabetes and diabetic retinopathy in a Mexican-American population: Proyecto VER. Diabetes Care. 2001;24:1204–9.
23. McKay R, McCarty CA, Taylor HR. Diabetic retinopathy in Victoria, Australia: the Visual Impairment Project. Br J Ophthalmol. 2000;84:865–70.
24. Toeller M, Buyken AE, Heitkamp G, Berg G, Scherbaum WA, EURODIAB Complications Study Group. Prevalence of chronic complications, metabolic control and nutritional intake in type 1 diabetes: comparison between different European regions. Horm Metab Res. 1999;31:680–5.
25. Leske MC, Wu SY, Hyman L, et al. Diabetic retinopathy in a black population: the Barbados Eye Study. Ophthalmology. 1999;106:1893–9.
26. Mitchell P, Smith W, Wang JJ, Attebo K. Prevalence of diabetic retinopathy in an older community: the Blue Mountains Eye Study. Ophthalmology. 1998;105:406–11.
27. Klein R, Klein BE, Moss SE, Linton KL. The Beaver Dam Eye Study. Retinopathy in adults with newly discovered and previously diagnosed diabetes mellitus. Ophthalmology. 1992;99:58–62.
28. Kempen JH, O'Colmain BJ, Leske MC, et al.. The prevalence of diabetic retinopathy among adults in the United States. Arch Ophthalmol. 2004;122:552–63.
29. Lecaire T, Palta M, Zhang H, Allen C, Klein R, D'Alessio D. Lower-than-expected prevalence and severity of retinopathy in an incident cohort followed during the first 4–14 years of type 1 diabetes: the Wisconsin Diabetes Registry Study. Am J Epidemiol. 2006;164:143–50.
30. Pambianco G, Costacou T, Ellis D, Becker DJ, Klein R, Orchard TJ. The 30-year natural history of type 1 diabetes complications: the Pittsburgh Epidemiology of Diabetes Complications Study experience. Diabetes. 2006;55:1463–9.
31. Dwyer MS, Melton LJ, III, Ballard DJ, Palumbo PJ, Trautmann JC, Chu CP. Incidence of diabetic retinopathy and blindness: a population-based study in Rochester, Minnesota. Diabetes Care. 1985;8:316–22.
32. Teuscher A, Schnell H, Wilson PW. Incidence of diabetic retinopathy and relationship to baseline plasma glucose and blood pressure. Diabetes Care. 1988;11:246–51.

33. Klein R, Klein BE, Moss SE, Davis MD, DeMets DL. The Wisconsin Epidemiologic Study of Diabetic Retinopathy. IX. Four-year incidence and progression of diabetic retinopathy when age at diagnosis is less than 30 years. Arch Ophthalmol. 1989;107:237–43.
34. Klein R, Klein BE, Moss SE, Davis MD, DeMets DL. The Wisconsin Epidemiologic Study of Diabetic Retinopathy. X. Four-year incidence and progression of diabetic retinopathy when age at diagnosis is 30 years or more. Arch Ophthalmol. 1989;107:244–9.
35. Klein R, Moss SE, Klein BE, Davis MD, DeMets DL. The Wisconsin Epidemiologic Study of Diabetic Retinopathy. XI. The incidence of macular edema. Ophthalmology. 1989;96:1501–10.
36. Klein R, Klein BE, Moss SE, Cruickshanks KJ. The Wisconsin Epidemiologic Study of Diabetic Retinopathy. XIV. Ten-year incidence and progression of diabetic retinopathy. Arch Ophthalmol. 1994;112:1217–28.
37. Henricsson M, Nystrom L, Blohme G, et al. The incidence of retinopathy 10 years after diagnosis in young adult people with diabetes: results from the nationwide population-based Diabetes Incidence Study in Sweden (DISS). Diabetes Care. 2003;26:349–54.
38. Lloyd CE, Becker D, Ellis D, Orchard TJ. Incidence of complications in insulin-dependent diabetes mellitus: a survival analysis. Am J Epidemiol. 1996;143:431–41.
39. Klein R, Palta M, Allen C, Shen G, Han DP, D'Alessio DJ. Incidence of retinopathy and associated risk factors from time of diagnosis of insulin-dependent diabetes. Arch Ophthalmol. 1997;115:351–6.
40. Tudor SM, Hamman RF, Baron A, Johnson DW, Shetterly SM. Incidence and progression of diabetic retinopathy in Hispanics and non-Hispanic whites with type 2 diabetes: San Luis Valley Diabetes Study, Colorado. Diabetes Care. 1998;21:53–61.
41. Klein R, Klein BE, Moss SE, Cruickshanks KJ. The Wisconsin Epidemiologic Study of Diabetic Retinopathy: XVII. The 14-year incidence and progression of diabetic retinopathy and associated risk factors in type 1 diabetes. Ophthalmology. 1998;105:1801–15.
42. Porta M, Sjoelie AK, Chaturvedi N, et al. Risk factors for progression to proliferative diabetic retinopathy in the EURODIAB Prospective Complications Study. Diabetologia. 2001;44:2203–9.
43. Ling R, Ramsewak V, Taylor D, Jacob J. Longitudinal study of a cohort of people with diabetes screened by the Exeter Diabetic Retinopathy Screening Programme. Eye. 2002;16:140–5.
44. Younis N, Broadbent DM, Vora JP, Harding SP. Incidence of sight-threatening retinopathy in patients with type 2 diabetes in the Liverpool Diabetic Eye Study: a cohort study. Lancet. 2003;361:195–200.
45. Klein R, Klein BE, Moss SE, Cruickshanks KJ. The Wisconsin Epidemiologic Study of Diabetic Retinopathy. XV. The long-term incidence of macular edema. Ophthalmology. 1995;102:7–16.
46. Hovind P, Tarnow L, Rossing K, et al. Decreasing incidence of severe diabetic microangiopathy in type 1 diabetes. Diabetes Care. 2003;26:1258–64.
47. Rabb MF, Gagliano DA, Sweeney HE. Diabetic retinopathy in blacks. Diabetes Care. 1990;13:1202–6.
48. Varma R, Torres M, Pena F, Klein R, Azen SP. Prevalence of diabetic retinopathy in adult Latinos: the Los Angeles Latino Eye Study. Ophthalmology. 2004;111:1298–306.
49. Roy MS. Diabetic retinopathy in African Americans with type 1 diabetes: The New Jersey 725: I. Methodology, population, frequency of retinopathy, and visual impairment. Arch Ophthalmol. 2000;118:97–104.
50. Roy MS, Klein R, O'Colmain BJ, Klein BE, Moss SE, Kempen JH. The prevalence of diabetic retinopathy among adult type 1 diabetic persons in the United States. Arch Ophthalmol. 2004;122:546–51.
51. Roy MS, Klein R. Macular edema and retinal hard exudates in African Americans with type 1 diabetes: the New Jersey 725. Arch Ophthalmol. 2001;119:251–9.
52. Roy MS, Affouf M. Six-year progression of retinopathy and associated risk factors in African American patients with type 1 diabetes mellitus: the New Jersey 725. Arch Ophthalmol. 2006;124:1297–306.
53. Klein R, Sharrett AR, Klein BE, et al. The association of atherosclerosis, vascular risk factors, and retinopathy in adults with diabetes: the Atherosclerosis Risk in Communities Study. Ophthalmology. 2002;109:1225–34.
54. Klein R, Marino EK, Kuller LH, et al. The relation of atherosclerotic cardiovascular disease to retinopathy in people with diabetes in the Cardiovascular Health Study. Br J Ophthalmol. 2002;86:84–90.
55. Harris MI, Klein R, Cowie CC, Rowland M, Byrd-Holt DD. Is the risk of diabetic retinopathy greater in non-Hispanic blacks and Mexican Americans than in non-Hispanic whites with type 2 diabetes? A U.S. population study. Diabetes Care. 1998;21:1230–5.

56. Wong TY, Klein R, Islam FM, et al. Diabetic retinopathy in a multi-ethnic cohort in the United States. Am J Ophthalmol. 2006;141:446–55.
57. Berinstein DM, Stahn RM, Welty TK, Leonardson GR, Herlihy JJ. The prevalence of diabetic retinopathy and associated risk factors among Sioux Indians. Diabetes Care. 1997;20:757–9.
58. Lee ET, Lu M, Bennett PH, Keen H. Vascular disease in younger-onset diabetes: comparison of European, Asian and American Indian cohorts of the WHO Multinational Study of Vascular Disease in Diabetes. Diabetologia. 2001;44 Suppl 2:S78–81.
59. Looker HC, Krakoff J, Knowler WC, Bennett PH, Klein R, Hanson RL. Longitudinal studies of incidence and progression of diabetic retinopathy assessed by retinal photography in Pima Indians. Diabetes Care. 2003;26:320–6.
60. McNeely MJ, Boyko EJ. Diabetes-related comorbidities in Asian Americans: results of a national health survey. J Diabetes Complications. 2005;19:101–6.
61. Donaghue KC, Fairchild JM, Craig ME, et al. Do all prepubertal years of diabetes duration contribute equally to diabetes complications? Diabetes Care. 2003;26:1224–9.
62. Klein BE, Moss SE, Klein R. Is menarche associated with diabetic retinopathy? Diabetes Care. 1990;13:1034–8.
63. Hanis CL, Hallman D. Genetics of diabetic retinopathy. Curr Diab Rep. 2006;6:155–61.
64. Uhlmann K, Kovacs P, Boettcher Y, Hammes HP, Paschke R. Genetics of diabetic retinopathy. Exp Clin Endocrinol Diabetes. 2006;114:275–94.
65. Klein R, Klein BE, Moss SE, Cruickshanks KJ. Relationship of hyperglycemia to the long-term incidence and progression of diabetic retinopathy. Arch Intern Med. 1994;154:2169–78.
66. Diabetes Control and Complications Trial Research Group. Progression of retinopathy with intensive versus conventional treatment in the Diabetes Control and Complications Trial. Ophthalmology. 1995;102:647–61.
67. Colagiuri S, Cull CA, Holman RR. Are lower fasting plasma glucose levels at diagnosis of type 2 diabetes associated with improved outcomes? U.K. Prospective Diabetes Study 61. Diabetes Care. 2002;25:1410–7.
68. Klein R, Klein BE, Moss SE. Relation of glycemic control to diabetic microvascular complications in diabetes mellitus. Ann Intern Med. 1996;124:90–6.
69. Diabetes Control and Complications Trial Research Group. The absence of a glycemic threshold for the development of long-term complications: the perspective of the Diabetes Control and Complications Trial. Diabetes. 1996;45:1289–98.
70. The Kroc Collaborative Study Group. Diabetic retinopathy after two years of intensified insulin treatment. Follow-up of the Kroc Collaborative Study. JAMA. 1988;260:37–41.
71. Lauritzen T, Frost-Larsen K, Larsen HW, Deckert T. Effect of 1 year of near-normal blood glucose levels on retinopathy in insulin-dependent diabetics. Lancet. 1983;1:200–4.
72. Lauritzen T, Frost-Larsen K, Larsen HW, Deckert T. Two-year experience with continuous subcutaneous insulin infusion in relation to retinopathy and neuropathy. Diabetes. 1985;34 Suppl 3:74–9.
73. Dahl-Jorgensen K, Brinchmann-Hansen O, Hanssen KF, et al. Effect of near normoglycaemia for two years on progression of early diabetic retinopathy, nephropathy, and neuropathy: the Oslo study. Br Med J (Clin Res Ed). 1986;293:1195–9.
74. Dahl-Jorgensen K, Brinchmann-Hansen O, Hanssen KF, Sandvik L, Aagenaes O. Rapid tightening of blood glucose control leads to transient deterioration of retinopathy in insulin dependent diabetes mellitus: the Oslo study. Br Med J (Clin Res Ed). 1985;290:811–5.
75. The Diabetes Control and Complications Trial Research Group. Lifetime benefits and costs of intensive therapy as practiced in the diabetes control and complications trial. JAMA. 1996;276:1409–15.
76. Writing Team for the Diabetes Control and Complications Trial/Epidemiology of Diabetes Interventions and Complications Research Group. Effect of intensive therapy on the microvascular complications of type 1 diabetes mellitus. JAMA. 2002;287:2563–9.
77. UK Prospective Diabetes Study (UKPDS) Group. Effect of intensive blood-glucose control with metformin on complications in overweight patients with type 2 diabetes (UKPDS 34). Lancet. 1998;352:854–65.
78. Gray A, Raikou M, McGuire A, et al., United Kingdom Prospective Diabetes Study Group. Cost effectiveness of an intensive blood glucose control policy in patients with type 2 diabetes: economic analysis alongside randomised controlled trial (UKPDS 41). BMJ. 2000;320:1373–8.

79. Duckworth WC, McCarren M, Abraira C. Glucose control and cardiovascular complications: the VA Diabetes Trial. Diabetes Care. 2001;24:942–5.
80. American Diabetes Association. Standards of medical care for patients with diabetes mellitus. Diabetes Care. 1994;17:616–23.
81. Klein R, Klein BE, Moss SE, Cruickshanks KJ. The medical management of hyperglycemia over a 10-year period in people with diabetes. Diabetes Care. 1996;19:744–50.
82. Harris MI. Health care and health status and outcomes for patients with type 2 diabetes. Diabetes Care. 2000;23:754–8.
83. Wagener HP, Dry TJ, Wilder RM. Retinitis in diabetes. N Engl J Med. 1934;211:1131–7.
84. Kohner EM. Diabetic retinopathy. Br Med Bull. 1989;45:148–73.
85. Patel V, Rassam SM, Chen HC, Jones M, Kohner EM. Effect of angiotensin-converting enzyme inhibition with perindopril and beta-blockade with atenolol on retinal blood flow in hypertensive diabetic subjects. Metabolism. 1998;47:28–33.
86. Dorf A, Ballintine EJ, Bennett PH, Miller M. Retinopathy in Pima Indians. Relationships to glucose level, duration of diabetes, age at diagnosis of diabetes, and age at examination in a population with a high prevalence of diabetes mellitus. Diabetes. 1976;25:554–60.
87. West KM, Erdreich LJ, Stober JA. A detailed study of risk factors for retinopathy and nephropathy in diabetes. Diabetes. 1980;29:501–8.
88. Ballard DJ, Melton LJ, III, Dwyer MS, et al. Risk factors for diabetic retinopathy: a population-based study in Rochester, Minnesota. Diabetes Care. 1986;9:334–42.
89. Knuiman MW, Welborn TA, McCann VJ, Stanton KG, Constable IJ. Prevalence of diabetic complications in relation to risk factors. Diabetes. 1986;35:1332–9.
90. Sjolie AK. Ocular complications in insulin treated diabetes mellitus. An epidemiological study. Acta Ophthalmol Suppl. 1985;172:1–77.
91. Haffner SM, Fong D, Stern MP, et al. Diabetic retinopathy in Mexican Americans and non-Hispanic whites. Diabetes. 1988;37:878–84.
92. Hamman RF, Mayer EJ, Moo-Young GA, Hildebrandt W, Marshall JA, Baxter J. Prevalence and risk factors of diabetic retinopathy in non-Hispanic whites and Hispanics with NIDDM: San Luis Valley Diabetes Study. Diabetes. 1989;38:1231–7.
93. McLeod BK, Thompson JR, Rosenthal AR. The prevalence of retinopathy in the insulin-requiring diabetic patients of an English country town. Eye. 1988;2 (Pt 4):424–30.
94. Kostraba JN, Klein R, Dorman JS, et al. The Epidemiology of Diabetes Complications Study. IV. Correlates of diabetic background and proliferative retinopathy. Am J Epidemiol. 1991;133:381–91.
95. Lee ET, Lee VS, Lu M, Russell D. Development of proliferative retinopathy in NIDDM. A follow-up study of American Indians in Oklahoma. Diabetes. 1992;41:359–67.
96. Lee ET, Lee VS, Kingsley RM, et al. Diabetic retinopathy in Oklahoma Indians with NIDDM. Incidence and risk factors. Diabetes Care. 1992;15:1620–7.
97. Klein R, Klein BE, Moss SE, Davis MD, DeMets DL. Is blood pressure a predictor of the incidence or progression of diabetic retinopathy? Arch Intern Med. 1989;149:2427–32.
98. Klein BE, Klein R, Moss SE, Palta M. A cohort study of the relationship of diabetic retinopathy to blood pressure. Arch Ophthalmol. 1995;113:601–6.
99. Klein R, Moss SE, Sinaiko AR, et al. The relation of ambulatory blood pressure and pulse rate to retinopathy in type 1 diabetes mellitus: the Renin-Angiotensin System Study. Ophthalmology. 2006;113:2231–6.
100. Adler AI, Stratton IM, Neil HA, et al. Association of systolic blood pressure with macrovascular and microvascular complications of type 2 diabetes (UKPDS 36): prospective observational study. BMJ. 2000;321:412–9.
101. Stratton IM, Cull CA, Adler AI, Matthews DR, Neil HA, Holman RR. Additive effects of glycaemia and blood pressure exposure on risk of complications in type 2 diabetes: a prospective observational study (UKPDS 75). Diabetologia. 2006;49:1761–9.
102. Chaturvedi N, Sjolie AK, Stephenson JM, et al., The EUCLID Study Group. Effect of lisinopril on progression of retinopathy in normotensive people with type 1 diabetes. EURODIAB controlled trial of lisinopril in insulin-dependent diabetes mellitus. Lancet. 1998;351:28–31.
103. Matthews DR, Stratton IM, Aldington SJ, Holman RR, Kohner EM. Risks of progression of retinopathy and vision loss related to tight blood pressure control in type 2 diabetes mellitus: UKPDS 69. Arch Ophthalmol. 2004;122:1631–40.

104. Estacio RO, Jeffers BW, Gifford N, Schrier RW. Effect of blood pressure control on diabetic microvascular complications in patients with hypertension and type 2 diabetes. Diabetes Care. 2000;23 Suppl 2:B54–64.
105. Gaede P, Vedel P, Parving HH, Pedersen O. Intensified multifactorial intervention in patients with type 2 diabetes mellitus and microalbuminuria: the Steno Type 2 Randomised Study. Lancet. 1999;353:617–22.
106. Chaturvedi N, Sjoelie AK, Svensson A. The Diabetic Retinopathy Candesartan Trials (DIRECT) Programme, rationale and study design. J Renin Angiotensin Aldosterone Syst. 2002;3:255–61.
107. American Diabetes Association. Clinical Practice Recommendations 2005. Diabetes Care. 2005;28 Suppl 1:S1–79.
108. Singer GM, Izhar M, Black HR. Goal-oriented hypertension management: translating clinical trials to practice. Hypertension. 2002;40:464–9.
109. Resnick HE, Foster GL, Bardsley J, Ratner RE. Achievement of American Diabetes Association clinical practice recommendations among U.S. adults with diabetes, 1999–2002: the National Health and Nutrition Examination Survey. Diabetes Care. 2006;29:531–7.
110. Saydah SH, Fradkin J, Cowie CC. Poor control of risk factors for vascular disease among adults with previously diagnosed diabetes. JAMA. 2004;291:335–42.
111. Klein BE, Moss SE, Klein R, Surawicz TS. The Wisconsin Epidemiologic Study of Diabetic Retinopathy. XIII. Relationship of serum cholesterol to retinopathy and hard exudate. Ophthalmology. 1991;98:1261–5.
112. Chew EY, Klein ML, Ferris FL, III, et al. Association of elevated serum lipid levels with retinal hard exudate in diabetic retinopathy: Early Treatment Diabetic Retinopathy Study (ETDRS) Report 22. Arch Ophthalmol. 1996;114:1079–84.
113. van Leiden HA, Dekker JM, Moll AC, et al. Blood pressure, lipids, and obesity are associated with retinopathy: the Hoorn Study. Diabetes Care. 2002;25:1320–5.
114. Miljanovic B, Glynn RJ, Nathan DM, Manson JE, Schaumberg DA. A prospective study of serum lipids and risk of diabetic macular edema in type 1 diabetes. Diabetes. 2004;53:2883–92.
115. Santos A, Salguero ML, Gurrola C, Munoz F, Roig-Melo E, Panduro A. The epsilon4 allele of apolipoprotein E gene is a potential risk factor for the severity of macular edema in type 2 diabetic Mexican patients. Ophthalmic Genet. 2002;23:13–9.
116. Duncan LJ, Cullen JF, Ireland JT, Nolan J, Clarke BF, Oliver MF. A three-year trial of atromid therapy in exudative diabetic retinopathy. Diabetes. 1968;17:458–67.
117. Gordon B, Chang S, Kavanagh M, et al. The effects of lipid lowering on diabetic retinopathy. Am J Ophthalmol. 1991;112:385–91.
118. Freyberger H, Schifferdecker E, Schatz H. [Regression of hard exudates in diabetic background retinopathy in therapy with etofibrate antilipemic agent]. Med Klin (Munich). 1994;89:594–7, 633.
119. Dale J, Farmer J, Jones AF, Gibson JM, Dodson PM. Diabetic ischaemic and exudative maculopathy: are their risk factors different? Diab Med. 2000;17:47.
120. Jerneld B. Prevalence of diabetic retinopathy. A population study from the Swedish island of Gotland. Acta Ophthalmol Suppl. 1988;188:3–32.
121. Cruickshanks KJ, Ritter LL, Klein R, Moss SE. The association of microalbuminuria with diabetic retinopathy: The Wisconsin Epidemiologic Study of Diabetic Retinopathy. Ophthalmology. 1993;100:862–7.
122. Klein R, Moss SE, Klein BE. Is gross proteinuria a risk factor for the incidence of proliferative diabetic retinopathy? Ophthalmology. 1993;100:1140–6.
123. Klein R. Diabetic retinopathy and nephropathy. In: Cortes P, Morgensen CE, eds. The diabetic kidney. Totowa, NJ: Humana Press; 2006.
124. Parving HH, Hommel E, Mathiesen E, et al. Prevalence of microalbuminuria, arterial hypertension, retinopathy and neuropathy in patients with insulin dependent diabetes. Br Med J (Clin Res Ed). 1988;296:156–60.
125. Jensen T, Deckert T. Diabetic retinopathy, nephropathy and neuropathy. Generalized vascular damage in insulin-dependent diabetic patients. Horm Metab Res Suppl. 1992;26:68–70.
126. Gilbert RE, Tsalamandris C, Allen TJ, Colville D, Jerums G. Early nephropathy predicts vision-threatening retinal disease in patients with type I diabetes mellitus. J Am Soc Nephrol. 1998;9:85–9.

127. Lloyd CE, Klein R, Maser RE, Kuller LH, Becker DJ, Orchard TJ. The progression of retinopathy over 2 years: the Pittsburgh Epidemiology of Diabetes Complications (EDC) Study. J Diabetes Complications. 1995;9:140–8.
128. Lloyd CE, Orchard TJ. Diabetes complications: the renal-retinal link. An epidemiological perspective. Diabetes Care. 1995;18:1034–6.
129. Estacio RO, McFarling E, Biggerstaff S, Jeffers BW, Johnson D, Schrier RW. Overt albuminuria predicts diabetic retinopathy in Hispanics with NIDDM. Am J Kidney Dis. 1998;31:947–53.
130. Kofoed-Enevoldsen A, Jensen T, Borch-Johnsen K, Deckert T. Incidence of retinopathy in type I (insulin-dependent) diabetes: association with clinical nephropathy. J Diabet Complications. 1987;1:96–9.
131. Nelson RG, Newman JM, Knowler WC, et al. Incidence of end-stage renal disease in type 2 (non-insulin-dependent) diabetes mellitus in Pima Indians. Diabetologia. 1988;31:730–6.
132. Klein R, Zinman B, Gardiner R, et al. The relationship of diabetic retinopathy to preclinical diabetic glomerulopathy lesions in type 1 diabetic patients: the Renin-Angiotensin System Study. Diabetes. 2005;54:527–33.
133. Goldsmith JR, Landaw SA. Carbon monoxide and human health. Science. 1968;162:1352–9.
134. Hawkins RI. Smoking, platelets and thrombosis. Nature. 1972;236:450–2.
135. Klein R, Klein BE, Davis MD. Is cigarette smoking associated with diabetic retinopathy? Am J Epidemiol. 1983;118:228–38.
136. Moss SE, Klein R, Klein BE. Association of cigarette smoking with diabetic retinopathy. Diabetes Care. 1991;14:119–26.
137. Moss SE, Klein R, Klein BE. Cigarette smoking and ten-year progression of diabetic retinopathy. Ophthalmology. 1996;103:1438–42.
138. Klein R, Moss SE, Klein BE, DeMets DL. Relation of ocular and systemic factors to survival in diabetes. Arch Intern Med. 1989;149:266–72.
139. Jakubowski JA, Vaillancourt R, Deykin D. Interaction of ethanol, prostacyclin, and aspirin in determining human platelet reactivity in vitro. Arteriosclerosis. 1988;8:436–41.
140. Kingsley LA, Dorman JS, Doft BH, et al. An epidemiologic approach to the study of retinopathy: the Pittsburgh Diabetic Morbidity and Retinopathy Studies. Diabetes Res Clin Pract. 1988;4:99–109.
141. Young RJ, McCulloch DK, Prescott RJ, Clarke BF. Alcohol: another risk factor for diabetic retinopathy? Br Med J (Clin Res Ed). 1984;288:1035–7.
142. Kohner EM, Aldington SJ, Stratton IM, et al. United Kingdom Prospective Diabetes Study, 30: diabetic retinopathy at diagnosis of non-insulin-dependent diabetes mellitus and associated risk factors. Arch Ophthalmol. 1998;116:297–303.
143. Moss SE, Klein R, Klein BE. The association of alcohol consumption with the incidence and progression of diabetic retinopathy. Ophthalmology. 1994;101:1962–8.
144. Valmadrid CT, Klein R, Moss SE, Klein BE, Cruickshanks KJ. Alcohol intake and the risk of coronary heart disease mortality in persons with older-onset diabetes mellitus. JAMA. 1999;282:239–46.
145. Adamis AP. Is diabetic retinopathy an inflammatory disease? Br J Ophthalmol. 2002;86:363–5.
146. Lechleitner M, Koch T, Herold M, Dzien A, Hoppichler F. Tumour necrosis factor-alpha plasma level in patients with type 1 diabetes mellitus and its association with glycaemic control and cardiovascular risk factors. J Intern Med. 2000;248:67–76.
147. Schmidt AM, Hori O, Chen JX, et al. Advanced glycation endproducts interacting with their endothelial receptor induce expression of vascular cell adhesion molecule-1 (VCAM-1) in cultured human endothelial cells and in mice. A potential mechanism for the accelerated vasculopathy of diabetes. J Clin Invest. 1995;96:1395–403.
148. Schram MT, Chaturvedi N, Schalkwijk C, et al. Vascular risk factors and markers of endothelial function as determinants of inflammatory markers in type 1 diabetes: the EURODIAB Prospective Complications Study. Diabetes Care. 2003;26:2165–73.
149. Schalkwijk CG, Chaturvedi N, Twaafhoven H, van Hinsbergh VW, Stehouwer CD. Amadori-albumin correlates with microvascular complications and precedes nephropathy in type 1 diabetic patients. Eur J Clin Invest. 2002;32:500–6.
150. Powell ED, Field RA. Diabetic retinopathy and rheumatoid arthritis. Lancet. 1964;41:17–8.

151. Yuuki T, Kanda T, Kimura Y, et al. Inflammatory cytokines in vitreous fluid and serum of patients with diabetic vitreoretinopathy. J Diabetes Complications. 2001;15:257–9.
152. Funatsu H, Yamashita H, Ikeda T, Mimura T, Shimizu E, Hori S. Relation of diabetic macular edema to cytokines and posterior vitreous detachment. Am J Ophthalmol. 2003;135:321–7.
153. Meleth AD, Agron E, Chan CC, et al. Serum inflammatory markers in diabetic retinopathy. Invest Ophthalmol Vis Sci. 2005;46:4295–301.
154. van Hecke MV, Dekker JM, Nijpels G, et al. Inflammation and endothelial dysfunction are associated with retinopathy: the Hoorn Study. Diabetologia. 2005;48:1300–6.
155. Poston L, Taylor PD. Glaxo/MRS Young Investigator Prize. Endothelium-mediated vascular function in insulin-dependent diabetes mellitus. Clin Sci (Lond). 1995;88:245–55.
156. Taverna MJ, Sola A, Guyot-Argenton C, et al. eNOS4 polymorphism of the endothelial nitric oxide synthase predicts risk for severe diabetic retinopathy. Diabet Med. 2002;19:240–5.
157. Shibuki H, Katai N, Yodoi J, Uchida K, Yoshimura N. Lipid peroxidation and peroxynitrite in retinal ischemia-reperfusion injury. Invest Ophthalmol Vis Sci. 2000;41:3607–14.
158. Hartnett ME, Stratton RD, Browne RW, Rosner BA, Lanham RJ, Armstrong D. Serum markers of oxidative stress and severity of diabetic retinopathy. Diabetes Care. 2000;23:234–40.
159. Tilton RG, Chang KC, LeJeune WS, Stephan CC, Brock TA, Williamson JR. Role for nitric oxide in the hyperpermeability and hemodynamic changes induced by intravenous VEGF. Invest Ophthalmol Vis Sci. 1999;40:689–96.
160. Papapetropoulos A, Garcia-Cardena G, Madri JA, Sessa WC. Nitric oxide production contributes to the angiogenic properties of vascular endothelial growth factor in human endothelial cells. J Clin Invest. 1997;100:3131–9.
161. Fukumura D, Gohongi T, Kadambi A, et al. Predominant role of endothelial nitric oxide synthase in vascular endothelial growth factor-induced angiogenesis and vascular permeability. Proc Natl Acad Sci U S A. 2001;98:2604–9.
162. Starkebaum G, Harlan JM. Endothelial cell injury due to copper-catalyzed hydrogen peroxide generation from homocysteine. J Clin Invest. 1986;77:1370–6.
163. Hofmann MA, Kohl B, Zumbach MS, et al. Hyperhomocyst(e)inemia and endothelial dysfunction in IDDM. Diabetes Care. 1997;20:1880–6.
164. Agardh CD, Agardh E, Andersson A, Hultberg B. Lack of association between plasma homocysteine levels and microangiopathy in type 1 diabetes mellitus. Scand J Clin Lab Invest. 1994;54:637–41.
165. Hoogeveen EK, Kostense PJ, Eysink PE, et al. Hyperhomocysteinemia is associated with the presence of retinopathy in type 2 diabetes mellitus: the Hoorn study. Arch Intern Med. 2000;160:2984–90.
166. Looker HC, Fagot-Campagna A, Gunter EW, et al. Homocysteine as a risk factor for nephropathy and retinopathy in type 2 diabetes. Diabetologia. 2003;46:766–72.
167. Vaccaro O, Perna AF, Mancini FP, et al. Plasma homocysteine and microvascular complications in type 1 diabetes. Nutr Metab Cardiovasc Dis. 2000;10:297–304.
168. Chiarelli F, Pomilio M, Mohn A, et al. Homocysteine levels during fasting and after methionine loading in adolescents with diabetic retinopathy and nephropathy. J Pediatr. 2000;137:386–92.
169. Hultberg B, Agardh E, Andersson A, et al. Increased levels of plasma homocysteine are associated with nephropathy, but not severe retinopathy in type 1 diabetes mellitus. Scand J Clin Lab Invest. 1991;51:277–82.
170. Hultberg B, Agardh CD, Agardh E, Lovestam-Adrian M. Poor metabolic control, early age at onset, and marginal folate deficiency are associated with increasing levels of plasma homocysteine in insulin-dependent diabetes mellitus. A five-year follow-up study. Scand J Clin Lab Invest. 1997;57:595–600.
171. Gaede P, Vedel P, Parving HH, Pedersen O. Elevated levels of plasma von Willebrand factor and the risk of macro- and microvascular disease in type 2 diabetic patients with microalbuminuria. Nephrol Dial Transplant. 2001;16:2028–33.
172. Lip PL, Belgore F, Blann AD, Hope-Ross MW, Gibson JM, Lip GY. Plasma VEGF and soluble VEGF receptor FLT-1 in proliferative retinopathy: relationship to endothelial dysfunction and laser treatment. Invest Ophthalmol Vis Sci. 2000;41:2115–9.
173. Olson JA, Whitelaw CM, McHardy KC, Pearson DW, Forrester JV. Soluble leucocyte adhesion molecules in diabetic retinopathy stimulate retinal capillary endothelial cell migration. Diabetologia. 1997;40:1166–71.

174. Miyamoto K, Khosrof S, Bursell SE, et al. Prevention of leukostasis and vascular leakage in streptozotocin-induced diabetic retinopathy via intercellular adhesion molecule-1 inhibition. Proc Natl Acad Sci U S A. 1999;96:10836–41.
175. Schroder S, Palinski W, Schmid-Schonbein GW. Activated monocytes and granulocytes, capillary nonperfusion, and neovascularization in diabetic retinopathy. Am J Pathol. 1991;139:81–100.
176. Tanaka Y, Adams DH, Shaw S. Proteoglycans on endothelial cells present adhesion-inducing cytokines to leukocytes. Immunol Today. 1993;14:111–5.
177. Adams DH, Shaw S. Leucocyte-endothelial interactions and regulation of leucocyte migration. Lancet. 1994;343:831–6.
178. Gearing AJ, Hemingway I, Pigott R, Hughes J, Rees AJ, Cashman SJ. Soluble forms of vascular adhesion molecules, E-selectin, ICAM-1, and VCAM-1: pathological significance. Ann N Y Acad Sci. 1992;667:324–31.
179. Szmitko PE, Wang CH, Weisel RD, de Almeida JR, Anderson TJ, Verma S. New markers of inflammation and endothelial cell activation: Part I. Circulation. 2003;108:1917–23.
180. Matsumoto K, Sera Y, Ueki Y, Inukai G, Niiro E, Miyake S. Comparison of serum concentrations of soluble adhesion molecules in diabetic microangiopathy and macroangiopathy. Diabet Med. 2002;19:822–6.
181. Diabetes Drafting Group. Prevalence of small vessel and large vessel disease in diabetic patients from 14 centres: the World Health Organisation Multinational Study of Vascular Disease in Diabetics. Diabetologia. 1985;28 Suppl:615–40.
182. LaPorte RE, Dorman JS, Tajima N, et al. Pittsburgh Insulin-Dependent Diabetes Mellitus Morbidity and Mortality Study: physical activity and diabetic complications. Pediatrics. 1986;78:1027–33.
183. van Leiden HA, Dekker JM, Moll AC, et al. Risk factors for incident retinopathy in a diabetic and nondiabetic population: the Hoorn study. Arch Ophthalmol. 2003;121:245–51.
184. Klein R, Klein BE, Moss SE. Is obesity related to microvascular and macrovascular complications in diabetes? The Wisconsin Epidemiologic Study of Diabetic Retinopathy. Arch Intern Med. 1997;157:650–6.
185. Orchard TJ, Dorman JS, Maser RE, et al. Factors associated with avoidance of severe complications after 25 yr of IDDM: Pittsburgh Epidemiology of Diabetes Complications Study I. Diabetes Care. 1990;13:741–7.
186. Kriska AM, LaPorte RE, Patrick SL, Kuller LH, Orchard TJ. The association of physical activity and diabetic complications in individuals with insulin-dependent diabetes mellitus: the Epidemiology of Diabetes Complications Study–VII. J Clin Epidemiol. 1991;44:1207–14.
187. Cruickshanks KJ, Moss SE, Klein R, Klein BE. Physical activity and proliferative retinopathy in people diagnosed with diabetes before age 30 yr. Diabetes Care. 1992;15:1267–72.
188. Klein BE, Moss SE, Klein R. Oral contraceptives in women with diabetes. Diabetes Care. 1990;13:895–8.
189. Klein BE, Klein R, Moss SE. Exogenous estrogen exposures and changes in diabetic retinopathy: the Wisconsin Epidemiologic Study of Diabetic Retinopathy. Diabetes Care. 1999;22:1984–7.
190. Temple RC, Aldridge VA, Sampson MJ, Greenwood RH, Heyburn PJ, Glenn A. Impact of pregnancy on the progression of diabetic retinopathy in Type 1 diabetes. Diabet Med. 2001;18:573–7.
191. Lauszus F, Klebe JG, Bek T. Diabetic retinopathy in pregnancy during tight metabolic control. Acta Obstet Gynecol Scand. 2000;79:367–70.
192. Klein BE, Moss SE, Klein R. Effect of pregnancy on progression of diabetic retinopathy. Diabetes Care. 1990;13:34–40.
193. Chew EY, Mills JL, Metzger BE, et al. Metabolic control and progression of retinopathy: The Diabetes in Early Pregnancy Study. National Institute of Child Health and Human Development Diabetes in Early Pregnancy Study. Diabetes Care. 1995;18:631–7.
194. Hemachandra A, Ellis D, Lloyd CE, Orchard TJ. The influence of pregnancy on IDDM complications. Diabetes Care. 1995;18:950–4.
195. Vaarasmaki M, Anttila M, Pirttiaho H, Hartikainen AL. Are recurrent pregnancies a risk in type 1 diabetes? Acta Obstet Gynecol Scand. 2002;81:1110–5.
196. Moss SE, Klein R, Klein BE. Ten-year incidence of visual loss in a diabetic population. Ophthalmology. 1994;101:1061–70.

197. Moss SE, Klein R, Klein BE. The 14-year incidence of visual loss in a diabetic population. Ophthalmology. 1998;105:998–1003.
198. Klein R, Klein BE. Vision disorders in diabetes. In: Harris MI, Cowie CC, Stern MP, Boyko EJ, Reiber GE, Bennett PH, eds. Diabetes in America, 2nd ed. Springfield, VA: National Institutes of Health. NIH Publication No. 95–1468; 1995:293–338.
199. Congdon N, O'Colmain B, Klaver CC, et al. Causes and prevalence of visual impairment among adults in the United States. Arch Ophthalmol. 2004;122:477–85.
200. Hove MN, Kristensen JK, Lauritzen T, Bek T. The prevalence of retinopathy in an unselected population of type 2 diabetes patients from Arhus County, Denmark. Acta Ophthalmol Scand. 2004;82:443–8.
201. Klein R, Klein BE, Lee KE, Cruickshanks KJ, Gangnon RE. Changes in visual acuity in a population over a 15-year period: the Beaver Dam Eye Study. Am J Ophthalmol. 2006;142:539–49.
202. Klein R, Klein BE, Moss SE, Davis MD, DeMets DL. Glycosylated hemoglobin predicts the incidence and progression of diabetic retinopathy. JAMA. 1988;260:2864–71.
203. Chase HP, Jackson WE, Hoops SL, Cockerham RS, Archer PG, O'Brien D. Glucose control and the renal and retinal complications of insulin-dependent diabetes. JAMA. 1989;261:1155–60.
204. The Diabetes Control and Complications Trial Research Group. Hypoglycemia in the Diabetes Control and Complications Trial. Diabetes. 1997;46:271–86.
205. Klein R, Klein BEK, Moss SE. Risk factors for retinopathy. In: Feman SS (ed). Ocular problems in diabetes mellitus. Boston: Blackwell Publishing; 1992:39.
206. Klein R. Diabetes mellitus: oculopathy. In: Degroot LJ, Jameson JL, eds. Endocrinology, 4th ed. Philadelphia, PA: WB Saunders; 1995:857–67.
207. Klein R, Klein BEK, Moss SE. Visual impairment in diabetes. Ophthalmology. 1984;91:1–9.

4 Diagnostic Modalities in Diabetic Retinopathy

Ron Margolis and Peter K. Kaiser

CONTENTS

ABSTRACT

In addition to ophthalmologic examination and retinal fundus photography, diagnostic modalities including fluorescein angiography (FA) and optical coherence tomography (OCT) currently play important roles in the evaluation of patients with diabetic retinopathy (DR). Fluorescein angiography has been a major diagnostic procedure in the clinical evaluation of DR for several decades. This chapter will review the principles and methodology underlying fluorescein angiography, as well as its specific application to the evaluation of diabetic retinopathy and especially retinal vascular permeability. Although fluorescein angiography provides valuable anatomic and functional information pertaining to the retinal vasculature, it does not provide ultrastructural anatomic detail and does not allow quantification of retinal thickness. Optical coherence tomography has emerged in recent years as an additional modality that provides clinically valuable information. This chapter details the principles and methodology of OCT. In addition, the application of OCT to the assessment of diabetic macular edema is discussed, including the value of OCT in providing quantitative information regarding retinal thickness. The different morphologic patterns of diabetic macular edema seen in

From: *Contemporary Diabetes: Diabetic Retinopathy*
Edited by: E. Duh © Humana Press, Totowa, NJ

OCT are presented, as well as a discussion of the application of OCT to clinical management of diabetic retinopathy. Finally, additional diagnostic modalities of potential benefit in evaluating DR are presented, including the retinal thickness analyzer (RTA) and scanning laser ophthalmoscopy (SLO). The detection of retinal abnormalities in diabetic patients is vital for preventing the associated complications and subsequent loss of vision. FA and OCT provide information essential to the optimal treatment and management of diabetic retinopathy.

Key Words: Diabetic retinopathy; macular edema, fluorescein angiography; optical coherence tomography; retinal thickness analyzer; scanning laser ophthalmoscopy.

INTRODUCTION

The majority of significant visual loss in patients with diabetic retinopathy (DR) is associated with three conditions: macular edema, macular ischemia, and retinal or optic disc neovascularization. These complications of DR have been diagnosed with funduscopic examination and fluorescein angiography (FA) for over four decades. In recent years, innovative new technologies have been developed to detect DR earlier and more accurately, particularly diabetic macular edema.

Diabetic macular edema is the most common cause of visual loss in diabetic patients, affecting up to one quarter of these patients *(1–4)*. Retinal thickening results from fluid leakage due to breakdown of the blood–retina barrier *(5)*. The gold standard treatment of diabetic macular edema consists of focal laser photocoagulation, which reduces moderate visual loss by 50% *(2)*. However, visual loss persists in a significant proportion of patients after laser treatment as irreversible damage to the retina has occurred. New medical therapies are currently being studied that prevent or reduce the progression of diabetic macular edema. These treatments have necessitated earlier and more quantitative detection of retinal thickening.

Clinically significant macular edema (CSME), as defined in the Early Treatment Diabetic Retinopathy Study (ETDRS), is a clinical diagnosis made at the slit lamp with stereoscopic biomicroscopy *(2)*. Although it is convenient and readily available, this technique is subjective and insensitive to small changes in retinal thickness, making early detection and follow-up for subtle changes after therapy difficult *(6, 7)*. Furthermore, slit lamp biomicroscopy does not quantify the severity or extent of foveal thickening, the retinal layers involved, or allow the physician to visualize ischemia. Similarly, stereo fundus photography is limited by the amount of stereopsis and by the threshold for thickening adopted by individual observers *(8, 9)*. Although stereo fundus photography has been used to follow for changes after treatment, its current use in clinical trials is greatly diminished.

Fluorescein angiography has been used for over 40 years in the evaluation of chorioretinal diseases. It is a dynamic modality that enables the ophthalmologist to assess both the anatomy and function of the retinal and choroidal vasculature. However, FA does not provide ultrastructural anatomic detail, and does not allow quantification of retinal thickness. Due to these limitations, several novel imaging techniques have been developed. The most sensitive, reproducible, and widely used modality has been optical coherence tomography (OCT).

FLUORESCEIN ANGIOGRAPHY

Properties

Fluorescein angiography was first attempted by MacLean and Maumenee in 1960 *(10)*, but it was not until the advent of the electronic flash that Novotny and Alvis were able to perform the first successful fluorescein angiogram *(11)*. This procedure has since been instrumental to our knowledge and treatment of chorioretinal diseases.

Sodium fluorescein is a yellow–red dye with a molecular weight of 376.67 kDa, a spectrum of absorption at 465–490 nm (blue), and excitation at 520–530 nm (yellow–green) *(12)*. The dye, either 2–3 ml of 25% concentration or 5 ml of 10% concentration, is injected as a bolus into a peripheral vein. Once injected, 80% of the dye binds with plasma proteins, particularly albumin. It is metabolized by the liver and kidney within 24–36 h and is eliminated in the urine. Under normal conditions, fluorescein is retained within the capillary walls due to the tight blood–retinal barrier. Conditions leading to the breakdown of the blood–retinal barrier lead to the leakage of fluorescein into the retina and vitreous.

Side Effects

The most common side effect of fluorescein is the temporary yellowing of the skin and conjunctiva lasting up to 12 h after injection, as well as an orange–yellow discoloration of the urine that lasts from 24 to 36 h *(13, 14)*. Other side effects include nausea, vomiting, or vasovagal reaction, which occurs in approximately 10% of patients. Severe vasovagal reactions resulting in bradycardia and hypotension are rare. Dye extravasation may cause pain, local tissue necrosis, subcutaneous granuloma, or toxic neuritis, although these are rare. Urticarial reactions occur in about 1% of cases, and can be avoided by premedicating the patient with antihistamines and/or corticosteroids. True anaphylaxis occurs in less than 1 in 100,000 cases. Although no teratogenic effects have been identified, the use of fluorescein in pregnant or lactating women in general should be avoided unless absolutely necessary.

Normal Fluorescein Angiography

A choroidal flush and optic nerve head fluorescence appear in 10–15 s after injection of dye (arm-to-eye circulation time) (Fig. 1a) *(15)*. In 10–15% of patients, a cilioretinal artery stemming from the choroidal circulation is present and will fluoresce simultaneously with the choroid. Since choroidal vessels are fenestrated, fluorescein molecules diffuse out of the choriocapillaris, giving the appearance of generalized choroidal fluorescence, which may be mottled or patchy due to the overlying retinal pigment epithelium.

Unlike choroidal vessels, normal retinal vessels and capillaries are impermeable to fluorescein due to endothelial tight junctions. The path of the dye as it travels through the retinal vasculature is therefore quite demarcated. Fluorescein filling of retinal arteries begins approximately 1 s after choroidal fluorescence (Fig. 1a). The arteriovenous phase is characterized by complete filling of the arteries and capillaries, with laminar filling of the veins (Fig. 1b). This has been attributed to the faster flow of blood as well

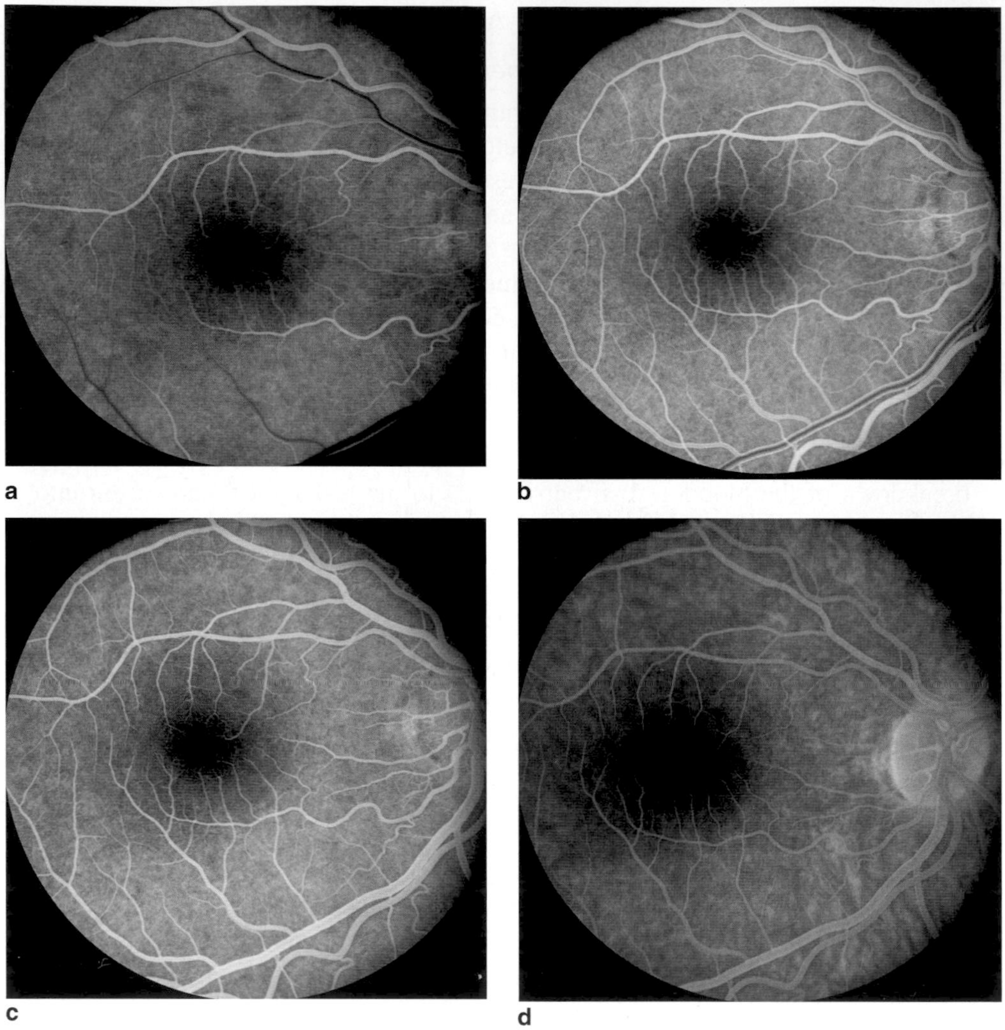

Fig. 1. Normal fluorescein angiography. (**a**) Choroidal filling is followed by arterial filling. (**b**) The arteriovenous phase is characterized by appearance of dye in a laminar pattern in the retinal veins. (**c**) The recirculation phase demonstrates declining fluorescence. (**d**) Late frames show staining of the disc, choroid, and Bruch's membrane.

as a higher concentration of erythrocytes in the central venous lumen. By 30 s, the first pass, or transit phase, of fluorescein through the retinal and choroidal vasculature is complete (Fig. 1c). This is followed by recirculation phases where there is intermittent mild fluorescence. At 10 min, both circulations are generally devoid of fluorescein. The late angiogram is characterized by staining of Bruch's membrane, the choroid, sclera, and margins of the optic nerve head (Fig. 1d).

A dark background in the macula is created by blockage of choroidal fluorescence by xanthophyll pigment and a high density of retinal pigment epithelial cells. The normal capillary free zone or foveal avascular zone (FAZ) is 300–500 μm.

Terminology

Several terms are commonly used to describe fluorescence abnormalities that aid in clinical correlation *(15, 16)*. Angiographic lesions may be hypofluorescent or hyperfluorescent. Hypofluorescence can be categorized into *blockage* (masking of fluorescence) such as with blood, or vascular *filling defect* due to deficient circulation, as in macular ischemia. Hyperfluorescence is caused by an increase in normal fluorescence or presence of abnormal fluorescence. *Autofluorescence* is seen in preinjection photographs and is caused by highly reflective substances such as optic disc drusen. *Transmission window defects* occur due to a decrease or absence of the retinal pigment epithelium, and appear as sharply defined hyperfluorescence that appears early and does not change through the angiograms. *Leakage* refers to the gradual increase in fluorescence throughout the angiogram due to fluorescein diffusing through the RPE into the subretinal space or neurosensory retina, out of retinal vessels into the retinal interstitium, or from retinal neovascularization into the vitreous. The borders of hyperfluorescence become increasingly blurred, and the greatest intensity occurs in the late frames of the angiogram. *Staining* results from fluorescein entry into a solid tissue that retains the dye, and appears as fluorescence that gradually increases in intensity through transit views and persists in late views, but its borders remain fixed throughout the angiogram. *Pooling* refers to the accumulation of fluorescein in a fluid-filled space in the retina or choroid with distinct margins.

Fluorescein Angiography in the Evaluation of Diabetic Retinopathy

FA has provided great understanding of the microvascular changes caused by diabetes. In diabetic retinopathy, endothelial tight junctions are destroyed, so that fluorescein can diffuse out of retinal vessels. The development of microaneurysms and increased capillary permeability are the earliest detectable changes (Fig. 2) *(17–19)*. These can often be

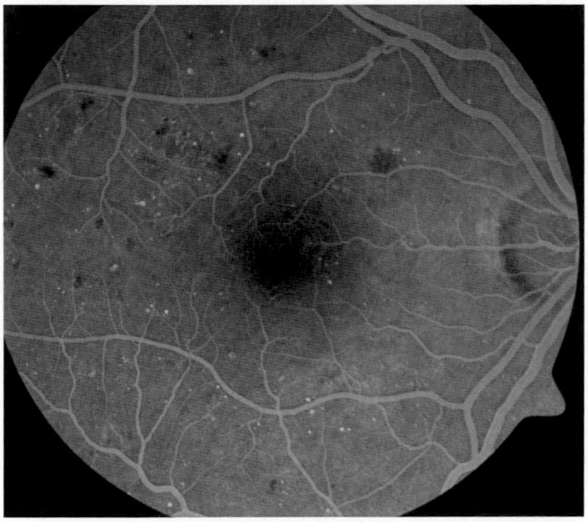

Fig. 2. Fluorescein angiography of background diabetic retinopathy is characterized by blocking defects appearing as local hypofluorescence and corresponding to intraretinal blood, and by small, round, or fusiform areas of hyperfluorescent corresponding to microaneurysms.

visualized on FA prior to being detected by funduscopic examination. The microaneurysms are predominantly on the venous side of the capillary bed. Microaneurysms may be round or fusiform, and scattered in the macular and perimacular regions, with no particular relationship to the distribution of the major retinal vessels. The dot and blot hemorrhages characteristic of DR block out fluorescence locally. Extensive macular microaneurysms may be seen without significant loss of visual acuity.

Focal areas of capillary closure may develop within the capillary bed affected by marked aneurysmal formation *(20, 21)*. Capillary closure occurs much more frequently and to a greater extent initially in the midperipheral fundus and generally increases toward the periphery (Fig. 3) *(22)*. Extensive midperipheral and peripheral capillary closure may not be apparent ophthalmoscopically. When nonperfusion results in deformation of the outline of the FAZ, it is termed macular ischemia (Fig. 4). Some enlargement of the FAZ occurs commonly in diabetes, but is usually not associated with visual loss until the FAZ approaches 1,000 μm in diameter *(17, 23–26)*. Dilated, tortuous, shunt capillaries may be evident in the ischemic peripheral retina. There is typically no angiographic evidence of choroidal vascular disease.

Neovascular proliferation is characterized by dye leakage into the vitreous (Fig. 5). Retinal neovascularization is often first seen at the junction of nonischemic and ischemic retina *(18, 27)*. Optic disc neovascularization is a reflection of widespread capillary nonperfusion. The new blood vessels on the optic disc tend to fill before the normal retinal arteries, suggesting that the choroid may be the source of blood for new vessels.

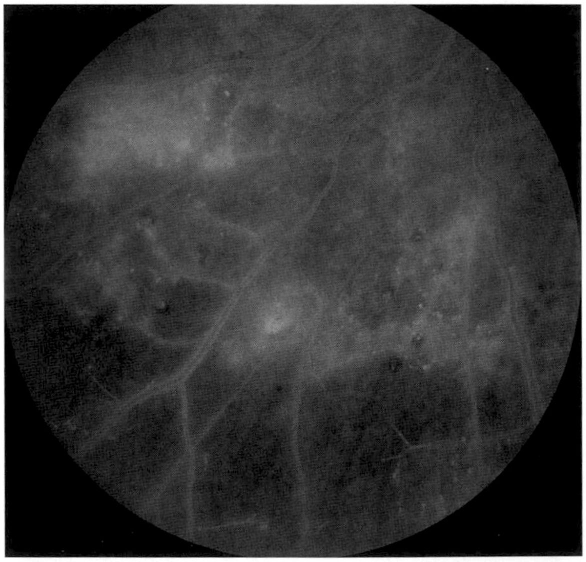

Fig. 3. Peripheral capillary nonperfusion appearing as hypofluorescence due to vascular filling defects. Adjacent to the zone of ischemia are areas of hyperfluorescence representing microaneurysms and leaking vessels.

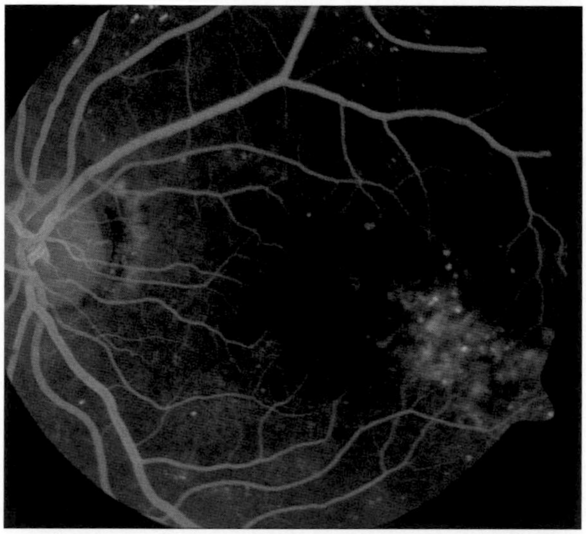

Fig. 4. Extensive capillary nonperfusion appearing as widespread vascular filling defects and enlargement of the foveal avascular zone. Microaneurysms and surrounding retinal edema appear as hyperfluorescence.

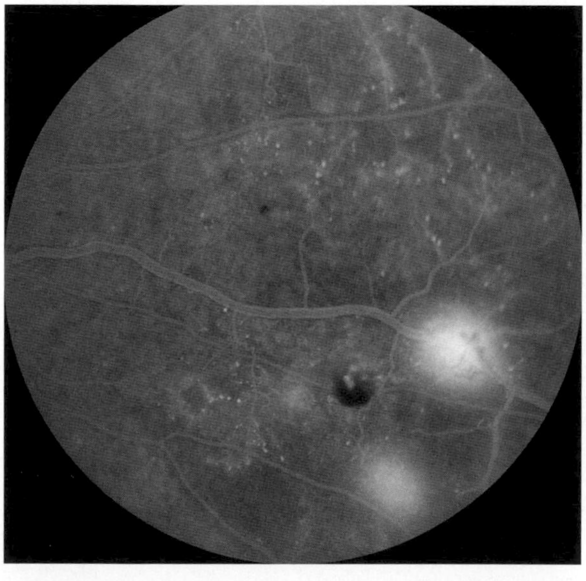

Fig. 5. Retinal neovascularization is characterized by dye leakage into the vitreous. Note multiple microaneurysms, blocking defect from preretinal hemorrhage, and diffuse pruning of the capillary tree.

Fluorescein Angiography in the Evaluation of Diabetic Macular Edema

FA findings in the macula can be organized into three patterns *(7)*. Focal leakage results from microaneurysms and dilated capillary segments, and causes focal macular edema (Fig. 6). Late ill-defined leakage of fluorescein results from a generalized breakdown of inner blood–retinal barrier and causes diffuse macular edema (Fig. 7). Late staining of

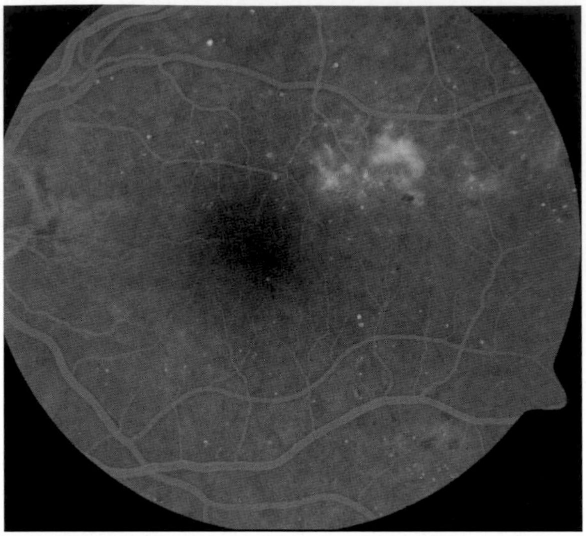

Fig. 6. Focal leakage from microaneurysms and dilated capillary segments causes focal macular edema.

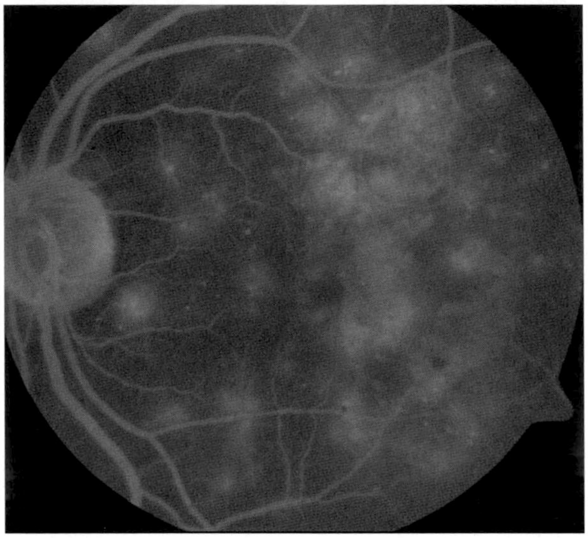

Fig. 7. Diffuse macular edema in late frames appears as ill-defined leakage of fluorescein from a generalized breakdown of inner blood retinal barrier.

fovea with pooling of the dye into parafoveal cyst-like spaces in a petalloid pattern is named cystoid macular edema (Fig. 8). These patterns may be found alone or concurrently. Due to the ability to visualize the source and/or area of leakage, FA is often used to guide focal or grid macular photocoagulation in the treatment of diabetic macular edema *(28)*.

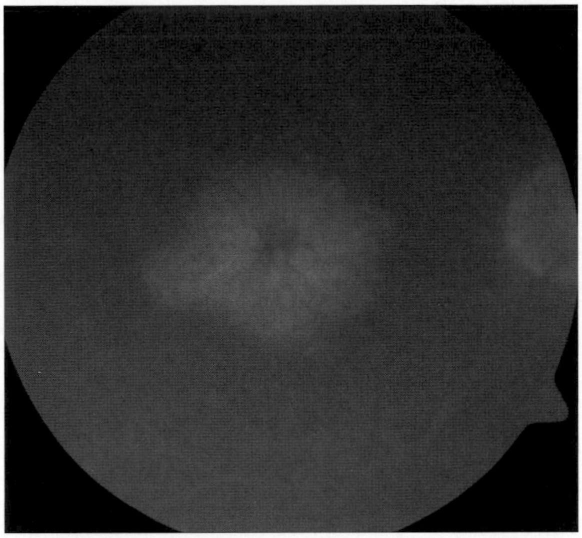

Fig. 8. Cystoid macular edema appears as late staining of fovea with pooling of the dye into parafoveal cyst-like spaces in a petalloid pattern.

Ozdek and colleagues attempted to correlate FA patterns of diabetic macular edema with described OCT patterns *(7)*. Mean foveal thickness as determined by OCT was the least in the no leakage group and progressively increased in order for focal, diffuse, and combined leakage groups. In addition, 63.3% of eyes that showed evidence of cystoid macular edema by OCT were not detected by FA. OCT also showed serous retinal detachment in 9.7% of eyes, none of which were detected by FA. Kang et al. showed that focal leakage correlated closely with homogeneous focal thickening on OCT *(29)*. Focal leakage showed the least foveal thickness and the best visual acuity among FA types. The proportion of focal leakage type decreased as diabetic retinopathy progressed. Diffuse or cystoid leakage correlated closely with outer retinal layer or subretinal fluid accumulation.

OPTICAL COHERENCE TOMOGRAPHY

Low-Coherence Interferometry

Since its first clinical application in 1991 *(30)*, OCT has dramatically increased our understanding of the morphological changes associated with many macular diseases, including diabetic macular edema *(31)*. Using noncontact, noninvasive scanning, OCT produces high-resolution two-dimensional cross-sectional images of ocular tissues *(32–34)*. Analogous to B-scan ultrasonography which uses sound echoes, OCT is based on reflections of light from the retinal tissue to produce a cross-sectional image. By using light instead of sound, OCT offers considerably higher axial resolution and faster acquisition times. When light is directed into the eye, it is reflected at the boundaries of tissues with different optical properties, as well as being scattered and absorbed by the ocular tissue. Low-coherence interferometry is used to measure the time-of-flight delay of light reflected from structures within the retina.

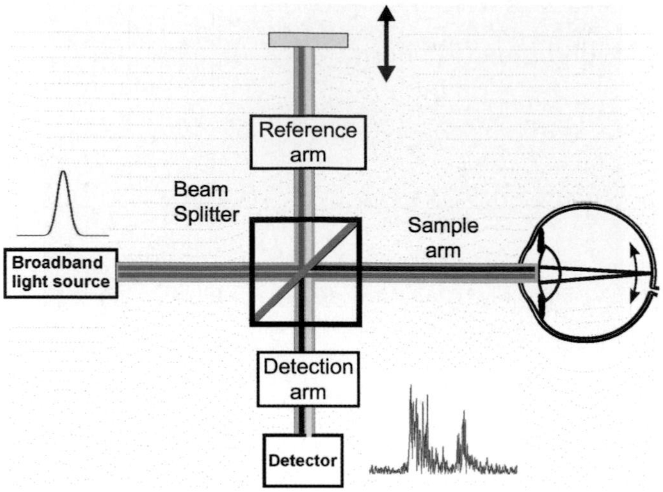

Fig. 9. Schematic diagram of a classic optical coherence tomography system. An interferometer splits the light source into a probe beam and a reference beam. The probe beam is reflected by retinal structures whose echoes result in a signal.

Current time-domain based OCT scanners use an infrared 200 μW, 830 nm wavelength probe light from a continuous-wave superluminescent diode source that is coupled into a fiberoptic Michelson interferometer (Fig. 9). The interferometer splits the light source into a probe beam and a reference beam. The probe beam is directed into the eye and is reflected from retinal structures at different distances. The reflected probe beam is composed of multiple echoes that give information about the distance and thickness of the retinal structures. The reference beam is projected at a known distance. In order for the reference beam and the backscattered light of the probe beam to combine at a detector, the reference beam must be altered. The amount that the reference beam is altered compared to its baseline results in a signal. Software manipulations of the raw OCT image data produce a false-color map representing three-dimensional topographic retinal features and quantitative retinal thickness measurements. The images are stored on digital media to enable comparison of serial evaluations and for archiving purposes.

OCT Image Interpretation

The resulting OCT image closely approximates the histologic appearance of the retina (Fig. 10). The top of the image corresponds to the vitreous cavity. In a normal patient, this will be optically silent, or may show the posterior hyaloidal face in an eye with a posterior vitreous detachment. The posterior vitreous face appears as a thin horizontal or oblique greenish line above or inserting into the retina. The anterior surface of the retina demonstrates high reflectivity, and in the fovea of normal eyes, demonstrates the central foveal depression. The horizontally aligned nerve fiber layer demonstrates higher tissue signal strength and is thicker closer to the optic nerve. The internal structure of the retina consists of heterogeneous reflections, corresponding to the varying

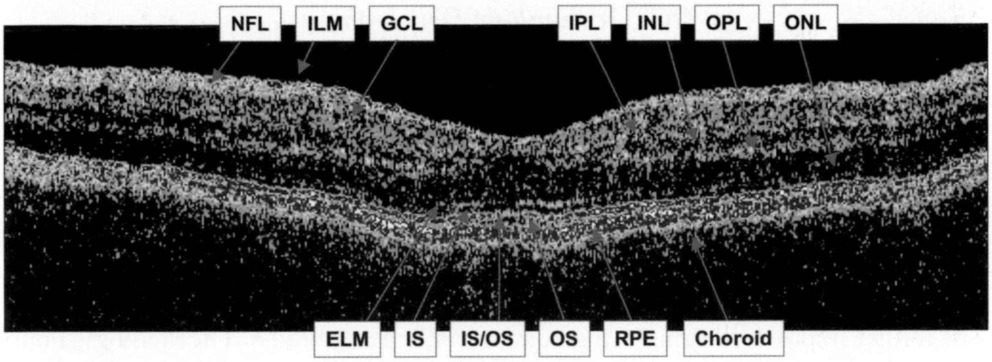

NFL: Nerve Fiber Layer
ILM: Inner Limiting Membrane
GCL: Ganglion Cell Layer
IPL: Inner Plexiform Layer
INL: Inner Nuclear Layer
OPL: Outer Plexiform Layer
ONL: Outer Nuclear Layer
ELM: External limiting membrane
IS: Photoreceptor Inner Segment
IS/OS: Junction of inner and outer photoreceptor segments
OS: Photoreceptor Outer Segment
RPE: Retinal Pigment Epithelium

Fig. 10. OCT of a normal human macula showing the characteristic foveal contour. The nerve fiber layer (NFL) is highly backscattering. The inner and outer plexiform layers (IPL, OPL) are more hyperreflective than the inner and outer nuclear layers (INL, ONL). There is a reflection from the boundary between the inner and outer segments of the photoreceptors (IS, OS). The RPE and choriocapillaris appear as the highly backscattering boundary beyond the posterior retina.

ultrastructural anatomy. The axially aligned cellular layers of the retina (inner nuclear, outer nuclear, and ganglion cell layers) demonstrate less backscattering and back-reflection of incident OCT light, and thus appear with a lower tissue signal (darker), compared to horizontally aligned structures (internal limiting membrane, Henle's layer, and NFL) that appear brighter. The retinal pigment epithelium, Bruch's membrane, and choriocapillaris complex collectively comprise the highly reflective external band. Just anterior to this band is another highly reflective line representing the junction between the photoreceptors' inner and outer segments. Reproducible patterns of retinal morphology seen by OCT have been shown to correspond to the location of retinal layers seen on light microscopic overlays in both normal and pathologic retinas *(17, 35–37, 40)*.

Image-processing software can quantify retinal thickness from the OCT tomograms as the distance between the anterior and posterior highly reflective boundaries of the retina *(38)*. A software algorithm known as segmentation uses the processes of smoothing, edge detection, and error correction to facilitate this process. Retinal thickness can therefore be determined at any transverse location. Hee et al. *(33)* developed a standardized mapping OCT protocol, consisting of six radial tomograms, each 6 mm in length, in a spoke pattern centered on the fovea. Retinal thickness is then displayed in two different manners: first as a two-dimensional color-coded map of retinal thickness in the posterior pole; and secondly as a numeric average of nine parafoveal areas corresponding the ETDRS subfields. Additional acquisition algorithms include the fast macular mapping protocol, which allows six radial scans to be performed in a single session of 1.92 s; and the high-density scan protocol consisting of six separate 6-mm radial lines, acquired in 7.32 s.

OCT Technology Development

Over the last decade, the development of OCT has progressed rapidly *(34)*. The first and second generations of commercial OCT instruments had an axial resolution of 10–15 μm. Third generation OCT (Stratus OCT; Carl Zeiss Meditec, Dublin, California, USA) provides an axial resolution of 8–10 μm. Because axial resolution depends on the "coherence length" of the light source, ultrahigh resolution images using a femtosecond titanium:sapphire laser light source can deliver resolutions of 1–3 μm, approaching the theoretical limit of OCT imaging *(37, 39)*. However, these ultrahigh resolution scanners are not yet available commercially.

To further improve imaging using commercially available OCT technology, Fourier or spectral-domain technology has been employed that delivers almost a 100-fold improvement in acquisition speed over current time-domain OCT scanners since the moving reference arm is eliminated and all data points can be analyzed at the same time. High-speed Fourier-domain OCT was first described by Wojtkowski and colleagues *(40, 41)*, and then by Nassif and associates *(42)*. Instead of a single detector, the detector arm of the Michelson interferometer uses a spectrometer, which measures spectral modulations produced by interference between the sample and reference reflections. A waveform that represents the amplitude of sample reflections as a function of depth is then produced. The spectrometer measurement is superior to time-domain OCT because no physical movement of the reference mirror is required, and data is therefore acquired at a much faster rate. Furthermore, this technique is able to simultaneous detect reflections from a broad range of depths, whereas time-domain OCT acquires signals from various depths sequentially. This improves the signal-to-noise ratio by a factor proportional to the number of detector elements in the spectrometer (typically 1024 or 2048). With increased imaging speed and greater signal to noise ratio, the Fourier-domain OCT scanners produce more detailed and brighter images (Fig. 11).

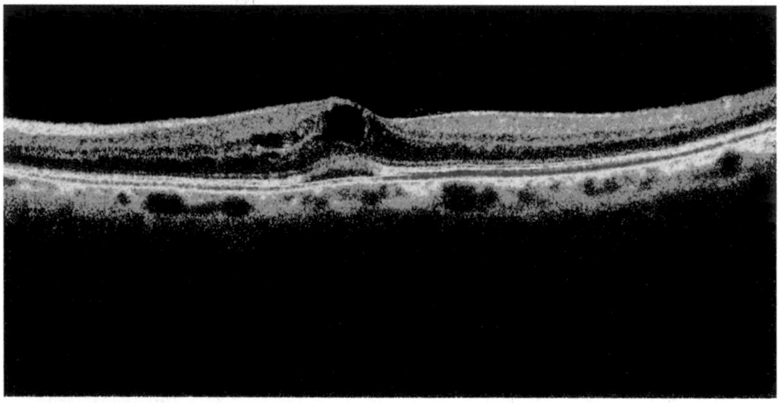

Fig. 11. (**a**) Fourier-domain OCT of a patient with diabetic macular edema. Figure courtesy of Jay Duker, MD. (**b**) Ultrahigh-resolution OCT of a patient with diabetic macular edema using an experimental unit at New England Eye Center, Boston, MA. Figure courtesy of Jay Duker, MD. (**c**) Three-dimensional reconstruction of patient with diabetic macular edema with Fourier-domain OCT. Figure courtesy of Jason Slakter, MD.

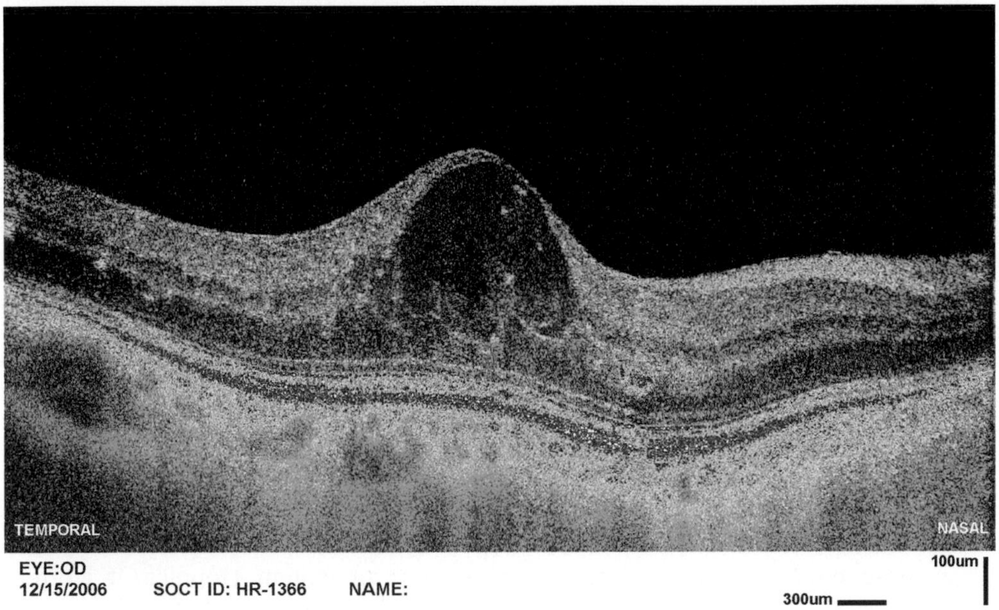

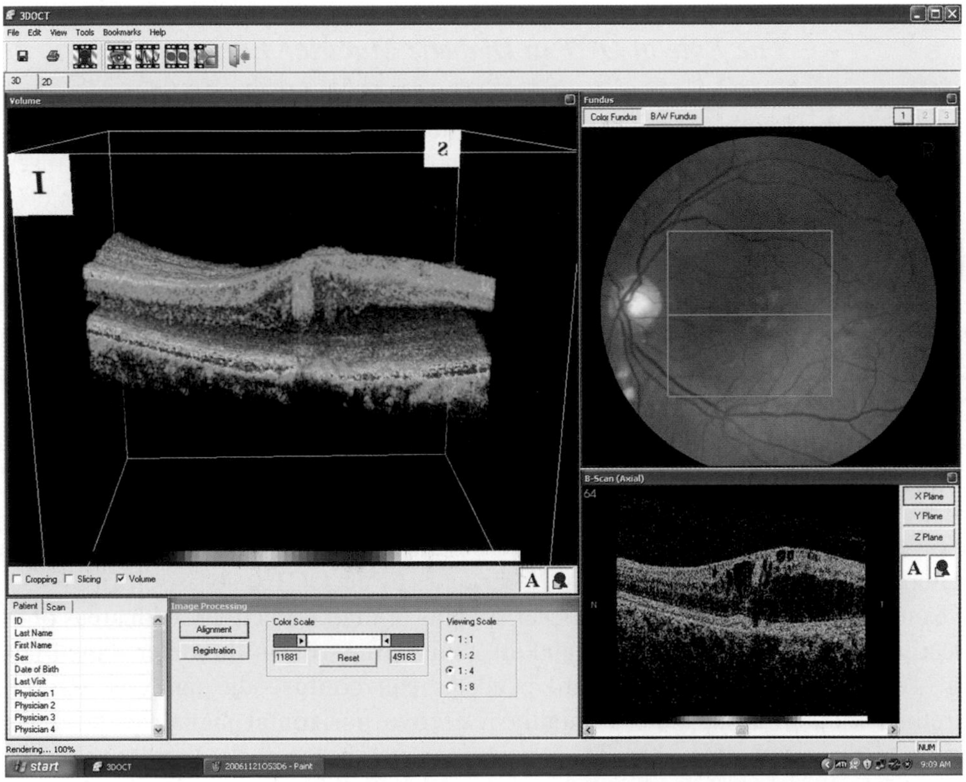

Fig. 11. (*continued*)

Fourier-domain OCT of the macula has been shown to provide greater detail (1125 A-scans vs. 512 A-scans) than commercially available time-domain OCT systems image in a shorter period of time (0.072 vs. 1.23 s) *(43)*. This dramatically decreases motion artifact, which appears as undulating of the retina in the slower time-domain OCT image. Because motion-correcting algorithms are not required, the images better represent the true topography of the retina. Moreover, the faster scanning time allow a larger area to be scanned and offers more precise registration. It is also possible to acquire three-dimentional OCT data that achieve comprehensive retinal coverage and allow correlation between OCT images and clinical fundus features *(44)*. The significant advantages of the Fourier-domain OCT will likely be the basis of the next generation of retinal OCT systems.

Doppler OCT has been used for measurement of blood flow using both time-domain *(45, 46)*. and Fourier-domain OCTs *(47, 48)*. The Doppler shift is localized in depth by use of joint time–frequency analysis algorithms, which generate depth-resolved Doppler frequency spectra of the reflected light. Rapid acquisition of retinal flow data in a few milliseconds allows the extraction of dynamic flow properties, such as the retinal vascular response to changes in perfusion pressure or oxygen content. Doppler OCT offers superior spatial resolution compared with Doppler ultrasound and Doppler scanning laser ophthalmoscopy. Unlike angiography, Doppler OCT is more quantitative and does not require injection of a contrast agent.

The Role of OCT in Diabetic Macular Edema

OCT retinal thickness measurements in diabetic patients have been shown in a number of studies to be highly reproducible. Retinal thickness measurements reproducible to within ±5% and ±6% were found for normal and diabetes subjects with diabetic macular edema, respectively *(49)*[-24] Thus, changes in central retinal thickness greater than 6% for healthy patients and greater than 10% for diabetic patients are likely to be due to true changes in retinal thickness rather than inconsistencies in the OCT measurements.

Changes in macular thickness may be reported in absolute values before and after treatment or in percentage change. However, no uniform method currently exists for reporting changes in macular thickness. Chan and Duker suggested a standardized method for reporting changes in macular thickness as a percentage of total possible change based on normative OCT data *(50)*. Standardizing reported changes in macular thickening may be required to better evaluate the efficacy of therapeutic intervention, as well as to compare various treatment strategies.

Some variability in retinal thickness measurements may be observed due to artifacts that impair the correct detection of retinal boundaries by the OCT analysis software *(49, 51)*. For example, intraretinal exudates appear as spots of high reflectivity with areas of low-reflective shadowing behind them, and are found primarily in the outer retinal layers (Fig. 12). Large collections of hard exudates can confuse the analysis algorithm. Epiretinal membrane appears as highly reflective horizontal signal at the anterior surface of the retina (Fig. 13). Thus, epiretinal membranes or a low lying posterior hyaloidal face can confuse the analysis algorithm and incorrectly increase reported retinal thickness *(52)*.

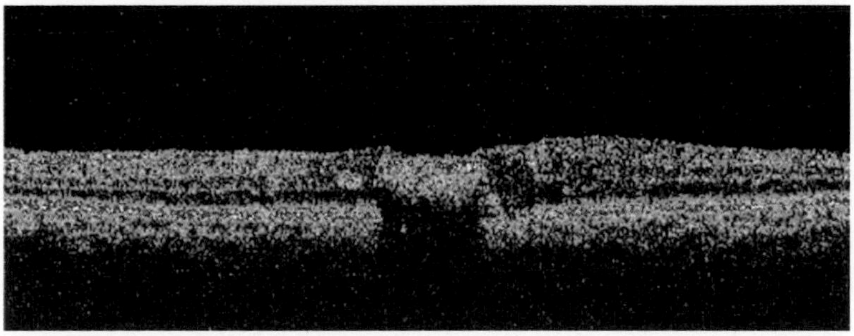

Fig. 12. OCT scan of intraretinal exudates appearing as spots of high reflectivity with areas of low-reflective shadowing behind them.

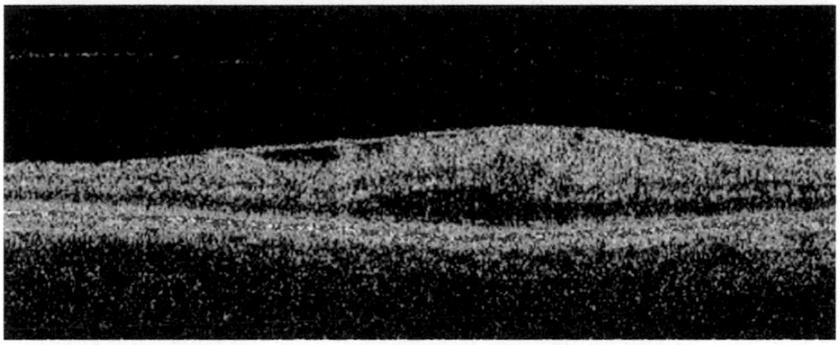

Fig. 13. OCT scan of epiretinal membrane appearing as highly reflective horizontal signal on the inner surface of the retina, with irregularities of the retinal surface beneath.

Morphologic Patterns of Diabetic Macular Edema

Studies have described the presence of at least five different morphologic patterns of diabetic macular edema seen on OCT *(7, 29, 53–55)*. *Diffuse retinal thickening* appears as increased sponge-like retinal thickness greater than 200 µm with reduced intraretinal reflectivity, particularly in the outer retinal layers (Fig. 14). *Cystoid macular edema* appears as small, round or oval, hyporeflective lacunae with highly reflective septae bridging the retinal layers and separating the cystoid-like cavities (Fig. 15). The cystoid spaces are located primarily in the outer retinal layers, leaving a thin outer layer in the fovea. Some morphologic differences exist between newly developed and long-standing cystoid macular edema *(53)*. In early cystoid macular edema, cystoid spaces primarily are located in the outer retinal layers, and the inner retinal layers are relatively preserved. In chronic cystoid macular edema, the septa of each cystoid space disappear, forming confluent large cystoid cavities (Fig. 16). Large cystoid spaces may involve the entire retinal layer, appearing as retinoschisis.

Posterior hyaloidal traction is defined as a highly reflective signal arising from the inner retinal surface and extending toward the optic nerve or peripherally (Fig. 17) *(54)*. *Subretinal fluid* or serous retinal detachment appears as a shallow elevation of the retina resembling a dome, with an optically clear space between the retina and the RPE, and

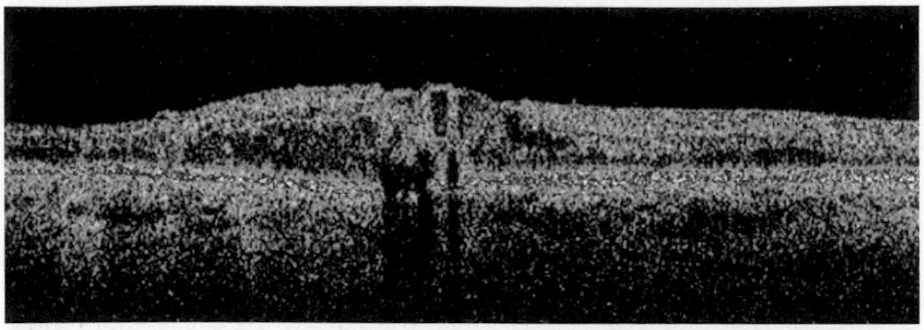

Fig. 14. OCT scan of diffuse macular edema appearing as increased sponge-like retinal thickening with reduced intraretinal reflectivity, particularly in the outer retinal layers. Note the intraretinal exudates.

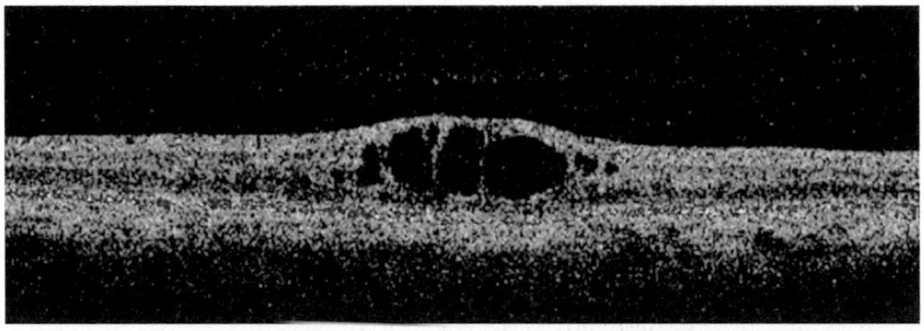

Fig. 15. OCT scan of cystoid macular edema appearing as round or oval, hyporeflective cystoid-like intraretinal spaces with septae bridging the retinal layers and separating the cavities. The cystoid spaces are located primarily in the outer retinal layers.

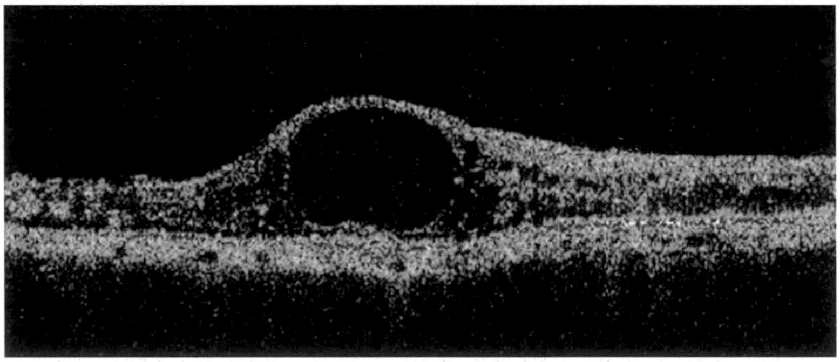

Fig. 16. OCT scan of chronic cystoid macular edema showing a large intraretinal cystoid cavity with loss of septae.

a distinct outer border of the detached retina (Fig. 18). The identification of the highly reflective posterior border of detached retina distinguishes subretinal from intraretinal fluid. Finally, *tractional retinal detachment* is defined as a peak-shaped detachment of the retina with an area of low signal underlying the highly reflective border of the neurosensory retina, and is accompanied by posterior hyaloidal traction (Fig. 19).

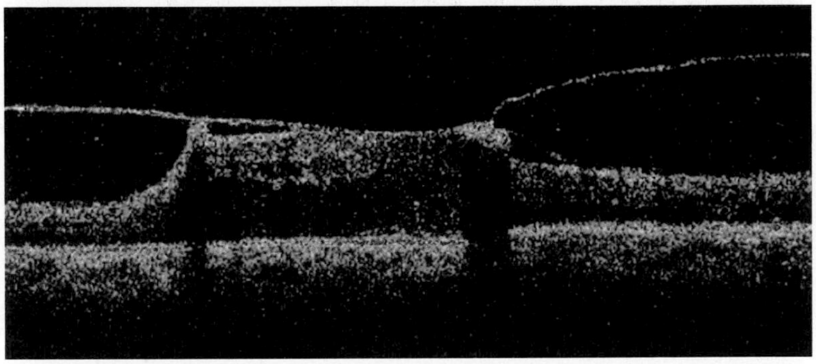

Fig. 17. OCT scan of posterior hyaloidal traction showing a highly reflective signal arising from the inner retinal surface and extending in an anterior–posterior direction. Note the diffuse macular edema.

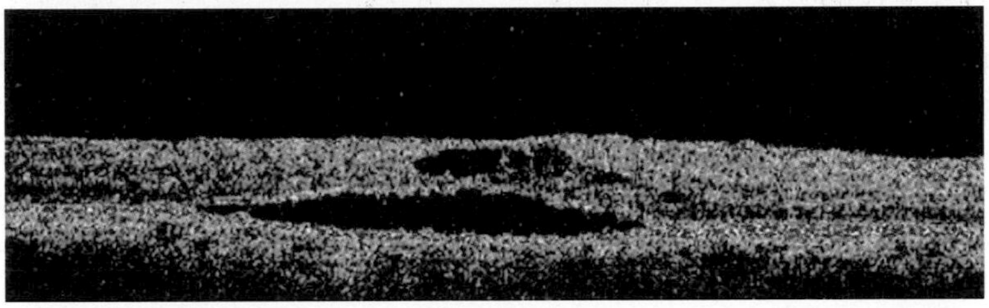

Fig. 18. OCT scan of subretinal fluid appearing as a shallow elevation of the retina with an optically clear space between the retina and the RPE. Cystoid macular edema is seen as well.

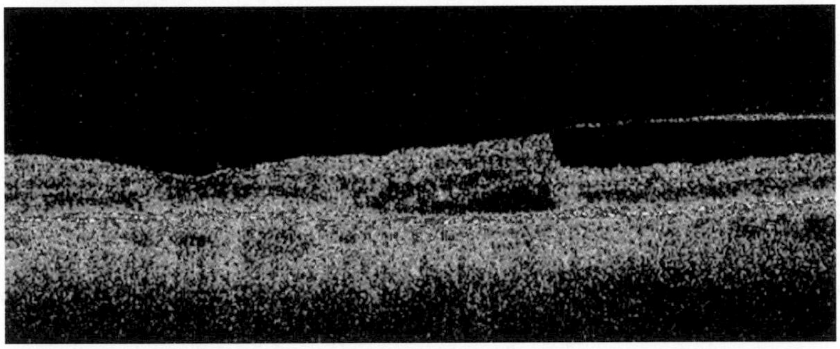

Fig. 19. OCT scan of a shallow tractional retinal detachment with posterior hyaloidal traction. A highly reflective signal corresponding to posterior hyaloidal traction arises from the inner retinal surface. A peak-shaped detachment of the retina can be seen with a hyporeflective area underneath the highly reflective border of the neurosensory retina.

While diffuse retinal thickening and cystoid macular edema may be detected by biomicroscopy, OCT seems particularly helpful in the analysis of the vitreomacular relationship. OCT is much more accurate than biomicroscopy in determining the status of the posterior hyaloid when it is only slightly detached from the macular surface *(35, 56–58)*. Evidence of posterior hyaloidal traction on OCT indicates vitreomacular traction as described by Lewis et al. *(59)*. In these cases, vitrectomy is beneficial. In other cases, the posterior hyaloid appears to be slightly reflective, detached from the retinal surface in the perifoveal area and attached at the foveal center. This aspect is quite common, and corresponds to early posterior vitreous detachment *(57, 58)*.

Clinical Applications of OCT in Diabetic Macular Edema

Several reports have studied the incidence of individual OCT patterns in diabetic macular edema and their clinical significance in an attempt to predict response to treatment and visual outcomes. In a study of 164 eyes with diabetic macular edema, the most common OCT pattern of cystoid macular edema was diabetic macular edema, which was found alone in 39.5% of eyes and in combination with other patterns in 97% of eyes *(54)*. Other authors reported an incidence of diffuse retinal thickening of 60–88% *(7, 53, 60)*. Cystoid macular edema has been reported to be present in 15–55% of eyes with diabetic macular edema *(7, 53, 54, 60)*. Cystoid macular edema in the absence of other patterns was found in 11.9% of cases *(53)*. Kim et al. found posterior hyaloidal traction in 15.6% of eyes *(54)*. Interestingly, the majority (81.4%) of eyes with posterior hyaloidal traction did not show evidence of a traction retinal detachment. However, it is possible that with longer follow-up, posterior hyaloidal traction may eventually lead to tractional retinal detachment. Serous or traction retinal detachments occur less frequently than the other three OCT patterns. Serous retinal detachment without posterior hyaloidal traction has been reported in 7–15% of eyes with diabetic macular edema *(7, 53, 54)*. Tractional retinal detachment due to posterior hyaloidal traction has been reported in less than 4% of cases *(7, 29, 54)*.

Although diffuse retinal thickening is often found as a single pattern of diabetic macular edema, the remaining OCT patterns usually do not appear alone. The most common combination described is diffuse retinal thickening with cystoid macular edema, seen in 29% of cases *(54)*. Other common patterns include: diffuse retinal thickening, cystoid macular edema, and posterior hyaloidal traction (7.3%); diffuse retinal thickening, cystoid macular edema, and serous retinal detachment (6.9%) (Fig. 20); diffuse retinal thickening and posterior hyaloidal traction (5.8%) (Fig. 21); diffuse retinal thickening, cystoid macular edema, posterior hyaloidal traction, and tractional retinal detachment (0.7%); and diffuse retinal thickening, posterior hyaloidal traction, and tractional retinal detachment (0.4%). Retinal detachment alone, either serous or tractional, has not been described.

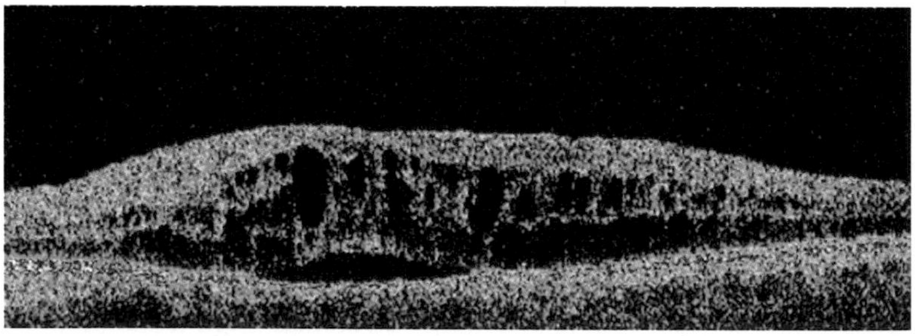

Fig. 20. OCT scan showing diffuse macular edema, cystoid macular edema, and subretinal fluid.

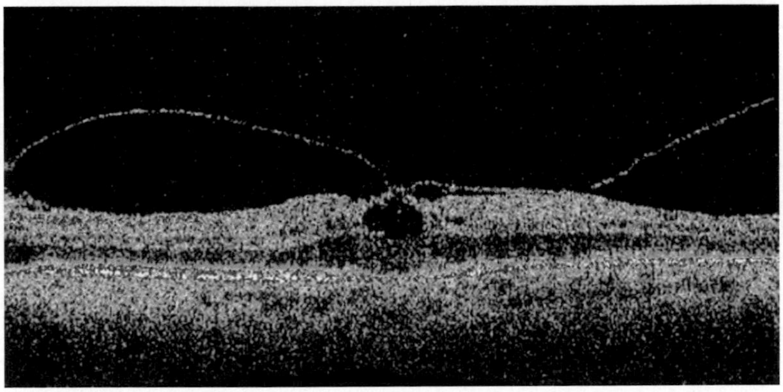

Fig. 21. OCT scan showing diffuse retinal thickening and posterior hyaloidal traction. An intraretinal cystoid cavity is present as well.

Compared with normal foveal thickness values, which range from 150 to 200 μm, mean retinal thickness in patients with diabetic macular edema has been reported between 400 and 500 μm, and range as high as 1,000 μm *(7, 53, 54, 60)*. OCT has also been used to demonstrate daily variation in the severity macular edema *(61)*. In addition, retinal thickness varies depending on the OCT pattern present. Although mean retinal thickness is elevated in each of the five diabetic macular edema patterns, patients with a retinal detachment, either serous or tractional, have the greatest retinal thickness *(53, 54)*. Patients with cystoid macular edema, posterior hyaloidal traction without tractional retinal detachment, and diffuse retinal thickening have increased retinal thickness but not to the same degree as patients with retinal detachment. Patients with cystoid macular edema have a greater increase in retinal thickness compared with patients with diffuse retinal thickening alone.

Several studies have demonstrated that foveal thickness measured by OCT is correlated with visual acuity in patients with DR *(7, 29, 33, 53–55, 62, 63)*. In particular, cystoid macular edema and posterior hyaloidal traction without tractional retinal detachment have been associated with worse visual acuity *(54)*. Kim et al. found that OCT patterns containing cystoid macular edema had the most profound effect on visual acuity, especially at lower retinal thickness *(54)*. Similarly, the presence of vitreomacular traction in the setting of diabetic macular edema has been associated with worse visual outcomes *(29, 54)*. Conversely, the presence of serous retinal detachment was not correlated with poorer visual acuity. However, other studies have not shown this correlation. A likely explanation for this disparity is the fact that the OCT cannot visualize photoreceptor function, so patients with longstanding diabetic retinopathy may have poor vision due to retinal abnormalities not visible with the scanner.

In recent years, OCT has been used extensively in the evaluation of treatment response of diabetic macular edema. Progression of macular thickening and its response to treatment with laser photocoagulation *(64, 65)*, subtenon's or intravitreal injection of triamcinolone acetonide *(66–68)*, or vitrectomy *(56, 69, 70)* have been monitored using serial OCT examinations. Retinal thickness measurement by OCT has been a main outcome studied by the Diabetic Retinopathy Clinical Research (DRCR) Network, a collaborative multicenter research effort that was formed in 2002. In one recent study, OCT was used to conclude that peribulbar injection of triamcinolone acetonide is unlikely to have any significant benefit in the treatment of diabetic macular edema in patients with good visual acuity *(71)*. Clearly, the ability to monitor changes in retinal thickness by OCT as a response to treatment has become invaluable to the assessment of the effects of current and new treatments.

A number of studies compared the use of OCT with slit-lamp biomicroscopy and stereo fundus photography in the detection of macular thickening. OCT was found to be sensitive to small changes in retinal thickness despite normal findings by slit-lamp biomicroscopy *(33, 38)*. Brown et al. reported good agreement between OCT and contact lens examination for the presence or absence of foveal edema when OCT thickness was considered normal (≤ 200 µm) or significantly increased (> 300 µm) *(6)*. However, when OCT foveal thickness was mildly increased (201–300 µm), slit-lamp biomicroscopy was sensitive in only 14% of cases.

Since guidelines for treatment of diabetic macular edema are based on stereoscopic diagnosis of "clinically significant" macular edema as defined by the ETDRS *(2)*, the value of treatment of early, or "subclinical" retinal thickening detected by OCT is still unknown. Furthermore, the best criteria for detecting subtle changes in retinal thickness remain to be defined and validated. Similarly, OCT criteria for evaluating the progression of nonclinically significant diabetic macular edema have not yet been clearly defined.

Prior to the development of OCT, stereo fundus photography had been the accepted gold standard for the evaluation of diabetic macular edema. Although stereo fundus photography has high resolution over the whole photographic field, quantifying retinal thickness is difficult using this method as it is dependent on the stereopsis of the observer and the quality of the fundus photographs. Strom et al. found a significant degree of agreement between stereo fundus photographs and OCT for both foveal and central macular area (1,000 µm in diameter) thickening *(72)*. Exact agreement on location was found in 89.4% of cases. When comparing measurements of the area of retinal thickening, exact agreement was found in 84.1% of cases. However, stereo fundus photographs tended to be more sensitive than OCT for the detection of retinal thickening in peripheral ETDRS fields. Goebel et al. found a good correlation between stereo fundus photographs and OCT ($r = 0.77$), although OCT was able to detect 12.6% of eyes with macular edema that were missed by stereo fundus photographs *(73)*.

OTHER RETINAL IMAGING MODALITIES IN DIABETIC RETINOPATHY

The *retinal thickness analyzer* (RTA) uses a single vertical narrow green He–Ne (543.3 nm) laser slit beam that is projected at an angle on the retina while a camera records the backscattered light *(74)*. Due to the oblique projection of the beam and the transparency of the retina, the backscattered light returns two peaks corresponding to the vitreoretinal and the chorioretinal interfaces. The calculated distance between the two light peaks determines the retinal thickness at a given point. During scanning, the

RTA acquires a red-free fundus image. Using blood vessels as guidelines, the registration software automatically overlays the map on the fundus image, enhancing reproducibility and measurement accuracy.

A number of studies *(75–77)* have compared the OCT and RTA in the detection of retinal thickening. Both instruments can detect small increases in retinal thickness of 20–40 μm and have been reported to yield reproducible measurements of foveal thickness *(75)*. Pires et al. *(76)* found OCT to be less sensitive than the RTA in detecting localized increases in retinal thickness in the early stages of diabetic retinal disease. Goebel et al. showed that retinal thickness values by RTA are lower than those by OCT for the same patient population *(73)*. Agreement of stereo fundus photography was consistently better with OCT than with RTA. The authors suggested that the algorithm in the RTA gets less accurate signal with greater retinal thickness because the video signal from the pigment epithelium is attenuated and blurred. The RTA may therefore be more appropriate in initial diabetic retinal disease rather than in more advanced stages with severe morphological alterations. Polito et al. reported a much lower rate of successful foveal thickness reading for the RTA (62%) than for OCT (98%) *(77)*. Neubauer et al. indicated that a greater proportion of falsely high thickness values might be present in RTA measurements *(75)*.

Scanning laser ophthalmoscopy (SLO) measures retinal topography and maps the retinal surface *(78)*. In the SLO, a narrow 1 mm beam of laser traverses the optical axis to a single 10 μm point on the fundus. A fundus image is then generated by scanning the laser over the retina in a raster fashion and detecting the reflected light with an avalanche photodetector. This signal is synchronously decoded to form a digital image. The capacity to carry out confocal imaging is a significant advantage of the SLO. By moving a confocal aperture between two end points chosen by the operator a large number of tomographic slices of the retina can be acquired. From this data, depth information on retinal features can be derived *(79)*. Tong et al. suggested that this technology may be potentially useful in screening for asymptomatic diabetic macular edema using a new scoring system *(80)*. Studies comparing OCT and SLO have not been performed to date.

CONCLUSIONS

The detection of retinal abnormalities in diabetic patients is vital for preventing the associated complications and subsequent loss of vision. With the emergence of new treatments for the prevention of diabetes-induced damage to the retinal microvasculature, early discovery of diabetic retinopathy is of primary importance. Fluorescein angiography remains an indispensable procedure for the diagnosis of macular edema, retinal ischemia, and proliferative diabetic retinopathy. Optical coherence tomography has become the gold standard test in the early detection of macular edema, vitreomacular traction, and subretinal fluid that are not detectable by biomicroscopy or fluorescein angiography. Technological advances such as the ultrahigh-resolution OCT will certainly provide ophthalmologists with greater understanding of retinal pathology in diabetic retinopathy. These diagnostic modalities will likely change how and when patients are treated, and may lead to the development of more effective therapies and improved outcomes.

REFERENCES

1. Klein R, Klein BE, Moss SE, Cruickshanks KJ. The Wisconsin Epidemiologic Study of Diabetic Retinopathy. XV. The long-term incidence of macular edema. Ophthalmology 1995;102(1):7–16.
2. Photocoagulation for diabetic macular edema. Early Treatment Diabetic Retinopathy Study report number 1. Early Treatment Diabetic Retinopathy Study research group. Arch Ophthalmol 1985;103(12): 1796–806.
3. Moss SE, Klein R, Klein BE. The incidence of vision loss in a diabetic population. Ophthalmology 1988;95(10):1340–8.
4. Fong DS, Ferris FL, 3rd, Davis MD, Chew EY. Causes of severe visual loss in the early treatment diabetic retinopathy study: ETDRS report no. 24. Early Treatment Diabetic Retinopathy Study Research Group. Am J Ophthalmol 1999;127(2):137–41.
5. Gardner TW, Antonetti DA, Barber AJ, LaNoue KF, Levison SW. Diabetic retinopathy: more than meets the eye. Surv Ophthalmol 2002;47 Suppl 2:S253–62.
6. Brown JC, Solomon SD, Bressler SB, Schachat AP, DiBernardo C, Bressler NM. Detection of diabetic foveal edema: contact lens biomicroscopy compared with optical coherence tomography. Arch Ophthalmol 2004;122(3):330–5.
7. Ozdek SC, Erdinc MA, Gurelik G, Aydin B, Bahceci U, Hasanreisoglu B. Optical coherence tomographic assessment of diabetic macular edema: comparison with fluorescein angiographic and clinical findings. Ophthalmologica 2005;219(2):86–92.
8. Kinyoun J, Barton F, Fisher M, Hubbard L, Aiello L, Ferris F, 3rd. Detection of diabetic macular edema. Ophthalmoscopy versus photography–Early Treatment Diabetic Retinopathy Study Report Number 5. The ETDRS Research Group. Ophthalmology 1989;96(6):746–50; discussion 50–1.
9. Yang Y, Vitale S, Ding Y, et al. A comparison of quantitative mapping and stereoscopic fundus photography grading of retinal thickness in diabetic eyes with macular edema. Ophthalmic Surg Lasers Imaging 2003;34(1):7–16.
10. Maclean AL, Maumenee AE. Hemangioma of the choroid. Am J Ophthalmol 1960;50:3–11.
11. Novotny HR, Alvis DL. A method of photographing fluorescence in circulating blood in the human retina. Circulation 1961;24:82–6.
12. Delori F, Ben-Sira I, Trempe C. Fluorescein angiography with an optimized filter combination. Am J Ophthalmol 1976;82(4):559–66.
13. Yannuzzi LA, Rohrer KT, Tindel LJ, et al. Fluorescein angiography complication survey. Ophthalmology 1986;93(5):611–7.
14. Kwan AS, Barry C, McAllister IL, Constable I. Fluorescein angiography and adverse drug reactions revisited: the Lions Eye experience. Clin Experiment Ophthalmol 2006;34(1):33–8.
15. Rabb MF, Burton TC, Schatz H, Yannuzzi LA. Fluorescein angiography of the fundus: a schematic approach to interpretation. Surv Ophthalmol 1978;22(6):387–403.
16. Brancato R, Trabucchi G. Fluorescein and indocyanine green angiography in vascular chorioretinal diseases. Semin Ophthalmol 1998;13(4):189–98.
17. Gass JD. A fluorescein angiographic study of macular dysfunction secondary to retinal vascular disease. IV. Diabetic retinal angiopathy. Arch Ophthalmol 1968;80(5):583–91.
18. Kohner EM, Dollery CT. Fluorescein angiography of the fundus in diabetic retinopathy. Br Med Bull 1970;26(2):166–70.
19. Norton EW, Gutman F. Diabetic retinopathy studied by fluorescein angiography. Ophthalmologica 1965;150(1):5–17.
20. Bresnick GH, Engerman R, Davis MD, de Venecia G, Myers FL. Patterns of ischemia in diabetic retinopathy. Trans Sect Ophthalmol Am Acad Ophthalmol Otolaryngol 1976;81(4 Pt 1):OP694–709.
21. Bresnick GH, De Venecia G, Myers FL, Harris JA, Davis MD. Retinal ischemia in diabetic retinopathy. Arch Ophthalmol 1975;93(12):1300–10.
22. Shimizu K, Kobayashi Y, Muraoka K. Midperipheral fundus involvement in diabetic retinopathy. Ophthalmology 1981;88(7):601–12.
23. Bresnick GH, Condit R, Syrjala S, Palta M, Groo A, Korth K. Abnormalities of the foveal avascular zone in diabetic retinopathy. Arch Ophthalmol 1984;102(9):1286–93.

24. Mansour AM, Schachat A, Bodiford G, Haymond R. Foveal avascular zone in diabetes mellitus. Retina 1993;13(2):125–8.
25. Ticho U, Patz A. The role of capillary perfusion in the management of diabetic macular edema. Am J Ophthalmol 1973;76(6):880–6.
26. Sigelman J. Diabetic macular edema in juvenile- and adult-onset diabetes. Am J Ophthalmol 1980;90(3):287–96.
27. Muraoka K, Shimizu K. Intraretinal neovascularization in diabetic retinopathy. Ophthalmology 1984;91(12):1440–6.
28. Kylstra JA, Brown JC, Jaffe GJ, et al. The importance of fluorescein angiography in planning laser treatment of diabetic macular edema. Ophthalmology 1999;106(11):2068–73.
29. Kang SW, Park CY, Ham DI. The correlation between fluorescein angiographic and optical coherence tomographic features in clinically significant diabetic macular edema. Am J Ophthalmol 2004;137(2): 313–22.
30. Huang D, Swanson EA, Lin CP, et al. Optical coherence tomography. Science 1991;254(5035): 1178–81.
31. Panozzo G, Gusson E, Parolini B, Mercanti A. Role of OCT in the diagnosis and follow up of diabetic macular edema. Semin Ophthalmol 2003;18(2):74–81.
32. Baumal CR. Clinical applications of optical coherence tomography. Curr Opin Ophthalmol 1999;10(3):182–8.
33. Hee MR, Puliafito CA, Duker JS, et al. Topography of diabetic macular edema with optical coherence tomography. Ophthalmology 1998;105(2):360–70.
34. Ripandelli G, Coppe AM, Capaldo A, Stirpe M. Optical coherence tomography. Semin Ophthalmol 1998;13(4):199–202.
35. Toth CA, Narayan DG, Boppart SA, et al. A comparison of retinal morphology viewed by optical coherence tomography and by light microscopy. Arch Ophthalmol 1997;115(11):1425–8.
36. Huang Y, Cideciyan AV, Papastergiou GI, et al. Relation of optical coherence tomography to microanatomy in normal and rd chickens. Invest Ophthalmol Vis Sci 1998;39(12):2405–16.
37. Drexler W. Ultrahigh-resolution optical coherence tomography. J Biomed Opt 2004;9(1):47–74.
38. Hee MR, Puliafito CA, Wong C, et al. Quantitative assessment of macular edema with optical coherence tomography. Arch Ophthalmol 1995;113(8):1019–29.
39. Drexler W, Sattmann H, Hermann B, et al. Enhanced visualization of macular pathology with the use of ultrahigh-resolution optical coherence tomography. Arch Ophthalmol 2003;121(5):695–706.
40. Wojtkowski M, Bajraszewski T, Targowski P, Kowalczyk A. Real-time in vivo imaging by high-speed spectral optical coherence tomography. Opt Lett 2003;28(19):1745–7.
41. Wojtkowski M, Leitgeb R, Kowalczyk A, Bajraszewski T, Fercher AF. In vivo human retinal imaging by Fourier domain optical coherence tomography. J Biomed Opt 2002;7(3):457–63.
42. Nassif N, Cense B, Park BH, et al. In vivo human retinal imaging by ultrahigh-speed spectral domain optical coherence tomography. Opt Lett 2004;29(5):480–2.
43. Srinivasan VJ, Wojtkowski M, Witkin AJ, et al. High-definition and 3-dimensional imaging of macular pathologies with high-speed ultrahigh-resolution optical coherence tomography. Ophthalmology 2006;113(11):2054 e1–14.
44. Wojtkowski M, Srinivasan V, Fujimoto JG, et al. Three-dimensional retinal imaging with high-speed ultrahigh-resolution optical coherence tomography. Ophthalmology 2005;112(10):1734–46.
45. Yazdanfar S, Rollins AM, Izatt JA. In vivo imaging of human retinal flow dynamics by color Doppler optical coherence tomography. Arch Ophthalmol 2003;121(2):235–9.
46. Rollins AM, Yazdanfar S, Barton JK, Izatt JA. Real-time in vivo color Doppler optical coherence tomography. J Biomed Opt 2002;7(1):123–9.
47. Leitgeb RA, Schmetterer L, Hitzenberger CK, et al. Real-time measurement of in vitro flow by Fourier-domain color Doppler optical coherence tomography. Opt Lett 2004;29(2):171–3.
48. Cense B, Chen TC, Nassif N, et al. Ultra-high speed and ultra-high resolution spectral-domain optical coherence tomography and optical Doppler tomography in ophthalmology. Bull Soc Belge Ophtalmol 2006(302):123–32.
49. Massin P, Vicaut E, Haouchine B, Erginay A, Paques M, Gaudric A. Reproducibility of retinal mapping using optical coherence tomography. Arch Ophthalmol 2001;119(8):1135–42.

50. Chan A, Duker JS. A standardized method for reporting changes in macular thickening using optical coherence tomography. Arch Ophthalmol 2005;123(7):939–43.
51. Polito A, Del Borrello M, Isola M, Zemella N, Bandello F. Repeatability and reproducibility of fast macular thickness mapping with stratus optical coherence tomography. Arch Ophthalmol 2005;123(10):1330–7.
52. Pierre-Kahn V, Tadayoni R, Haouchine B, Massin P, Gaudric A. Comparison of optical coherence tomography models OCT1 and Stratus OCT for macular retinal thickness measurement. Br J Ophthalmol 2005;89(12):1581–5.
53. Otani T, Kishi S, Maruyama Y. Patterns of diabetic macular edema with optical coherence tomography. Am J Ophthalmol 1999;127(6):688–93.
54. Kim BY, Smith SD, Kaiser PK. Optical coherence tomographic patterns of diabetic macular edema. Am J Ophthalmol 2006;142(3):405–12.
55. Alkuraya H, Kangave D, Abu El-Asrar AM. The correlation between optical coherence tomographic features and severity of retinopathy, macular thickness and visual acuity in diabetic macular edema. Int Ophthalmol 2005;26(3):93–9.
56. Massin P, Duguid G, Erginay A, Haouchine B, Gaudric A. Optical coherence tomography for evaluating diabetic macular edema before and after vitrectomy. Am J Ophthalmol 2003;135(2):169–77.
57. Uchino E, Uemura A, Ohba N. Initial stages of posterior vitreous detachment in healthy eyes of older persons evaluated by optical coherence tomography. Arch Ophthalmol 2001;119(10):1475–9.
58. Gaucher D, Tadayoni R, Erginay A, Haouchine B, Gaudric A, Massin P. Optical coherence tomography assessment of the vitreoretinal relationship in diabetic macular edema. Am J Ophthalmol 2005;139(5):807–13.
59. Lewis H, Abrams GW, Blumenkranz MS, Campo RV. Vitrectomy for diabetic macular traction and edema associated with posterior hyaloidal traction. Ophthalmology 1992;99(5):753–9.
60. Yamamoto S, Yamamoto T, Hayashi M, Takeuchi S. Morphological and functional analyses of diabetic macular edema by optical coherence tomography and multifocal electroretinograms. Graefes Arch Clin Exp Ophthalmol 2001;239(2):96–101.
61. Frank RN, Schulz L, Abe K, Iezzi R. Temporal variation in diabetic macular edema measured by optical coherence tomography. Ophthalmology 2004;111(2):211–7.
62. Yang CS, Cheng CY, Lee FL, Hsu WM, Liu JH. Quantitative assessment of retinal thickness in diabetic patients with and without clinically significant macular edema using optical coherence tomography. Acta Ophthalmol Scand 2001;79(3):266–70.
63. Catier A, Tadayoni R, Paques M, et al. Characterization of macular edema from various etiologies by optical coherence tomography. Am J Ophthalmol 2005;140(2):200–6.
64. Bandello F, Polito A, Del Borrello M, Zemella N, Isola M. "Light" versus "classic" laser treatment for clinically significant diabetic macular oedema. Br J Ophthalmol 2005;89(7):864–70.
65. Shimura M, Yasuda K, Nakazawa T, Ota S, Tamai M. Effective treatment of diffuse diabetic macular edema by temporal grid pattern photocoagulation. Ophthalmic Surg Lasers Imaging 2004;35(4):270–80.
66. Audren F, Lecleire-Collet A, Erginay A, et al. Intravitreal triamcinolone acetonide for diffuse diabetic macular edema: phase 2 trial comparing 4 mg vs 2 mg. Am J Ophthalmol 2006;142(5):794–99.
67. Ozdek S, Bahceci UA, Gurelik G, Hasanreisoglu B. Posterior subtenon and intravitreal triamcinolone acetonide for diabetic macular edema. J Diabetes Complications 2006;20(4):246–51.
68. Ciardella AP, Klancnik J, Schiff W, Barile G, Langton K, Chang S. Intravitreal triamcinolone for the treatment of refractory diabetic macular oedema with hard exudates: an optical coherence tomography study. Br J Ophthalmol 2004;88(9):1131–6.
69. Recchia FM, Ruby AJ, Carvalho Recchia CA. Pars plana vitrectomy with removal of the internal limiting membrane in the treatment of persistent diabetic macular edema. Am J Ophthalmol 2005;139(3):447–54.
70. Parolini B, Panozzo G, Gusson E, et al. Diode laser, vitrectomy and intravitreal triamcinolone. A comparative study for the treatment of diffuse non tractional diabetic macular edema. Semin Ophthalmol 2004;19(1–2):1–12.

71. Chew E, Strauber S, Beck R, et al. Randomized trial of peribulbar triamcinolone acetonide with and without focal photocoagulation for mild diabetic macular edema: a pilot study. Ophthalmology 2007;114(6):1190–6.
72. Strom C, Sander B, Larsen N, Larsen M, Lund-Andersen H. Diabetic macular edema assessed with optical coherence tomography and stereo fundus photography. Invest Ophthalmol Vis Sci 2002;43(1):241–5.
73. Goebel W, Franke R. Retinal thickness in diabetic retinopathy: comparison of optical coherence tomography, the retinal thickness analyzer, and fundus photography. Retina 2006;26(1):49–57.
74. Zeimer R, Shahidi M, Mori M, Zou S, Asrani S. A new method for rapid mapping of the retinal thickness at the posterior pole. Invest Ophthalmol Vis Sci 1996;37(10):1994–2001.
75. Neubauer AS, Priglinger S, Ullrich S, et al. Comparison of foveal thickness measured with the retinal thickness analyzer and optical coherence tomography. Retina 2001;21(6):596–601.
76. Pires I, Bernardes RC, Lobo CL, Soares MA, Cunha-Vaz JG. Retinal thickness in eyes with mild nonproliferative retinopathy in patients with type 2 diabetes mellitus: comparison of measurements obtained by retinal thickness analysis and optical coherence tomography. Arch Ophthalmol 2002;120(10):1301–6.
77. Polito A, Shah SM, Haller JA, et al. Comparison between retinal thickness analyzer and optical coherence tomography for assessment of foveal thickness in eyes with macular disease. Am J Ophthalmol 2002;134(2):240–51.
78. Vieira P, Manivannan A, Sharp PF, Forrester JV. True colour imaging of the fundus using a scanning laser ophthalmoscope. Physiol Meas 2002;23(1):1–10.
79. Konno S, Takeda M, Yanagiya N, Akiba J, Yoshida A. Three-dimensional analysis of macular diseases with a scanning retinal thickness analyzer and a confocal scanning laser ophthalmoscope. Ophthalmic Surg Lasers 2001;32(2):95–9.
80. Tong L, Ang A, Vernon SA, et al. Sensitivity and specificity of a new scoring system for diabetic macular oedema detection using a confocal laser imaging system. Br J Ophthalmol 2001;85(1):34–9.

II Pathophysiology/Basic Research

5 In Vivo Models of Diabetic Retinopathy

Timothy S. Kern

CONTENTS

ABSTRACT

Animal models are being used by numerous investigators to study the pathogenesis of diabetic retinopathy. Each of the different animal models has advantages and disadvantages that should be kept in mind when selecting which model to use. This chapter will summarize the histopathology of animal models of diabetic retinopathy and will address four important topics for each model (type of diabetes, histopathology and rate of development of retinopathy, therapies or gene modifications studied in this model, and advantages and disadvantages of the model). Each of the diabetic models studied to date reproduces the capillary degeneration that characterizes the early stages of the retinopathy, but neurodegeneration has been studied only in diabetic rodents. Although none of the available models has been found to reliably develop preretinal neovascularization to date, this deficiency could be due to insufficient durations of diabetes (resulting in insufficient obliteration of retinal capillaries) rather than an intrinsic difference between humans and animal models.

From: *Contemporary Diabetes: Diabetic Retinopathy*
Edited by: E. Duh © Humana Press, Totowa, NJ

Key Words: Diabetic retinopathy; animal models; retina; pathogenesis.

The mechanisms leading to the development of diabetic retinopathy remain under investigation. Animal models of diabetic retinopathy remain a critical part of our efforts to understand the pathogenesis of the process and to identify promising ways to inhibit the retinal disease. This chapter will summarize the histopathology of animal models of diabetic retinopathy. For each animal model, we will address four pertinent questions that are relevant to the use of different species as a model of diabetic retinopathy (type of diabetes, histopathology and rate of development of retinopathy, therapies or gene modifications studied in this model, and advantages and disadvantages of the model).

WHAT DEFINES A GOOD ANIMAL MODEL OF DIABETIC RETINOPATHY?

The value of any animal model depends in large part on how well the model reproduces lesions of the human disease. There have been some who said that there were no "good" or "appropriate" animal models of diabetic retinopathy, because available models have not been found to progress to the advanced lesions of the retinopathy. However, as desirable as that would be, is it necessary for each animal model to develop the full spectrum of lesions that characterize diabetic retinopathy? What is the value of models that develop the early stages of the retinopathy, but might not develop the more advanced lesions? These and other questions will be examined after summarizing the most utilized animal models.

Table 1 summarizes the types of lesions of retinopathy in diabetic humans and diabetic animals, and an approximate duration when the nonproliferative changes begin to

Table 1
Types of Lesions of Retinopathy in Diabetic Humans and Diabetic Animals

Pathology apparent	*Human* *7 + years*	*Primate* *7 + years*	*Dog* *3 + years*	*Cat* *4 + years*	*Rat* *½ + years*	*Mouse* *½ + years*
Background						
Microaneurysms	+	+	+	+	±	0
Degenerate capillaries	+	+	+	+	+	+
Pericyte loss	+	+	+	+	+	+
IRMA	+	+	+	+	0	0
Hemorrhages	+	?	+	+	0	0
BM thickening	+	+	+	+	+	+
Neurodegeneration	+	?	?	?	+	±
Retinal edema	+	+	+	?	?	?
Neovascularization						
Intraretinal	+	?	+	?	?	?
Preretinal	+	0	0	0	±	0

Adapted with permission from Springer *(156)*

be manifest. As can be seen, the shorter-lived models develop considerably less pathology than is characteristic of diabetic patients, likely due in part to shorter lifespan. Available evidence suggests that the earlier stages of the retinopathy (notably capillary degeneration) can contribute to the later development of later stages of the retinopathy. Since diabetes-induced degeneration of retinal capillaries has been found to occur in all species studied to date, and progressive deterioration of those capillaries can contribute to retinal ischemia and likely neovascularization over long periods of time, the data suggest that even species that develop only the earliest stages of the retinopathy can offer valuable insight regarding events at various points along the spectrum of events that ultimately leads to the advanced stages of the retinopathy.

DIABETIC PRIMATES

Type of Diabetes

Type 1 diabetes. The development of diabetic retinopathy has been studied in rhesus monkeys by alloxan, streptozotocin, or total pancreatectomy.

Type 2 diabetes. Aging primates commonly become obese and develop insulin resistance, and in some cases, also hypertension. The development of retinopathy has been studied in obese rhesus monkeys (Macaca mulatta) and cynomolgus monkeys (Macaca fascicularis) that developed diabetes spontaneously.

Histopathology and Rate of Development of the Retinopathy

Studies to date have revealed a very slowly developing retinopathy in diabetic primates. Retinal microaneurysms were found to develop infrequently in a group of 12 alloxan diabetic rhesus monkeys studied through 10–15 years of chronic glycosuria *(1,2)*. Microaneurysms occurred in only five of the diabetic monkeys, never during the first 7 years of diabetes, and no more than four microaneurysms occurred in any eye. A dot hemorrhage occasionally was encountered ophthalmoscopically, and occurred also in nondiabetic monkeys studied for comparison, and unlike microaneurysms, the red dots showed no fluorescence during angiography and disappeared within a few days. An ischemic retinopathy with macular edema appeared in two of the monkeys, but microaneurysms were few and the relative role of diabetes or vascular hypertension in its development is uncertain *(2)*. Microaneurysms were said to occur in three rhesus monkeys alloxan diabetic 2 to 4 years, but no photographic or other evidence was provided *(3)*. Monkeys studied up to 15 years after induction of diabetes by streptozotocin or pancreatectomy likewise had a relative absence of vascular lesions of diabetic retinopathy, although retinal ischemia and defects in the blood-retinal barrier and macula did appear *(4,5)*.

Retinas from the primates with type 2 diabetes show a retinopathy that seems somewhat different from the picture described for the primates with type 1 diabetes, but the duration of diabetes commonly is unknown in the spontaneous diabetes. These primates developed hemorrhages, large areas of retinal capillary nonperfusion, cotton-wool spots, intraretinal hemorrhages, and hard exudates in the macula. Formation of small IRMAs and microaneurysms was associated with the areas of nonperfusion, and some aged spontaneously diabetic monkeys developed macular edema *(6–8)*.

Retinal neovascularization has not been observed to date in diabetic primates. Whether or not retinal neurons degenerate in diabetic primates has not been reported.

Therapies Studied in this Model

None.

Advantages and Disadvantages of the Model

A major advantage of the primate model is the presence of a macula, which is lacking in nonprimate models. As can be seen from the studies conducted to date, however, the development of retinopathy is slow and variable between animals. The retinopathy that has been detected is most similar to the early to midstages of retinopathy in patients, and neovascularization has not been observed. The ethical issues related to use of primates, the expenses associated with their maintenance, slow development of pathology, and lack of availability of molecular regents have not favored use of this model.

DIABETIC DOGS

Type of Diabetes

Studies to date of diabetic dogs have focused on type 1 diabetes, the diabetes being induced by injections of alloxan, streptozotocin, or growth hormone, or by pancreatectomy. No long-term studies have been reported using dogs having type 2 diabetes.

Histopathology and Rate of Development of Retinopathy

The retinopathy which develops in diabetic dogs includes saccular capillary microaneurysms (MA), degenerate (acellular and nonperfused) capillaries (AC), pericyte ghosts (PG), varicose and dilated capillaries (or intraretinal microvascular abnormalities (IRMAs)), and dot and blot hemorrhages *(9–12)*. Several of these vascular lesions are illustrated in Fig. 1. Arteriolar smooth muscle cell loss also has been observed in diabetic dogs *(13, 14)*, just as it has been described in diabetic humans. There is a long interval before retinopathy becomes manifest in diabetic dogs (just as in diabetic humans), but in general, dogs do seem to develop retinal histopathology in diabetes sooner than do diabetic patients. After about 2 years of hyperglycemia in diabetic dogs, increasing numbers of retinal capillaries come to possess endothelial cells but few or no pericytes, and microaneurysms begin to appear soon after. Within 5 years of insulin-deficient diabetes, all dogs with chemically induced diabetes have retinopathy.

Neovascularization has been observed to develop in diabetic dogs, albeit only within the retina and not in preretinal vitreous *(15)*. Whether or not retinal neurons die in diabetes has not been reported.

Therapies Studied in this Model

Improved glycemic control from the onset of diabetes (for 5 years) was found to significantly inhibit the development of retinopathy in diabetic dogs *(16, 17)*. Instituting good glycemic control after a prior period of poor glycemic control, however, was

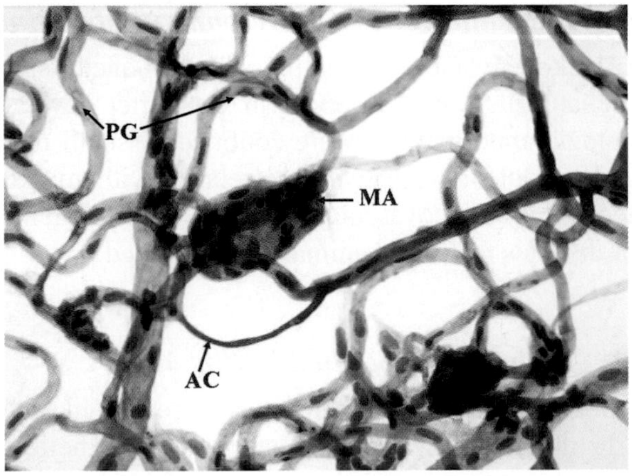

Fig. 1. Vascular histopathology characteristic of the retinopathy that develops in diabetic dogs (5 years diabetes). Lesions visible include a saccular capillary microaneurysm (MA), degenerate and acellular capillaries (AC), and pericyte ghosts (PG).

found to be less effective *(17)*, similar to findings in diabetic patients *(18)*. Administration of aminoguanidine from the onset of diabetes (also for 5 years) significantly inhibited the development of retinal microaneurysms, acellular capillaries, and pericyte ghosts in diabetic dogs, and administration of moderate doses of aspirin for an equal duration significantly inhibited the development of retinal hemorrhages and acellular capillaries over the 5 years of study *(19)*. Diabetic dogs treated with the nonsteroidal anti-inflammatory drug, Sulindac, had less retinal capillary basement membrane volume than did untreated diabetic dogs *(20)*. Administration of an aldose reductase inhibitor in doses sufficient to totally prevent the diabetes-induced accumulation of sorbitol had no effect on the development of retinal histopathology in diabetic dogs *(12)*.

Advantages and Disadvantages of the Model

The retinal histopathology that develops in this animal model is very similar to that which develops in diabetic patients, and the severity of the retinopathy can become more severe than develops in shorter-lived models such as rodents. Nonetheless, preretinal neovascularization has not been observed to develop in the 5–8 years of diabetes that this model has been studied. In addition, the cost, slow development of lesions, and lack of availability of antibodies or molecular biology reagents have made dog models less popular as models for the study of diabetic complications in recent years.

DIABETIC CATS

Type of Diabetes

Studies of diabetic cats to date have focused on type 1 diabetes, the diabetes being induced by pancreatectomy with or without alloxan *(21)*. One cat with long-standing spontaneous diabetes also was studied.

Histopathology and Rate of Development of Retinopathy

Microaneurysms, leukocyte and platelet plugging of aneurysms and venules, and degenerating endothelial cells were observed in cats after several years of diabetes *(22, 23)*. These histologic abnormalities were confined to small regions; some areas of histologic abnormalities could be positively correlated with markedly abnormal PO2 profiles *(23)*. Neither preretinal neovascularization nor neurodegeneration was reported during the 9 years of diabetes that these animals were studied.

Therapies Studied in this Model

Retinal capillary basement membrane thickness increased in diabetic cats compared to normal cats, and the thickening was significantly less in diabetic cats treated with the anti-inflammatory sulindac compared to the untreated diabetic cats *(24)*.

Advantages and Disadvantages of the Model

The retinopathy that develops in this animal model seems very similar to that which develops in diabetic patients and diabetic dogs. The major advantage of the cat over the dog is the reported resistance of cats to develop cataract in diabetes *(25)*. Like the dog, preretinal neovascularization has not been observed to develop in the several years of diabetes that this model has been studied, and the cost, slow development of lesions, and lack of availability of antibodies or molecular biology regents likewise have made this model less popular.

DIABETIC RATS

Type of Diabetes

Type 1 diabetes

Streptozotocin-diabetic or alloxan-diabetic rats have been a primary model for research into the pathogenesis of diabetic retinopathy *(26–45)*. Other strains that spontaneously develop an insulin-deficient diabetes, including the diabetic BB (BioBreeding) or BBW (BioBreeding Wistar) rat *(46)*, the Torii (SDT) rat *(47)*, and the WBN/Kob rat *(48)*, also have been studied with respect to development of retinopathy.

Type 2 diabetes

Some models of type 2 diabetes have been studied with respect to their susceptibility to develop retinal lesions in diabetes (Zucker diabetic fatty rat, ZDF/Gmi-fa, Goto-Kakizaki rat, Otsuka Long-Evans Tokushima fatty (OLETF) rat, BBZDP/Wor, Obese Koletsky (SHROB) rat, spontaneously hypertensive/NIH-corpulent rat strain (SHR/N-cp). Most of these strains show some degree of hyperglycemia, impaired glucose tolerance, and defective insulin response to glucose, with or without obesity and hypertension.

Histopathology and Rate of Development of Retinopathy

Vascular disease

The models in which diabetes has been induced chemically reproducibly develop acellular, degenerate capillaries, pericyte loss and basement membrane thickening. Acellular capillaries in the diabetics have been found to become significantly more numerous than in nondiabetic rats at about 6 months of diabetes. Immunohistochemical methods have demonstrated a significant loss of pericytes after as little as 2 months of diabetes *(49)*, whereas numbers of pericyte ghosts (a different way to assess pericyte loss) have not been significantly increased above normal until about 6 months of diabetes *(37, 50–52)*. More advanced stages of the retinopathy (microaneurysms, IRMA (intraretinal microvascular abnormalities), and hemorrhages) have not been reported to develop reproducibly, although some of these abnormalities have been reported at very long durations of diabetes *(53)*. Vascular abnormalities consistent with possible intraretinal neovascularization also have been reported *(53)*, but have not been observed in the preretinal vitreous.

The retinal vascular disease in spontaneous models of type 1 models seems consistent with that reported in chemically induced diabetes. Diabetic BB rats exhibit retinal lesions similar to those observed in rats having chemically induced diabetes, including pericyte loss, basement membrane thickening, "microinfarctions with areas of nonperfusion" (i.e., capillary degeneration), and an absence of microaneurysms after 8–11 months of diabetes *(54–58)*. Pancreas transplantation inhibited development of the retinal microvascular lesions *(59)*. Studies of vascular histopathology in Torii (SDT) rat retina seem contradictory. Histology and fluorescein angiography reportedly demonstrated nonperfusion and neovascularization in the retina at the extraordinarily short duration of 5–10 weeks of diabetes *(60)*, but another report claimed that Torii rats at age of 50 weeks show proliferative retinopathy without vascular nonperfusion *(61)*. Photomicrographs published demonstrating neovascularization have not been convincing. Degeneration of retinal capillaries and preretinal neovascularization has been claimed also in male WBN/Kob rats at 19 and 24 months of age, respectively *(62)*, but photographic documentation of the new vessels has been equivocal. Retinal degeneration (not typical of diabetes) also occurred in this model *(63–65)*.

Retinal vascular pathology in type 2 models of diabetes has been less well studied. Zucker fatty rats diabetic approximately 5 months had thickening of retinal capillary basement membrane, but the expected capillary degeneration was not apparent *(66)*. In fact, nuclear density of retinal capillary cells was *greater* than normal in diabetic animals *(66, 67)*. Likewise, mild or no retinal vascular changes were detected in Goto-Kakizaki (GK) rats; the ratio of retinal capillary endothelial cells to pericytes was greater than normal at 8 months of age *(33)*, but neither pericyte ghosts nor acellular (degenerate) capillaries were detected *(33)*.

Otsuka Long-Evans Tokushima fatty (OLETF) rats had retinal capillary basement membrane thickening at 14 months of age *(36)*, as well as loss of cells from the inner nuclear and photoreceptor layers of the retina, ultrastructural evidence of endothelial degeneration and microaneurysm-like lesions *(43)*. In contrast, other investigators found no pericyte ghosts and no increase in number of degenerate, acellular capillaries in 45-week-old OLETF rats, and those authors concluded that this strain of rat was not a good model of diabetic retinopathy *(68)*.

Examination of the retinal vasculature in Obese Koletsky (SHROB) rats demonstrated degeneration and loss of intramural pericytes and extensive capillary dropout after 3 months of age in lean and obese rats, with more frequent pathology in the obese rat *(69, 70)*. Retinal capillary dropout is severe and progressive, resulting in some cases in preretinal neovascularization after 6–12 months of age *(70)*. No microaneurysms and retinal hemorrhages were found. These reports were only descriptive, with no quantitative or mechanistic studies to explain the histopathology.

After 24 weeks consuming a 54% sucrose diet, increased numbers of pericyte ghosts and endothelial cells were detected in the obese, spontaneously hypertensive/NIH-corpulent rat strain (SHR/N-cp) compared to lean, nondiabetic controls fed with sucrose diet *(71)*. At 6 months of age, the males of the spontaneously hypertensive/McCune-corpulent rat (SHR/N:Mcc-cp) showed increased E/P ratio, increased basement membrane thickness, and capillary obstruction *(35)*. Acellular capillaries and pericyte ghosts also were detected in these animals but were not quantified in this study. The BBZDP/Wor strain has been reported to develop pericyte loss and retinal capillary basement thickening *(58)*.

Neuronal disease

Rats having insulin-deficient diabetes lose retinal ganglion cells *(39, 56, 72–81)*, and this neurodegeneration has been detected as early as 1 month of diabetes *(75)*. It has been postulated that this early neurodegeneration might contribute to the pathogenesis of the vascular pathology, but Nepafenac, a COX inhibitor, inhibited diabetes-induced degeneration of retinal capillaries while having no effect on the loss of retinal ganglion cells *(81)*. Neurodegeneration has not been studied in models of type 2 diabetes to date.

Therapies or Gene Modifications Studied in this Model

Rats have been used in a variety of studies on the effects of therapy on development of diabetic retinopathy (Table 2). Most of these studies have been conducted using chemically induced diabetic models, and for durations of diabetes of less than one year.

Advantages and Disadvantages of the Model

Rats have been the most commonly used models of diabetic retinopathy. They develop at least the early stages of the retinopathy within only months of diabetes, are inexpensive to house, and easy to handle, and reagents (including antibodies) are widely available. Potential disadvantages of this model are the rapid onset of cataract which develops in diabetes and can limit visibility of the fundus, and the inability to genetically modify rats at present.

DIABETIC MICE

Type of Diabetes

Type 1 diabetes

Studies of retinopathy using mouse models of type 1 diabetes have utilized chemically induced diabetes or, recently, the spontaneous diabetes of the Ins2^{Akita} mouse. The Ins2^{Akita} mouse contains a dominant point mutation in the insulin 2 gene that induces spontaneous type 1 diabetes, especially in males *(88)*.

Table 2
Effects of Therapies on Development of Diabetic Retinopathy in Rats

Therapy	*Defect corrected by therapy*	*Reference*
Aminoguanidine	Capillary degeneration, pericyte loss	*(50, 82, 83)*
Aldose reductase inhibitor	Capillary degeneration	*(39, 44)*
Pyridoxamine	Capillary degeneration	*(38)*
Antioxidants	Capillary degeneration, pericyte loss	*(34, 37)*
Nepafenac	Capillary degeneration, pericyte loss, but no effect on loss of retinal ganglion cells	*(81)*
Salicylates	Capillary degeneration, pericyte loss, loss of retinal ganglion cells	*(84–86)*
PARP inhibitor	Capillary degeneration, pericyte loss	*(51)*
Nerve growth factor	Capillary degeneration, apoptosis of retinal ganglion cells	*(74)*
Benfotiamine	Capillary degeneration	*(41)*
Sigma factor	Loss of retinal ganglion cells	*(87)*

Type 2 diabetes

db/db mice develop a type 2 diabetes due to loss of function mutation in the leptin receptor gene. The C57Bl/KsJ *db/db* has early hyperinsulinemia, obesity, and progressive hyperglycemia. Diabetes in the C57Bl/6J *db/db* strain is less severe. The KK mouse strain exhibits glucose intolerance and insulin resistance, and becomes obese with aging *(89)*. Introduction of lethal yellow *agouti* gene (A^y) into KK mice resulted in KKA^y mice *(90)*, which are characterized by early onset and prolongation of severe levels of hyperinsulinemia, hyperglycemia, obesity, and yellow coat color *(91)*, accompanied by pathological changes in a variety of tissues *(92)*.

Histopathology and Rate of Development of Retinopathy

Vascular disease

C57B1/6J mice made diabetic with streptozotocin develop retinal vascular pathology characteristic of the early stages of diabetic retinopathy (degenerate, acellular capillaries (AC) and pericyte ghosts (PG); Fig. 2) beginning at about 6 months of diabetes. The degenerate capillaries and pericyte ghosts become more numerous with increasing duration of diabetes *(93–95)*. $Ins2^{Akita}$ mice develop similar retinal vascular pathology with increasing duration of diabetes, becoming also significantly greater than in nondiabetic controls by 6 months of diabetes. J129sv/B16 mice having streptozotocin-induced diabetes of 4 months' duration have been reported to develop neovascularization *(96)*, but the claimed "neovascularization" has been poorly demonstrated and seems more likely to be only increased retinal vascular density.

The capillary disease that develops in type 2 models of diabetes seems quite similar to that seen in type 1 models. Compared to that in nondiabetic controls, genetically diabetic *db/db* mice have been observed to develop pericyte loss, strand-like and relatively acellular capillaries, thickening of retinal capillary basement membranes, as well

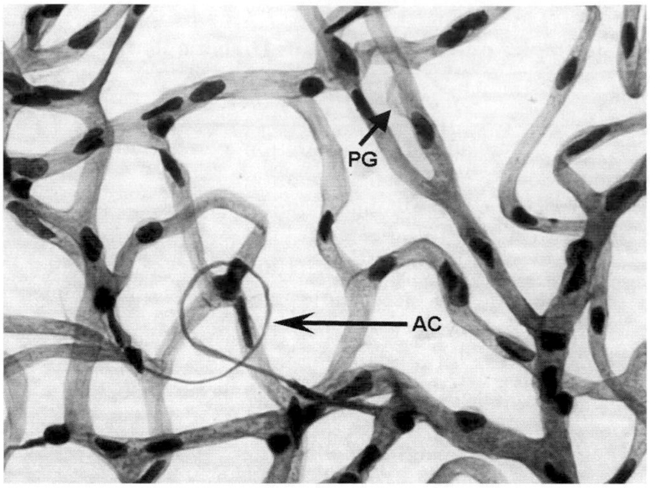

Fig. 2. Vascular histopathology characteristic of the retinopathy that develops in diabetic rats (8 months diabetes). Lesions visible include a degenerate, acellular capillary (AC) and a pericyte ghost (PG).

as blood-retinal barrier breakdown *(97–99)*. These animals also showed increased density of retinal capillaries in the inner nuclear layer, which was interpreted as vessel proliferation (but not preretinal neovascularization). *db/db* mice crossed with apolipoprotein E-deficient mice, resulting in both hyperglycemia and hyperlipidemia, exhibited accelerated development of acellular capillaries and pericyte ghosts compared with littermate control diabetic animals, demonstrating hyperlipidemia can accelerate the degeneration of retinal capillaries in diabetes *(100)*.

Pericyte ghosts and acellular capillaries with occasional microaneurysms have been reported between 20 and 64 weeks of age in the KK mouse *(101)*. After 3 months of diabetes, the major changes in the retinal capillaries involved mitochondria, with endothelial cell hyperplasia, basement membrane thickening, and some edema and vacuolar degeneration of capillary cells *(102)*.

Neural disease

Whether or not neurodegeneration occurs in the diabetic C57Bl/6 model is controversial. Some investigators have reported a 20–25% loss of cells in the ganglion cell layer after only 14 weeks of diabetes *(103)*, whereas others have detected no evidence of ganglion cell loss after as long as a year of diabetes *(93)*. Diabetic C57Bl/6 mice have not been found to show Müller glial cell activation (based on GFAP induction) *(39, 104)*, other than a transient increase that disappears soon after induction of diabetes *(93)*. In contrast, heterozygous $Ins2^{Akita}$ male mice developed significant reductions in the thickness of the inner plexiform and inner nuclear layers and in the number of cell bodies in the retinal ganglion cell layer after 22 weeks of hyperglycemia *(105)*. After 1 month of diabetes, the numbers of apoptotic cells in the retinal ganglion cell and inner nuclear layers of diabetic KKA^y mice were significantly greater than in nondiabetic controls, and the rate of cell death increased with duration of diabetes *(102)*. Fifteen-month-old *db/db* mice were reported to have increased apoptosis of retinal ganglion cells and other cells of the neural retina. Glial cells showed evidence of concurrent degeneration, proliferation, and activation *(99)*.

Therapies or Gene Modifications Studied in this Model

The list of therapies or genes studied with respect to their role in the pathogenesis of diabetic retinopathy in mice is rapidly growing (see Table 3). This model continues to provide new insight into the pathogenesis of retinopathy, especially via genetic manipulation.

Advantages and Disadvantages of the Model

Advantages of mice are that genetic modifications are becoming relatively easy to achieve, reagents and antibodies are readily available, housing is inexpensive, and the histopathology develops relatively quickly (at a rate similar to that in diabetic rats). A concern about the model mainly is related to the very early (and modest) histopathology that has been found to develop within the lifespan of diabetic animals. Whether or not C57Bl/6J mice are protected from diabetes-induced neurodegeneration also needs to be resolved.

OTHER RODENTS

Diabetic hamsters have been reported to develop the usual spectrum of lesions, including acellular capillaries, pericyte loss, and endothelial proliferation, but they have not been found to develop microaneurysms or neovascularization *(108)*.

NONDIABETIC MODELS THAT DEVELOP ASPECTS OF DIABETIC-LIKE RETINOPATHY

Galactose Feeding

Nondiabetic dogs fed a diet enriched with 30% galactose developed a retinopathy that was indistinguishable from that of diabetic dogs and patients, including microaneurysms, vaso-obliteration, pericyte ghosts, and hemorrhages *(12, 30, 109–119)*. Likewise,

Table 3
Therapies or Genes Studied in Mouse Diabetic Retinopathy Models

Gene or therapy	*Defect corrected by therapy or gene manipulation*	*Reference*
ICAM-$1^{-/-}$	Leukostasis, permeability, capillary degeneration	*(52)*
CD-$18^{-/-}$	Leukostasis, permeability, capillary degeneration	*(52)*
Minocycline	Permeability, neurodegeneration, cytokine production	*(106)*
	Capillary degeneration	*(94)*
sRAGE	Capillary degeneration, retinal function	*(100)*
IL-1β receptor$^{-/-}$	Capillary degeneration	*(94)*
iNOS$^{-/-}$	Capillary degeneration	*(95)*
5-Lipoxygenase$^{-/-}$	Capillary degeneration	*(107)*

experimental galactosemia has been shown to cause diabetic-like retinal lesions also in rats *(30, 37, 50, 120–123)* and mice *(52, 124)*. The galactose-retinopathy model was utilized extensively for studies of the role of aldose reductase in the pathogenesis of diabetic-like retinopathy *(12, 30, 111–123)*, but numerous other biochemical sequelae of hyperglycemia including nonenzymatic glycation, protein kinase C activity, and oxidative stress *(125–133)* also occur in galactosemia. The galactose-fed model has been used also in studies of the role of leukostasis and interleukin-1β in the development of retinopathy *(52, 94)*, and the abilities of aminoguanidine, antioxidants, minocycline, and antisense against fibronectin and other basement membrane components to inhibit the retinopathy *(37, 50, 94, 134, 135)*.

Experimental galactosemia can be an easy model of diabetic-like pathology, and the animals require less nursing care than experimental diabetes. Not to be overlooked, however, is the expense of the galactose diet, which can be costly if animals are large or numerous. Moreover, the pathogenesis of galactose-induced retinopathy seems to differ from that of diabetic retinopathy in some manner, since aminoguanidine inhibits the retinal microvascular disease in diabetic rats *(19, 50, 82, 83)* but not in galactose-fed rats *(50, 136)*, and caspases activated in diabetic mice differ from those induced in galactose-fed mice *(137)*.

Nondiabetic Models in Which Growth Factors are Altered

VEGF overexpression

Vascular endothelial growth factor 165 was injected into the eyes of normal cynomolgus monkeys, and as a result, capillaries became nonperfused, dilated, and tortuous *(138)*. Preretinal neovascularization was observed throughout peripheral retina, but not in the posterior pole. Arterioles demonstrated endothelial cell hyperplasia and microaneurysmal dilations. Overexpression of VEGF in retinal photoreceptors results in neovascularization, demonstrating the role of the growth factor in the neovascular response *(139–144)*. This neovascular response, however, differs from that in diabetic retinopathy in that the abnormal blood vessel growth is toward the photoreceptors (the source of overexpressed VEGF), rather than toward the inner retina and vitreous.

IGF overexpression

Nondiabetic mice overexpressing IGF-1 in the retina developed several vascular alterations characteristic of diabetic retinopathy, including nonproliferative lesions (pericyte loss, thickened capillary basement membrane, intraretinal microvascular abnormalities), proliferative retinopathy, and retinal detachment *(145)*. Likewise, injection of a single dose of hrIGF-1 into the vitreous cavity of pigs resulted in an angiopathy that included increased endothelial density, basement membrane thickening, vascular leakage, and microaneurysms *(146)*.

PDGF-B-deficient mice

PDGF (platelet-derived growth factor-B) has major effects on pericyte activation, survival, and growth *(147)*. Mice with a genetic ablation of PDGF-B exhibit several vascular phenotypes characteristic of diabetic retinopathy, including a reduction in the number of pericytes and increase in the numbers of acellular capillaries *(148)*. In chronic hyperglycemia, PDGF-B-deficient mice developed aggravated retinopathy, including high numbers of acellular capillaries and the formation of microaneurysms *(149)*.

Oxygen-Induced Retinopathy

Probably the most utilized animal model of preretinal neovascularization is the oxygen-induced retinopathy (OIR) model *(150)*. In this model, exposure of neonatal animals to elevated concentrations of oxygen impairs development of the normal retinal vasculature and causes regression of many existing vessels. After removal from the high oxygen environment, the lack of retinal blood vessels results in profound retinal ischemia and neovascularization. The neovascularization in this model differs from diabetic retinopathy in that the neovascularization in the OIR model occurs acutely in a retina that is not fully differentiated, as compared to the progressive capillary obliteration that develops in the fully differentiated retina in diabetes.

Sympathectomy

Several retinal lesions consistent with diabetic retinopathy also have been detected after sympathectomy in rats *(151)*. Experimental elimination of sympathetic innervation to the eye resulted in increases in expression of basement membrane proteins, capillary basement membrane thickness, and glial fibrillary acidic protein (GFAP) staining, and reduced number of capillary pericytes *(151, 152)*. There was a significant reduction in photoreceptor numbers due to apoptosis and changes of choroidal vascularity in the sympathectomized eye *(153)*.

Retinal Ischemia–Reperfusion

Ischemia and reperfusion injury to the retina has been known for many years to cause degeneration of retinal neurons. Subsequent to the neuronal injury, however, retinal capillaries also begin to degenerate, a fact that was only recently demonstrated *(154)*. The capillary degeneration is morphologically similar to that which develops in diabetes, but occurs over a period of only days (instead of months to years in diabetes). Aminoguanidine, a nonspecific inhibitor of iNOS, inhibited the degeneration of both neuronal and vascular cells of the retina. This study raises a possibility that damage to the neural retina contributes to capillary degeneration, and perhaps does so also in diabetes.

AREN'T THERE ANY "GOOD" MODELS OF DIABETIC RETINOPATHY?

Some have claimed that there are no "good" or "appropriate" animal models of diabetic retinopathy because diabetic animal models have failed to reproduce the advanced (neovascular) stages of diabetic retinopathy. The statement that animal models have not developed the advanced lesions of diabetic retinopathy seems accurate, but is that because the animals do not live long enough, or because the animals lack some critical biochemical feature that would allow the neovascular response? Moreover, some diabetic or galactosemic animals *have* been demonstrated to develop intraretinal vessel structures that are characteristic of endothelial proliferation or intraretinal neovascularization after prolonged study *(15, 115, 155)*.

A critical component of diabetic retinopathy that is commonly overlooked is duration of diabetes. Vaso-obliteration and subsequent retinal ischemia are believed to be major causes of neovascularization in the retina, and one likely reason that the diabetic models have not developed preretinal neovascularization is that much less retinal vaso-obliteration develops during the short duration of diabetes that the animal models are studied (as compared to the more extensive vaso-obliteration that develops over many years in diabetic patients). Efforts to reduce the length of research studies, usually by using models that develop complications "faster," likely will not provide much insight into how the early stages of diabetic retinopathy progress to the neovascular stages in humans, and why animals seem not to duplicate this. On the other hand, identifying causes of capillary obliteration in diabetes, and using models where those processes are especially accelerated are likely to provide a perspective that is directly relevant to understanding and developing therapies to inhibit the progression of diabetic retinopathy.

SUMMARY

Animal models of diabetic retinopathy have provided a wealth of information pertaining to biochemical, physiological, and histopathologic abnormalities that contribute to the development of diabetic retinopathy, and additional insight from the models can be expected to continue. Nevertheless, the advantages and deficiencies of the various models need to be recognized in order to utilize them to their fullest potential. The early stages of diabetic retinopathy have been found to develop in essentially all species studied who have had diabetes for sufficiently long durations. It does seem that animal models develop at least the early stages of the retinopathy faster than what occurs in diabetic humans (rodents < dogs and cats < humans and nonhuman primates). Rats and genetically modified mice are likely to remain the most utilized models to study the pathogenesis of the retinopathy and in efforts to develop pharmacological therapies to inhibit it. There remains considerable value, however, in the use also of larger animals as models of diabetic retinopathy, since the rate at which the retinopathy develops, the life span of the animals, and the size of eye are more comparable in large animals to that of humans. Only primates have the macula, an important site of damage in diabetic retinopathy.

REFERENCES

1. Engerman RL. Development of retinopathy in diabetic monkeys. In: Excerpta Medican International Congress Series No 481: Tenth Congress of the International Diabetes Federation; 1979:58.
2. Bresnick G, Engerman R, Davis MD, de Venecia G, Myers FL. Patterns of ischemia in diabetic retinopathy. Trans Am Acad Ophthalmol Otolaryngol 1976;81:694–709.
3. Gibbs GE, Wilson RB, Gifford H. Glomerulosclerosis in the long-term alloxan diabetic monkey. Diabetes 1966;15:258–61.
4. Jonasson O, Jones CW, Bauman A, John E, Manaligod J, Tso MO. The pathophysiology of experimental insulin-deficient diabetes in the monkey. Ann Surg 1985;201:27–39.
5. Tso MOM, Kurosawa A, Benhamou E, Bauman A, Jeffrey J, Jonasson O. Microangiopathic retinopathy in experimental diabetic monkeys. Trans Am Ophthalmol Soc 1988;86:390–418.
6. Kim SY, Johnson MA, McLeod DS, et al. Retinopathy in monkeys with spontaneous type 2 diabetes. Invest Ophthalmol Vis Sci 2004;45(12):4543–53.

7. Johnson MA, Lutty GA, McLeod DS, et al. Ocular structure and function in an aged monkey with spontaneous diabetes mellitus. Exp Eye Res 2005;80(1):37–42.
8. Laver N, Robison WG, Jr., Hansen BC. Spontaneously diabetic monkeys as a model for diabetic retinopathy. (ARVO abstract). Invest Ophthalmol Vis Sci 1994;35(Suppl):1733.
9. Engerman RL, Bloodworth JMB, Jr. Experimental diabetic retinopathy in dogs. Arch Ophthalmol 1965;73:205–10.
10. Engerman RL, Finkelstein D, Aguirre G, et al. Appropriate animal models for research on human diabetes mellitus and its complications. Ocular complicat Diabetes 1982;31(Suppl. 1):82–8.
11. Engerman RL. Pathogenesis of diabetic retinopathy. Diabetes 1989;38:1203–6.
12. Engerman RL, Kern TS. Aldose reductase inhibition fails to prevent retinopathy in diabetic and galactosemic dogs. Diabetes 1993;42:820–5.
13. Ashton N. Arteriolar involvement in diabetic retinopathy. Brit J Ophthal 1953;37:282–92.
14. Gardiner TA, Stitt AW, Anderson HR, Archer DB. Selective loss of vascular smooth muscle cells in the retinal microcirculation of diabetic dogs. Brit J Ophthal 1994;78:54–60.
15. Wallow IH, Engerman RL. Permeability and patency of retinal blood vessels in experimental diabetes. Invest Ophthalmol 1977;16:447–61.
16. Engerman RL, Bloodworth JMB, Jr, Nelson S. Relationship of microvascular disease in diabetes to metabolic control. Diabetes 1977;26:760–9.
17. Engerman RL, Kern TS. Progression of incipient diabetic retinopathy during good glycemic control. Diabetes 1987;36:808–12.
18. Diabetes Control and Complications Trial Research Group. The effect of intensive treatment of diabetes on the development of long-term complications in insulin-dependent diabetes mellitus. N Engl J Med 1993;329:977–86.
19. Kern TS, Engerman RL. Pharmacologic inhibition of diabetic retinopathy: Aminoguanidine and aspirin. Diabetes 2001;50:1636–42.
20. Gardiner TA, Anderson HR, Degenhardt T, et al. Prevention of retinal capillary basement membrane thickening in diabetic dogs by a non-steroidal anti-inflammatory drug. Diabetologia 2003;46(9):1269–75.
21. Reiser HJ, Whitworth UG, Jr., Hatchell DL, et al. Experimental diabetes in cats induced by partial pancreatectomy alone or combined with local injection of alloxan. Lab Anim Sci 1987;37(4):449–52.
22. Hatchell DL, Braun RD, Lutty GA, McLeod DS, Toth CA. Progression of diabetic retinopathy in a cat. Invest Ophthalmol Vis Sci 1995;36:S1067.
23. Linsenmeier RA, Braun RD, McRipley MA, et al. Retinal hypoxia in long-term diabetic cats. Invest Ophthalmol Vis Sci 1998;39(9):1647–57.
24. Mansour SZ, Hatchell DL, Chandler D, Saloupis P, Hatchell MC. Reduction of basement membrane thickening in diabetic cat retina by sulindac. Invest Ophthalmol Vis Sci 1990;31(3):457–63.
25. Salgado D, Reusch C, Spiess B. Diabetic cataracts: different incidence between dogs and cats. Schweiz Arch Tierheilkd 2000;142(6):349–53.
26. Hammes H-P, Klinzing I, Wiegand S, Bretzel RG, Cohen AM, Federlin K. Islet transplantation inhibits diabetic retinopathy in the sucrose-fed diabetic Cohen diabetic rat. Invest Ophthalmol Vis Sci 1993;34:2092–6.
27. Kern TS, Engerman RL. Comparison of retinal lesions in alloxan-diabetic rats and galactose-fed rats. Curr Eye Res 1994;13:863–7.
28. Hammes H-P, Syed S, Uhlmann M, et al. Aminoguanidine does not inhibit the initial phase of experimental diabetic retinopathy in rats. Diabetologia 1995;38:269–73.
29. Hammes HP, Strodter D, Weiss A, Bretzel RG, Federlin K, Brownlee M. Secondary intervention with aminoguanidine retards the progression of diabetic retinopathy in rat model. Diabetologia 1995;38:656–60.
30. Kern TS, Engerman RL. Galactose-induced retinal microangiopathy in rats. Invest Ophthalmol Vis Sci 1995;36:490–6.
31. Hammes HP, Weiss A, Fuhrer D, Kramer HJ, Papavassilis C, Grimminger F. Acceleration of experimental diabetic retinopathy in the rat by omega-3 fatty acids. Diabetologia 1996;39(3):251–5.
32. Kern TS, Kowluru R, Engerman RL. Dog and rat models of diabetic retinopathy. In: Shafrir E, ed. Lessons from Animal Diabetes. London: Smith-Gordon; 1996:395–408.
33. Agardh CD, Agardh E, Zhang H, Ostenson CG. Altered endothelial/pericyte ratio in Goto-Kakizaki rat retina. J Diabetes Complicat 1997;11(3):158–62.

34. Hammes HP, Bartmann A, Engel L, Wulfroth P. Antioxidant treatment of experimental diabetic retinopathy in rats with nicanartine. Diabetologia 1997;40:629–34.
35. Kim SH, Chu YK, Kwon OW, McCune SA, Davidorf FH. Morphologic studies of the retina in a new diabetic model; SHR/N:Mcc-cp rat. Yonsei Med J 1998;39(5):453–62.
36. Miyamura N, Bhutto IA, Amemiya T. Retinal capillary changes in Otsuka Long-Evans Tokushima fatty rats (spontaneously diabetic strain). Electron-microscopic study. Ophthalmic Res 1999;31(5):358–66.
37. Kowluru RA, Tang J, Kern TS. Abnormalities of retinal metabolism in diabetes and experimental galactosemia. VII. Effect of long-term administration of antioxidants on the development of retinopathy. Diabetes 2001;50(8):1938–42.
38. Stitt A, Gardiner TA, Alderson NL, et al. The AGE inhibitor pyridoxamine inhibits development of retinopathy in experimental diabetes. Diabetes 2002;51(9):2826–32.
39. Asnaghi V, Gerhardinger C, Hoehn T, Adeboje A, Lorenzi M. A role for the polyol pathway in the early neuroretinal apoptosis and glial changes induced by diabetes in the rat. Diabetes 2003;52(2):506–11.
40. Gardiner TA, Anderson HR, Stitt AW. Inhibition of advanced glycation end-products protects against retinal capillary basement membrane expansion during long-term diabetes. J Pathol 2003;201(2):328–33.
41. Hammes HP, Du X, Edelstein D, et al. Benfotiamine blocks three major pathways of hyperglycemic damage and prevents experimental diabetic retinopathy. Nat Med 2003;9(3):294–9.
42. Kato N, Yashima S, Suzuki T, Nakayama Y, Jomori T. Long-term treatment with fidarestat suppresses the development of diabetic retinopathy in STZ-induced diabetic rats. J Diabetes Complicat 2003;17(6):374–9.
43. Lu ZY, Bhutto IA, Amemiya T. Retinal changes in Otsuka long-evans Tokushima Fatty rats (spontaneously diabetic rat)–possibility of a new experimental model for diabetic retinopathy. Jpn J Ophthalmol 2003;47(1):28–35.
44. Dagher Z, Park YS, Asnaghi V, Hoehn T, Gerhardinger C, Lorenzi M. Studies of rat and human retinas predict a role for the polyol pathway in human diabetic retinopathy. Diabetes 2004;53(9):2404–11.
45. Kowluru RA, Kowluru A, Chakrabarti S, Khan Z. Potential contributory role of H-Ras, a small G-protein, in the development of retinopathy in diabetic rats. Diabetes 2004;53(3):775–83.
46. Marliss EB, Nakhooda AF, Poussier P, Sima AA. The diabetic syndrome of the 'BB' Wistar rat: possible relevance to type 1 (insulin-dependent) diabetes in man. Diabetologia 1982;22(4):225–32.
47. Shinohara M, Masuyama T, Shoda T, et al. A new spontaneously diabetic non-obese Torii rat strain with severe ocular complications. Int J Exp Diabetes Res 2000;1(2):89–100.
48. Nakama K, Shichinohe K, Kobayashi K, et al. Spontaneous diabetes-like syndrome in WBN/KOB rats. Acta Diabetol Lat 1985;22(4):335–42.
49. Hammes HP, Lin J, Wagner P, et al. Angiopoietin-2 causes pericyte dropout in the normal retina: evidence for involvement in diabetic retinopathy. Diabetes 2004;53(4):1104–10.
50. Kern TS, Tang J, Mizutani M, et al. Response of capillary cell death to aminoguanidine predicts the development of retinopathy: comparison of diabetes and galactosemia. Invest Ophthalmol Vis Sci 2000;41(12):3972–8.
51. Zheng L, Szabo C, Kern TS. Poly(ADP-ribose) polymerase is involved in the development of diabetic retinopathy via regulation of nuclear factor-kappaB. Diabetes 2004;53(11):2960–7.
52. Joussen AM, Poulaki V, Le ML, et al. A central role for inflammation in the pathogenesis of diabetic retinopathy. Faseb J 2004;18:1450–2.
53. Yu DY, Cringle SJ, Su EN, Yu PK, Jerums G, Cooper ME. Pathogenesis and intervention strategies in diabetic retinopathy. Clin Exp Ophthalmol 2001;29(3):164–6.
54. Sima AAF, Garcia-Salinas R, Basu PK. The BB Wistar rat: an experimental model for the study of diabetic retinopathy. Metabolism 1983;32 (Suppl. 1):136–40.
55. Grant MB, Ellis EA, Wachowski MB, Murray FT. Free radical derived oxidant localization in retinas of BBZ/WOR diabetic rats. Diabetes 1996;45 (Suppl. 2):192A.
56. Sima AA, Zhang WX, Cherian PV, Chakrabarti S. Impaired visual evoked potential and primary axonopathy of the optic nerve in the diabetic BB/W-rat. Diabetologia 1992;35(7):602–7.
57. Sima AA, Chakrabarti S, Garcia-Salinas R, Basu PK. The BB-rat–an authentic model of human diabetic retinopathy. Curr Eye Res 1985;4(10):1087–92.
58. Murray F, Wachowski M, Diani A, Ellis E, Grant M. Intermediate and long term diabetic (type II) complications in the spontaneously diabetic (BBZ/Wor) rat (Abstract). Diabetes 1996;45:272.

59. Chakrabarti S, Sima AAF, Tze WJ, Tai J. Prevention of diabetic retinal capillary pericyte degeneration and loss by pancreatic islet allograft. Curr Eye Res 1987;6:649–58.
60. Miao G, Ito T, Uchikoshi F, et al. Stage-dependent effect of pancreatic transplantation on diabetic ocular complications in the Spontaneously Diabetic Torii rat. Transplantation 2004;77(5):658–63.
61. Yamada H, Yamada E, Higuchi A, Matsumura M. Retinal neovascularisation without ischaemia in the spontaneously diabetic Torii rat. Diabetologia 2005;48:1663–68.
62. Matsuura T, Horikiri K, Ozaki K, Narama I. Proliferative retinal changes in diabetic rats (WBN/Kob). Lab Anim Sci 1999;49(5):565–9.
63. Ogawa T, Ohira A, Amemiya T. Superoxide dismutases in retinal degeneration of WBN/Kob rat. Curr Eye Res 1998;17(11):1067–73.
64. Miyamura N, Amemiya T. Lens and retinal changes in the WBN/Kob rat (spontaneously diabetic strain). Electron-microscopic study. Ophthalmic Res 1998;30(4):221–32.
65. Azuma M, Sakamoto-Mizutani K, Nakajima T, Kanaami-Daibo S, Tamada Y, Shearer TR. Involvement of calpain isoforms in retinal degeneration in WBN/Kob rats. Comp Med 2004;54(5):533–42.
66. Yang YS, Danis RP, Peterson RG, Dolan PL, Wu YQ. Acarbose partially inhibits microvascular retinopathy in the Zucker Diabetic Fatty rat (ZDF/Gmi-fa). J Ocul Pharmacol Ther 2000;16(5):471–9.
67. Danis RP, Yang Y. Microvascular retinopathy in the Zucker diabetic fatty rat. Invest Ophthalmol Vis Sci 1993;34(7):2367–71.
68. Matsuura T, Yamagishi S, Kodama Y, Shibata R, Ueda S, Narama I. Otsuka Long-Evans Tokushima fatty (OLETF) rat is not a suitable animal model for the study of angiopathic diabetic retinopathy. Int J Tissue React 2005;27(2):59–62.
69. Huang SS, Khosrof SA, Koletsky RJ, Benetz BA, Ernsberger P. Characterization of retinal vascular abnormalities in lean and obese spontaneously hypertensive rats. Clin Exp Pharmacol Physiol 1995;22 (Suppl. 1):S129–S31.
70. Benetz B, Khosrof S, Huang S, et al. Age of onset of retinal vascular changes in the obese SHR. (ARVO abstract). Invest Ophthalmol Vis Sci 1996;37:S971.
71. Robison WG, Jr, McCaleb ML, Feld LG, Michaelis OE, IV, Laver N, Mercandetti M. Degenerated intramural pericytes ('ghost cells') in the retinal capillaries of diabetic rats. Curr Eye Res 1991;10:339–50.
72. Chakrabarti S, Zhang WX, Sima AA. Optic neuropathy in the diabetic BB-rat. Adv Exp Med Biol 1991;291:257–64.
73. Kamijo M, Cherian PV, Sima AAF. The preventive effect of aldose reductase inhibition on diabetic optic neuropathy in the BB/W rat. Diabetologia 1993;36:893–8.
74. Hammes H-P, Federoff HJ, Brownlee M. Nerve growth factor prevents both neuroretinal programmed cell death and capillary pathology in experimental diabetes. Mol Med 1995;1:527–34.
75. Barber AJ, Lieth E, Khin SA, Antonetti DA, Buchanan AG, Gardner TW. Neural apoptosis in the retina during experimental and human diabetes. Early onset and effect of insulin. J Clin Invest 1998;102:783–91.
76. Lieth E, Gardner TW, Barber AJ, Antonetti DA. Retinal neurodegeneration: early pathology in diabetes. Clin Exp Ophthalmol 2000;28(1):3–8.
77. Agardh E, Bruun A, Agardh CD. Retinal glial cell immunoreactivity and neuronal cell changes in rats with STZ-induced diabetes. Curr Eye Res 2001;23(4):276–84.
78. Aizu Y, Oyanagi K, Hu J, Nakagawa H. Degeneration of retinal neuronal processes and pigment epithelium in the early stage of the streptozotocin-diabetic rats. Neuropathology 2002;22(3):161–70.
79. Aizu Y, Katayama H, Takahama S, Hu J, Nakagawa H, Oyanagi K. Topical instillation of ciliary neurotrophic factor inhibits retinal degeneration in streptozotocin-induced diabetic rats. Neuroreport 2003;14(16):2067–71.
80. Park SH, Park JW, Park SJ, et al. Apoptotic death of photoreceptors in the streptozotocin-induced diabetic rat retina. Diabetologia 2003;46(9):1260–8.
81. Kern TS, Miller CM, Du Y, et al. Topical administration of nepafenac inhibits diabetes-induced retinal microvascular disease and underlying abnormalities of retinal metabolism and physiology. Diabetes 2007;56(2):373–9.
82. Hammes H-P, Martin S, Federlin K, Geisen K, Brownlee M. Aminoguanidine treatment inhibits the development of experimental diabetic retinopathy. Proc Natl Acad Sci USA 1991;88:11555–8.
83. Hammes H-P, Brownlee M, Edelstein D, Saleck M, Martin S, Federlin K. Aminoguanidine inhibits the development of accelerated diabetic retinopathy in the spontaneous hypertensive rat. Diabetologia 1994;37:32–5.

84. Sun W, Hoenh T, Gerhardinger C, Lorenzi M. Antiplatelet/Anti-Inflammatory drugs do not prevent early neuroretinal apoptosis and glial changes in diabetic rats (American Diabetes Association abstract). Diabetes 2004:899.
85. Sun W, Gerhardinger C, Dagher Z, Hoehn T, Lorenzi M. Aspirin at low-intermediate concentrations protects retinal vessels in experimental diabetic retinopathy through non-platelet-mediated effects. Diabetes 2005;54(12):3418–26.
86. Zheng L, Howell SJ, Hatala DA, Huang K, Kern TS. Salicylate-based anti-inflammatory drugs inhibit the early lesion of diabetic retinopathy. Diabetes 2007;56(2):337–45.
87. Smith SB, Jiang G, Mysona B, Martin-Studdard A, Roon P, Ganapathy V. The sigma receptor-1 (σR1) ligand Pentazocine (PTZ) affords marked protection against neuronal degeneration in the Ins2Akita mouse model of retinopathy. ARVO abstract 2007:Number 1541.
88. Yoshioka M, Kayo T, Ikeda T, Koizumi A. A novel locus, Mody4, distal to D7Mit189 on chromosome 7 determines early-onset NIDDM in nonobese C57BL/6 (Akita) mutant mice. Diabetes 1997;46(5):887–94.
89. Ikeda H. KK mouse. Diabetes Res Clin Pract 1994;24 Suppl:S313–6.
90. Iwatsuka H, Shino A, Suzuoki Z. General survey of diabetic features of yellow KK mice. Endocrinol Jpn 1970;17(1):23–35.
91. Siracusa LD. The agouti gene: turned on to yellow. Trends Genet 1994;10(12):423–8.
92. Herberg L, Coleman DL. Laboratory animals exhibiting obesity and diabetes syndromes. Metabolism 1977;26(1):59–99.
93. Feit-Leichman RA, Kinouchi R, Takeda M, et al. Vascular Damage in a Mouse Model of Diabetic Retinopathy: Relation to Neuronal and Glial Changes. Invest Ophthalmol Vis Sci 2005;46:4281–7.
94. Vincent JA, Mohr S. Inhibition of Caspase-1/Interleukin-1β Signaling Prevents Degeneration of Retinal Capillaries in Diabetes and Galactosemia. Diabetes 2007;56:224–30.
95. Zheng L, Du Y, Miller C, et al. Critical role of iNOS in degeneration of retinal capillaries in diabetes. Diabeteologia 2007;50:In press.
96. Ebrahimian TG, Tamarat R, Clergue M, Duriez M, Levy BI, Silvestre JS. Dual effect of angiotensin-converting enzyme inhibition on angiogenesis in type 1 diabetic mice. Arterioscler Thromb Vasc Biol 2005;25(1):65–70.
97. Midena E, Segato T, Radin S, et al. Studies on the retina of the diabetic db/db mouse. I. Endothelial cell-pericyte ratio. Ophthalmic Res 1989;21(2):106–11.
98. Clements RS, Jr., Robison WG, Jr., Cohen MP. Anti-glycated albumin therapy ameliorates early retinal microvascular pathology in db/db mice. J Diabetes Complicat 1998;12(1):28–33.
99. Cheung AK, Fung MK, Lo AC, et al. Aldose reductase deficiency prevents diabetes-induced blood-retinal barrier breakdown, apoptosis, and glial reactivation in the retina of db/db mice. Diabetes 2005;54(11):3119–25.
100. Barile GR, Pachydaki SI, Tari SR, et al. The RAGE axis in early diabetic retinopathy. Invest Ophthalmol Vis Sci 2005;46(8):2916–24.
101. Duhault J, Lebon F, Boulanger M. KK mice as a model of microangiopathic lesions in diabetes. In: 7th Europ Conf Microcirculation. Aberdeen: Karger; 1973:453–8.
102. Ning X, Baoyu Q, Yuzhen L, Shuli S, Reed E, Li QQ. Neuro-optic cell apoptosis and microangiopathy in KKAY mouse retina. Int J Mol Med 2004;13(1):87–92.
103. Martin PM, Roon P, Van Ells TK, Ganapathy V, Smith SB. Death of retinal neurons in streptozotocin-induced diabetic mice. Invest Ophthalmol Vis Sci 2004;45(9):3330–6.
104. Barber AJ, Antonetti DA, Reiter CEN, Stiller CA, Gardner TW, Bronson SK. The Ins2Akita mouse as a model of diabetic retinopathy (Abstract). Invest. Ophthalmol. Vis. Sci. 2004 45: E-Abstract 3245.
105. Barber AJ, Antonetti DA, Kern TS, et al. The Ins2Akita mouse as a model of early retinal complications in diabetes. Invest Ophthalmol Vis Sci 2005;46(6):2210–8.
106. Krady JK, Basu A, Allen CM, et al. Minocycline reduces proinflammatory cytokine expression, microglial activation, and caspase-3 activation in a rodent model of diabetic retinopathy. Diabetes 2005;54(5):1559–65.
107. Gubitosi-Klug R, Kern T. A role for 5-lipoxygenase in diabetic retinopathy. Diabetes 2006;55 (Suppl):Abstract 225.
108. Hammes HP, Wellensiek B, Kloting I, Sickel E, Bretzel RG, Brownlee M. The relationship of glycacmic level to advanced glycation end-product (AGE) accumulation and retinal pathology in the spontaneous diabetic hamster. Diabetologia 1998;41(2):165–70.

109. Engerman RL, Kern TS. Experimental galactosemia produces diabetic-like retinopathy. Diabetes 1982;31(Suppl):26A.
110. Engerman RL, Kern TS. Experimental galactosemia produces diabetic-like retinopathy. Diabetes 1984;33:97–100.
111. Kador PF, Akagi Y, Terubayashi H, Wyman M, Kinoshita JH. Prevention of pericyte ghost formation in retinal capillaries of galactose-fed dogs by aldose reductase inhibitors. Arch Ophthalmol 1988;106:1099–102.
112. Kador PF, Akagi Y, Takahashi Y, Ikebe H, Wyman M, Kinoshita JH. Prevention of retinal vessel changes associated with diabetic retinopathy in galactose-fed dogs by aldose reductase inhibitors. Arch Ophthalmol 1990;108:1301–9.
113. Frank RN. The galactosemic dog. A valid model for both early and late stages of diabetic retinopathy. Arch Ophthalmol 1995;113(3):275–6.
114. Engerman RL, Kern TS. Retinopathy in galactosemic dogs continues to progress after cessation of galactosemia. Arch Ophthalmol 1995;113:355–8.
115. Kador PF, Takahashi Y, Wyman M, Ferris F, III. Diabeteslike proliferative retinal changes in galactose-fed dogs. Arch Ophthalmol 1995;113:352–4.
116. Kern TS, Engerman RL. Vascular lesions in diabetes are distributed non-uniformly within the retina. Exp Eye Res 1995;60:545–9.
117. Neuenschwander H, Takahashi Y, Kador PF. Dose-dependent reduction of retinal vessel changes associated with diabetic retinopathy in galactose-fed dogs by the aldose reductase inhibitor M79175. J Ocul Pharmacol Ther 1997;13(6):517–28.
118. Kobayashi T, Kubo E, Takahashi Y, Kasahara T, Yonezawa H, Akagi Y. Retinal vessel changes in galactose-fed dogs. Arch Ophthalmol 1998;116(6):785–9.
119. Kador PF, Takahashi Y, Akagi Y, et al. Effect of galactose diet removal on the progression of retinal vessel changes in galactose-fed dogs. Invest Ophthalmol Vis Sci 2002;43(6):1916–21.
120. Robison WG, Jr, Nagata M, Laver N, Hohman TC, Kinoshita JH. Diabetic-like retinopathy in rats prevented with an aldose reductase inhibitor. Invest Ophthalmol Vis Sci 1989;30:2285–92.
121. Robison WG, Jr, Nagata M, Tillis TN, Laver N, Kinoshita JH. Aldose reductase and pericyte-endothelial cell contacts in retina and optic nerve. Invest Ophthalmol Vis Sci 1989;30:2293–9.
122. Robison WG, Jr., Laver NM, Jacot JL, Glover JP. Sorbinil prevention of diabetic-like retinopathy in the galactose-fed rat model. Invest Ophthalmol Vis Sci 1995;36:2368–80.
123. Robison WG, Jr. Diabetic retinopathy: galactose-fed rat model. Invest Ophthalmol Vis Sci 1995;36(9):4A, 1743–4.
124. Kern TS, Engerman RL. A mouse model of diabetic retinopathy. Arch Ophthalmol 1996;114:986–90.
125. Chiou SH, Chylack LT, Jr., Bunn HF, Kinoshita JH. Role of nonenzymatic glycosylation in experimental cataract formation. Biochem Biophys Res Commun 1980;95(2):894–901.
126. Monnier VM, Sell DR, Abdul-Karim FW, Emancipator SN. Collagen browning and cross-linking are increased in chronic experimental hyperglycemia: relevance to diabetes and aging. Diabetes 1988;37:867–72.
127. Kern TS, Kowluru R, Engerman RL. Abnormalities of retinal metabolism in diabetes or galactosemia. ATPases and glutathione. Invest Ophthalmol Vis Sci 1994;35:2962–7.
128. Kowluru R, Kern TS, Engerman RL. Abnormalities of retinal metabolism in diabetes or galactosemia II. Comparison of gamma-glutamyl transpeptidase in retina and cerebral cortex, and effects of antioxidant therapy. Curr Eye Res 1994;13:891–6.
129. Xia P, Inoguchi T, Kern TS, Engerman RL, Oates PJ, King GL. Characterization of the mechanism for the chronic activation of DAG-PKC pathway in diabetes and hypergalactosemia. Diabetes 1994;43:1122–9.
130. Kern TS, Kowluru RA, Engerman RL. Effect of antioxidants on the development of retinopathy in diabetes and galactosemia. Invest Ophthalmol Vis Sci 1996;37:S970.
131. Kowluru RA, Kern TS, Engerman RL. Abnormalities of retinal metabolism in diabetes or experimental galactosemia. IV. Antioxidant defense system. Free Radicals Biol Med 1996;22:587–92.
132. Kowluru RA, Jirousek MR, Stramm LE, Farid NA, Engerman RL, Kern TS. Abnormalities of retinal metabolism in diabetes or experimental galactosemia. V. Relationship between protein kinase C and ATPases. Diabetes 1998;47:464–9.
133. Kowluru RA, Engerman RL, Kern TS. Abnormalities of retinal metabolism in diabetes or experimental galactosemia. VI. Comparison of retinal and cerebral cortex metabolism, and effects of antioxidant therapy. Free Radic Biol Med 1999;26(3–4):371–8.

134. Roy S, Sato T, Paryani G, Kao R. Downregulation of fibronectin overexpression reduces basement membrane thickening and vascular lesions in retinas of galactose-fed rats. Diabetes 2003;52(5):1229–34.
135. Oshitari T, Polewski P, Chadda M, Li AF, Sato T, Roy S. Effect of combined antisense oligonucleotides against high-glucose- and diabetes-induced overexpression of extracellular matrix components and increased vascular permeability. Diabetes 2006;55(1):86–92.
136. Frank RN, Amin R, Kennedy A, Hohman TC. An aldose reductase inhibitor and aminoguanidine prevent vascular endothelial growth factor expression in rats with long-term galactosemia. Arch Ophthalmol 1997;115(8):1036–47.
137. Mohr S, Tang J, Kern TS. Caspase activation in retinas of diabetic and galactosemic mice and diabetic patients. Diabetes 2002;51:1172–79.
138. Tolentino MJ, Miller JW, Gragoudas ES, et al. Intravitreous injections of vascular endothelial growth factor produce retinal ischemia and microangiopathy in an adult primate. Ophthalmology 1996;103(11):1820–8.
139. Okamoto N, Tobe T, Hackett SF, et al. Transgenic mice with increased expression of vascular endothelial growth factor in the retina: a new model of intraretinal and subretinal neovascularization. Am J Pathol 1997;151(1):281–91.
140. Ohno-Matsui K, Hirose A, Yamamoto S, et al. Inducible expression of vascular endothelial growth factor in adult mice causes severe proliferative retinopathy and retinal detachment. Am J Pathol 2002;160(2):711–9.
141. van Eeden PE, Tee LB, Lukehurst S, et al. Early vascular and neuronal changes in a VEGF transgenic mouse model of retinal neovascularization. Invest Ophthalmol Vis Sci 2006;47(10):4638–45.
142. Shen WY, Lai YK, Lai CM, et al. Pathological heterogeneity of vasoproliferative retinopathy in transgenic mice overexpressing vascular endothelial growth factor in photoreceptors. Adv Exp Med Biol 2006;572:187–93.
143. van Eeden PE, Tee L, Shen WY, et al. Characterisation of a model for retinal neovascularisation. VEGF model characterisation. Adv Exp Med Biol 2006;572:163–8.
144. Lai CM, Dunlop SA, May LA, et al. Generation of transgenic mice with mild and severe retinal neovascularisation. Br J Ophthalmol 2005;89(7):911–6.
145. Ruberte J, Ayuso E, Navarro M, et al. Increased ocular levels of IGF-1 in transgenic mice lead to diabetes-like eye disease. J Clin Invest 2004;113(8):1149–57.
146. Danis RP, Bingaman DP. Insulin-like growth factor-1 retinal microangiopathy in the pig eye. Ophthalmology 1997;104(10):1661–9.
147. Benjamin LE, Hemo I, Keshet E. A plasticity window for blood vessel remodelling is defined by pericyte coverage of the preformed endothelial network and is regulated by PDGF-B and VEGF. Development 1998;125(9):1591–8.
148. Hammes HP, Lin J, Renner O, et al. Pericytes and the pathogenesis of diabetic retinopathy. Diabetes 2002;51(10):3107–12.
149. Enge M, Bjarnegard M, Gerhardt H, et al. Endothelium-specific platelet-derived growth factor-B ablation mimics diabetic retinopathy. Embo J 2002;21(16):4307–16.
150. Madan A, Penn JS. Animal models of oxygen-induced retinopathy. Front Biosci 2003;8:d1030–43.
151. Wiley LA, Steinle JJ. Sympathetic Innervation Regulates Basement Membrane Thickening, Pericyte Numbers and Müller Cell Reactivity in Rat Retina (ARVO abstract). Invest Ophthalmol Vis Sci 2004 45: E-Abstract 3258.
152. Steinle JJ, Smith PG. Sensory but not parasympathetic nerves are required for ocular vascular remodeling following chronic sympathectomy in rat. Auton Neurosci 2003;109(1–2):34–41.
153. Steinle JJ, Lindsay NL, Lashbrook BL. Cervical sympathectomy causes photoreceptor-specific cell death in the rat retina. Auton Neurosci 2005;120(1–2):46–51.
154. Zheng L, Gong B, Hatala DA, Kern TS. Retinal ischemia and reperfusion causes capillary degeneration: similarities to diabetes. Invest Ophthalmol Vis Sci 2007;48(1):361–7.
155. Moravski CJ, Skinner SL, Stubbs AJ, et al. The renin-angiotensin system influences ocular endothelial cell proliferation in diabetes: transgenic and interventional studies. Am J Pathol 2003;162(1):151–60.
156. Kern TS, Mohr, S. Nonproliferative stages of disbetic retinopathy: animal models and pathogenesis. pp. 303–16 in Retinal Vascular Disease (eds AM Joussen, TW Gardner, B. Kirchhof, SJ Ryan), 2007, Springer.

A Pathways of Hyperglycemia–Induced Damage

6 The Polyol Pathway and Diabetic Retinopathy

Mara Lorenzi and Peter J. Oates

CONTENTS

ABSTRACT

The polyol pathway is a two-step metabolic pathway in which glucose is reduced to sorbitol, which is then converted to fructose. Several biochemical features and a large body of data implicate the polyol pathway as a plausible and important contributor to diabetic retinopathy and other complications of diabetes. In both humans and experimental animals, all retinal cell types known to be affected by diabetes contain aldose reductase (AR), the first and rate-limiting enzyme of the pathway. Metabolism through the pathway is accelerated by elevated cytoplasmic glucose concentrations induced by hyperglycemia. The resulting altered concentrations of pathway products and cofactors can cause osmotic and oxidative stress, the latter through multiple mechanisms that include the generation of precursors of advanced glycation endproducts. These stresses eventually lead to apoptosis and proinflammatory events. In diabetic individuals, certain polymorphisms of the AR gene are associated with high AR expression levels and an accelerated or more severe course of retinopathy. Conversely, genetic ablation of AR in mice results in protection from diabetic retinopathy. In rats with experimental diabetes, drugs that inhibit AR are, as of today, the only

From: *Contemporary Diabetes: Diabetic Retinopathy*
Edited by: E. Duh © Humana Press, Totowa, NJ

drugs documented to prevent the whole spectrum of abnormalities induced by diabetes in glial cells, neurons, and vascular cells of the retina. This may have translational importance, because human diabetic retinopathy has recently become known to include glial and neuronal abnormalities.

The efficacy of AR inhibitors (ARIs) has been, for the most part, disappointing in humans. The major reason for the discrepant results in clinical vs. preclinical studies is likely discrepant doses; for example, in recent studies the ARI sorbinil proved successful in preventing retinopathy in diabetic rats when given at a dose 20-fold larger than the dose used unsuccessfully in a past clinical trial. It has become clear that larger doses of ARIs ensure that metabolic flux through both steps of the pathway is inhibited – as opposed to merely reducing sorbitol accumulation. A current hypothesis posits that normalization of glucose flux through the pathway is required in order to prevent excessive turnover of pathway cofactors and oxidative stress; and that the latter is a critical, if not the main, determinant of the tissue consequences of excess polyol pathway activity. Testing this concept in humans will become possible when new drugs, capable of inhibiting aldose reductase with higher in vivo efficacy and safety than the older ARIs, become available. It is reasonable and important to advocate, and work toward, the discovery of such drugs because some features of diabetic retinopathy appear best or uniquely approached via inhibition of excess polyol pathway activity.

Key Words: Diabetic retinopathy; polyol pathway; aldose reductase; sorbitol dehydrogenase; aldose reductase polymorphisms; sorbitol; fructose; osmotic stress; oxidative stress; advanced glycation endproducts; pericytes; endothelial cells; Müller glial cells; apoptosis; inflammation; aldose reductase inhibitors.

INTRODUCTION

Retinopathy is the most severe of the ocular complications of diabetes *(1)*. More than all other complications of diabetes, retinopathy may begin as a rather pure manifestation of glucose toxicity. This is suggested and supported by the demonstration that experimental galactosemia induces in animals a picture of retinal microangiopathy highly similar to that of nonproliferative diabetic retinopathy *(2, 3)*, while not mimicking fully complications of diabetes in other tissues *(4)*. Galactosemia induced by a galactose-rich diet results in elevated hexose levels in blood without the array of metabolic and hormonal changes characteristic of diabetes *(3)*. Hence, the galactosemic model provides a rigorous argument for the discrete role of hyperhexosemia in causing retinopathy. The role of hyperhexosemia is also suggested by the fact that the levels of glycated hemoglobin (HbA_{1c}) over time are the dominant predictor of retinopathy progression in diabetic patients *(5)*. This observation is less compelling in its pathogenic implications than the first because, while HbA_{1c} does reflect glycemic levels, glycemic levels reflect a multitude of metabolic and hormonal changes. However, the HbA_{1c} data are critically important because they are consistent with a role for glucose toxicity in human diabetic retinopathy.

The galactosemic model also points to a biochemical mechanism for how elevated hexose levels may lead to retinopathy: activation of the polyol pathway. The longest known consequence of polyol pathway activation is a rise in tissue polyol levels. For example, when blood galactose levels increase, many tissues accumulate galactitol, which is produced from galactose via the action of aldose reductase (AR), the first and rate-limiting enzyme in the polyol pathway. AR inhibitors prevent in most cases the rise in tissue polyol and, at sufficiently high dose, tissue damage observed in experimental galactosemia *(6)*. This does not mean that high glucose causes tissue damage via precisely the same mechanisms as high galactose, considering that glucose is substrate for several enzymatic and nonenzymatic reactions in addition to those of the polyol pathway, and is metabolized differently from galactose even in the polyol pathway. That is, galactose is metabolized by AR more avidly than glucose, and galactitol, the product of galactose metabolism through AR, is a very poor substrate for further metabolism by the second enzyme in the pathway, sorbitol dehydrogenase *(7–9)*; therefore, galactitol accumulates to an even greater degree than sorbitol. [Although galactitol is a poor substrate for the second step of the polyol pathway, galactose can cause a rise in NADH/NAD^+ by another pathway, likely the galactonate pathway *(10)*]. In any event, the galactosemic model – where hyperhexosemia in the presence of normal insulin action is the trigger, and aldose reductase is a key transducer from hyperhexosemia to retinal histopathology that closely resembles human diabetic retinopathy *(3, 11)* – has provided an important and testable paradigm for the pathogenesis of diabetic retinopathy.

Indeed, several experimental findings over the years have made the polyol pathway an attractive mechanism for the characteristic lesions of human diabetic retinopathy. As will be described in more detail below, certain polymorphisms in the promoter region of the aldose reductase gene are associated with susceptibility to, or more rapid progression of, diabetic retinopathy *(12)*. Polyol pathway activity can damage cells by multiple mechanisms (*(13)*, and later in this chapter), and all cell types that in the human retina are affected by diabetes contain AR *(14–16)*. The neuroglial abnormalities now known to be part of both human and experimental diabetic retinopathy *(17, 18)* are attributable in experimental animals to polyol pathway activity *(19, 20)*, as is the spectrum of early and late vascular abnormalities *(16)*. But the evidence necessary to implicate mechanistically the polyol pathway in the pathogenesis of human diabetic retinopathy is not yet in. In this chapter we aim to review in some detail the features of the polyol pathway, the reasons for its attractiveness as a mechanism and a target, and the steps that must be taken to prove or disprove that it is relevant to human diabetic retinopathy.

BIOCHEMISTRY AND GENETICS OF THE POLYOL PATHWAY

The polyol pathway consists of two soluble cytoplasmic enzymes, AR and sorbitol dehydrogenase (Fig. 1a and b, respectively). The first enzyme, AR, can convert intracellular glucose and NADPH to sorbitol and $NADP^+$, while the second enzyme, sorbitol dehydrogenase, reversibly changes sorbitol and NAD^+ into fructose and NADH. In the diabetic state, chronic hyperactivity of this pathway is driven by "hyperglysolia," i.e., chronically elevated cytosolic glucose concentration, and underlies shifts in cellular redox, osmotic, and antioxidant systems.

Aldose Reductase

The Aldose Reductase Enzyme

Aldose reductase (E.C. 1.1.1.21; abbreviated ALD2, AKR1B1, or in this chapter, AR) was first described by Hers *(21)* and belongs to the aldo-keto reductase superfamily *(22)*.

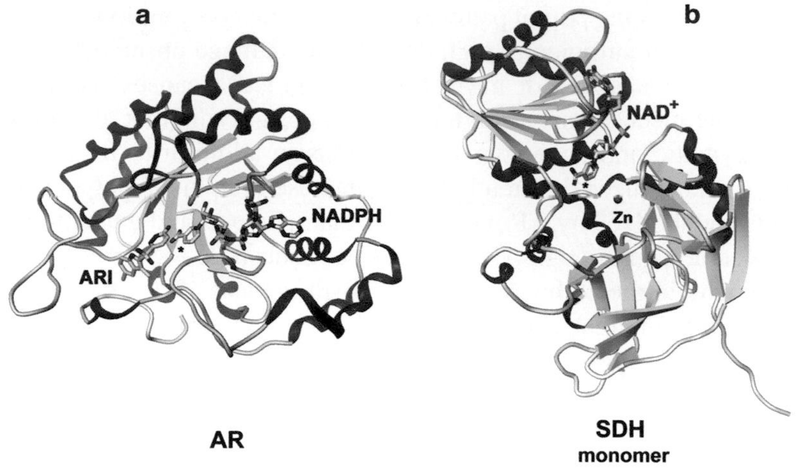

Fig. 1. X-Ray structures of the two enzymes of the polyol pathway, aldose reductase and sorbitol dehydrogenase. Shown in Fig. 1a is human aldose reductase (AR) with a bound molecule of nicotinamide-adenine dinucleotide phosphate (NADPH) cofactor as well as a molecule of aldose reductase inhibitor (ARI) ARI-809. The *asterisk* (*) designates the C4 carbon of the nicotinamide ring of NADPH, the site of the substrate hydride transfer from the C4 carbon of the nicotinamide ring to the C1 aldehydic carbon of the substrate, e.g., glucose (not shown). Prepared by PJO from Protein Data Bank (http://www.rcsb.org) entry 1Z89 *(177)* using MoVit v. 2.0. Shown in Fig. 1b is a human sorbitol dehydrogenase (SDH) monomer of an SDH tetramer with a bound molecule of oxidized nicotinamide-adenine dinucleotide (NAD^+) cofactor and a catalytic zinc atom (Zn) (sphere). The *asterisk* (*) designates the C4 carbon of the nicotinamide ring of NAD^+, the site of hydride transfer between the nicotinamide ring and the C2 carbon of the substrate, e.g., sorbitol or fructose (not shown). Prepared by PJO from Protein Data Bank (http://www.rcsb.org) entry 1PL8 and from data in *(50)*, using MoVit v. 2.0.

AR is a monomeric enzyme of ~35,900 Da with an $(\alpha/\beta)_8$ structure composed of eight beta-pleated sheet segments comprising a β-barrel surrounded by eight alpha-helices and two small accessory helices (Fig. 1a). AR is localized to cell cytoplasm and contains no metal ion or carbohydrate *(23, 24)*. The enzyme preferentially uses NADPH as a hydride donor to reduce aldehydic carbons to the corresponding alcohol, e.g., glucose to sorbitol.

Aldose reductase has broad substrate specificity, but its "natural" substrate in most tissues is unknown. Its kinetic constants are such that it functions primarily in the reductive direction, that is, to reduce aldehydes to corresponding alcohols *(25)*. Its kinetic mechanism is formally categorized as compulsory ordered bi–bi with coenzyme binding first, then binding of aldehyde followed by alcohol leaving first and oxidized coenzyme $NADP^+$ leaving last *(26)*. Although the K_m for glucose is often reported as 70–400 mM, AR acts catalytically only on the low abundance (0.0023%) aldehydic, straight-chain form of glucose, as opposed to the much more prevalent cyclic anomeric "boat" and "chair" forms of glucose *(27, 28)*; it transforms the straight-chain form of glucose with a K_m of 5 μM *(29)*. AR transforms glucose into sorbitol relatively slowly with a k_{cat} of ~30 min^{-1} *(29)*. For further details on the structure and enzymology of AR, the reader is referred to recent studies and previous reviews, e.g., *(26, 30, 31)*.

The Aldose Reductase Gene

Location and Structure of the AR Gene. The aldose reductase gene (*AKR1B1*) has been localized to human chromosome 7 locus q35 *(32)* and is distributed over ~18 kilobases (kb) that contain ten exons coding for 316 amino acids *(33, 34)* (Fig. 2).

Interestingly, the 7q35 genetic region was previously linked to diabetic complications by independent studies *(35, 36)*. The AR gene basal promoter has a TATA box at −37, a CCAAT box at −104, and an androgen-like response element at −396 to −382 *(33, 37)*. About 1,200 basepairs (bp) upstream of the transcription start site there is a 132 bp region that contains three osmotic response elements, labeled OreA, OreB, and OreC *(38)*.

The rat and mouse AR genes are 14.1 and 14.2 kb, respectively, i.e., slightly shorter than the ~18 kb human AR gene, but they are of similar overall organization to the human gene *(39, 40)*. However, transcriptional regulation is complex and may involve species-specific elements *(39)*.

Polymorphisms of the AR Gene

Three types of genetic polymorphisms have been identified in the human AR gene. The most studied is an $(AC)_n$ repeat microsatellite located ~2.1 kb upstream of the transcription start site *(41)* (Fig. 2). The number of AC repeats varies in different

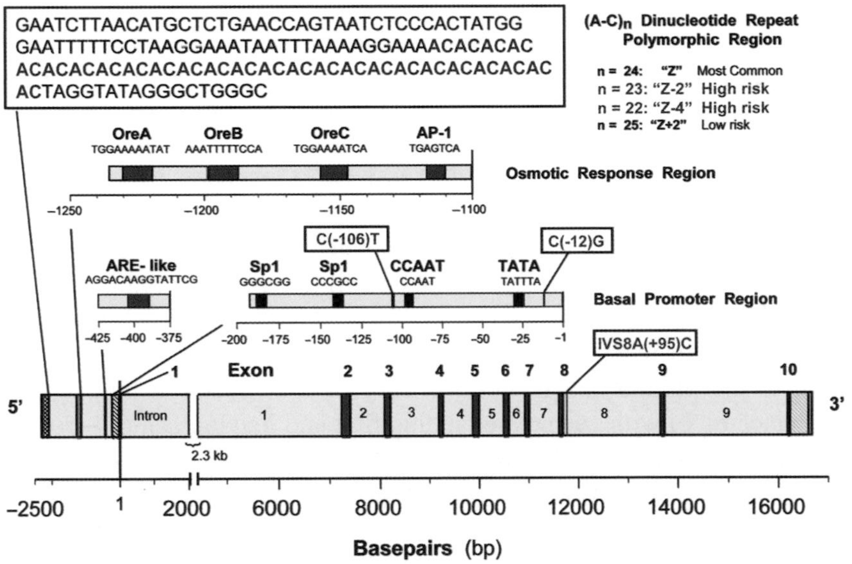

Fig. 2. Structure of the human aldose reductase (*AKR1B1*) gene. Starting from position 1 ("Basepairs," *x*-axis) and going to the right, the gene consists of nine introns (*numbered gray areas*) and ten exons (*bolded numbers* above *dark gray gene areas*) that code for the 316 amino acids of the AR polypeptide. A 2.3 kb part of intron 1 is omitted for illustrative purposes. Working upstream (to the *left*) from position 1, the Basal Promoter Region is shown to extend back to approximately bp −190 and contains TATA, CCAAT, and Sp1 elements (*shaded areas*). Further upstream there is an Androgen Response Element-like (ARE-like) sequence at ~−390 (*shaded area*) and in the Osmotic Response Region there is an AP-1 binding site at −1,110 and the three Osmotic Response Elements (Ore), OreC, B, and A in the −1,150 to −1,230 region. Finally, at approximately 2.1 kb upstream there is an (AC)n Dinucleotide Repeat microsatellite region with its polymorphic variants indicated. Additional single nucleotide polymorphisms in the gene include C(−106)T and C(−12)G in the basal promoter region, as well as the IVS8A(+95)C polymorphism in intron 8. These genetic polymorphisms have been linked to altered expression levels of the AR gene product and/or to altered retinopathy risk in human diabetics. See text for further discussion. Modified slightly with permission from *(178)*.

individuals with up to 13 different alleles in some populations. The most common allele in all populations is $n = 24$, called "Z." An allele with two fewer bases, i.e., one less $(AC)_n$ unit, viz., $n = 23$, is designated "Z–2." Similarly, a microsatellite allele with one additional AC unit compared to the most frequent, viz., $n = 25$, is referred to as "Z + 2," etc. A second polymorphism of the AR gene is a C(−106)T single nucleotide polymorphism (SNP) in the basal promoter region *(42)*. A third polymorphism is a BamHI site consisting of a single A to C substitution at the 95th nucleotide of intron 8 *(43, 44)* [IVS8A(+95)C in Fig. 2; also designated A(+11842)C *(12)*]. The $(AC)_n$ and C(−106)T polymorphisms are closely linked *(42, 45, 46)*. A C(−12)G SNP has also been described *(47)*.

Sorbitol Dehydrogenase

The Sorbitol Dehydrogenase Enzyme

Sorbitol dehydrogenase (SDH) *(48)* (EC 1.1.1.14) belongs to a superfamily of medium-chain dehydrogenase/reductases *(49)*, and the X-ray structure of human and rat SDH has been determined (Fig. 1b) *(50, 51)*. The native enzyme is 140,000–160,000 Da and has four identical subunits of 354–356 amino acids that each contain one catalytic zinc and one NAD(H) binding site *(29, 52, 53)* (Fig. 1b). The N-terminal amino acid of human and sheep SDH is acetylated, e.g., *(54)*. Interestingly, the tip of the "tail" of the SDH monomer (Fig. 1b) is predominantly hydrophobic, suggesting it could interact with a lipid environment. Although the subcellular localization of SDH is primarily cytosolic *(55, 56)*, some of the SDH in human liver is found to be associated with the microsomal fraction *(57)* and multiple SDH isoforms have been reported *(9, 58)*.

Each independent monomer of SDH stereospecifically oxidizes a spectrum of secondary alcohols *(59, 60)*, including sorbitol which it reversibly oxidizes to fructose using coenzyme NAD^+ *(60)*. SDH likely binds and releases the straight-chain form of fructose *(61)*; this conformer exists at ~0.8% of the total ketose *(62)*. Galactitol is metabolized weakly or negligibly by SDH, e.g., *(7, 9, 63)*. Kinetic analysis of the mechanism of SDH reveals that it has a compulsory ordered reaction that is classified as Theorell-Chance bi–bi with coenzyme binding first and leaving last *(64–66)*. The K_m of SDH for sorbitol is 1–4 mM and its k_{cat} is ~100 s^{-1} at pH 7.1 *(29, 63, 67, 68)*. Thus, the catalytic rate constant, k_{cat}, of SDH is approximately three times higher than for AR.

The Sorbitol Dehydrogenase Gene

Location and Structure of the SDH Gene. The SDH gene, *SORD,* resides on human chromosome 15 *(69)*. Its position on this chromosome is reported at 15q15 *(70, 71)* or 15q21.1 *(72)*. The human *SORD* gene has nine exons and eight introns and extends approximately 30 kb *(73)*. Three Sp1 sites (CCCGCCCC) and a CACCC box were found in the 5′ noncoding region, but classical TATAA or CCAAT elements were absent, although a unique repetitive $(CAAA)_5$ sequence was observed. In all tissues analyzed, two transcriptional initiation signals occur at 16 and 89 bp upstream of the translation initiation site for SDH. As seen for rat SDH mRNA *(74)*, human SDH mRNA has an open reading frame that codes for 356 amino acids *(73)*. In addition, a second ATG translation start site codon 126 bp upstream from the first start site was detected in sequencing rat testis SDH cDNA; in principle this could code for an additional 42 amino acid N-terminal peptides in a pre-SDH *(75)*. However, this peptide is probably removed in post-translational processing since pre-SDH has not yet been detected experimentally.

LEVEL OF EXPRESSION OF POLYOL PATHWAY ENZYMES AND DIABETIC RETINOPATHY

Natural Variations in Polyol Pathway Enzyme Levels and Diabetic Retinopathy

AR Polymorphisms and Risk of Diabetic Retinopathy

Certain polymorphisms of the AR gene have been linked in numerous, but not all, genotypic studies to faster or slower rates of development of diabetic retinopathy and other diabetic complications, e.g., *(12, 76)*. In particular, the "Z–2" $(AC)_n$ microsatellite polymorphism, i.e., $(AC)_{23}$ (Fig. 2), was originally discovered in association with rapid progression of diabetic retinopathy; i.e., Z–2 occurred in higher than expected frequencies in patients with type 2 diabetes who had retinopathy after a relatively short (~5 years) duration of known diabetes *(41)*. Subsequent studies in both type 1 and type 2 diabetic patients across different ethnic groups have found a positive association of Z–2, C(−106) T, and A(+11842)C polymorphisms of the AR gene (Fig. 2) with diabetic retinopathy *(12, 77)*. One report found an association between C(−12)G, elevated AR transcription rate, and diabetic retinopathy *(47)*. Negative studies may be attributable to differences in the sample size, patients' characteristics such as duration of disease and genetic complexities in certain populations. For example, the CC genotype of the C(−106)T polymorphism, which caused higher AR transcriptional rates in vitro *(78)*, was found associated with an approximately twofold increased risk of having proliferative retinopathy independent of other risk factors in Caucasian Brazilians, but not in African Brazilians *(79)*.

The Z–2 allele of the AR gene was also found to be associated with approximately twofold higher levels of AR mRNA in peripheral blood monocytes of diabetic patients with nephropathy vs. diabetic patients without nephropathy or nephropathic patients without diabetes *(80)*. In studies in vitro, constructs containing the Z–2 variant of the AR microsatellite resulted in rates of AR gene transcription 1.6- to 6-fold higher than constructs containing the Z + 2 or other variants of the microsatellite *(78)*. In Japanese patients with type 2 diabetes, the Z–4, not the Z–2, polymorphism was found associated with proliferative retinopathy and with higher AR protein levels in the erythrocytes; while the Z + 2 allele was associated with absence of diabetic retinopathy *(81)*. Likewise, the prevalence of diabetic retinopathy was observed to increase significantly with elevated erythrocyte AR levels in type 2 diabetic patients with duration of known diabetes of less than 10 years, but not with longer durations *(82)*, another suggestion that increased AR expression may work to accelerate the development of retinopathy.

Conversely, several reports have linked polymorphisms associated with low expression of AR with lower than average frequencies of diabetic retinopathy, e.g., *(81)*. Consistent with these and the aforementioned data, Zou and coworkers reported a twofold higher AR activity level in erythrocytes from Z–2/Z–2 patients than in erythrocytes from Z + 2/Z + 2 patients, although confirmation of the specificity of the enzyme activity assay (vs. aldehyde reductase activity) is warranted *(83)*.

SDH Polymorphisms and Diabetic Retinopathy

Although variations in the human SDH gene sequence have been detected, the impact of such variations on the expression of the gene or the prevalence and course of diabetic complications has not been determined *(70)*.

Experimental Manipulations of Polyol Pathway Enzyme Levels and Retinopathy

AR Overexpression

Overexpression of human AR in diabetic mice accelerated diabetic neuropathy as manifested by a significantly increased drop in nerve conduction velocity and increased severity of nerve fiber atrophy in diabetic transgenic mice compared to nontransgenic diabetic littermates *(84)*. However, no data for retinal endpoints in these AR transgenic diabetic mice are yet available. Another set of transgenic mice carrying human AR was studied after receiving for only 5–7 days diets high in glucose or galactose; in mice fed a diet containing 20% galactose for 7 days, the ocular pathology observed was cataract and occlusion of the retinal-choroidal vessels *(85)*. However, in these transgenic mice no data for retinal endpoints were reported at later times or at any time in which diabetes was also present.

SDH Overexpression

Bovine retinal capillary pericytes that were exposed to 30 mM glucose had modestly increased reactive oxygen species (ROS) generation, reduced DNA synthesis, and upregulated VEGF expression; under the same conditions, SDH overexpression significantly stimulated ROS generation and accentuated the cytopathic effects of glucose in an ARI- and antioxidant sensitive manner *(86)*. These data strongly suggest that elevated metabolic flux through the SDH step of the polyol pathway, as well as through the AR step of the polyol pathway, can contribute to ROS generation in retinal cells exposed to high glucose levels.

Transgenic mice that overexpress SDH have not been described to date.

AR "Knockout" Mice

Signs of diabetic retinopathy that include blood-retinal barrier breakdown, loss of pericytes, neuroretinal apoptosis, glial activation, and proliferation of blood vessels, were observed in 15-month-old *db/db* mice, and were all attenuated or prevented in *db/db* mice with an AR null mutation ($AR^{-/-}$ *db/db*) *(87)*. In the same study, AR deficiency also prevented diabetes-induced increased retinal nitrotyrosine staining, a marker of oxidative-nitrosative stress, reduction of platelet/endothelial cell adhesion molecule-1 expression, and increased expression of vascular endothelial growth factor, suggesting that AR is responsible for this spectrum of early events in the pathogenesis of diabetic retinopathy. The same group recently reported that AR deficiency prevented neuroretinal damage and glial activation induced by carotid artery transient ischemia *(88)*, consistent with similar findings in cardiac tissue *(89)*.

SDH-Deficient Mice

No retinal endpoint data have been reported for C57BL/LiA SDH-deficient strain of mice that can be rendered diabetic with streptozotocin treatment *(90)*.

MECHANISMS OF CELLULAR TOXICITY OF THE POLYOL PATHWAY AND RELEVANCE TO DIABETIC RETINOPATHY

To begin entertaining a connection of the polyol pathway with diabetic retinopathy, it must be known that some critical cell types in the retina contain the enzymes of the pathway. This condition is well satisfied for AR, which is present in the vascular pericytes, endothelial cells, ganglion cells, and Müller glial cells of all species studied, including human *(14–16, 91–93)*.

Chronic polyol pathway hyperactivity can impose on cells a variety of stresses, notably osmotic and oxidative stress, increased protein kinase C activation, and enhanced glycation via fructose and its metabolites leading to formation of advanced glycation endproducts (AGEs) (Fig. 3). Activation of the polyol pathway is also tightly coupled to activation of the pentose phosphate pathway (PPP) *(7)* which produces, among other metabolites, NADPH and glyceraldehyde-3-phosphate, the latter also strongly implicated in AGE formation *(94, 95)* (Fig. 3). Eventually, it will be important to know which of these stresses are operative in the individual retinal cell types that contain AR and undergo damage or death in diabetes. This knowledge may have therapeutic implications related to effective doses of AR inhibitors and identification of alternative drugs. For the moment, however, individual retinal cell types are not accessible with the rapidity required for direct biochemical and metabolic studies. We thus illustrate the biochemical and metabolic consequences of polyol pathway activation using data obtained in the whole retina and, mostly, in other tissues.

Osmotic Stress

AR reduces cytosolic glucose to sorbitol using NADPH as a cofactor. Sorbitol is an alcohol, polyhydroxylated and strongly hydrophilic, and therefore does not diffuse readily through cell membranes and can accumulate intracellularly with possible osmotic consequences *(96)*. Of note, production of intracellular osmolytes to counterbalance extracellular hypertonicity is a physiological role of AR in the kidney medulla *(97)*. Insofar as accumulation of 1 μmol of membrane-impermeant solute per gram of intracellular tissue water will increase osmotic pressure by 1 mOsm per liter, elevation of intracellular sorbitol will trigger osmotic regulatory mechanisms *(98)*. When such mechanisms, relatively unexplored in the retina, fail to fully compensate for increased intracellular sorbitol in the diabetic state, osmotic stress will result (Fig. 3). Probably only tissues and organs that accumulate concentrations of sorbitol in excess of 5 μmol per gram will suffer osmotic consequences *(99, 100)*. The increase in sorbitol concentrations measured in the whole retina of diabetic rats is not in the range that would generate osmotic stress *(19, 101)*, but measurements performed in the whole organ may not be informative of events in discrete cell types. For example, a cell type that had an especially high ratio of AR to SDH could accumulate sorbitol to the point of generating intracellular hypertonicity, and yet the amount of sorbitol would be diluted substantially if the measurement, performed in the whole retina, included cell types not accumulating sorbitol. Additional studies are required to ascertain the susceptibility of individual retinal cell types to polyol pathway-induced osmotic stress.

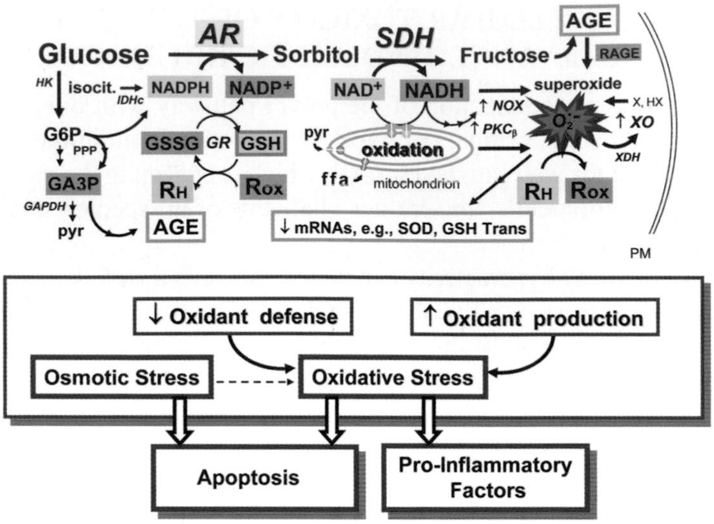

Fig. 3. Biochemical mechanisms linking the polyol pathway to apoptosis and proinflammatory responses. Elevated cytosolic glucose (*upper left*) causes accelerated transformation of glucose to sorbitol by aldose reductase (AR), with consumption of free cytosolic NADPH and production of $NADP^+$. $NADP^+$ triggers the pentose phosphate pathway (PPP) and other NADPH-synthesizing enzymes, e.g., $NADP^+$-dependent cytoplasmic isocitrate (isocit.) dehydrogenase (IDHc) and malic enzyme (not shown), to replenish NADPH. NADPH is essential for glutathione reductase (GR) to reduce oxidized glutathione (GSSG) back to reduced glutathione (GSH), and GSH is in turn essential for restoring oxidized cellular biomolecules (Rox) to their reduced state (RH). Thus, an increased rate of NADPH utilization reduces cellular antioxidant defenses and can enhance vulnerability to oxidative stress (*text box*). In the second step of the polyol pathway, sorbitol is oxidized to fructose by sorbitol dehydrogenase (SDH), with concomitant reduction of free cytosolic NAD^+ to NADH. Increased intracellular sorbitol and fructose concentrations can cause osmotic stress (*text box, lower left*) which can contribute importantly to apoptosis (*text box, lower left*). Elevation of free cytosolic NADH relative to NAD^+ contributes to increased superoxide (Fig. 3: $O_2^{\cdot -}$) generation via a variety of pathways, including provision of substrate for NAD(P)H oxidase (NOX) and for mitochondrial oxidation (mitochondrion). Oxidative stress (*textbox*) can be further amplified by oxidation of xanthine dehydrogenase (XDH) to xanthine oxidase (XO) which produces superoxide from xanthine (X), hypoxanthine (HX) and oxygen; it can also impair the synthesis of mRNAs for antioxidant enzymes (*textbox*). Finally, fructose produced in the second step of the polyol pathway is a precursor of advanced glycation endproducts (AGEs) which interact with the receptor for AGEs (RAGE) to also contribute to oxidant production (*upper right*). AGEs also result from reactions of triose phosphates such as glyceraldehyde-3-phosphate (GA3P) (*left side*) that are elevated because of oxidative-stress-related reduced activity of glyceraldehyde-3-phosphate dehydrogenase (GAPDH). Thus, the second reaction of the polyol pathway triggers production of oxidant from multiple sources and impairs antioxidant defenses, with the consequence of generating oxidative stress (and nitrative stress, not shown) that can activate both proapoptotic and proinflammatory signals (*textboxes*). Additional abbreviations: *ffa* free fatty acids; *G6P* glucose-6-phosphate; *GSH Trans.* glutathione transferase; *HK* hexokinase; *PM* plasma membrane; *pyr* pyruvate; *SOD* superoxide dismutase.

Oxidative Stress

Linkage of the polyol pathway activity with the generation of oxidative stress begins in principle with consumption of NADPH by AR, as this could result in less NADPH cofactor being available for glutathione reductase, an enzyme critical for maintaining the intracellular pool of reduced glutathione (GSH) (Fig. 3). Nuclear magnetic resonance studies of rat lens exposed in vitro to both high glucose levels and oxidants indicate competition between the polyol pathway and the glutathione reductase pathway for NADPH *(102)*. However, in some tissues, rapid regeneration of NADPH is possible through the action of the pentose phosphate pathway (PPP) *(103)*, as well as by cytoplasmic malic enzyme and $NADP^+$-dependent isocitrate dehydrogenase, e.g., *(104)*. The latter two enzyme activities are reported to be "high" in rat retinal tissue, with $NADP^+$-dependent isocitrate dehydrogenase activity (Fig. 3) ~8-fold higher per retina than malic enzyme *(105)*. Depletion of NADPH or GSH has not been observed in the retina of rats with a short (6 weeks) duration of diabetes *(101)*. It must be noted, however, that after such short diabetes duration there is also no evidence of diabetes-induced toxicity for relevant retinal cell types. Apoptosis of retinal capillary cells is not yet detectable *(106)*, and Müller glial cells do not show reactive characteristics (C. Gerhardinger, unpublished observations).

In the second step of the pathway, persistent utilization of NAD^+ by SDH can lead to an increased ratio of NADH/NAD^+, a condition that has been termed "pseudohypoxia" *(107)*. Numerous investigators have observed increased free cytoplasmic NADH/NAD^+ (calculated from retinal lactate/pyruvate) in retinas from diabetic rats and retinas exposed to high glucose in vitro when compared to normal retinas *(108–112)*. Discordant results *(113, 114)* seem likely to be due to methodological differences. Elevated free cytoplasmic NADH/NAD^+ has been linked to a multitude of metabolic and signaling changes that contribute to oxidative stress and changes in gene expression *(115, 116)*. For example, excess NADH can provide substrate for NAD(P)H oxidase, which, in the presence of oxygen, generates superoxide and related intracellular oxidant species *(117)* (Fig. 3). Superoxide reacts nonenzymatically with nitric oxide to produce the powerful oxidant, peroxynitrite *(118)* (for simplicity not shown in Fig. 3); thus, nitric oxide levels also play a key role in retinopathy *(119)*. Elevated cytoplasmic unbound NADH as well as cytoplasmic pyruvate can also transmit reducing equivalents into the mitochondrion via mitochondrial transporters and shuttles and accelerate electron transport within the mitochondrial membrane, a process also linked to superoxide production *(120)* (Fig. 3). In addition increased oxidative stress can reversibly convert xanthine dehydrogenase to superoxide-generating xanthine oxidase (Fig. 3) *(121)*, an enzyme found in human and bovine inner retinal capillaries and in human cones *(122)*.

Excess polyol pathway activity can contribute to oxidative stress also by interfering with upregulation of antioxidant defenses. Peripheral white blood cells or fibroblasts from diabetic patients with retinopathy and nephropathy, but not from uncomplicated diabetic patients or healthy individuals, when exposed to high glucose in vitro failed to induce mRNAs for antioxidant defense enzymes including catalase, glutathione peroxidase, and cytoplasmic superoxide dismutase *(123, 124)*. In white blood cells, the defect correlated inversely with the AR genotype, i.e., the high AR expression genotype manifested low antioxidant mRNA induction. Moreover, an essentially normal response of antioxidant mRNAs was restored by treatment in vitro with ARI zopolrestat *(124)*. Thus, it appears that increased flux through the polyol pathway can interfere with the induction or upregulation of antioxidant defense enzymes (Fig. 3), especially in cells from individuals prone to the complications of diabetes. Consistent with these findings in human cells, treatment with fidarestat, an ARI structurally distinct from zopolrestat, prevented oxidative stress and allowed upregulation of antioxidant defense enzymes in the retina of diabetic rats *(101)*. Importantly, fidarestat did not prevent oxidative stress caused in cultured retinal endothelial cells by three different pro-oxidants under normal glucose conditions, demonstrating that the ARI did not have direct antioxidant activity. Rather, the antioxidant effect of the ARI in the diabetic rat retina results in all likelihood from inhibiting elevated metabolic flux through retinal aldose reductase (see also the sections "AR Knockout Mice" and "Effects of ARIs in Experimental Diabetic Retinopathy").

Activation of Protein Kinase C

Sustained elevation of NADH/NAD$^+$ under hyperglysolic conditions coupled with oxidative and poly(ADP-ribose) polymerase-mediated inhibition of glyceraldehyde-3-phosphate dehydrogenase *(125)*, favors production of diacylglycerol which activates protein kinase C (PKC). Accordingly, AR inhibition prevents high glucose-induced diacylglycerol production and PKC activation in vascular smooth muscle cells *(126)* and rat glomeruli *(127)*, and glucose-induced PKC activation in human mesangial cells *(128)*. PKC can further activate the superoxide-producing NAD(P)H oxidase complex *(129)* (Fig. 3).

Generation of AGE Precursors

The fructose produced by the polyol pathway, which can directly fructosylate proteins and induce cross-linking more rapidly than glucose *(130)*, can enter in the formation of fructose-3-phosphate and 3-deoxyglucosone. These are powerful glycating agents and AGE precursors *(131)*, and their formation is prevented by ARI treatment in both the erythrocytes of diabetic patients *(132, 133)* and the lens of diabetic rats *(134)*. Moreover, 3-deoxyglucosone has been shown to inactivate intracellular enzymes important in the detoxification of oxidant species *(133)*. The retina of experimentally diabetic rats shows accumulation of AGEs colocalized with AGE receptors *(135)*, and interaction of AGEs with their receptor generates oxidative stress *(136, 137)*. Excess polyol pathway activity may thus contribute to oxidative stress also through the generation of AGE precursors.

Proinflammatory Events and Apoptosis

Reactive oxygen species, functioning both as signaling and damaging molecules, are known to trigger proinflammatory responses *(138)* as well as apoptosis *(139)* (Fig. 3). It may thus be expected that chronically enhanced polyol pathway activity in diabetes will contribute to both these types of events. Of the proinflammatory events described in diabetic retinopathy, a few have been examined in relation to polyol pathway activity. AR inhibitors have shown thus far to prevent in experimentally diabetic rats increased expression of leukocyte adhesion molecules *(140)* and complement activation *(16)*. Apoptosis is a prominent phenomenon in the diabetic retina *(141, 142)*, and AR inhibitors have successfully prevented in diabetic rats apoptosis of both retinal neurons and vascular cells *(16, 19, 140)*.

Polyol pathway activity appears thus sufficient to initiate the oxidative stress that is observed in the diabetic retina and to account for cellular consequences that have the potential to shape the development and progression of diabetic retinopathy. To prove or disprove a causative role of the polyol pathway in the lesions of diabetic retinopathy, studies have been undertaken over the years using AR inhibitors (ARIs). These drugs have been useful tools and have provided results that justify a continuing interest in the polyol pathway. However, the results also urge the development of new types of drugs and the testing of new hypotheses. We provide below highlights of studies with ARIs used to date that are instrumental to the well-informed interpretation of the results obtained in diabetic retinopathy.

ARI STRUCTURES AND PROPERTIES

ARIs have been reviewed on numerous occasions, and the reader is directed to the published reviews for details, e.g., *(6, 96, 143–146)*. Selected ARIs of current interest or of particular historical interest to diabetic retinopathy are shown in Fig. 4. There have been three major chemical classes of ARIs (1) spiro-imides, exemplified in Fig. 4 by sorbinil, fidarestat, and ranirestat; (2) carboxylic acids, illustrated by tolrestat, zopolrestat, zenarestat, and epalrestat; and (3) pyridazinones, represented by ARI-809. Each class has had distinctive strengths and limitations in terms of in vitro potency, in vivo potency, pharmacokinetic properties, and safety. With few exceptions, toxicity has been unique for each ARI and apparently not related to AR inhibition.

For reasons of cost, speed, and presumed tissue sensitivity, most ARI clinical trials have been conducted against diabetic neuropathy. Epalrestat (Fig. 4) is commercially available (only) in Japan for this indication, and a multiyear study has recently reported a protective effect of chronic epalrestat use on diabetic nerve function *(147)*, although the study was not double blinded *(148)*. Fidarestat and ranirestat (Fig. 4) have been studied for improvement of diabetic neuropathy, but have given disappointing results in their Phase 2 *(149)* and Phase 3 *(150)* trials, respectively. However, Phase 3 study of ranirestat for prevention of progression of diabetic neuropathy and retinopathy is currently ongoing *(150)*. A recent analysis based on translational pharmacology data in preclinical models of diabetic neuropathy, suggests that most ARIs have been used in human neuropathy trials at doses that were of inadequate functional potency against the endpoints tested *(151)*. This appears to have resulted from relying on nerve sorbitol levels as the primary biomarker of tissue effect, which caused an ~20- to 40-fold overestimation of in vivo potency. Thus, despite early encouraging results, sorbinil, tolrestat, zopolrestat, and zenarestat (Fig. 4) are no longer in development. Nor is the newly discovered pyridazinone ARI-809 *(152)*, recently found to absorb UV-A and UV-B and to cause exacerbation of spontaneous light-induced retinal damage in albino rats after 6 months of dosing *(153)*. However, the discovery of the pyridazinone class demonstrated that it is possible to find new classes of ARIs with in vivo potencies high enough to exert robust in vivo antioxidant activity as opposed to simply lowering tissue sorbitol *(151)*.

ARIs that penetrate lens have shown in most cases robust activity against retinopathy when given at relatively high doses in preclinical models (see later), but there has been only one major ARI trial for diabetic retinopathy, the Sorbinil Retinopathy Trial, which was unsuccessful and will be discussed further below.

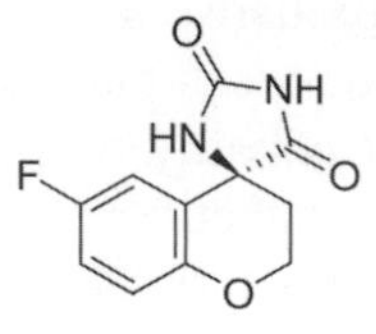

Sorbinil

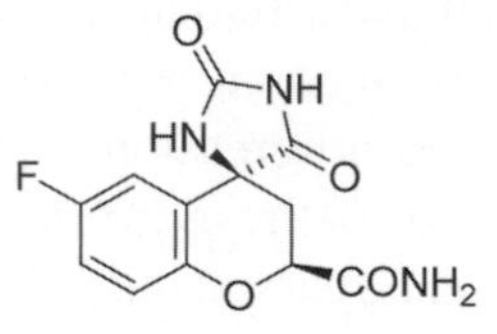

Fidarestat, SNK-860

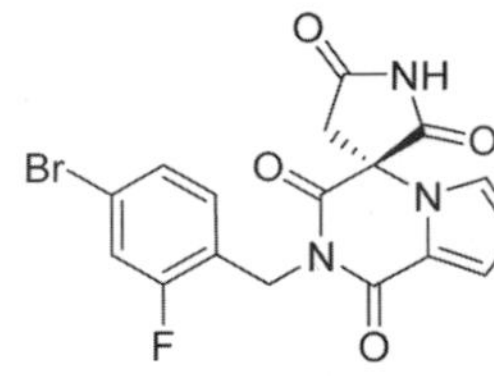

Ranirestat, AS-3201

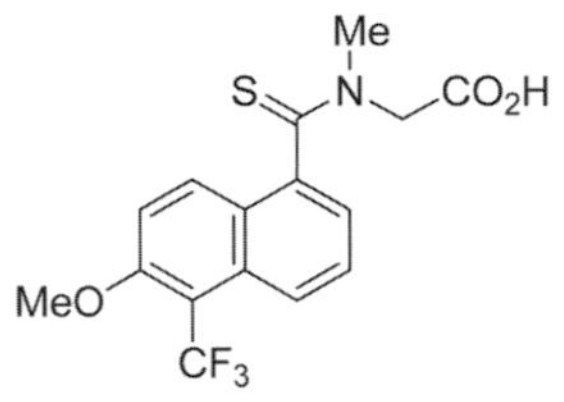

Tolrestat

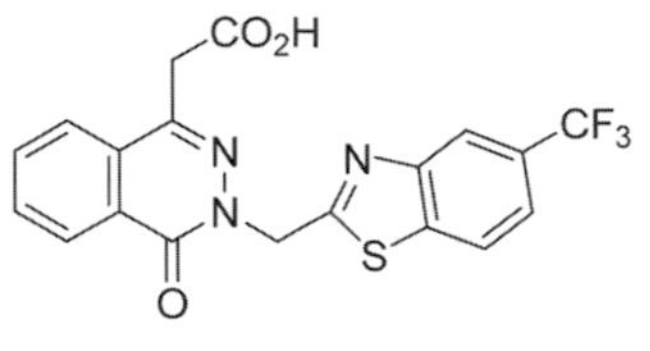

Zopolrestat

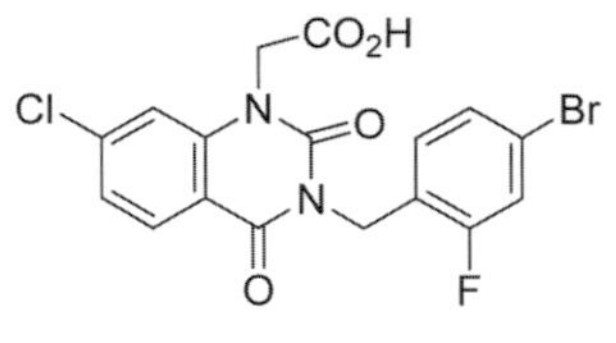

Zenarestat

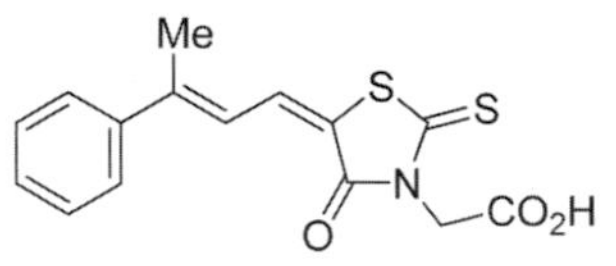

Epalrestat

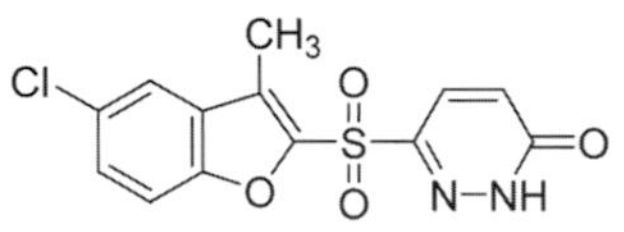

ARI-809, CP-744,809

Fig. 4. Structures of selected aldose reductase inhibitors (ARIs). See text for further discussion.

EFFECTS OF ARIS IN EXPERIMENTAL DIABETIC RETINOPATHY

It has become evident over the years that the species of the experimental animal model and the dose of ARI are important determinants of the effect on retinopathy. Whether induced by galactosemia or diabetes, retinopathy is more consistently susceptible to prevention by ARIs in the rat than in the dog model (reviewed in *(154)*). The reasons have not been investigated systematically, but may relate, at least in part, to the doses of ARIs used in the two species and relevant pharmacokinetics. In diabetic dogs, the ARI sorbinil used at a dose of 20 mg/kg/day failed to prevent the typical vascular lesions of retinopathy *(155)*. This could not be attributed to absent activity of the polyol pathway in the retina of diabetic dogs, insofar as the retinal concentration of sorbitol increased by the approximately threefold observed in most models, and the increase was prevented by the dose of sorbinil used *(155)*. Studies on the role of the polyol pathway in the neuropathy of diabetic rats made clear that inhibition of tissue fructose accumulation predicted the efficacy of ARIs on outcomes related to neuropathy better than inhibition of sorbitol accumulation *(151, 156, 157)*. This is consistent with the hypothesis that tissue damage is a consequence of the flux of glucose through the pathway altering homeostasis at several levels (see earlier), rather than of the amount of tissue sorbitol measurable at any given time *(29, 102)*. The reason normalization of abnormal metabolic flux through the polyol pathway – as opposed to normalization of tissue sorbitol – is essential in order to prevent tissue damage is because the abnormal flux is closely linked to the generation of oxidative stress (Fig. 3) *(151, 158)*.

When tested on functional abnormalities of the retina or retinal vessels in diabetic rats, sorbinil at a dose of 10 mg/kg/day reduced but did not prevent deterioration of the electroretinogram *(159)*, and different ARIs prevented in a dose-related manner albumin permeation *(160)*. Among the characteristic structural changes of retinal vessels, basement membrane thickening was only partially prevented in diabetic rats by ponalrestat in experiments that did not however document the effect of the dose used on polyol pathway metabolites *(161)*; fidarestat prevented basement membrane thickening in a dose-related manner, while pericyte loss appeared sensitive to all doses of fidarestat tested *(162)*.

Studies performed more recently in the diabetic rat have taken such dose considerations into account and used doses of ARIs documented in advance to prevent or decrease substantially retinal fructose accumulation. It is of note that for both sorbinil and ARI-809, two structurally different ARIs, the doses used to normalize retinal fructose in diabetic rats (65 and 50 mg/kg/day, respectively) led to lowering of sorbitol below control levels *(19, 140)*. This is consistent with the pattern seen with functionally efficacious doses in diabetic rat nerve, e.g., *(156, 157)*, and confirms that doses targeting fructose levels inhibit the pathway to a greater extent than doses targeting, and often not even normalizing, sorbitol levels.

The streptozocin diabetic rat is currently the most comprehensive model for human diabetic retinopathy. Like diabetic humans, diabetic rats show in the retinal capillaries apoptosis of pericytes and endothelial cells *(141)*, deposition of complement *(163)*, and ultimately development of pericyte ghosts and acellular capillaries *(16, 141)*. Diabetic rats also show the Müller cell reactivity *(18)* and apoptosis of neurons in the ganglion cell layer *(142)* observed in human diabetes. All these abnormalities are prevented in the diabetic rat by different ARIs administered at doses that inhibit retinal polyol pathway activity *(16, 19, 140)*.

The recent results in diabetic rats are not only proving a role for the polyol pathway in the spectrum of vascular, glial, and neural abnormalities that diabetes induces in the retina; they are also showing that ARIs are, to date, the only drugs that can prevent the whole spectrum of abnormalities (Fig. 5). When sorbinil and aspirin were compared to each other in the same experiments, both prevented the development of acellular capillaries, but only sorbinil prevented neuronal apoptosis and Müller cell reactivity *(20)*. This could have translational importance if we were to learn that the early neural and/or glial abnormalities occurring in the diabetic retina impact on clinically important aspects of retinopathy. For example, proper Müller cell function may be critical to the prevention and/or resolution of macular edema *(164)*, and there is evidence that diabetes affects the regulation of water channels in these cells *(165)*.

New observations are also defining with increasing precision the mechanisms whereby the polyol pathway causes the retinal abnormalities. ARIs inhibit AR preferentially, and can inhibit also aldehyde reductase, another enzyme in the aldo–keto reductase superfamily that plays a role in the detoxification of reactive aldehydes. This has generated the question of whether inhibition of aldehyde reductase *(166)* contributes to the beneficial or to the unwanted effects of ARIs, especially at the higher doses *(167)*. Availability of ARI-809 (Fig. 4), characterized as one of the most potent and selective ARIs yet described with an IC_{50} for aldehyde reductase of 930 nM as compared to 1 nM

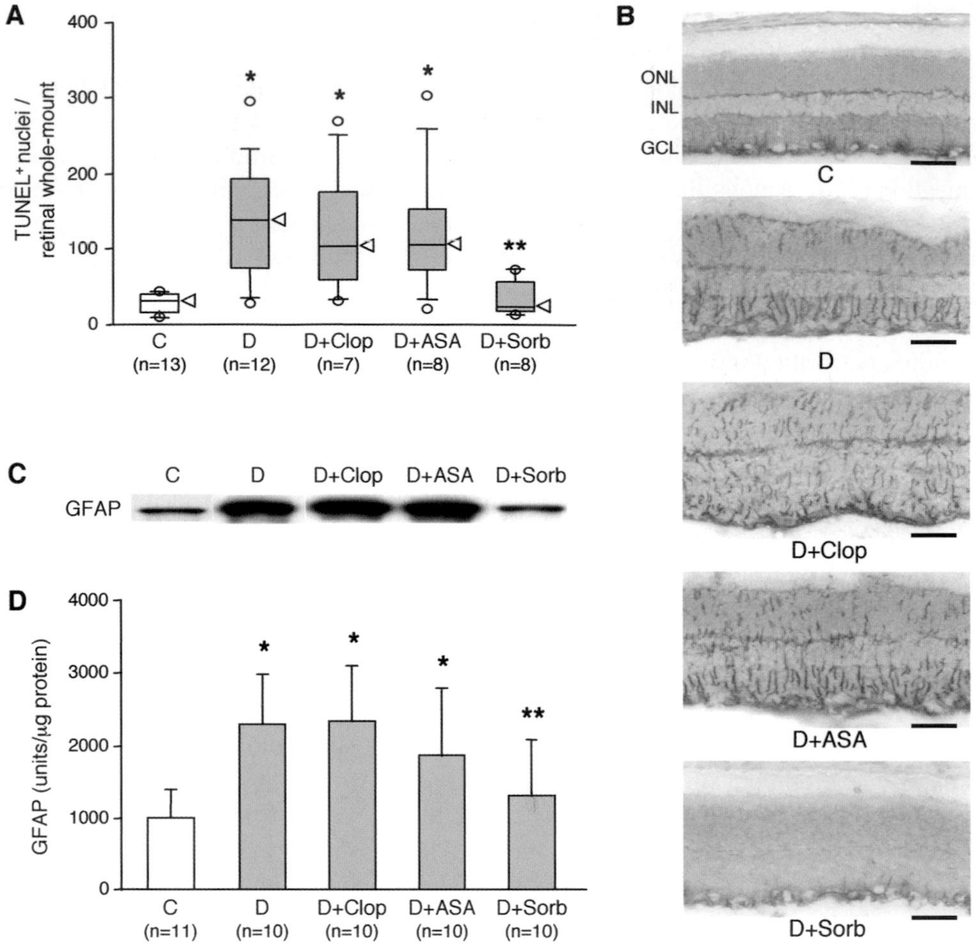

Fig. 5. Comparison of the effects of clopidogrel, aspirin, and ARI sorbinil on neuronal apoptosis and glial reactivity in the retina of rats with 2.5 months of streptozotocin-induced diabetes. In these experiments, rats were randomized from the time of diabetes induction to treatment with clopidogrel (Clop) (10 mg/kg/day), used as a selective antiplatelet agent, aspirin (ASA) (30 mg/kg/day) used as anti-inflammatory and antiplatelet agent, and ARI sorbinil (Sorb) (65 mg/kg/day) to test the effects of the three drugs on early and late vascular, neuronal, and glial abnormalities caused by diabetes in the retina. Clopidogrel had no effect on any abnormality tested, aspirin prevented all capillary abnormalities (results not shown in this figure), but only sorbinil prevented both the capillary and the neuroglial abnormalities. Neuronal apoptosis (**A**) was measured by counting TUNEL-positive nonvascular nuclei in whole retinas mounted and observed vitreal side up. In the boxplots, the bars encompass from the 90th to the 10th percentile of the scores and the box from the 75th to the 25th percentile; *arrows* point to the median. Glial reactivity was assessed by observing (**B**) the pattern of glial fibrillary acidic protein (GFAP) immunostaining in retinal sections (diabetes causes GFAP to be prominently expressed in the processes of the Müller glial cells that span the thickness of the retina; *GCL* ganglion cell layer; *INL* inner nuclear layer; *ONL* outer nuclear layer), and by measuring the levels of retinal GFAP by immunoblot ((**C**) shows a representative immunoblot, and (**D**) the quantitation of the signals from immunoblots of retinal GFAP). *C* control rats, *D* diabetic rats. $^{*}P < 0.006$ vs. control rats; $^{**}P < 0.002$ vs. diabetic rats. Copyright © 2005 American Diabetes Association (from *(20)* reprinted with permission from the *American Diabetes Association*).

for AR *(152)*, has made it possible to target specifically the role of the polyol pathway in the early stages of the development of experimental diabetic retinopathy. ARI-809 administered to diabetic rats at doses documented to inhibit both sorbitol and fructose accumulation in the retina, reproduced exactly all preventative effects on retinopathy *(16, 19, 20)* observed with the less specific *(168)* ARI sorbinil *(140)*. On this basis, it can be stated that aldose reductase is itself the key relay that converts hyperglycemia into glucotoxicity for specific cell types in the retina. This conclusion is bolstered by the robust protection against the effects of diabetes observed in the retinas of 15-month-old *db/db* mice lacking the AR gene product *(87)*.

As to the nature of the glucotoxicity generated through AR activity in the retinal vessels and leading to the characteristic histopathology of diabetic retinopathy, gene expression profiling points to the concurrence of multiple events, but identifies oxidative stress and proinflammatory changes as uniquely induced by excessive polyol pathway activity *(169)*. This "signature" may become a useful reference when seeking evidence for polyol pathway activity in human diabetic retinopathy.

THE POLYOL PATHWAY IN HUMAN DIABETIC RETINOPATHY

The Sorbinil Trial

The Sorbinil Retinopathy Trial has been the only major clinical trial testing an AR inhibitor on diabetic retinopathy. In this multicenter, randomized, placebo-controlled, double-blind study, 497 patients with insulin-dependent diabetes and absent to mild retinopathy were followed for a median of 41 months. The sorbinil-treated (250 mg/day) group was found not to differ from the placebo-treated group in terms of progression of retinopathy, although the number of microaneurysms increased at a slightly slower rate in the sorbinil-treated group *(170)*. Knowledge gained since the trial warns that the findings are not readily interpretable. First, the efficacy of sorbinil was monitored by measuring in erythrocytes the levels of sorbitol, an imprecise indicator of flux, and now known to be a poor predictor of the functional benefits of ARIs *(156)*. Moreover, erythrocyte sorbitol levels remained 26% above normal, and there was no information of an effect of sorbinil on the polyol pathway in retinal target cells. Although sorbinil could not have been used in larger doses on account of the risk of side effects in humans, the drug was given at a dose corresponding to 3.5 mg/kg/day, almost 20-fold lower than the dose effective in prevention of retinopathy in diabetic rats *(16)*. It is therefore probable that the dose of sorbinil used in the Sorbinil Trial was insufficient to silence the polyol pathway and did not permit testing the role of the pathway in diabetic retinopathy. Additionally, approximately half of the study population had some degree of retinopathy, and the treatment lasted a little over 3 years. We have since learned from the Diabetes Control and Complications Trial (DCCT) that in diabetic retinopathy prevention is much more effective than intervention, and that 3 years are grossly insufficient to demonstrate the efficacy even of treatments, such as improved glycemic control, that have a priori a high likelihood of success *(171)*.

Evidence Supporting Polyol Pathway Activity and Functional Importance in Human Diabetic Retinopathy

The negative results of the Sorbinil Trial could be falsely negative, or may instead reflect that the polyol pathway is not active and/or not pathogenic in human diabetes.

Only the appropriate tools, i.e., new ARIs with a therapeutic index higher than those of the older drugs, and clinical trials better controlled and better designed than the Sorbinil trial will finally, bring the polyol pathway hypothesis to rigorous testing in human diabetic retinopathy.

Several observations support a continuing interest in testing the hypothesis. Studies in postmortem human eyes have shown in retinas from diabetic patients with retinopathy more abundant AR immunoreactivity in ganglion cells, nerve fibers, and Müller cells, as compared to retinas from nondiabetic individuals *(172)*. After negative findings by several investigators in the past, we have documented unequivocally that human retinal endothelial cells contain AR *(16)* (Fig. 6). Insofar as the good health of endothelial cells is critical to the highly regulated permeability and structural integrity of the retinal capillaries, excess glucose flux through the AR of retinal endothelial cells becomes a strong candidate mechanism for the disruption of barrier properties and the capillary obliteration characteristic of human diabetic retinopathy. We have reviewed above the presence of AR in other retinal cell types, such as pericytes and Müller cells, also affected in human diabetes. Finally, human retinas from nondiabetic eye donors accumulate sorbitol when exposed to high glucose in organ culture *(16)* (Fig. 7). The extent of accumulation is quite comparable to that occurring

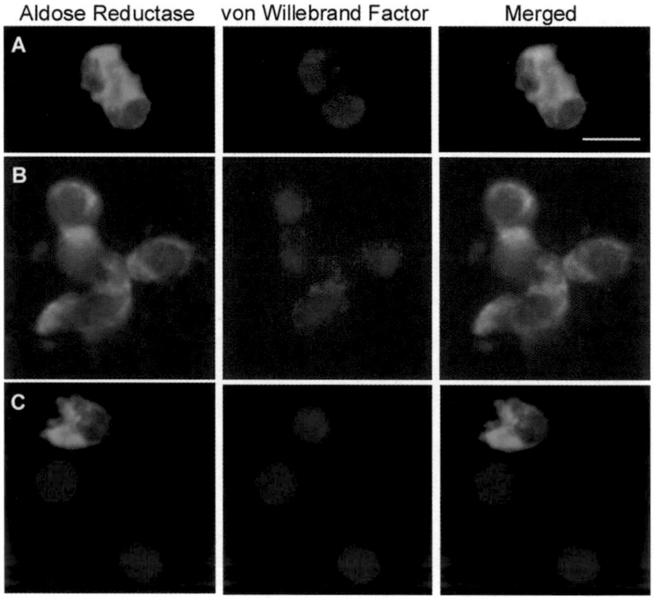

Fig. 6. Aldose reductase in human retinal endothelial cells. Fresh retinas obtained from postmortem eyes of nondiabetic donors were incubated with collagenase type 1, and the dissociated cells were fixed briefly with acetone and immunostained with antibodies to AR and von Willebrand factor. (**A**) and (**B**) show AR immunoreactivity (*green*) in cells manifesting the granular perinuclear fluorescence of von Willebrand factor (*red*) characteristically seen in retinal endothelial cells in situ *(179)*. The AR antibodies used in (**A**) were a gift from D. Carper, those used in (**B**) from R. Sorenson. Panel (**C**) shows cells from the same preparations staining only for AR or for neither protein. Bar = 20 μm. Copyright © 2004 American Diabetes Association (from *(16)* reprinted with permission from the *American Diabetes Association)*.

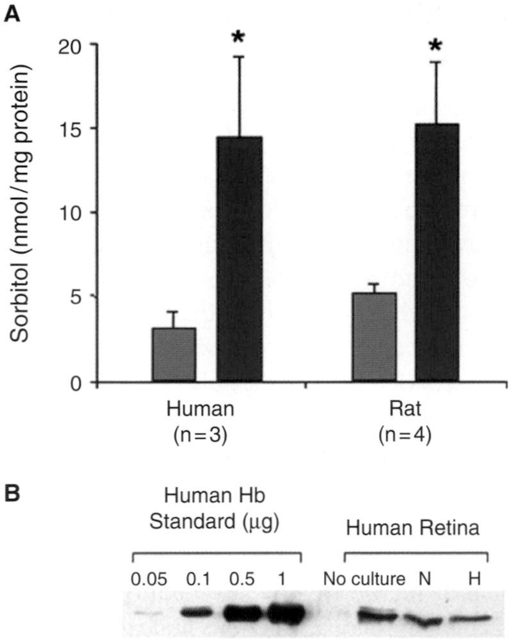

Fig. 7. Aldose reductase activity in human retina. Fresh retinas obtained from postmortem eyes of nondiabetic donors were exposed for 24 h in organ culture to normal (5 mmol/l, *blue bar*) or high (30 mmol/l, *red bar*) glucose, and sorbitol levels were measured. Fresh retinas obtained from normal rats were tested in parallel. In (**A**), the bars represent the mean ± SD of the measurements performed in the indicated number of individuals. $^*P < 0.01$ vs. normal glucose. (**B**) Presents a hemoglobin (Hb) immunoblot performed to assess the quantity of erythrocytes trapped in the blood vessels of the human retinas and potentially contributing to sorbitol accumulation. Protein lysate (20 μg/lane) from fresh human retina or retina incubated in normal (N) or high (H) glucose was subjected to SDS–PAGE together with human Hb standards and probed with antibodies to Hb. Hb levels in the whole human retina did not exceed 40 μg, whereas both the basal and stimulated levels of sorbitol were of the magnitude measured per gram Hb in human erythrocytes. This documented that resident cells of the human retina metabolize glucose to sorbitol when exposed to high glucose. Copyright © 2004 American Diabetes Association (from *(16)* reprinted with permission from the *American Diabetes Association*).

in the normal rat retina incubated in parallel, indicating that human retinal AR is readily responsive to hyperglycemia. The human enzyme is in fact widely used as a transgene in mice to confer susceptibility to diabetic complications, from cataract *(100)*, to atherosclerosis *(173)*. The evidence that the polyol pathway can be activated in the human retina in the presence of high glucose permits anticipation of tissue consequences, and complements in this respect the information from the human genetic studies reported earlier (see the sections "Polymorphisms of the AR Gene" and "AR Polymorphisms and Risk of Diabetic Retinopathy") that alleles associated with elevated AR expression are also associated with accelerated development or progression of human diabetic retinopathy.

PERSPECTIVE AND NEEDS

Rationale for Defining the Pathogenic Role of the Polyol Pathway

We see at least three reasons, connected to therapeutic opportunities, for continuing the quest for the role of the polyol pathway in human diabetic retinopathy. The overarching reason is the persistent need for adjunct treatments to pre-empt in diabetic patients the damaging effects of residual hyperglycemia on tissues. The strategies available to control hyperglycemia have improved dramatically over the last 15 years, but the means available remain imperfect and most often do not ensure sustained normoglycemia. Hence, knowing conclusively that the polyol pathway is operative and pathogenic in the human retina when hyperglycemia develops, would provide a rational target toward prevention of tissue damage. ARIs are not the sole type of drugs that may become useful as adjunct treatment for diabetic retinopathy *(174)*. However, the nature of the cellular stresses that the polyol pathway can engender may make ARIs the most rational or even the only approach to some abnormalities. Specifically, if glucose flux through the pathway generates oxidative stress by a multitude of mechanisms – from generation of ROS and AGEs to decreased antioxidant defenses (Fig. 3) – prevention will likely be much more effective if directed to the upstream causal catalytic trigger with an ARI than to multiple downstream effectors through exogenous noncatalytic antioxidants. Furthermore, if glucose flux through the pathway indeed also generates osmotic stress, the need to know is even more compelling because other types of adjunct drugs would not likely be able to prevent or cure such occurrence. The third reason for defining precisely the contribution of the polyol pathway to retinopathy is its candidacy to be a unique player in the causation of diabetic macular edema. Cytotoxic effects of the pathway in endothelial cells could initiate capillary leakage, and in Müller cells could generate intracellular edema and/or compromise the reabsorption of fluid in the inner retina. It is noteworthy that ARIs are the only type of drug, among those tested to date, able to prevent in diabetic rats the reactive features of Müller cells *(20)* (Fig. 5), and that a recent anecdotal statement reports clinical benefits of an ARI on macular edema in diabetic patients *(175)*.

Needs to be Met to Arrive at Anti-Polyol Pathway Therapy

Several needs must be met to make polyol pathway inhibition a viable therapeutic alternative in diabetic retinopathy. The first type of need is quantitative data on the activity and consequences of the polyol pathway in specific retinal cell types, complemented by modeling in genetically engineered mice to arrive at a detailed reconstruction of the contribution of the pathway to discrete features of diabetic retinopathy. These data will help us address the second type of need, which is the development of informative surrogate endpoints for polyol pathway activity in the human retina. In view of the duration and cost of clinical trials targeting prevention or early intervention in retinopathy in the era of intensive treatment of diabetes, it is likely that only drugs that have given encouraging results when pilot-tested on surrogate endpoints will be brought to full trial. This practice will lessen the risk of false negative trials, because experimentation on the long-term clinical features of retinopathy will be initiated only upon verification of drug efficacy on relevant shorter-term outcomes.

The final and crucial type of need is the availability of new, more potent, and better tolerated ARIs. Heretofore ARIs were designed on the basis of the osmotic theory of diabetic complications to lower tissue sorbitol, a theory that has been confirmed in the diabetic lens *(100)*. However, recent data reviewed earlier in this chapter indicate that oxidative stress and subtle proinflammatory events can be initiated by the polyol pathway and are critical components of the pathogenesis of diabetic retinopathy *(174, 176)*. Data from the experimental and human diabetic nerve indicate that higher doses of ARIs are needed to prevent oxidant stress than to normalize tissue sorbitol *(151)*; a similar relationship may apply in the diabetic retina. Therefore, now is the time to attempt to identify new classes of well-tolerated ARIs whose efficacy is based, not on lowering tissue sorbitol, but on lowering oxidative stress markers. The multiple molecular interactions depicted in Fig. 3 highlight the concept that the cellular consequences of the polyol pathway are likely to be the balance of the demands imposed by excess pathway activity and the responses available within, or mounted by, the cells. It may thus be indicated to develop dose–response data for the cell types of interest, comparing systematically the doses of ARIs that inhibit sorbitol accumulation, oxidative stress, AGE formation, and retinal functional and histological outcomes, respectively. Doses for particular endpoints may differ in the different cell types, and one would want to use the minimal dose to achieve efficacy on the designated critical target. The next few years of experiments will determine whether and how ARIs will be included in tomorrow's prescription for the prevention of diabetic retinopathy and its sight-threatening features. After courting the polyol pathway for so many years, an empowering verdict would be welcomed by all.

REFERENCES

1. Frank RN. Diabetic retinopathy. N Engl J Med 2004;350:48–58.
2. Robison WG, Jr., Kador PF, Kinoshita JH. Retinal capillaries: Basement membrane thickening by galactosemia prevented with aldose reductase inhibitor. Science 1983;221:1177–1179.
3. Engerman RL, Kern TS. Experimental galactosemia produces diabetic-like retinopathy. Diabetes 1984;33:97–100.
4. Engerman RL, Kern TS. Hyperglycemia and development of glomerular pathology: Diabetes compared with galactosemia. Kid Int 1989;36:41–45.
5. The Diabetes Control and Complications Trial Research Group. The relationship of glycemic exposure (HbA1c) to the risk of development and progression of retinopathy in the Diabetes Control and Complications Trial. Diabetes 1995;44:968–983.
6. Sarges R, Oates PJ. Aldose reductase inhibitors: Recent developments. Prog Drug Res 1993;40:99–161.
7. Kinoshita JH, Futterman S, Satoh K, Merola LO. Factors affecting the formation of sugar alcohols in ocular lens. Biochim Biophys Acta 1963;74:340–350.
8. Barretto OC, Beutler E. The sorbitol-oxidizing enzyme of red blood cells. J Lab Clin Med 1975;85:645–649.
9. Maret W, Auld DS. Purification and characterization of human liver sorbitol dehydrogenase. Biochemistry 1988;27:1622–1628.
10. Berry GT, Wehrli S, Reynolds R, et al. Elevation of erythrocyte redox potential linked to galactonate biosynthesis: Elimination by tolrestat. Metab Clin Exp 1998;47:1423–1428.
11. Robison WG, Jr., Nagata M, Laver N, Hohman TC, Kinoshita JH. Diabetic-like retinopathy in rats prevented with an aldose reductase inhibitor. Invest Ophthalmol Vis Sci 1989;30:2285–2292.
12. Demaine AG. Polymorphisms of the aldose reductase gene and susceptibility to diabetic microvascular complications. Curr Med Chem 2003;10:1389–1398.
13. Chung SS, Chung SK. Aldose reductase in diabetic microvascular complications. Curr Drug Targets 2005;6:475–486.
14. Akagi Y, Yajima Y, Kador PF, Kuwabara T, Kinoshita JH. Localization of aldose reductase in the human eye. Diabetes 1984;33:562–566.

15. Akagi Y, Kador PF, Kuwabara T, Kinoshita JH. Aldose reductase localization in human retinal mural cells. Invest Ophthalmol Vis Sci 1983;24:1516–1519.
16. Dagher Z, Park YS, Asnaghi V, Hoehn T, Gerhardinger C, Lorenzi M. Studies of rat and human retinas predict a role for the polyol pathway in human diabetic retinopathy. Diabetes 2004;53:2404–2411.
17. Mizutani M, Gerhardinger C, Lorenzi M. Müller cell changes in human diabetic retinopathy. Diabetes 1998;47:445–449.
18. Gerhardinger C, Costa MB, Coulombe MC, Toth I, Hoehn T, Grosu P. Expression of acute-phase response proteins in retinal Müller cells in diabetes. Invest Ophthalmol Vis Sci 2005;46:349–357.
19. Asnaghi V, Gerhardinger C, Hoehn T, Adeboje A, Lorenzi M. A role for the polyol pathway in the early neuroretinal apoptosis and glial changes induced by diabetes in the rat. Diabetes 2003;52:506–511.
20. Sun W, Gerhardinger C, Dagher Z, Hoehn T, Lorenzi M. Aspirin at low-intermediate concentrations protects retinal vessels in experimental diabetic retinopathy through non-platelet-mediated effects. Diabetes 2005;54:3418–3426.
21. Hers HG. L'aldose-reductase. Biochim Biophys Acta 1960;37:120–126.
22. Penning TM, Drury JE. Human aldo-keto reductases: Function, gene regulation, and single nucleotide polymorphisms. Arch Biochem Biophys 2007;464:241.
23. Ludvigson MA, Sorenson RL. Immunohistochemical localization of aldose reductase. I. Enzyme purification and antibody preparation: Localization in peripheral nerve, artery, and testis. Diabetes 1980;29:438–449.
24. Clements RS, Jr., Weaver JP, Winegrad AI. The distribution of polyol: NADP oxidoreductase in mammalian tissues. Biochem Biophys Res Commun 1969;37:347–353.
25. Grimshaw CE. Aldose reductase: Model for a new paradigm of enzymic perfection in detoxification catalysts. Biochemistry 1992;31:10139–10145.
26. Grimshaw CE, Bohren KM, Lai CJ, Gabbay KH. Human aldose reductase: Rate constants for a mechanism including interconversion of ternary complexes by recombinant wild-type enzyme. Biochemistry 1995;34:14356–14365.
27. Grimshaw CE. Direct measurement of the rate of ring opening of D-glucose by enzyme-catalyzed reduction. Carbohydr Res 1986;148:345–348.
28. Inagaki K, Miwa I, Okuda J. Affinity purification and glucose specificity of aldose reductase from bovine lens. Arch Biochem Biophys 1982;216:337–344.
29. Oates PJ. Polyol pathway and diabetic peripheral neuropathy. Int Rev Neurobiol 2002;50:325–392.
30. Biadene M, Hazemann I, Cousido A, et al. The atomic resolution structure of human aldose reductase reveals that rearrangement of a bound ligand allows the opening of the safety-belt loop. Acta Chrystallogr Sect D Biol Crystallogr 2007;63:665–672.
31. Petrash JM, Tarle I, Wilson DK, Quiocho FA. Aldose reductase catalysis and crystallography: Insights from recent advances in enzyme structure and function. Diabetes 1994;43:955–959.
32. Graham A, Heath P, Morten JEN, Markham AF. The human aldose reductase gene maps to chromosome region 7q35. Hum Genet 1991;86:509–514.
33. Graham A, Brown L, Hedge PJ, Gammack AJ, Markham AF. Structure of the human aldose reductase gene. J Biol Chem 1991;266:6872–6877.
34. Chung S, LaMendola J. Cloning and sequence determination of human placental aldose reductase gene. J Biol Chem 1989;264:14775–14777.
35. Imperatore G, Hanson RI, Pettitt DJ, Kobes S, Bennett PH, Knowler WC. Sib-pair linkage analysis for susceptibility genes for microvascular complications among Pima Indians with type 2 diabetes. Diabetes 1998;47:821–830.
36. Patel A, Hibberd ML, Millward BA, Demaine AG. Chromosome 7q35 and susceptibility to diabetic microvascular complications. J Diabetes Complications 1996;10:62–67.
37. Wang K, Bohren KM, Gabbay KH. Characterization of the human aldose reductase gene promoter. J Biol Chem 1993;268:16052–16058.
38. Ko BCB, Ruepp B, Bohren KM, Gabbay KH, Chung SS. Identification and characterization of multiple osmotic response sequences in the human aldose reductase gene. J Biol Chem 1997;272:16431–16437.
39. McGowan MH, Iwata T, Carper DA. Characterization of the mouse aldose reductase gene and promoter in a lens epithelial cell line. Mol Vis 1998;4:2, http://www.emory.edu/molvis/v4/p2.

40. Graham C, Szpirer C, Levan G, Carper D. Characterization of the aldose reductase-encoding gene family in rat. Gene 1991;107:259–267.
41. Ko BC, Lam KS, Wat NM, Chung SS. An (A-C)n dinucleotide repeat polymorphic marker at the 5′- end of the aldose reductase gene is associated with early-onset diabetic retinopathy in NIDDM patients. Diabetes 1995;44:727–732.
42. Kao YL, Donaghue K, Chan A, Knight J, Silink M. A novel polymorphism in the aldose reductase gene promoter region is strongly associated with diabetic retinopathy in adolescents with Type 1 diabetes. Diabetes 1999;48:1338–1340.
43. Patel A, Ratanachaiyavong S, Millward BA, Demaine AG. Polymorphisms of the aldose reductase locus (ALR2) and susceptibility to diabetic microvascular complications. Adv Exp Med Biol 1993;328:325–332.
44. Kao YL, Donaghue K, Chan A, Knight J, Silink M. An aldose reductase intragenic polymorphism associated with diabetic retinopathy. Diabetes Res Clin Pract 1999;46:155–160.
45. Demaine A, Cross D, Millward A. Polymorphisms of the aldose reductase gene and susceptibility to retinopathy in Type 1 diabetes mellitus. Invest Ophthalmol Vis Sci 2000;41:4064–4068.
46. Moczulski DK, Scott L, Antonellis A, et al. Aldose reductase gene polymorphisms and susceptibility to diabetic nephropathy in Type 1 diabetes mellitus. Diabet Med 2000;17:111–118.
47. Li Q, Xie P, Huang J, Gu Y, Zeng W, Song H. Polymorphisms and functions of the aldose reductase gene 5′-regulatory region in Chinese patients with Type 2 diabetes mellitus. Chin Med J (Engl) 2002;115:209–213.
48. Blakley RL. The metabolism and antiketogenic effects of sorbitol. Sorbitol dehydrogenase. Biochem J 1951;49:257–271.
49. Persson B, Zigler JS, Jörnvall H. A super-family of medium-chain dehydrogenases/reductases (MDR) - sub-lines including Xi-crystallin, alcohol and polyol dehydrogenases, quinone oxidoreductases, enoyl reductases, VAT-1 and other proteins. Eur J Biochem 1994;226:15–22.
50. Pauly TA, Ekstrom JL, Beebe DA, et al. X-ray crystallographic and kinetic studies of human sorbitol dehydrogenase. Structure (Cambridge) 2003;11:1071–1085.
51. Johansson K, El-Ahmad M, Kaiser C, et al. Crystal structure of sorbitol dehydrogenase. Chem Biol Interact 2001;130–132:351–358.
52. Moriyama T, Nakano T, Wada T, et al. Crystallization and properties of liver sorbitol dehydrogenase (EC 1.1.1.14) (Japanese). J Nara Med Assoc 1973;24:356–362.
53. Jeffery J, Jörnvall H. Sorbitol dehydrogenase. Adv Enzymol Relat Areas Mol Biol 1988;61:47–106.
54. Karlsson C, Maret W, Auld DS, Höög J-O, Jörnvall H. Variability within mammalian sorbitol dehydrogenases: The primary structure of the human liver enzyme. Eur J Biochem 1989;186:543–550.
55. Chida K, Yamamoto N, Yasuda K. Histochemical study of polyol dehydrogenase: Localization of sorbitol dehydrogenase in mouse-liver and kidney. Acta Histochem Cytochem 1975;8:234–246.
56. Cohen RB. Studies on a polyhydric alcohol dehydrogenase system utilizing a histochemical method. Lab Invest 1961;10:459–465.
57. Maret W. Novel substrates and inhibitors of human liver sorbitol dehydrogenase. Adv Exp Med Biol 1991;284:327–336.
58. Murray RK, Gadacz I, Bach M, Hardin S, Morris HP. Metabolic and electrophoretic studies of rat liver sorbitol dehydrogenase. Can J Biochem 1969;47:587–593.
59. Lindstad RI, Koll P, McKinley-McKee JS. Substrate specificity of sheep liver sorbitol dehydrogenase. Biochem J 1998;330:479–487.
60. Lindstad RI, McKinley-McKee JS. Methylglyoxal and the polyol pathway: Three-carbon compounds are substrates for sheep liver sorbitol dehydrogenase. FEBS Lett 1993;330:31–35.
61. Maret W. Human sorbitol dehydrogenase: A secondary alcohol dehydrogenase with distinct pathophysiological roles. pH-dependent kinetic studies. Adv Exp Med Biol 1996;414:383–393.
62. Angyal SJ. The composition of reducing sugars in solution. Adv Carbohydr Chem Biochem 1984;42:15–68.
63. Smith MG. Polyol dehydrogenases. Crystallization of the L-iditol dehydrogenase of sheep liver. Biochem J 1962;83:135–144.
64. Marini I, Bucchioni L, Borella P, DelCorso A, Mura U. Sorbitol dehydrogenase from bovine lens: Purification and properties. Arch Biochem Biophys 1997;340:383–391.

65. Lindstad RI, Hermansen LF, McKinley-McKee JS. The kinetic mechanism of sheep liver sorbitol dehydrogenase. Eur J Biochem 1992;210:641–647.
66. Lindstad RI, McKinley-McKee JS. Effect of pH on sheep liver sorbitol dehydrogenase steady-state kinetics. Eur J Biochem 1995;233:891–898.
67. Karlsson C. Mammalian sorbitol dehydrogenase. Stockholm: Karolinska Institutet; 1994.
68. Burnell JN, Holmes RS. Purification and properties of sorbitol dehydrogenase from mouse liver. Int J Biochem 1983;15:507–511.
69. Donald LJ, Wang HS, Hamerton JL. Assignment of the sorbitol dehydrogenase locus to human chromosome 15 pter leads to q21. Biochem Genet 1980;18:425–431.
70. Carr IM, Markham AF. Molecular genetic analysis of the human sorbitol dehydrogenase gene. Mamm Genome 1995;6:645–652.
71. Lee FK, Cheung MC, Chung S. The human sorbitol dehydrogenase gene: cDNA cloning, sequence determination, and mapping by fluorescence in situ hybridization. Genomics 1994;21:354–358.
72. Iwata T, Carper D. Human sorbitol dehydrogenase gene. cDNA sequence and expression. Adv Exp Med Biol 1995;372:373–381.
73. Iwata T, Popescu NC, Zimonjic DB, et al. Structural organization of the human sorbitol dehydrogenase gene (SORD). Genomics 1995;26:55–62.
74. Karlsson C, Jörnvall H, Höög J-O. Sorbitol dehydrogenase: cDNA coding for the rat enzyme. Variations within the alcohol dehydrogenase family independent of quaternary structure and metal content. Eur J Biochem 1991;198:761–765.
75. Wen Y, Bekhor I. Sorbitol dehydrogenase. Full-length cDNA sequencing reveals a mRNA coding for a protein containing an additional 42 amino acids at the N-terminal end. Eur J Biochem 1993;217:83–87.
76. Warpeha KM, Chakravarthy U. Molecular genetics of microvascular disease in diabetic retinopathy. Eye 2003;17:305–311.
77. Demaine A, Cross D. Genetics of aldose reductase and susceptibility to diabetic retinopathy. Appl Genomics Proteomics 2002;3:137–149.
78. Yang B, Millward A, Demaine A. Functional differences between the susceptibility Z−2/C−106 and protective Z + 2/T−106 promoter region polymorphisms of the aldose reductase gene may account for the association with diabetic microvascular complications. Biochim Biophys Acta 2003;1639:1–7.
79. Santos KG, Canani LH, Gross JL, Tschiedel B, Souto KE, Roisenberg I. The −106CC genotype of the aldose reductase gene is associated with an increased risk of proliferative diabetic retinopathy in Caucasian-Brazilians with Type 2 diabetes. Mol Genet Metab 2006;88:280–284.
80. Shah VO, Dorin RI, Sun Y, Braun M, Zager PG. Aldose reductase gene expression is increased in diabetic nephropathy. J Clin Endocrinol Metab 1997;82:2294–2298.
81. Ikegishi Y, Tawata M, Aida K, Onaya T. Z–4 allele upstream of the aldose reductase gene is associated with proliferative retinopathy in Japanese patients with NIDDM, and elevated luciferase gene transcription in vitro. Life Sci 1999;65:2061–2070.
82. Oishi N, Kubo E, Takamura Y, Maekawa K, Tanimoto T, Akagi Y. Correlation between erythrocyte aldose reductase level and human diabetic retinopathy. Brit J Ophthalmol 2002;86:1363–1366.
83. Zou X, Lu J, Pan C. Effect of polymorphism of (AC)n in the 5′-end of aldose reductase gene on erythrocyte aldose reductase activity in patients with type 2 diabetes mellitus. Chin J Endocrinol Metabol 2000;16:346–349.
84. Yagihashi S, Yamagishi SI, Wada Ri R, et al. Neuropathy in diabetic mice overexpressing human aldose reductase and effects of aldose reductase inhibitor. Brain 2001;124:2448–2458.
85. Yamaoka T, Nishimura C, Yamashita K, et al. Acute onset of diabetic pathological changes in transgenic mice with human aldose reductase cDNA. Diabetologia 1995;38:255–261.
86. Amano S, Yamagishi S, Kato N, et al. Sorbitol dehydrogenase overexpression potentiates glucose toxicity to cultured retinal pericytes. Biochem Biophys Res Commun 2002;299:183–188.
87. Cheung AK, Fung MK, Lo AC, et al. Aldose reductase deficiency prevents diabetes-induced blood-retinal barrier breakdown, apoptosis, and glial reactivation in the retina of db/db mice. Diabetes 2005;54:3119–3125.
88. Cheung AKH, Lo ACY, Chung SSM, Chung SK. Aldose reductase-deficient mice were protected from the neuro-retinal injury after carotid artery transient ischemia. FASEB J 2006;20:A639.

89. Hwang YC, Kaneko M, Bakr S, et al. Central role for aldose reductase pathway in myocardial ischemic injury. FASEB J 2004;18:1192–1199.
90. Ng TF, Lee FK, Song ZT, et al. Effects of sorbitol dehydrogenase deficiency on nerve conduction in experimental diabetic mice. Diabetes 1998;47:961–966.
91. Ludvigson MA, Sorenson RL. Immunohistochemical localization of aldose reductase. Ii. Rat eye and kidney. Diabetes 1980;29:450–459.
92. Chakrabarti S, Sima AA, Nakajima T, Yagihashi S, Greene DA. Aldose reductase in the BB rat: Isolation, immunological identification and localization in the retina and peripheral nerve. Diabetologia 1987;30:244–251.
93. Kern TS, Engerman RL. Distribution of aldose reductase in ocular tissues. Exp Eye Res 1981;33:175–182.
94. Hamada Y, Araki N, Koh N, Nakamura J, Horiuchi S, Hotta N. Rapid formation of advanced glycation end products by intermediate metabolites of glycolytic pathway and polyol pathway. Biochem Biophys Res Commun 1996;228:539–543.
95. Ahmed N, Thornalley PJ. Advanced glycation endproducts: What is their relevance to diabetic complications? Diabetes Obes Metab 2007;9:233–245.
96. Kador PF, Kinoshita JH, Sharpless NE. Aldose reductase inhibitors: A potential new class of agents for the pharmacological control of certain diabetic complications. J Med Chem 1985;28:841–849.
97. Burg MB, Kwon ED, Kultz D. Regulation of gene expression by hypertonicity. Annu Rev Physiol 1997;59:437–455.
98. Burg MB. Coordinate regulation of organic osmolytes in renal cells. Kid Int 1996;49:1684–1685.
99. Gabbay KH. The sorbitol pathway and the complications of diabetes. N Engl J Med 1973;288:831–836.
100. Lee AY, Chung SK, Chung SS. Demonstration that polyol accumulation is responsible for diabetic cataract by the use of transgenic mice expressing the aldose reductase gene in the lens. Proc Natl Acad Sci USA 1995;92:2780–2784.
101. Obrosova IG, Minchenko AG, Vasupuram R, et al. Aldose reductase inhibitor fidarestat prevents retinal oxidative stress and vascular endothelial growth factor overexpression in streptozotocin-diabetic rats. Diabetes 2003;52:864–871.
102. Barnett PA, Gonzalez RG, Chylack LT, Jr., Cheng HM. The effect of oxidation on sorbitol pathway kinetics. Diabetes 1986;35:426–432.
103. Newsholme EA, Start C. Regulation in metabolism. Chichester: John Wiley & Sons Ltd.; 1973.
104. Kil IS, Lee YS, Bae YS, Huh TL, Park JW. Modulation of NADP(+)-dependent isocitrate dehydrogenase in aging. Redox Rep 2004;9:271–277.
105. Winkler BS, DeSantis N, Solomon F. Multiple NADPH-producing pathways control glutathione (GSH) content in retina. Exp Eye Res 1986;43:829–847.
106. Gerhardinger C, McClure KD, Romeo G, Podesta F, Lorenzi M. IGF-i mRNA and signaling in the diabetic retina. Diabetes 2001;50:175–183.
107. Williamson JR, Chang K, Frangos M, et al. Hyperglycemic pseudohypoxia and diabetic complications. Diabetes 1993;42:801–813.
108. Graymore CN, Towlson MJ. The metabolism of the retina of the normal and alloxan diabetic rat. The levels of oxidised and reduced pyridine nucleotides and the oxidation of the carbon-1 and carbon-6 of glucose. Vision Res 1966;5:379–389.
109. Heath H, Kang SS, Philippou D. Glucose, glucose-6-phosphate, lactate and pyruvate content of the retina, blood and liver of streptozotocin-diabetic rats fed sucrose- or starch-rich diets. Diabetologia 1975;11:57–62.
110. Tilton RG, Chang K, Nyengaard JR, Van den Enden M, Ido Y, Williamson JR. Inhibition of sorbitol dehydrogenase: Effects on vascular and neural dysfunction in streptozocin-induced diabetic rats. Diabetes 1995;44:234–242.
111. Salceda R, Vilchis C, Coffe V, Hernandez-Munoz R. Changes in the redox state in the retina and brain during the onset of diabetes in rats. Neurochem Res 1998;23:893–897.
112. Nyengaard JR, Ido Y, Kilo C, Williamson JR. Interactions between hyperglycemia and hypoxia: Implications for diabetic retinopathy. Diabetes 2004;53:2931–2938.
113. Diederen RM, Starnes CA, Berkowitz BA, Winkler BS. Reexamining the hyperglycemic pseudohypoxia hypothesis of diabetic oculopathy. Invest Ophthalmol Vis Sci 2006;47:2726–2731.

114. Ola MS, Berkich DA, Xu Y, et al. Analysis of glucose metabolism in diabetic rat retinas. Am J Physiol 2006;290:E1057–E1067.
115. Williamson JR, Ido Y, Kilo C, Tilton RG. Hyperglycemic pseudohypoxia and Diabetes Complications: Sorbitol pathway–generated NADHc mediates Diabetes Complications. In: Robertson RP, ed. Commentaries on perspectives in Diabetes, vol. 2. Alexandria, VA: Am Diabetes Assoc 2006:39–41.
116. Ido Y. Pyridine nucleotide redox abnormalities in diabetes. Antiox Redox Signal 2007;9:931–942.
117. Griendling KK, Sorescu D, Ushio-Fukai M. NAD(P)H oxidase: Role in cardiovascular biology and disease. Circ Res 2000;86:494–501.
118. Pacher P, Beckman JS, Liaudet L. Nitric oxide and peroxynitrite in health and disease. Physiol Rev 2007;87:315–424.
119. Zheng L, Du Y, Miller C, et al. Critical role of inducible nitric oxide synthase in degeneration of retinal capillaries in mice with streptozotocin-induced diabetes. Diabetologia 2007;50:1987–1996.
120. Brownlee M. The pathobiology of diabetic complications: A unifying mechanism. Diabetes 2005;54:1615–1625.
121. Berry CE, Hare JM. Xanthine oxidoreductase and cardiovascular disease: Molecular mechanisms and pathophysiological implications. J Physiol 2004;555:589–606.
122. Fox NE, van Kuijk FJ. Immunohistochemical localization of xanthine oxidase in human retina. Free Radic Biol Med 1998;24:900–905.
123. Ceriello A, Morocutti A, Mercuri F, et al. Defective intracellular antioxidant enzyme production in type 1 diabetic patients with nephropathy. Diabetes 2000;49:2170–2177.
124. Hodgkinson AD, Bartlett T, Oates PJ, Millward BA, Demaine AG. The response of antioxidant genes to hyperglycemia is abnormal in patients with type 1 diabetes and diabetic nephropathy. Diabetes 2003;52:846–851.
125. Du X, Matsumura T, Edelstein D, et al. Inhibition of GAPDH activity by poly(ADP-ribose) polymerase activates three major pathways of hyperglycemic damage in endothelial cells. J Clin Invest 2003;112:1049–1057.
126. Ramana KV, Friedrich B, Tammali R, West MB, Bhatnagar A, Srivastava SK. Requirement of aldose reductase for the hyperglycemic activation of protein kinase C and formation of diacylglycerol in vascular smooth muscle cells. Diabetes 2005;54:818–829.
127. Keogh RJ, Dunlop ME, Larkins RG. Effect of inhibition of aldose reductase on glucose flux, diacylgylcerol formation, protein kinase C, and phospholipase A–2 activation. Metab Clin Exp 1997;46:41–47.
128. Ishii H, Tada H, Isogai S. An aldose reductase inhibitor prevents glucose-induced increase in transforming growth factor-beta and protein kinase C activity in cultured human mesangial cells. Diabetologia 1998;41:362–364.
129. Inoguchi T, Li P, Umeda F, et al. High glucose level and free fatty acid stimulate reactive oxygen species production through protein kinase C-dependent activation of NAD(P)H oxidase in cultured vascular cells. Diabetes 2000;49:1939–1945.
130. McPherson JD, Shilton BH, Walton DJ. Role of fructose in glycation and cross-linking of proteins. Biochemistry 1988;27:1901–1907.
131. Szwergold BS, Kappler F, Brown TR. Identification of fructose 3-phosphate in the lens of diabetic rats. Science 1990;247:451–454.
132. Hamada Y, Nakamura J, Naruse K, et al. Epalrestat, an aldose reductase ihibitor, reduces the levels of N-epsilon-(carboxymethyl)lysine protein adducts and their precursors in erythrocytes from diabetic patients. Diabetes Care 2000;23:1539–1544.
133. Niwa T, Tsukushi S. 3-deoxyglucosone and AGEs in uremic complications: Inactivation of glutathione peroxidase by 3-deoxyglucosone. Kid Int 2001;59 (Suppl 78):S37–S41.
134. Gonzalez RG, Miglior S, Von SI, Buckley L, Neuringer LJ, Cheng HM. 31P NMR studies of the diabetic lens. Magn Reson Med 1988;6:435–444.
135. Stitt AW, Li YM, Gardiner TA, Bucala R, Archer DB, Vlassara H. Advanced glycation end products (AGEs) co-localize with AGE receptors in the retinal vasculature of diabetic and of AGE-infused rats. Am J Pathol 1997;150:523–531.
136. Yan SD, Schmidt AM, Anderson GM, et al. Enhanced cellular oxidant stress by the interaction of advanced glycation end products with their receptors/binding proteins. J Biol Chem 1994;269:9889–9897.

137. Wautier MP, Chappey O, Corda S, Stern DM, Schmidt AM, Wautier JL. Activation of NADPH oxidase by AGE links oxidant stress to altered gene expression via RAGE. Am J Physiol 2001;280: E685–E694.
138. Zhao W, Diz DI, Robbins ME. Oxidative damage pathways in relation to normal tissue injury. Br J Radiol 2007;80 Spec No 1:S23–S31.
139. Wang X, Martindale JL, Liu Y, Holbrook NJ. The cellular response to oxidative stress: Influences of mitogen-activated protein kinase signalling pathways on cell survival. Biochem J 1998;333: 291–300.
140. Sun W, Oates PJ, Coutcher JB, Gerhardinger C, Lorenzi M. A selective aldose reductase inhibitor of a new structural class prevents or reverses early retinal abnormalities in experimental diabetic retinopathy. Diabetes 2006;55:2757–2762.
141. Mizutani M, Kern TS, Lorenzi M. Accelerated death of retinal microvascular cells in human and experimental diabetic retinopathy. J Clin Invest 1996;97:2883–2890.
142. Barber AJ, Lieth E, Khin SA, Antonetti DA, Buchanan AG, Gardner TW. Neural apoptosis in the retina during experimental and human diabetes. Early onset and effect of insulin. J Clin Invest 1998;102:783–791.
143. Suzen S, Buyukbingol E. Recent studies of aldose reductase enzyme inhibition for diabetic complications. Curr Med Chem 2003;10:1329–1352.
144. Matsuda H, Morikawa T, Toguchida I, Yoshikawa M. Structural requirements of flavonoids and related compounds for aldose reductase inhibitory activity. Chem Pharm Bull (Tokyo) 2002;50:788–795.
145. Eggler JF, Larson ER, Lipinski CA, Mylari BL, Urban FJ. A perspective of aldose reductase inhibitors. Adv Med Chem 1993;2:197–246.
146. Larson ER, Lipinski CA, Sarges R. Medicinal chemistry of aldose reductase inhibitors. Med Res Rev 1988;8:159–186.
147. Matsuoka K, Sakamoto N, Akanuma Y, et al. A long-term effect of epalrestat on motor conduction velocity of diabetic patients: ARI-Diabetes Complications Trial (ADCT). Diabetes Res Clin Pract 2007;77:S263–S268.
148. Tesfaye S. Is epalrestat an effective treatment for diabetic peripheral neuropathy? Nature Clin Pract Endocrinol Metab 2007;3:84.
149. Daiichi Sankyo Co. Ltd. Group Research & Development Pipeline. 2006 March.
150. Eisai Co. Ltd. Investor's meetings. Tokyo, Japan; 2007 July, Oct; 2008 July.
151. Oates PJ. Aldose reductase: Still a compelling target for diabetic neuropathy. Current Drug Targets 2008;9:14–36.
152. Mylari BL, Armento SJ, Beebe DA, et al. A novel series of non-carboxylic acid, non-hydantoin inhibitors of aldose reductase with potent oral activity in diabetic rat models: 6-(5-chloro-3-methylbenzofuran-2-sulfonyl)-2H-pyridazin-3-one and congeners. J Med Chem 2005;48:6326–6339.
153. Singh J, Isobe Y, Brees D, et al. Retinal effects of aldose reductase inhibitor (ARI), PFE-ARI. Proc Int Congr Toxicol 2007:83.
154. Lorenzi M. The polyol pathway as a mechanism for diabetic retinopathy: Attractive, elusive, and resilient. Experimental Diabetes Research 2007;Article ID 61038.
155. Engerman RL, Kern TS. Aldose reductase inhibition fails to prevent retinopathy in diabetic and galactosemic dogs. Diabetes 1993;42:820–825.
156. Cameron NE, Cotter MA. Dissociation between biochemical and functional effects of the aldose reductase inhibitor, ponalrestat, on peripheral nerve in diabetic rats. Br J Pharmacol 1992;107: 939–944.
157. Cameron NE, Cotter MA, Dines KC, Maxfield EK, Carey F, Mirrlees DJ. Aldose reductase inhibition, nerve perfusion, oxygenation and function in streptozotocin-diabetic rats: Dose-response considerations and independence from a myo-inositol mechanism. Diabetologia 1994;37:651–663.
158. Obrosova IG, Szabo C, Stevens MJ, Pacher P. Aldose reductase inhibitor fidarestat alleviates diabetes-induced retinal oxidative-nitrosative stress and poly(ADP-ribose) polymerase activation. Invest Ophthalmol Vis Sci 2005;46:4704.
159. MacGregor LC, Matschinsky FM. Treatment with aldose reductase inhibitor or with myo-inositol arrests deterioration of the electroretinogram of diabetic rats. J Clin Invest 1985;76:887–889.

160. Tilton RG, Chang K, Pugliese G, et al. Prevention of hemodynamic and vascular albumin filtration changes in diabetic rats by aldose reductase inhibitors. Diabetes 1989;37:1258–1270.
161. Chakrabarti S, Sima AAF. Effect of aldose reductase inhibition and insulin treatment on retinal capillary basement membrane thickening in BB rats. Diabetes 1989;38:1181–1186.
162. Kato N, Yashima S, Suzuki T, Nakayama Y, Jomori T. Long-term treatment with fidarestat suppresses the development of diabetic retinopathy in STZ-induced diabetic rats. J Diabetes Complicat 2003;17:374–379.
163. Zhang J, Gerhardinger C, Lorenzi M. Early complement activation and decreased levels of glycosylphosphatidylinositol-anchored complement inhibitors in human and experimental diabetic retinopathy. Diabetes 2002;51:3499–3504.
164. Bringmann A, Uckermann O, Pannicke T, Iandiev I, Reichenbach A, Wiedemann P. Neuronal versus glial cell swelling in the ischaemic retina. Acta Ophthalmol Scand 2005;83:528–538.
165. Iandiev I, Pannicke T, Reichenbach A, Wiedemann P, Bringmann A. Diabetes alters the localization of glial aquaporins in rat retina. Neurosci Lett 2007;421:132–136.
166. Koh YH, Park YS, Takahashi M, Suzuki K, Taniguchi N. Aldehyde reductase gene expression is induced by lipid peroxidation end products, MDA and HNE. Free Radic Res 2000;33:739–746.
167. El-Kabbani O, Podjarny A. Selectivity determinants of the aldose and aldehyde reductase inhibitor-binding sites. Cell Mol Life Sci 2007;DOI 10.1007/s00018–007–6514–3:1–9.
168. Barski OA, Gabbay KH, Grimshaw CE, Bohren KM. Mechanism of human aldehyde reductase: Characterization of the active site pocket. Biochemistry 1995;34:11264–11275.
169. Gerhardinger C, Dagher Z, Sebastiani P, Park YS, Lorenzi M. Overexpression of genes of the TGF-beta pathway in retinal capillaries is the common target of drugs that prevent diabetic retinopathy. Diabetes 2007;56 (Suppl 1):A212.
170. Sorbinil Retinopathy Trial Research Group. A randomized trial of sorbinil, an aldose reductase inhibitor, in diabetic retinopathy. Arch Ophthalmol 1990;108:1234–1244.
171. The Diabetes Control and Complications Trial Research Group. The effect of intensive treatment of diabetes on the development and progression of long-term complications in insulin-dependent diabetes mellitus. N Engl J Med 1993;329:977–986.
172. Vinores SA, Campochiaro PA, Williams EH, May EE, Green WR, Sorenson RL. Aldose reductase expression in human diabetic retina and retinal pigment epithelium. Diabetes 1988;37:1658–1664.
173. Vikramadithyan RK, Hu Y, Noh HL, et al. Human aldose reductase expression accelerates diabetic atherosclerosis in transgenic mice. J Clin Invest 2005;115:2434–2443.
174. Lorenzi M. Mechanisms and strategies for prevention in diabetic retinopathy. Curr Diab Rep 2006;6:102–107.
175. Kador PF. Ocular pathology of Diabetes mellitus. In: Tasman W, Jaeger EA, eds. Duane's Ophthalmology. Philadelphia: Lippincott Williams & Wilkins, 2007.
176. Williams MD, Nadler JL. Inflammatory mechanisms of diabetic complications. Curr Diab Rep 2007;7:242–248.
177. Steuber H, Zentgraf M, Podjarny A, Heine A, Klebe G. High-resolution crystal structure of aldose reductase complexed with the novel sulfony-pyridazinone inhibitor exhibiting an alternative active site anchoring group. J Mol Biol 2006;356:45–56.
178. Oates PJ, Mylari BL. Exp Opin Invest Drugs 1999;8(12):2095–2119.
179. Boeri D, Cagliero E, Podesta F, Lorenzi M. Vascular wall von Willebrand factor in human diabetic retinopathy. Invest Ophthalmol Vis Sci 1994;35:600–607.

7 The Role of Advanced Glycation in Diabetic Retinopathy

Alan W. Stitt

CONTENTS

ABSTRACT

Through intensive laboratory and clinic-based research the complex nature of diabetic retinopathy pathogenesis is becoming better appreciated. Nevertheless, further research is needed to achieve a clear understanding of the cellular and molecular basis of disease initiation and progression. Such advances may lead to effective treatments that not only preserve vision at the late stages of disease but can also prevent retinopathy progression from the point of diabetes diagnosis. This chapter discusses the role that formation and accumulation of advanced glycation endproducts (AGEs) play in diabetic retinopathy. In particular, it will outline our current knowledge about how AGE adducts influence retinal function in diabetes. There will be emphasis placed on the modulatory role of AGE receptors and useful new therapeutic approaches to inhibit AGE formation or harmful receptor interactions in order to prevent diabetic retinopathy.

Key Words: Diabetic retinopathy; pathogenesis; advanced glycation endproducts (AGEs); receptor for AGEs (RAGE); retina; microvasculopathy; AGE inhibitors; therapy

From: *Contemporary Diabetes*: *Diabetic Retinopathy*
Edited by: E. Duh © Humana Press, Totowa, NJ

INTRODUCTION TO DIABETIC RETINOPATHY

In humans the central retinal artery branches into a unique microvascular system that plays a major role in embryological development of the retina and other intraocular structures *(1)*. In maturity this microvasculature serves the peculiar metabolic requirements of the unique neuroglial configuration of the retina. Within the vascular unit itself, there is complex crosstalk between the component cells which maintains cell function/survival, blood flow, and the inner blood-retinal barrier (iBRB). For example, the end-artery vascular network of the retina lacks any obvious autonomic nerve supply, and blood flow into the capillary beds is tightly regulated in response to the metabolic needs of the retinal parenchyma. This is achieved, in large part, by the regulatory capacity of the component smooth muscle cells in the retinal arteries and arterioles which are highly sensitive to endothelial-generated vasodilators and vasoconstrictors *(2)*. When these cell relationships are disrupted, as in some pathological situations such as diabetes, the vasculature can become dysfunctional, losing the ability to tightly regulate flow and maintain barrier properties. Vascular cells may eventually die and this leads to progressive nonperfusion of the retina.

Diabetic retinopathy is widely regarded as a quintessential disease of the intraretinal microvasculature, although as diabetes progresses changes may also occur in the choroidal vessels. The vascular-centric view of this disease has led to its clinical classification into two forms: nonproliferative diabetic retinopathy (NPDR) and proliferative diabetic retinopathy (PDR). The nonproliferative form is by far the most common, and in a significant number of cases it progresses to sight-threatening PDR *(3)*. The greatest risk of vision loss occurs in the later phases of diabetic retinopathy with the development of macular edema and/or retinal neovascularization, the former being a direct consequence of iBRB breakdown and the latter to widespread retinal ischemia *(4)*. Retinopathy is the most common microvascular complication suffered by patients with diabetes, and it remains a major cause of visual impairment worldwide *(5)*.

Measurable dysfunction of the retinal microvasculature commences within weeks of diabetes onset in both patients and animal models of diabetic retinopathy. This is characterized by changes to retinal blood flow, impaired autoregulation, and abnormal vasopermeability to plasma proteins *(2, 6)*. As disease duration increases, the nonproliferative phase of diabetic retinopathy is associated with excessive capillary permeability leading to iBRB dysfunction *(7)*, capillary basement membrane (BM) thickening *(8)*, and pericyte/smooth muscle depletion *(9)*. Weakness of capillary walls (perhaps because of pericyte loss) and increased intraluminal pressure probably lead to the formation of microaneurysms which provide a clinically visible, quantifiable lesion in the fundus of diabetic patients. These are often associated with large areas of nonperfusion at the arterial side of the circulation *(10, 11)* (Fig. 1). Progression to the proliferative stage of diabetic retinopathy is linked to widespread ischemia and subsequent upregulation of potent angiogenic growth factors such as VEGF that drive preretinal neovascularization. Presence of new vessels on the retinal surface may lead to retraction of the vitreous from sites of firm fibrovascular adhesion and, if left untreated, can lead to tractional retinal detachment. Also associated with retinal vasodegeneration, diabetic macular edema (DME) is caused by wholesale breakdown of the iBRB and constitutes a major cause of vision loss associated with diabetic retinopathy.

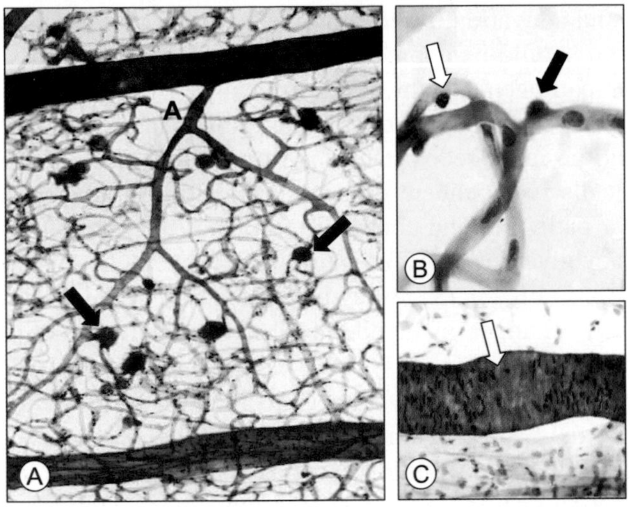

Fig. 1. Histopathology in diabetic retinopathy. (**A**) Trypsin digest prepared from a type-2 diabetic patient indicating widespread demise of smooth muscle from a precapillary arteriole (A), numerous microaneurysms and acellular vessels in the capillary bed downstream of this vessel (*arrows*). Note that the microaneurysms are located at the arterial side of the circulation. (**B**) Trypsin digest of 4-year diabetic dog showing a pericyte ghost stained red by the PAS technique (*black arrow*). A viable pericyte staining strongly with hematoxylin is also apparent on the capillary wall (*white arrow*). (**C**) Diabetes also results in loss of smooth muscle (*arrow*) from arteries and arterioles in the central retina.

Diabetic retinopathy is a progressive disorder, and epidemiological investigations, such as the Wisconsin Epidemiologic Study of Diabetic Retinopathy (WESDR), have demonstrated that patients with more severe baseline lesions show faster progress to vision-threatening retinopathy *(12)*. Failure to regulate blood glucose leads to biochemical abnormalities in diabetic cells and tissues, and the range of pathologic lesions in retina and other vascular beds are indicative of a complex interplay between hyperglycemia-induced metabolic and hemodynamic pathways. Therefore it is important to establish the cellular and molecular basis of disease initiation and progression. Such advances may lead to effective treatments that not only preserve vision at the late stages but also can prevent retinopathy from the point of diabetes diagnosis.

While microvascular dysfunction remains a central tenet of diabetic retinopathy, it should be appreciated that these vessels are intimately linked to retinal neuroglia function. A concurrent retinal "neuropathy" occurs during diabetes that is characterized by early electroretinogram (ERG) defects *(13)*, decreased color contrast sensitivity, neuronal/glial abnormalities and eventual depletion of neurons *(14, 15)*. It is therefore important to always view diabetic retinopathy from the perspective of the entire retina, including both the microvessels and the neuropile they serve *(16)*.

PATHOGENESIS OF DIABETIC RETINOPATHY

Acute or chronic exposure to the diabetic milieu results in a raft of biochemical and metabolic abnormalities, and many related pathogenic mechanisms have been implicated in the progression of diabetic retinopathy. The formation of advanced glycation endproducts (AGEs) and activation of receptors for AGEs constitute the main focus of this chapter, although it should be appreciated that hyperglycemia can simultaneously provoke several other pathogenic pathways in retinal cells. One such mechanism is linked to increased flux through the polyol or hexosamine pathways which is associated with subsequent alterations in the redox state of pyridine nucleotides *(17)*. Accumulation of sorbitol in retinal cells is dependent on activity of aldose reductase, and this may impinge on a range of pathways and contribute to diabetic retinopathy *(18)*. Also, de novo synthesis of diacylglycerol (DAG) leading to the overactivation of several isoforms of protein kinase C (PKC) *(19)*, excessive production of free radicals leading to oxidative stress *(20, 21)*, changes in blood rheology and hemodynamics *(2, 22)*, and overactivation of the renin-angiotensin system (RAS) *(23)* contribute significantly to retinopathy as diabetes progresses. These mechanisms have formed a basis for therapeutic intervention, and the PKC β inhibitor ruboxistaurin holds promise for preventing progression of diabetic retinopathy. While protection was not observed for some aspects of pathology in a recent clinical trial, ruboxistaurin did achieve significant reduction in the vision loss through DME *(24)*.

Pathogenic pathways to diabetic retinopathy continue to be elucidated, but these should not necessarily be viewed as independent phenomena. As an exemplar for this, Brownlee has proposed a unifying concept whereby hyperglycemia increases superoxide production (via the mitochondrial electron transport chain) which in turn initiates accelerated AGE formation and also exacerbates many of the aforementioned pathogenic mechanisms *(25)*. This hypothesis has been reinforced in the field of retinopathy, in which three biochemical abnormalities involving AGE formation, flux through the hexosamine pathway, and DAG-mediated activation of PKC-β have been attenuated using the thiamine derivative benfotiamine. Treatment of diabetic animals with benfotiamine showed a convergent protective effect on three pathways and also inhibited proinflammatory NFκB activation, culminating in effective prevention of key diabetes-related retinal lesions *(26)*. More recently, benefits of this drug have also been demonstrated in retinal microvascular cells exposed to high glucose *in vitro (27)*.

BIOCHEMISTRY OF AGE FORMATION

Excess glucose in cells leads to enhanced nonenzymatic glycation reactions between reducing sugars and the free amino groups on proteins, lipids, and DNA. This is an inevitable consequence of the reactivity of aldehydes and as a consequence nearly all body proteins carry some "burden" of chemically attached carbohydrate. The nature of this chemistry was established as early as 1912 when the food chemist Louis Camille Maillard reported formation of yellow brown products on heating mixtures of amino acids and sugars. The so-called Maillard reaction begins with the formation of a Schiff base between glucose and ε-amino groups (e.g., lysine) that slowly rearranges to relatively stable Amadori adducts (Fig. 2). The most widely known Amadori product is a modification of hemoglobin (HbA1c) which is used clinically as an indicator for cumulative exposure to elevated blood glucose. Both the Schiff base and the Amadori compound can undergo further oxidation and dehydration so that their concentrations ultimately depend on both forward and reverse reactions. The forward reactions give rise to additional protein-bound compounds collectively termed AGEs. During diabetes

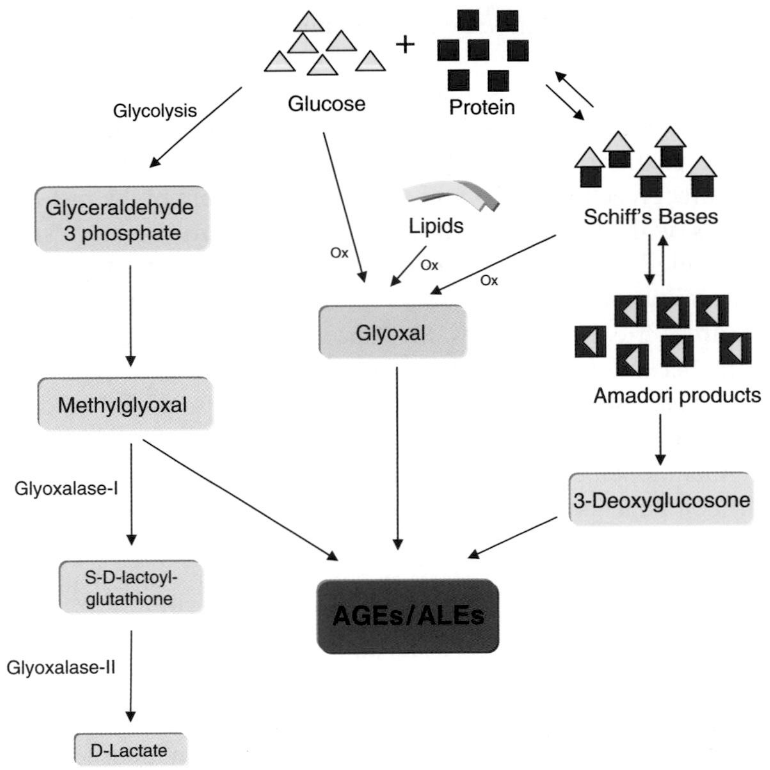

Fig. 2. Simple schematic of AGE formation. AGEs and so-called advanced lipoxidation endproducts (ALEs) can form from glucose or through reactive carbonyl intermediates. Reducing sugars (*triangle*) react with protein amino groups (*square*) to form Schiff bases which may undergo further rearrangements to form Amadori products. These products are reversible but may progress to more stable, irreversible AGEs which may then accumulate. Reactive oxygen and/or nitrogen species can oxidize free or protein-bound carbohydrates and lead to dicarbonyl compounds (examples of which are methylglyoxal and 3-deoxyglucosone – see main text body for details) that can subsequently react with lysine and arginine residues on protein to form AGEs or, if lipid-derived, ALEs.

the rate of formation of AGEs exceeds that predicted by first-order kinetics; thus, over time even modest hyperglycemic events can result in significant accumulation of AGEs on long-lived macromolecules *(28)*.

AGE adducts are irreversible, and their rate of accumulation in tissues depends on a number of factors including longevity of the modified protein, availability of metal ions, and redox balances. AGE formation often leads to crosslinking, pigmentation, and fluorescence of proteins, and their origin from an array of precursor molecules contributes to the heterogeneity of these chemical structures *(28)*. Many AGE adducts have been identified *in vivo* including Nε-(carboxy-methyl) lysine (CML), crossline, pentosidine, furoyl-furanyl imidazole (FFI), hydroimidazolone, 1-alkyl-2-formyl-3,4-glycosyl-pyrrole (AFGP), argpyrimidine, glyoxal lysine dimer (GOLD), and methyl glyoxal lysine dimer (MOLD) *(28, 29)*.

Glucose is much less reactive than α-oxaloaldehydes such as glyoxal (GO), methylglyoxal (MGO), and 3-deoxyglucosone (3-DG) that arise from glycolytic metabolism *(28, 30)* (Fig. 2). The concentrations of these dicarbonyls are significantly raised in cells exposed to high glucose, and they are also elevated in diabetic plasma *(31)*. Dicarbonyls can react directly with protein to yield many of the same structures derived from the Amadori product, and they constitute an important source of intra- and extracellular AGEs *(32)*. For example, fructose-lysine can undergo metal-catalyzed oxidative cleavage giving rise to the irreversible "glycoxidation" product, CML which can also be formed from direct reaction of GO with lysine, independent of the presence of glucose. GO also reacts with arginine residues on protein to form carboxymcthyl-arginine (CMA) *(33)*, while MGO can give rise to the AGEs N(-(carboxyethyl)lysine (CEL) and arginine-hydroimidazolone *(28, 32)*. MGO is also derived from spontaneous elimination of phosphate from triose phosphates, the concentrations of which are increased during hyperglycemia because of the increased flux of glucose through glycolysis.

Cells may have endogenous protection against intracellular reactivity of AGE-forming dicarbonyls and several such "detoxifying" enzymes have been identified. For example, a glutathione-dependent glyoxalase complex (formed from glyoxalase I and glyoxalase II components) acts as an effective detoxification system for GO and MGO *(34)*. The enzyme system catalyzes conversion of MGO to S-D-lactoylglutathione which is subsequently converted to D-lactate by glyoxalase II. Cells that overexpress this enzyme show less accumulation of MGO-derived AGEs *(35)*.

Dyslipidemia is often overlooked as a pathogenic force in diabetic retinopathy *(36)*. Lipid peroxidation reactions can also form a class of Maillard products called advanced lipoxidation endproducts (ALEs), and these are linked to diabetes and dyslipidemia *(37)* (Fig. 2). ALEs may represent an important source of protein modification especially in lipid-rich, highly oxidative environments, such as in the retina. Although understanding about the role of ALEs in diabetic retinopathy lags far behind that which is known about AGEs, these pathogenic adducts deserve more investigation.

PATHOGENIC ROLE OF AGES IN DIABETIC RETINOPATHY

AGEs and Clinical Correlation of Diabetic Retinopathy

The methods for AGE quantification in biological systems are based on analytical and/or immunocytochemical analysis that differ between researchers, and this has produced variable outcomes in a wide range of studies. With this proviso, patient-based studies have demonstrated that the levels of AGEs in serum correlate with the clinical progression of diabetic retinopathy *(38)*. While many reported studies measured a range of ill-defined AGE moieties, others evaluated specific adducts such as CML, pentosidine, crossline, or hydroimidazolone *(39–41)* and found association with diabetic retinopathy. At the same time, some studies have reported no correlation between AGE levels and retinopathy in diabetic patients *(39, 42)*, although the apparent disparity with other studies may be related to variations in patient populations, presence of nephropathy, and/or the nonuniform assays for plasma AGE quantification.

AGE-modified proteins in serum get readily cleared (except during renal dysfunction) and thus may not always provide robust biomarkers for disease. By contrast, modification of extracellular matrix proteins isolated from skin biopsies often provides more meaningful data *(43)*. This is well illustrated by recent investigation of skin AGEs by the Diabetic Control and Complications Trial (DCCT) skin collagen ancillary study group

(44) which has added weight to the assertion that glycation and AGE modifications on long-lived proteins could be associated with progression of diabetic retinopathy. This study followed over 200 patients from the original DCCT for a further 10 years under the auspices of the Epidemiology of Diabetes Interventions and Complications (EDIC) trial *(45)*. It revealed that levels of diabetic retinopathy were significantly less in the group initially maintained under "tight" glycemic control and that these benefits extended far beyond the period of intensive insulin therapy *(45)*. The patients under "conventional" control for the first 10 years maintained a so-called hyperglycemic or metabolic memory and retained a strong association with retinopathic progression. Interestingly, the same memory phenomenon was also shown for retinopathy nearly 20 years previously by Engerman and Kern in variously controlled diabetic dogs *(46)*. CML-modified skin collagen significantly predicted the progression of retinopathy (and nephropathy) even after initiation of intensive insulin therapy *(45)*. Furthermore, the predictive effect of hemoglobin A1c (HbA1c) vanished after adjustment for furosine and CML, suggesting that accumulation of these adducts is an excellent marker for retinopathic progression and could offer a basis for the metabolic memory phenomenon *(44)*.

AGE Accumulation in the Eye

AGEs have been extensively quantified in ocular tissues and shown to be elevated in diabetics when compared to nondiabetic controls. This includes cornea *(47)* and vitreous *(48)*, where the levels of adducts may form an association with diabetic retinopathy *(49)*. In the retina, AGEs and/or late Amadori products have been localized to vascular cells, neurons, and glia of diabetics *(50–55)*. This would be expected to have pathogenic implications for the individual cells and retinal function. Although differential accumulation of AGEs exists in the diabetic retina over the course of life, diabetes significantly enhances the occurrence of these adducts in the vascular and neural tissue components *(54)*.

Effect of AGEs on Retinal Cells

Demise of the retinal microvasculature remains a hallmark lesion of retinopathy in both diabetic animal models and patients *(11)*. Retinal capillaries could be the principal targets for AGE-induced toxicity by several routes (Fig. 3). AGEs induce toxic effects on retinal pericytes by inducing apoptotic death linked to increased oxidative stress *(56)* and depleted superoxide dismutase (SOD) activity. Increases in such oxidative stress along with enhanced levels of ceramide and DAG further contribute to pericyte loss in the retinal capillaries *(57)*. In addition, some studies have indicated that AGEs cause osteoblastic differentiation and calcification in retinal pericytes by the activation of alkaline phosphatases eventually leading to apoptosis *(58)*. Pericytes exposed to AGE-modified basement membrane undergo MAPK-dependent apoptosis *(59)* and show acute attenuation in endothelin-1 (ETA receptor mediated)-induced contraction with subsequent downregulation of ETA receptor signaling suggesting that substrate-derived AGE cross-links could influence pericyte physiology *(60)*. A more recent study shows that the intrinsic glyoxalase I detoxification system is critical for pericyte survival, and under high glucose conditions these cells may undergo rapid apoptosis possibly by the inactivation of glyoxalase by nitric oxide (NO) *(61)*.

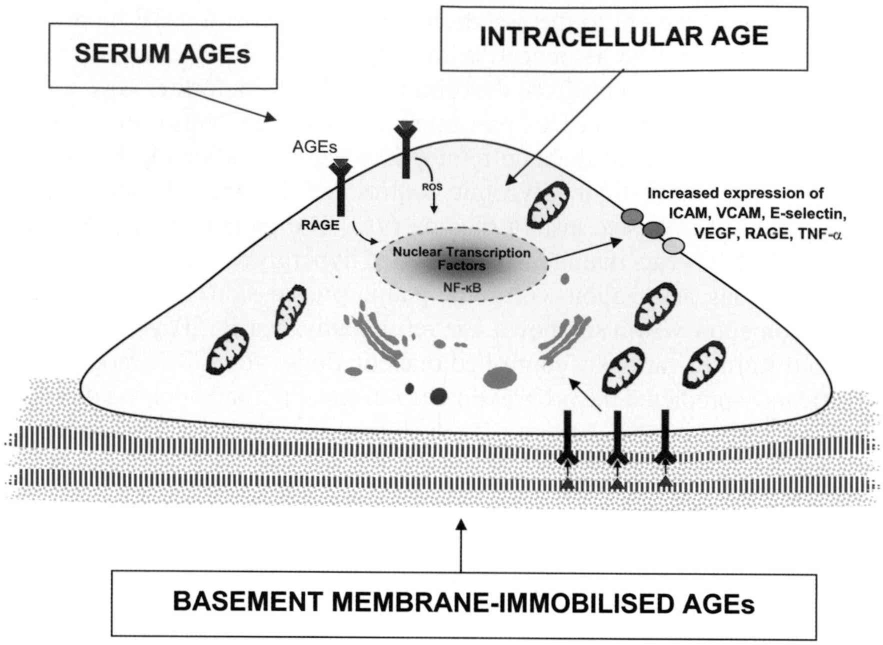

Fig. 3. AGEs interact with vascular cells from three main routes. High glucose can precipitate rapid AGE formation through reaction of intracellular proteins with dicarbonyls or through complex interplay with superoxide radicals released from the mitochondria. AGE-modified serum proteins may interact with vascular endothelium via AGE receptors like RAGE which can activate NFκB transcription leading to enhanced expression of adhesion molecules, TNF-α and VEGF. Serum-derived AGEs reach pericytes via transendothelial trafficking or as a result of blood-retinal barrier dysfunction. These serum AGEs may also interact directly with cell surface glycoproteins with potentially damaging effects on membrane integrity and function. Sedentary cells like endothelium encounter AGEs immobilized on basement membrane where they may influence cell attachment through disruption of integrin signaling. Integrins of various subunit combinations are important for function and ongoing survival cues, and disruption of signaling contributes to dysfunction and death. There are many uncertainties about how AGE adducts immobilized in the basement membrane could interact with RAGE (or other AGE receptors) expressed on the basal plasma membrane, but this may be a significant mode of cell dysfunction.

Retinal microvascular endothelial cells show proangiogenic responses to AGEs at lower concentrations by the involvement of MAPK, PKC, and NF-κB signaling pathways *(62)*, although at higher concentrations these adducts are toxic to endothelial cells *(63)* and in vivo may eventually lead to enhanced microvascular closure *(64)*. Under hyperglycemic conditions retinal endothelial cells accumulate MGO and MGO-derived AGE adducts (such as hydroimidazolone and argpyrimidine) which *in vivo* would contribute to premature closure of capillaries *(65)*. AGEs cause upregulation of ICAM expression, increasing leukocyte adherence and inducing iBRB dysfunction *(66)* (Fig. 3). Exposure of retinal cells to AGEs significantly upregulates expression of VEGF *(67)* and leads to the activation of the hypoxia inducible factor-1 *(68)*.

Beyond microvasculopathy, diabetes also leads to progressive retinal neurovascular dysfunction, and there is accumulating evidence that advanced glycation could play an important role in this pathophysiology. AGEs induce toxicity and subsequent apoptosis in retinal neurons by the activation of inducible nitric oxide synthase (iNOS) *(69)*. In particular, retinal ganglion cells seem sensitive to AGE-induced damage *(70)*. Independent of the complexities of the diabetic milieu, non-diabetic rats which are exposed to “diabetic-like” levels of exogenously formed AGEs show increased retinal VEGF mRNA expression which is linked to concomitant breakdown of the blood-retinal barrier *(66, 71)* (Fig. 4). Similar treatments may cause loss of pericytes *(72)*, and taken together this suggests that high serum levels of AGE-modified proteins may induce lesions that are comparable to those occurring during diabetic retinopathy.

RECEPTORS FOR AGES

It is established that AGEs interact with cell surface receptors and binding proteins to evoke downstream proinflammatory responses that could play a critical role in pathogenesis of diabetic complications *(73–75)*. Depending on the receptor type involved, these proteins may also be involved in important homeostatic functions by clearing/ detoxifying AGE-modified macromolecules from serum and tissues.

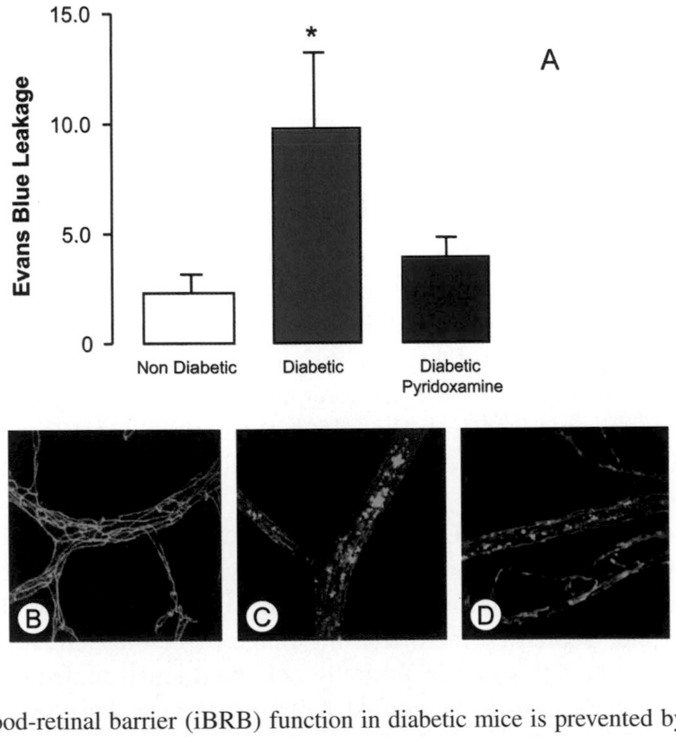

Fig. 4. Inner blood-retinal barrier (iBRB) function in diabetic mice is prevented by AGE inhibition. (**A**) The Evans blue assay for retinal vasopermeability shows that diabetic animals demonstrate an increased BRB dysfunction when compared to nondiabetic controls ($*p < 0.05$). Diabetic mice treated with the AGE inhibitor, pyridoxamine, do not show this vasopermeability response and are comparable to nondiabetic controls. (**B**) Fluorescent immunostaining for occludin-1 of retinal flatmounts from nondiabetic mice shows plasma membrane localization at the tight junctions of the endothelium. (**C**) Diabetics show the same gross amounts of occludin-1, but the protein appears aggregated in the cytoplasm of endothelial cells rather than at the plasma membrane. (**D**) Pyridoxamine-treated diabetic mice partially prevent disruption of the tight junction integrity (original magnification ×200).

The 35-kDa receptor for AGE (RAGE) is the best characterized AGE-receptor protein and was originally identified in endothelium, although it is now known to be present in multiple vascular, neural, and cardiac tissues *(76)*. RAGE acts as a signaling receptor for at least two distinct AGEs: CML *(77)* and hydroimidazolone adducts *(29)*. These ligands can evoke proinflammatory signaling cascades mediated through NF-κB transcriptional activation and leading to oxidative stress and upstream expression of molecules such as ICAM-1/VCAM-1 *(78, 79)*. A naturally occurring soluble fragment of RAGE (sRAGE) can block AGE receptor binding and effectively suppress vasculopathy. This may form an important endogenous regulatory mechanism for RAGE-mediated inflammation since it has been shown that patients with coronary artery disease *(80)* and diabetic complications *(81)* have low endogenous sRAGE.

It should be appreciated that RAGE is a promiscuous receptor and can bind many non-AGE ligands, including amphoterin *(82)* and amyloid beta peptide *(83)*. RAGE also binds to members of the S100/calgranulin family whose interaction on endothelium, mononuclear phagocytes, and lymphocytes trigger cellular activation and inflammation *(84)*. S100A12 (Extracellular novel RAGE binding protein (EN-RAGE)) acts as an important ligand for RAGE with these interactions reported to be increased in patients with type 2 diabetes *(85)*. EN-RAGE is induced by IL-6 exposure via the JAK-STAT kinase pathway, while activation of the peroxisome proliferators activator receptor gamma (PPARγ) inhibits its production of EN-RAGE in macrophages *(86)*. Binding of EN-RAGE to RAGE induces strong inflammatory stimuli by producing cytokines like IL-8, TNF-α *(87)* which are linked to atherosclerosis *(88)* and vascular hyperplasia *(89)*.

RAGE in Diabetic Retinopathy

There appears to be significant activation of the proinflammatory RAGE axis among the patients with PDR and proliferative vitreoretinopathy which may be associated with concurrent presence of AGE ligands *(90)*. Hyperglycemic mice exhibit enhanced RAGE expression in the inner retina, particularly in Muller cells, which show elevated receptor levels at the vitreoretinal surface *(91)*. This opens a further new paradigm for possible RAGE-mediated involvement in retinal neuropathic abnormalities during diabetes, and recent studies have indicated a role for the receptor in Muller cell dysfunction *(92)*.

Modulation of the AGE-RAGE axis has therapeutic potential as demonstrated by sRAGE efficacy against diabetes-related neuronal dysfunction and vascular lesions in mice *(92)*. The clinical potential for reducing RAGE signaling in the cells of the diabetic retina is further underscored by the increasing range of new RAGE-regulating agents. One such agent is TTP488 which is an orally delivered small molecule that has completed a Phase IIa study in patients with Alzheimer's disease. This "RAGE-blocker" is also being evaluated in the Phase II trial for the patients with diabetic nephropathy, while another large molecule TTP4000 may soon enter Phase I clinical trials *(93)*. These agents are exciting because they directly address RAGE-ligand binding and show great potential for diabetic complications although their role in retinopathy requires assessment.

Some commonly used diabetes drugs such as thiazolidinediones (Rosiglitazone) *(94)* or calcium channel blockers like nifedipine *(95)* reduce RAGE expression in endothelial cells and could serve to limit proinflammatory effects of AGEs. In particular,

Rosiglitazone can inhibit neointimal hyperplasia via downregulation of RAGE expression in aortic smooth muscle cells *(96)*. 3-Hydroxy-3-methylglutaryl coenzyme A reductase inhibitors (statins) may also lead to a reduction in AGE-RAGE elicited angiogenesis via suppression of VEGF *(97)*. Moreover, angiotensin II receptor blockers (ARB) can reduce RAGE expression which should be factored into the benefit that these agents have in preventing diabetic retinopathy *(98)*. This observation is further elucidated by recent work which suggests AGEs activate chymase-dependent alternative pathway contributing to more than 70% of production of angiotensin II production which was inhibited by the use of neutralizing antibodies for RAGE *(99)*. In addition to the downregulation of RAGE and concomitant reduction in oxidative stress, an important ARB, Telmisartan, also acts as selective modulator of PPARγ which suggests some crosstalk between AGE-RAGE system and PPARγ modulation *(100)*. Thus a complex interplay between enhanced levels of AGEs, suppressed antioxidant status, and upregulation of RAGE axis may together play a pivotal role in the progression of diabetic retinopathy.

Other AGE Receptors in Diabetic Retinopathy

While RAGE biology is well established, other AGE receptors may also play an important pathogenic role in diabetic complications in general and retinopathy in particular. So-called AGE-R1 and AGE-R2 are expressed on the plasma membrane of endothelium, monocytes/macrophages, T lymphocytes, neurons, glia, renal cells, and smooth muscle *(101)*. AGE-R1 serves as both cell surface and intracellular binding/transporting protein and may have a negative regulatory influence on RAGE and therefore serve to reduce proinflammatory responses *(102)*. AGE-R2 may act as a substrate for PKC *(103)* and have role in intracellular signaling leading to cytokine and growth factor secretion associated with AGE receptor binding *(104)*. Galectin-3, also termed AGE-R3, is a member of beta-galactoside-binding lectin family present in foam cells of the atherosclerotic lesion *(105)*. AGE-R3 is capable of promoting high molecular weight complex formation with AGE ligands and with other membrane receptor molecules on the cell surface *(106)*. AGE-R3 lacks a signal sequence indicating that this protein probably requires association with other members of the complex (AGE-R1 and AGE-R2) to operate *(106)*. AGE-R3-deficient mice develop more severe renal lesions in the presence of diabetes as compared to wild-type counterparts suggesting an important protective role for this protein in AGE-induced tissue injury *(107, 108)*. This response may be tissue-specific since AGE-R3 shows an opposing response in the context of retinal angiogenic repair mechanisms. AGE-treated wild-type diabetic mice show enhanced retinal ischemia, an effect which is abolished in AGE-R3 knock out animals *(64)*.

AGE-modified proteins may also bind to the class A scavenger receptor (SR-A), class B scavenger receptors like CD36, SR-BI, Type D scavenger receptor LOX-1 and the fasciclin EGF-like, laminin-type EGF-like, and link domain-containing scavenger receptor-1 (FEEL-1) *(109, 110)*. CD36 mediates endocytic uptake of AGEs and subsequent degradation and in addition to AGE interactions may serve as a major receptor for oxidized LDL in macrophages and smooth-muscle-derived foam cells in atherosclerotic lesions *(111)*. The role of CD36 in diabetic retinopathy remains largely unknown.

ANTI-AGE STRATEGIES FOR DIABETIC RETINOPATHY

In recent years there have been many approaches to protect against AGE formation, reduce AGE receptor signaling cascades, or sever established AGE crosslinks. These treatments not only offer an important insight into the pathogenic role of AGEs in diabetic retinopathy but also have translational potential for the treatment of patients.

Amadori product formation is an important basis of Maillard chemistry in biological systems because progression to AGE formation requires chemical rearrangement to create reactive intermediates. An important pharmacological strategy for the inhibition of this process commenced with the small nucleophilic hydrazine compound aminoguanidine (Pimagedine) *(112)* (Fig. 5). This drug is a potent inhibitor

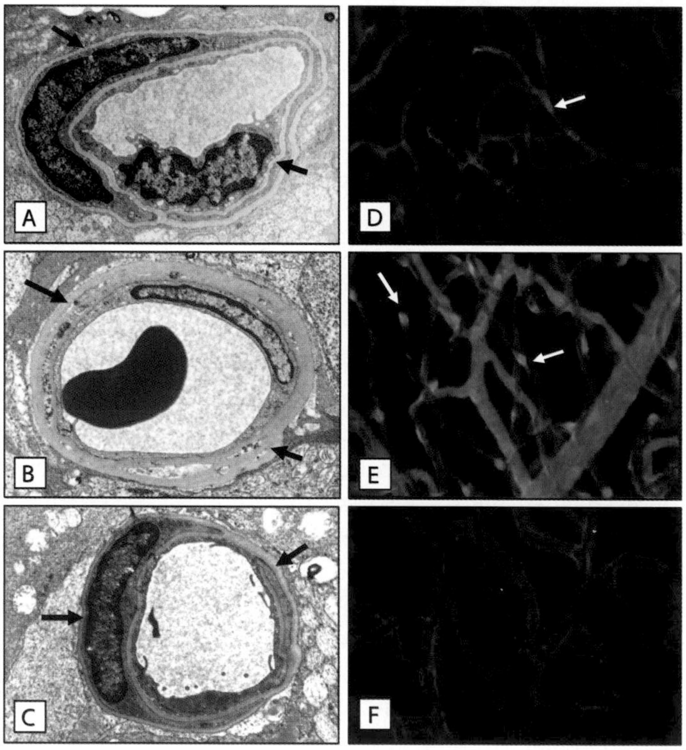

Fig. 5. Basement membrane thickening and AGE immunoreactivity in diabetic rat retina. Transmission electron microscopy (TEM) of rat retina shows that retinal capillary basement membranes (BMs) (*arrows*) are susceptible to thickening during 12 months of diabetes (compare nondiabetic (**A**), with diabetic (**B**)). Treatment of diabetic rat with the AGE inhibitor aminoguanidine protects against diabetes-related BM thickening (**C**)). Trypsin digest preparations were evaluated for AGE immunoreactivity using an AGE-specific monoclonal antibody. The retinal microvasculature of 12-month-old nondiabetic rats demonstrates some AGE immunoreactivity which is largely within the vascular BM, as indicated by diffuse fluorescence (*arrow*) (**D**). Twelve-month diabetic rat retinal vessels show intense AGE immunoreactivity, localized particularly in the retinal arteries and arterioles (**E**). The cell bodies of the retinal pericytes show high levels of AGEs when compared to controls (*arrows*). Treatment of diabetic rats with aminoguanidine for the duration of diabetes reduces AGE immunoreactivity within the cells and vessel walls (**F**).

of AGE-mediated crosslinking and has been shown to prevent diabetic vascular complications in experimental animals *(113)*, including diabetic retinopathy *(50, 114–117)*. Aminoguanidine has been evaluated in a multicenter clinical trial where it failed to achieve statistically significant lowering of serum creatinine, but showed positive signs toward slowing the progression of overt nephropathy and retinopathy progression *(118)*.

For many patients there will have been extensive AGE formation at the time of diabetes diagnosis. Therefore it would be beneficial to attack established AGE crosslinks in tissues. This constitutes an exciting approach since it would "break" pre-accumulated AGEs and subsequently allow their clearance via the kidney. An AGE crosslink "breaker" prototype has been described to attack dicarbonyl-derived crosslinks in vitro *(119)*, and there are now at least two such (related) chemical agents with reported ability to reduce tissue AGEs in experimental diabetes *(120, 121)*. The compound ALT-711 has been shown to ameliorate myocardial stiffness in aged dogs *(122)* and improve the ability of carotid arteries to expand during systole in diabetic rats *(121)*. In preliminary clinical trials, ALT-711 modestly improved arterial compliance in aged patients with measurable cardiovascular stiffening *(113)*. The effects of ALT-711 on retinopathy have yet to be evaluated.

Compounds with post-Amadori product scavenging potential offer therapeutic potential since this is an important route for AGE formation in vivo. So-called Amadorins have an ability to scavenge reactive carbonyls and therefore inhibit the conversion of Amadori intermediates to AGEs and also ALEs *(37, 123)*. Aminoguanidine possesses no scavenging properties *(123, 124)*, but it has been found that the derivative of vitamin B6, pyridoxamine (Pyridorin™), is an efficacious and specific post-Amadori inhibitor *(37, 124, 125)*, with the ability to prevent renal dysfunction in diabetic rats *(126)*. Also in rats, pyridoxamine successfully reduced retinal AGE accumulation and also prevented upregulation of BM-associated genes and diabetes-associated capillary acellularity *(127)*.

CONCLUSION

Initiation and progression of retinopathy reflect the multifactorial nature of metabolic upset within the diabetic milieu leading to activation of many inter-related pathogenic pathways. Long-term management of retinopathy in the ever-expanding number of diabetic patients will involve precise regulation of their glycemic, vasotensive, and lipidemic profiles, hopefully in combination with drugs that ameliorate an array of biochemical and metabolic abnormalities. Experimental work suggests that AGE formation and activation of AGE receptors represent a key pathogenic mechanism in diabetic retinopathy, and inhibition of these pathways presents a valid avenue for therapeutic exploitation (Fig. 6). As our knowledge of Maillard chemistry and its biological impact improves, alongside clear elucidation of AGE-receptor signaling, there are likely to be exciting new opportunities for therapeutic management of diabetic retinopathy at all stages of the disease.

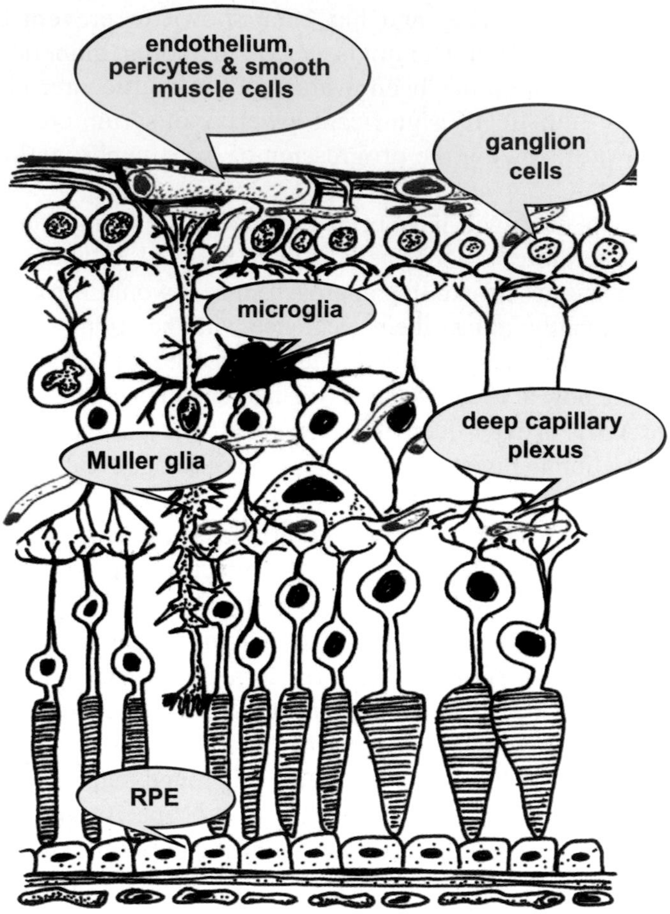

Fig. 6. Potential targets for AGE accumulation and RAGE activation in retina AGE accumulation and RAGE (mRNA and protein) expression has been shown in numerous cell types in the mammalian retina. This stylized retina indicates the various component cells that could represent possible pathogenic targets for AGE accumulation and resultant cell dysfunction. They may also represent the therapeutic targets for agents that can prevent RAGE ligand binding and/or signaling cascades. All cell types depicted have shown AGE accumulation in retina (or in comparable cells in brain, e.g., microglia) and have the potential to be activated by several RAGE ligands (not just AGEs). This could evoke prooxidant or proinflammatory pathogenic responses that are relevant to diabetic retinopathy.

REFERENCES

1. Saint-Geniez M, D'Amore PA. Development and pathology of the hyaloid, choroidal and retinal vasculature. Int J Dev Biol 2004;48(8–9):1045–58.
2. Schmetterer L, Wolzt M. Ocular blood flow and associated functional deviations in diabetic retinopathy. Diabetologia 1999;42(4):387–405.
3. Klein R, Klein BE, Moss SE. Epidemiology of proliferative diabetic retinopathy. Diabetes Care 1992;15(12):1875–91.
4. Frank RN. Diabetic retinopathy. N Engl J Med 2004;350(1):48–58.
5. Marshall SM, Flyvbjerg A. Prevention and early detection of vascular complications of diabetes. BMJ 2006;333(7566):475–80.

6. McMillan DE. The microcirculation in diabetes. Microcirc Endothelium Lymphatics 1984;1(1):3–24.
7. Antonetti DA, Lieth E, Barber AJ, Gardner TW. Molecular mechanisms of vascular permeability in diabetic retinopathy. Semin Ophthalmol 1999;14(4):240–8.
8. Stitt AW, Anderson HR, Gardiner TA, Archer DB. Diabetic retinopathy: quantitative variation in capillary basement membrane thickening in arterial or venous environments. Br J Ophthalmol 1994;78(2):133–7.
9. vom Hagen F, Feng Y, Hillenbrand A, et al. Early loss of arteriolar smooth muscle cells: more than just a pericyte loss in diabetic retinopathy. Exp Clin Endocrinol Diabetes 2005;113(10):573–6.
10. Stitt AW, Gardiner TA, Archer DB. Histological and ultrastructural investigation of retinal microaneurysm development in diabetic patients. Br J Ophthalmol 1995;79(4):362–7.
11. Gardiner TA, Archer DB, Curtis TM, Stitt AW. Arteriolar involvement in the microvascular lesions of diabetic retinopathy: implications for pathogenesis. Microcirculation 2007;14(1):25–38.
12. Klein BE, Davis MD, Segal P, et al. Diabetic retinopathy. Assessment of severity and progression. Ophthalmology 1984;91(1):10–7.
13. Tzekov R, Arden GB. The electroretinogram in diabetic retinopathy. Surv Ophthalmol 1999;44(1):53–60.
14. Lieth E, Gardner TW, Barber AJ, Antonetti DA. Retinal neurodegeneration: early pathology in diabetes. Clin Experiment Ophthalmol 2000;28(1):3–8.
15. Garner A. Histopathology of diabetic retinopathy in man. Eye 1993;7(Pt 2):250–3.
16. Antonetti DA, Barber AJ, Bronson SK, et al. Diabetic retinopathy: seeing beyond glucose-induced microvascular disease. Diabetes 2006;55(9):2401–11.
17. Tilton RG CK, Pugliese G, Eades DM, Province MA, Sherman WR, Kilo C, Williamson JR. Prevention of hemodynamlemma and vascular albumin filtration changes in diabetic rats by aldose reductase inhibitors. Diabetes 1989;38(10):1258–70.
18. Sun W, Oates PJ, Coutcher JB, Gerhardinger C, Lorenzi M. A selective aldose reductase inhibitor of a new structural class prevents or reverses early retinal abnormalities in experimental diabetic retinopathy. Diabetes 2006;55(10):2757–62.
19. Curtis TM, Scholfield CN. The role of lipids and protein kinase Cs in the pathogenesis of diabetic retinopathy. Diabetes Metab Res Rev 2004;20(1):28–43.
20. Obrosova IG, Minchenko AG, Marinescu V, et al. Antioxidants attenuate early up regulation of retinal vascular endothelial growth factor in streptozotocin-diabetic rats. Diabetologia 2001;44(9):1102–10.
21. Kowluru RA, Atasi L, Ho YS. Role of mitochondrial superoxide dismutase in the development of diabetic retinopathy. Invest Ophthalmol Vis Sci 2006;47(4):1594–9.
22. Tooke J. Possible pathophysiological mechanisms for diabetic angiopathy in type 2 diabetes. J Diabetes Complicat 2000;14(4):197–200.
23. Miyata T, van Ypersele de Strihou C. Angiotensin II receptor blockers and angiotensin converting enzyme inhibitors: implication of radical scavenging and transition metal chelation in inhibition of advanced glycation end product formation. Arch Biochem Biophys 2003;419(1):50–4.
24. PKC-DRS2 Group, Aiello LP, Davis MD, et al. Effect of Ruboxistaurin on Visual Loss in Patients with Diabetic Retinopathy. Ophthalmology 2006.
25. Brownlee M. Biochemistry and molecular cell biology of diabetic complications. Nature 2001;414(6865):813–20.
26. Hammes HP, Du X, Edelstein D, et al. Benfotiamine blocks three major pathways of hyperglycemic damage and prevents experimental diabetic retinopathy. Nat Med 2003;9(3):294–9.
27. Berrone E, Beltramo E, Solimine C, Ape AU, Porta M. Regulation of intracellular glucose and polyol pathway by thiamine and benfotiamine in vascular cells cultured in high glucose. J Biol Chem 2006;281(14):9307–13.
28. Thorpe SR, Baynes JW. Maillard reaction products in tissue proteins: New products and new perspectives. Amino Acids 2003;25(3–4):275–81.
29. Goldin A, Beckman JA, Schmidt AM, Creager MA. Advanced glycation end products: sparking the development of diabetic vascular injury. Circulation 2006;114(6):597–605.
30. Lal S, Szwergold BS, Taylor AH, et al. Metabolism of fructose-3-phosphate in the diabetic rat lens. Arch Biochem Biophys 1995;318(1):191–9.

31. Odani H, Shinzato T, Matsumoto Y, Usami J, Maeda K. Increase in three alpha,beta-dicarbonyl compound levels in human uremic plasma: specific in vivo determination of intermediates in advanced Maillard reaction. Biochem Biophys Res Commun 1999;256(1):89–93.
32. Thornalley PJ, Langborg A, Minhas HS. Formation of glyoxal, methylglyoxal and 3-deoxyglucosone in the glycation of proteins by glucose. Biochem J 1999;344 (Pt 1):109–16.
33. Glomb MA, Pfahler C. Amides are novel protein modifications formed by physiological sugars. J Biol Chem 2001;276(45):41638–47.
34. Kuhla B, Luth HJ, Haferburg D, Boeck K, Arendt T, Munch G. Methylglyoxal, glyoxal, and their detoxification in Alzheimer's disease. Ann N Y Acad Sci 2005;1043:211–6.
35. Shinohara M, Thornalley PJ, Giardino I, et al. Overexpression of glyoxalase-I in bovine endothelial cells inhibits intracellular advanced glycation endproduct formation and prevents hyperglycemia-induced increases in macromolecular endocytosis. J Clin Invest 1998;101(5):1142–7.
36. Yu Y, Lyons TJ. A lethal tetrad in diabetes: hyperglycemia, dyslipidemia, oxidative stress, and endothelial dysfunction. Am J Med Sci 2005;330(5):227–32.
37. Onorato JM, Jenkins AJ, Thorpe SR, Baynes JW. Pyridoxamine, an inhibitor of advanced glycation reactions, also inhibits advanced lipoxidation reactions. Mechanism of action of pyridoxamine. J Biol Chem 2000;275(28):21177–84.
38. Ono Y, Aoki S, Ohnishi K, Yasuda T, Kawano K, Tsukada Y. Increased serum levels of advanced glycation end-products and diabetic complications. Diabetes Res Clin Pract 1998;41(2):131–7.
39. Sugiyama S, Miyata T, Ueda Y, et al. Plasma levels of pentosidine in diabetic patients: an advanced glycation end product. J Am Soc Nephrol 1998;9(9):1681–8.
40. Yamaguchi M, Nakamura N, Nakano K, et al. Immunochemical quantification of crossline as a fluorescent advanced glycation endproduct in erythrocyte membrane proteins from diabetic patients with or without retinopathy. Diabet Med 1998;15(6):458–62.
41. Fosmark DS, Torjesen PA, Kilhovd BK, et al. Increased serum levels of the specific advanced glycation end product methylglyoxal-derived hydroimidazolone are associated with retinopathy in patients with type 2 diabetes mellitus. Metabolism 2006;55(2):232–6.
42. Wagner Z, Wittmann I, Mazak I, et al. N(epsilon)-(carboxymethyl)lysine levels in patients with type 2 diabetes: role of renal function. Am J Kidney Dis 2001;38(4):785–91.
43. Sell DR, Lapolla A, Odetti P, Fogarty J, Monnier VM. Pentosidine formation in skin correlates with severity of complications in individuals with long-standing IDDM. Diabetes 1992;41(10):1286–92.
44. Genuth S, Sun W, Cleary P, et al. Glycation and carboxymethyllysine levels in skin collagen predict the risk of future 10-year progression of diabetic retinopathy and nephropathy in the diabetes control and complications trial and epidemiology of diabetes interventions and complications participants with type 1 diabetes. Diabetes 2005;54(11):3103–11.
45. Team W. Effect of intensive therapy on the microvascular complications of type 1 diabetes mellitus. Jama 2002;287(19):2563–9.
46. Engerman RL, Kern TS. Progression of incipient diabetic retinopathy during good glycemic control. Diabetes 1987;36(7):808–12.
47. Sato E, Mori F, Igarashi S, et al. Corneal advanced glycation end products increase in patients with proliferative diabetic retinopathy. Diabetes Care 2001;24(3):479–82.
48. Stitt AW, Moore JE, Sharkey JA, et al. Advanced glycation end products in vitreous: Structural and functional implications for diabetic vitreopathy. Invest Ophthalmol Vis Sci 1998;39(13):2517–23.
49. Fosmark DS, Bragadottir R, Stene-Johansen I, et al. Increased vitreous levels of hydroimidazolone in type 2 diabetes patients are associated with retinopathy: a case-control study. Acta Ophthalmol Scand 2007.
50. Gardiner TA, Anderson HR, Stitt AW. Inhibition of advanced glycation end-products protects against retinal capillary basement membrane expansion during long-term diabetes. J Pathol 2003;201(2):328–33.
51. Hammes HP, Alt A, Niwa T, et al. Differential accumulation of advanced glycation end products in the course of diabetic retinopathy. Diabetologia 1999;42(6):728–36.
52. Murata T, Nagai R, Ishibashi T, Inomuta H, Ikeda K, Horiuchi S. The relationship between accumulation of advanced glycation end products and expression of vascular endothelial growth factor in human diabetic retinas. Diabetologia 1997;40(7):764–9.

53. Schalkwijk CG, Ligtvoet N, Twaalfhoven H, et al. Amadori albumin in type 1 diabetic patients: correlation with markers of endothelial function, association with diabetic nephropathy, and localization in retinal capillaries. Diabetes 1999;48(12):2446–53.
54. Stitt AW, Li YM, Gardiner TA, Bucala R, Archer DB, Vlassara H. Advanced glycation end products (AGEs) co-localize with AGE receptors in the retinal vasculature of diabetic and of AGE-infused rats. Am J Pathol 1997;150(2):523–31.
55. Hammes HP, Brownlee M, Edelstein D, Saleck M, Martin S, Federlin K. Aminoguanidine inhibits the development of accelerated diabetic retinopathy in the spontaneous hypertensive rat. Diabetologia 1994;37(1):32–5.
56. Chen BH, Jiang DY, Tang LS. Advanced glycation end-products induce apoptosis involving the signaling pathways of oxidative stress in bovine retinal pericytes. Life Sci 2006;79(11):1040–8.
57. Denis U, Lecomte M, Paget C, Ruggiero D, Wiernsperger N, Lagarde M. Advanced glycation end-products induce apoptosis of bovine retinal pericytes in culture: involvement of diacylglycerol/ceramide production and oxidative stress induction. Free Radic Biol Med 2002;33(2):236–47.
58. Yamagishi S, Fujimori H, Yonekura H, Tanaka N, Yamamoto H. Advanced glycation endproducts accelerate calcification in microvascular pericytes. Biochem Biophys Res Commun 1999;258(2):353–7.
59. Liu B, Bhat M, Padival AK, Smith DG, Nagaraj RH. Effect of dicarbonyl modification of fibronectin on retinal capillary pericytes. Invest Ophthalmol Vis Sci 2004;45(6):1983–95.
60. Hughes SJ, Wall N, Scholfield CN, et al. Advanced glycation endproduct modified basement membrane attenuates endothelin-1 induced [Ca2+]i signalling and contraction in retinal microvascular pericytes. Mol Vis 2004;10:996–1004.
61. Miller AG, Smith DG, Bhat M, Nagaraj RH. Glyoxalase I is critical for human retinal capillary pericyte survival under hyperglycemic conditions. J Biol Chem 2006;281(17):11864–71.
62. Mamputu JC, Renier G. Signalling pathways involved in retinal endothelial cell proliferation induced by advanced glycation end products: inhibitory effect of gliclazide. Diabetes Obes Metab 2004;6(2):95–103.
63. Chibber R, Molinatti PA, Rosatto N, Lambourne B, Kohner EM. Toxic action of advanced glycation end products on cultured retinal capillary pericytes and endothelial cells: relevance to diabetic retinopathy. Diabetologia 1997;40(2):156–64.
64. Stitt AW, McGoldrick C, Rice-McCaldin A, et al. Impaired retinal angiogenesis in diabetes: role of advanced glycation end products and galectin-3. Diabetes 2005;54(3):785–94.
65. Padayatti PS, Jiang C, Glomb MA, Uchida K, Nagaraj RH. High concentrations of glucose induce synthesis of argpyrimidine in retinal endothelial cells. Curr Eye Res 2001;23(2):106–15.
66. Moore TC, Moore JE, Kaji Y, et al. The role of advanced glycation end products in retinal microvascular leukostasis. Invest Ophthalmol Vis Sci 2003;44(10):4457–64.
67. Lu M, Kuroki M, Amano S, et al. Advanced glycation end products increase retinal vascular endothelial growth factor expression. J Clin Invest 1998;101(6):1219–24.
68. Treins C, Giorgetti-Peraldi S, Murdaca J, Van Obberghen E. Regulation of vascular endothelial growth factor expression by advanced glycation end products. J Biol Chem 2001;276(47):43836–41.
69. Kobayashi T, Oku H, Komori A, et al. Advanced glycation end products induce death of retinal neurons via activation of nitric oxide synthase. Exp Eye Res 2005;81(6):647–54.
70. Lecleire-Collet A, Tessier LH, Massin P, et al. Advanced glycation end products can induce glial reaction and neuronal degeneration in retinal explants. Br J Ophthalmol 2005;89(12):1631–3.
71. Stitt AW, Bhaduri T, McMullen CB, Gardiner TA, Archer DB. Advanced glycation end products induce blood-retinal barrier dysfunction in normoglycemic rats. Mol Cell Biol Res Commun 2000;3(6):380–8.
72. Xu X, Li Z, Luo D, et al. Exogenous advanced glycosylation end products induce diabetes-like vascular dysfunction in normal rats: a factor in diabetic retinopathy. Graefes Arch Clin Exp Ophthalmol 2003;241(1):56–62.
73. Sano H, Nagai R, Matsumoto K, Horiuchi S. Receptors for proteins modified by advanced glycation endproducts (AGE)–their functional role in atherosclerosis. Mech Ageing Dev 1999;107(3):333–46.
74. Schmidt AM, Stern DM. RAGE: a new target for the prevention and treatment of the vascular and inflammatory complications of diabetes. Trends Endocrinol Metab 2000;11(9):368–75.

75. Vlassara H. The AGE-receptor in the pathogenesis of diabetic complications. Diabetes Metab Res Rev 2001;17(6):436–43.
76. Neeper M, Schmidt AM, Brett J, et al. Cloning and expression of a cell surface receptor for advanced glycosylation end products of proteins. J Biol Chem 1992;267(21):14998–5004.
77. Kislinger T, Fu C, Huber B, et al. N(epsilon)-(carboxymethyl)lysine adducts of proteins are ligands for receptor for advanced glycation end products that activate cell signaling pathways and modulate gene expression. J Biol Chem 1999;274(44):31740–9.
78. Yamagishi S, Fujimori H, Yonekura H, Yamamoto Y, Yamamoto H. Advanced glycation endproducts inhibit prostacyclin production and induce plasminogen activator inhibitor-1 in human microvascular endothelial cells. Diabetologia 1998;41(12):1435–41.
79. Wautier JL, Schmidt AM. Protein glycation: a firm link to endothelial cell dysfunction. Circ Res 2004;95(3):233–8.
80. Falcone C, Emanuele E, D'Angelo A, et al. Plasma levels of soluble receptor for advanced glycation end products and coronary artery disease in nondiabetic men. Arterioscler Thromb Vasc Biol 2005;25(5):1032–7.
81. Katakami N, Matsuhisa M, Kaneto H, et al. Decreased endogenous secretory advanced glycation end product receptor in type 1 diabetic patients: its possible association with diabetic vascular complications. Diabetes Care 2005;28(11):2716–21.
82. Hori O, Brett J, Slattery T, et al. The receptor for advanced glycation end products (RAGE) is a cellular binding site for amphoterin. Mediation of neurite outgrowth and co-expression of rage and amphoterin in the developing nervous system. J Biol Chem 1995;270(43):25752–61.
83. Chaney MO, Stine WB, Kokjohn TA, et al. RAGE and amyloid beta interactions: atomic force microscopy and molecular modeling. Biochim Biophys Acta 2005;1741(1–2):199–205.
84.Hofmann MA, Drury S, Fu C, et al. RAGE mediates a novel proinflammatory axis: a central cell surface receptor for S100/calgranulin polypeptides. Cell 1999;97(7):889–901.
85. Kosaki A, Hasegawa T, Kimura T, et al. Increased plasma S100A12 (EN-RAGE) levels in patients with type 2 diabetes. J Clin Endocrinol Metab 2004;89(11):5423–8.
86. Hasegawa T, Kosaki A, Kimura T, et al. The regulation of EN-RAGE (S100A12) gene expression in human THP-1 macrophages. Atherosclerosis 2003;171(2):211–8.
87. Kim MH, Choi YW, Choi HY, Myung KB, Cho SN. The expression of RAGE and EN-RAGE in leprosy. Br J Dermatol 2006;154(4):594–601.
88. Ehlermann P, Eggers K, Bierhaus A, et al. Increased proinflammatory endothelial response to S100A8/A9 after preactivation through advanced glycation end products. Cardiovasc Diabetol 2006;5:6.
89. Zhou Z, Wang K, Penn MS, et al. Receptor for AGE (RAGE) mediates neointimal formation in response to arterial injury. Circulation 2003;107(17):2238–43.
90. Pachydaki SI, Tari SR, Lee SE, et al. Upregulation of RAGE and its ligands in proliferative retinal disease. Exp Eye Res 2006;82(5):807–15.
91. Howes KA, Liu Y, Dunaief JL, et al. Receptor for advanced glycation end products and age-related macular degeneration. Invest Ophthalmol Vis Sci 2004;45(10):3713–20.
92. Barile GR, Pachydaki SI, Tari SR, et al. The RAGE axis in early diabetic retinopathy. Invest Ophthalmol Vis Sci 2005;46(8):2916–24.
93. Pfizer and TransTech Pharma Enter Into Agreement for the Development and Commercialization of RAGE Modulators. Transtech Pharma Inc, 2006. (Accessed at http://www.ttpharma.com/press_releases/20061809_pfizer.html
94. Marx N, Walcher D, Ivanova N, et al. Thiazolidinediones reduce endothelial expression of receptors for advanced glycation end products. Diabetes 2004;53(10):2662–8.
95. Yamagishi S, Takeuchi M. Nifedipine inhibits gene expression of receptor for advanced glycation end products (RAGE) in endothelial cells by suppressing reactive oxygen species generation. Drugs Exp Clin Res 2004;30(4):169–75.
96. Wang K, Zhou Z, Zhang M, et al. Peroxisome proliferator-activated receptor gamma down-regulates receptor for advanced glycation end products and inhibits smooth muscle cell proliferation in a diabetic and nondiabetic rat carotid artery injury model. J Pharmacol Exp Ther 2006;317(1):37–43.
97. Yamagishi S, Nakamura K, Matsui T, Sato T, Takeuchi M. Potential utility of statins, 3-hydroxy-3-methylglutaryl coenzyme A reductase inhibitors in diabetic retinopathy. Med Hypotheses 2006;66(5):1019–21.

98. Yamagishi S, Takeuchi M, Matsui T, Nakamura K, Imaizumi T, Inoue H. Angiotensin II augments advanced glycation end product-induced pericyte apoptosis through RAGE overexpression. FEBS Lett 2005;579(20):4265–70.
99. Koka V, Wang W, Huang XR, Kim-Mitsuyama S, Truong LD, Lan HY. Advanced glycation end products activate a chymase-dependent angiotensin II-generating pathway in diabetic complications. Circulation 2006;113(10):1353–60.
100. Nakamura K, Yamagishi S, Nakamura Y, et al. Telmisartan inhibits expression of a receptor for advanced glycation end products (RAGE) in angiotensin-II-exposed endothelial cells and decreases serum levels of soluble RAGE in patients with essential hypertension. Microvasc Res 2005;70(3):137–41.
101. Stitt AW, He C, Friedman S, et al. Elevated AGE-modified ApoB in sera of euglycemic, normolipidemic patients with atherosclerosis: relationship to tissue AGEs. Mol Med 1997;3(9):617–27.
102. Lu C, He JC, Cai W, Liu H, Zhu L, Vlassara H. Advanced glycation endproduct (AGE) receptor 1 is a negative regulator of the inflammatory response to AGE in mesangial cells. Proc Natl Acad Sci U S A 2004;101(32):11767–72.
103. Stitt AW, He C, Vlassara H. Characterization of the advanced glycation end-product receptor complex in human vascular endothelial cells. Biochem Biophys Res Commun 1999;256(3):549–56.
104. Wautier JL, Guillausseau PJ. Advanced glycation end products, their receptors and diabetic angiopathy. Diabetes Metab 2001;27(5 Pt 1):535–42.
105. Zhu W, Sano H, Nagai R, Fukuhara K, Miyazaki A, Horiuchi S. The role of galectin-3 in endocytosis of advanced glycation end products and modified low density lipoproteins. Biochem Biophys Res Commun 2001;280(4):1183–8.
106. Iacobini C, Amadio L, Oddi G, et al. Role of galectin-3 in diabetic nephropathy. J Am Soc Nephrol 2003;14(8 Suppl 3):S264–70.
107. Pugliese G, Pricci F, Iacobini C, et al. Accelerated diabetic glomerulopathy in galectin-3/AGE receptor 3 knockout mice. Faseb J 2001;15(13):2471–9.
108. Iacobini C, Menini S, Oddi G, et al. Galectin-3/AGE-receptor 3 knockout mice show accelerated AGE-induced glomerular injury: evidence for a protective role of galectin-3 as an AGE receptor. Faseb J 2004;18(14):1773–5.
109. Tamura Y, Adachi H, Osuga J, et al. FEEL-1 and FEEL-2 are endocytic receptors for advanced glycation end products. J Biol Chem 2003;278(15):12613–7.
110. Horiuchi S, Sakamoto Y, Sakai M. Scavenger receptors for oxidized and glycated proteins. Amino Acids 2003;25(3–4):283–92.
111. Ohgami N, Nagai R, Ikemoto M, et al. CD36, a member of class B scavenger receptor family, is a receptor for advanced glycation end products. Ann N Y Acad Sci 2001;947:350–5.
112. Brownlee M, Vlassara H, Kooney A, Ulrich P, Cerami A. Aminoguanidine prevents diabetes-induced arterial wall protein cross-linking. Science 1986;232(4758):1629–32.
113. Vasan S, Foiles P, Founds H. Therapeutic potential of breakers of advanced glycation end product-protein crosslinks. Arch Biochem Biophys 2003;419(1):89–96.
114. Hammes HP, Martin S, Federlin K, Geisen K, Brownlee M. Aminoguanidine treatment inhibits the development of experimental diabetic retinopathy. Proc Natl Acad Sci U S A 1991;88:11555–8.
115. Kern TS, Engerman RL. Pharmacological inhibition of diabetic retinopathy: aminoguanidine and aspirin. Diabetes 2001;50(7):1636–42.
116. Kern TS, Tang J, Mizutani M, et al. Response of capillary cell death to aminoguanidine predicts the development of retinopathy: comparison of diabetes and galactosemia. Invest Ophthalmol Vis Sci 2000;41(12):3972–8.
117. Agardh E, Hultberg B, Agardh C. Effects of inhibition of glycation and oxidative stress on the development of cataract and retinal vessel abnormalities in diabetic rats. Curr Eye Res 2000;21(1):543–9.
118. Bolton WK, Cattran DC, Williams ME, et al. Randomized trial of an inhibitor of formation of advanced glycation end products in diabetic nephropathy. Am J Nephrol 2004;24(1):32–40.
119. Vasan S, Zhang X, Kapurniotu A, et al. An agent cleaving glucose-derived protein crosslinks in vitro and in vivo. Nature 1996;382(6588):275–8.
120. Cooper ME, Thallas V, Forbes J, et al. The cross-link breaker, N-phenacylthiazolium bromide prevents vascular advanced glycation end-product accumulation. Diabetologia 2000;43(5):660–4.

121. Wolffenbuttel BH, Boulanger CM, Crijns FR, et al. Breakers of advanced glycation end products restore large artery properties in experimental diabetes. Proc Natl Acad Sci U S A 1998;95(8):4630–4.
122. Asif M, Egan J, Vasan S, et al. An advanced glycation endproduct cross-link breaker can reverse age-related increases in myocardial stiffness. Proc Natl Acad Sci U S A 2000;97(6):2809–13.
123. Khalifah RG, Baynes JW, Hudson BG. Amadorins: novel post-Amadori inhibitors of advanced glycation reactions. Biochem Biophys Res Commun 1999;257(2):251–8.
124. Voziyan PA, Metz TO, Baynes JW, Hudson BG. A post-Amadori inhibitor pyridoxamine also inhibits chemical modification of proteins by scavenging carbonyl intermediates of carbohydrate and lipid degradation. J Biol Chem 2002;277(5):3397–403.
125. Price DL RP, Thorpe SR, Baynes JW,. Chelating activity of advanced glycation end-product inhibitors. J Biol Chem 2001;276(52):48967–72.
126. Degenhardt TP, Alderson NL, Arrington DD, et al. Pyridoxamine inhibits early renal disease and dyslipidemia in the streptozotocin-diabetic rat. Kidney Int 2002;61(3):939–50.
127. Stitt AW, Gardiner TA, Alderson NL, et al. The AGE inhibitor pyridoxamine inhibits development of retinopathy in experimental diabetes. Diabetes 2002;51(9):2826–32.

8 The Role of Protein Kinase C in Diabetic Retinopathy

Manvi Prakash, Jennifer K. Sun, and George L. King

CONTENTS

ABSTRACT

The protein kinase C (PKC) molecule is part of a serine/threonine kinase family that catalyzes phosphorylation of key proteins involved in signal transduction. Conventional and novel PKC isoforms are upregulated by diacylglycerol (DAG), which in turn is increased by the hyperglycemia of diabetes. PKC isoforms are differentially expressed and activated in tissues throughout the body, including the aorta, kidney, heart, monocytes, and retina, but not in the brain or peripheral nerves. In the retina, PKC activation is associated with changes in retinal blood flow, possibly through effects on retinal pericytes, the expression of endothelium-derived growth factors, and/or leukostasis. The activation of PKC may also lead to basement membrane and extracellular matrix alterations within the retinal vasculature. Increases in retinal vascular permeability and angiogenesis are seen with PKC activation related to its actions on vascular endothelial growth factor. Inhibition of PKC, particularly PKC-beta isoforms, appears to ameliorate many of these effects on the retinal vasculature. Ruboxistaurin is a PKC inhibitor with a high affinity for PKC-beta isoforms. Human clinical studies with this drug are ongoing, but trials have already demonstrated its efficacy in preventing vision loss, decreasing the need for laser treatment, and decreasing the progression of macular edema in patients with diabetes.

From: *Contemporary Diabetes*: *Diabetic Retinopathy*
Edited by: E. Duh © Humana Press, Totowa, NJ

Key Words: Protein kinase C, diacylglycerol, diabetes, diabetic retinopathy, retinal blood flow, vascular permeability, angiogenesis, ruboxistaurin

INTRODUCTION

Numerous studies, including the Diabetes Control and Complications Trial (DCCT) and the United Kingdom Prospective Diabetes Study (UKPDS), have demonstrated a close correlation between increased blood glucose levels and diabetic complications affecting multiple organ systems, including the brain, cardiovascular system, kidneys, and eyes. Complications from this disease may be divided into macrovascular, including coronary artery disease, atherosclerosis, and peripheral vascular disease; and microvascular, including retinopathy, nephropathy, and neurovascular defects. Intensive control of blood glucose can successfully delay the onset, and slow the progression, of diabetic retinopathy, nephropathy, neuropathy, and cardiac abnormalities *(1)*.

In addition to systemic factors such as hyperglycemia, local tissue responses are equally important in the development of pathologies both in the type and the severity of complications. For example, some vascularized organs such as the pulmonary system do not manifest significant pathological functions even though they are exposed to the same levels of hyperglycemia and other systemic metabolites that exist in the diabetic condition. Another clear example of the importance of tissue response is in the area of angiogenic response. In the retina, excessive proliferation of endothelial cells is the hallmark of diabetic proliferative retinopathy. In contrast, myocardium and peripheral limbs exhibit too little neovascularization in response to hypoxia even though all the tissues are exposed to hyperglycemia, oxidative stress, or inflammatory cytokines. Thus, a complete understanding requires the clarification of changes in systemic and local factors.

Hyperglycemia has been shown to affect several signal transduction pathways including the elevation of diacylglycerol (DAG) levels and the activation of protein kinase C (PKC) and MAP kinases *(2, 3)*. We have focused on the effects of PKC activation since this pathway is involved in regulating vascular function in a variety of ways including endothelial permeability regulation, vasoconstriction, extracellular matrix synthesis and turnover, cell growth, angiogenesis, activating cytokines, and adherence of leukocytes. This chapter will review the role of PKC in diabetes and its complications, particularly in respect to PKC's actions affecting retinal blood flow, basement membrane and extracellular matrix changes, and vascular permeability and angiogenesis.

PKC

Protein kinase C (PKC) is part of a serine/threonine kinase family that phosphorylates key proteins involved in cardiovascular and endothelial function. It catalyzes the phosphate group transfer from ATP to other substrate proteins. PKC has individual isozymes, which are selectively activated in vascular tissues by diacylglycerol (DAG). Synthesis of DAG is in turn upregulated in vascular tissues by hyperglycemia. Differences in structure and substrate requirements have yielded approximately 12 different PKC isoforms. These differences allow classification of PKC into three different groups: Conventional (cPKC), novel (nPKC), and atypical PKCs (aPKC) (Table 1) *(4, 5–9)*.

Table 1
Protein Kinase C Subtypes

Conventional PKC (cPKC)	*Novel PKC (nPKC)*	*Atypical PKC (aPKC)*
α, βI, βII, γ	δ, ε, η, θ	ζ, ι/π
Ca^{2+} dependent	Ca^{2+} independent	Ca^{2+} independent
Activated by PS and DAG	Regulated by PS and DAG	Regulated by PS

PS phosphatidylserine

Each PKC molecule contains a single polypeptide chain with an N-terminal regulatory region and a C-terminal catalytic region. The different isoforms are products of separate genes (except for PKCβ1 and β2 which are same gene alternate splice variants).

The three PKC groups are characterized by differences in the four conserved domains, referred to as C1–C4. All PKC isozymes contain C3 and C4, which are located in the C-terminal catalytic portion of the molecule. The C3 site is involved in binding ATP, whereas the C4 site recognizes substrates to be phosphorylated by PKC *(5–9)*. The cPKC polypeptide structure contains all four conserved domains and five variable regions. The components required for interaction with DAG, phorbol esters, phosphatidylserine, and calcium are located in the C1 and C2 domains in the N-terminal portion of the molecule. In contrast to the cPKC subclass, both nPKC and aPKC possess C2-like regions, that do not bind calcium, so that only cPKC is calcium dependent (Table 1).

DAG-PKC PATHWAY

In cells, DAG is the physiologic activator of PKC. DAG, in turn, is derived from multiple pathways, including the hydrolysis of phosphatidylinositol (PI) by phospholipase C (PLC), and by synthesis from dihydroxyacetone phosphate and glycerol 3-phosphate. However, several studies have shown that PI hydrolysis does not lead to hyperglycemia-induced increases in DAG in vascular cells. De novo synthesis involving the metabolism of dihydroxyacetone phosphate into lysophosphatidic acid and then phosphatidic acid (PA) has been shown to lead to glucose-induced DAG formation *(10–12)*.

Hyperglycemia mediated upregulation of DAG causing corresponding increases in PKC activity has been demonstrated in the retina, aorta, heart, monocytes, and glomeruli from animals and humans with diabetes *(10–12)*. PKC isoforms are diffusely located in mammalian tissue and vary widely in regard to their tissue localization. These isoforms are differentially activated within these tissues (Table 2). Of all the isoforms, the largest fraction is that of PKCβ, which belongs to the cPKC family. This isoform family, as mentioned earlier, requires DAG for activation. Studies have shown that the PKCβ isoform demonstrates the most significant increase in a variety of vascularized tissues in hyperglycemic states. It is also one of the isoforms activated in hyperglycemic states in monocytes and leukocytes *(13–17)*. However, PKCα and δ isoforms have also been reported to be activated in several tissues including the retina, heart, kidney, and the monocytes.

Table 2
Differential Expression and Activation of PKC Isoforms in Tissues and Cultured Cells Under Normal and Hyperglycemic Conditions

Tissue/cultured cell type	*PKC isoforms in normal tissue*	*PKC isoforms activated by hyperglycemia/diabetes*	*References*
Rat aorta	α, βII	βII	(13)
Rat aortic smooth muscle cells	α, βII	βII	(15,16)
	α, βI, βII, δ	βII > δ	(18)
Rat kidney	α, βI, βII, δ, ε, ζ	α, ε	(19)
Rat glomeruli	α, βI, βII, δ, ε	α = βI	(20)
	α, βII, δ, ε	βII	(54)
	α, βII, δ, ε	ε > δ > α	(21)
Rat mesangial cells	α, δ, ε, ζ	ζ > α	(22)
Rat retina	α, βI, βII, ε	βII > ε > α > βI	(18)
Bovine retinal endothelial cells	α, βI, βII, δ, ε, ζ	δ > βII > α > βII	(17)
Rat corpus cavernosum	α, βI, βII, δ, ε	βII	(23)
Rat heart	α, βII	βII	(13)
	α, β, δ, ε, ζ	α > δ	(24)
	α, β, δ, ε, ζ	α	(19)
Rat cardiac myocytes	δ, ε	ε	(25)
Rat sciatic nerve	α, βI, βII, δ, ε	No difference	(26)

This preferential activation of different PKC isoforms in different tissues in hyperglycemic states is not fully understood. Several theories have been proposed. First, calcium levels may change the overall affinity of PKC isoforms to DAG. It has been suggested that the PKCβ isoform may be more sensitive to DAG than the nPKC or aPKC isoforms when low calcium levels are present (though the latter are overall calcium independent). Another possibility is that because of the specific subcellular location of some isoforms, they may be differentially activated in cases of hyperglycemia-induced increases in DAG. For example, because PKCβ is present intracellularly, rather than being membrane-bound, the mitochondrial-Golgi apparatus could preferentially activate it. Third, varying ratios of synthesis and degradation could contribute to different concentrations of isoform reported in different tissues *(29–31)*. Fourth, it is also possible that the activation of PKCβ isoform appears to be greater than other isoforms due to our ability to measure the changes between control and diabetic states.

DIABETES AND RETINAL BLOOD FLOW

Capillary pericyte loss is among the earliest and most specific features of clinical diabetic retinopathy. Retinal pericytes serve a key role in maintaining capillary integrity and function. Their loss can lead to vessel dysfunction, vascular permeability, increase in vessel diameter and loss of regulatory tone, endothelial cell proliferation, and formation of microaneurysms. All these changes may in turn alter retinal blood flow dynamics and result in retinal ischemia. This ischemia can cause release of growth factors that stimulate new, unhealthy blood vessel formation and proliferation. This stage of proliferative retinopathy can lead to hemorrhages and fibrosis, and eventually either vitreous hemorrhage or retinal detachment with poor visual outcome. The increased loss of pericytes is likely due to apoptosis as a response to diabetes-induced decreases in PDGF-B receptor's actions. We have shown that PDGF-β levels are actually increased in the retina of diabetic animals, suggesting that diabetes and possibly PKC activation may cause PDGF-B resistance in retinal pericytes, affecting permeability and blood flow *(30)*.

Some hemodynamic abnormalities are evident and can be recognized before any clinical signs of retinopathy are evident. Circulatory abnormalities have been reported in Type 1 diabetic patients with no clinical signs of retinopathy. Retinal blood flow is significantly decreased in these patients as shown by video fluorescein angiography (VFA) *(31)*. Laser Doppler methods have also shown decreased arterial blood velocity in diabetic patients with no-to-minimal retinopathy *(32)*. With longer duration of disease and progression to proliferative retinopathy, retinal blood flow will actually increase *(33–36)*. Proposed mechanisms to explain initial decreases in retinal blood flow include diabetes-related changes in vasoactive factors in concordance with the PKC signal transduction pathway resulting in increased resistance to blood flow in early stages of diabetes.

It has been reported that injection of the PKC activator, phorbol dibutyrate, into the vitreous of healthy rats resulted in a significant increase in arteriovenous passage time. This paralleled the increase noted in 2–4 week diabetic rats in the same study. In addition, intravitreal administration of R59949, a DAG kinase inhibitor, into healthy rats demonstrated increased levels of total retinal DAG and showed dose-dependent decreases in retinal blood flow *(37)*.

PKC could exert its effects on retinal vascular reactivity by changing the expression of certain endothelium-derived growth factors. One such factor is endothelin-1 (ET-1), a potent vasoconstrictor which has been identified in capillary endothelial cells, pericytes, and other retinal cells *(38, 39)*. Retina samples from diabetic rats showed increased mRNA levels of ET-1. If ET-1 is given as an intravitreal injection to nondiabetic rats, there is increased retinal vasoconstriction and resultant decreases in retinal blood flow. Taking another approach, injecting the ET-1 receptor antagonist, BQ-123, dose dependently increases retinal blood flow in diabetic rats. In addition, when bovine retinal capillary endothelial cells and pericytes are exposed to high glucose concentrations, both membranous PKC activity and ET-1 expression are increased *(17)*. Following the administration of two compounds, PKC inhibitor (GF 109203X) and mitogen-activated protein kinase inhibitor (PD 98059), the noted increase in ET-1 is inhibited. Another endothelium-derived growth factor altering vasoreactivity is nitric oxide (NO), which, in contrast to ET-1, is a vasodilator. In response to increased glucose levels, both expression and production of NO are decreased in cultured retinal endothelial cells *(40)*. This decrease can be partially restored by inhibiting PKC. The combined effects of an increase in ET-1 (a vasoconstrictor) and a decrease in NO (a vasodilator) could contribute to overall vasoconstriction and resulting increased resistance to blood flow. Therefore, these endothelium-derived growth factors may exert significant vasoactive effects to promote the initial decrease in retinal blood flow observed in early diabetes.

Leukostasis may also play a significant role in diabetic pathology, though it likely does not entirely explain the observed decrease in retinal blood flow. Leukocytes and monocytes show increased adhesion to retinal endothelial cells in response to the PKC activation seen in early diabetes *(41)*. This increased adhesion is more directly related to oxidative stress than to hyperglycemia and can be blocked by the administration of either *d*-α-tocopherol (a nonspecific PKC inhibitor) or ruboxistaurin (RBX) (a PKCβ-specific inhibitor).

BASEMENT MEMBRANE AND ECM CHANGES

Diabetic vasculature undergoes other early changes in the course of diabetes. Increased deposition of ECM causes capillary basement membrane thickening *(42)*. This in turn affects vascular permeability, cellular adhesion, proliferation, differentiation, and gene expression *(43)*. Increased expression of collagens, fibronectin, and laminin has been reported prior to basement membrane thickening *(44, 45)*. Expression and transcription of these substances have been shown to be reduced in response to administering PKC inhibitors.

Growth factors are also thought to play a role in basement membrane and ECM alterations. For example, transforming growth factor β (TGFβ) has been established as a regulator of ECM accumulation and increases expression of certain collagens and fibronectin. Studies show increased expression of TGFβ in response to hyperglycemia *(46)*. Another growth factor, connective tissue growth factor (CTGF), has also been shown to regulate ECM accumulation via TGFβ-dependent and TGFβ-independent mechanisms *(47)*. Hyperglycemia-induced increases in the expression of CTGF appear to be dependent on both TGFβ expression and the PKC signaling pathway, as increases are tempered by an anti-TGFβ antibody and by PKC inhibition *(48–49)*. PKC activation may play a role in this increase leading to the accumulation of ECM. Certain proto-oncogenes, c-fos and c-jun, are induced by PKC. They regulate gene expression via an AP-1 binding site whose consensus sequence is present in the promoter region of TGFβ, CTGF, fibronectin, and laminin *(50–53)*.

VASCULAR PERMEABILITY AND ANGIOGENESIS

Diabetes causes a marked increase in vascular permeability to macromolecules such as albumin *(54)*. This has been noted significantly in the retinal and renal vasculature. This change in permeability in the retinal vasculature leads to the clinical sequelae of transudation of fluid into the retina and subsequent visual loss from macular edema. Cultured endothelial cells have shown increased permeability in response to phorbol ester-activated PKC to macromolecules including albumin *(55–56)*. This increase is reduced by PKC inhibitors. It has been suggested that PKC causes the phosphorylation of certain cytoskeletal proteins (caldesmon, vimentin, talin, and vinculin), and through this mechanism, stimulates the endothelial cell contractile apparatus, resulting in increased vascular permeability *(57–59)*.

Increased levels of vascular endothelial growth factor (VEGF) have been demonstrated in vitreous fluid and aqueous in patients with proliferative diabetic retinopathy *(60)*. VEGF has mitogenic effects on endothelial cells and promotes vascular permeability. It is also a key factor in mediating hypoxia-induced angiogenesis. Increased expression of VEGF is reported in vascular smooth muscle cells in response to high glucose. PKC inhibition leads to a decrease in this increased VEGF expression. The nonisoform-specific PKC inhibitors GFX and H-7 prevent cellular proliferation in response to VEGF. In addition, LY333531 (ruboxistaurin), which selectively inhibits the PKCβ isoform, also decreases VEGF's mitogenic effects (versus the antisense PKCα oligonucleotide that did not reduce the mitogenic effects). This suggests an important role for PKCβ in VEGF-mediated cellular proliferation *(61, 62)*.

INHIBITION OF PKCβ

Many early PKC inhibitors were nonspecific and were associated with a variety of adverse clinical side effects. More recent PKC inhibitors proposed for clinical study, including ruboxistaurin (RBX), which inhibits PKCβ, have targeted specific PKC isoforms. The PKCβ isoform is of particular clinical interest because it demonstrates increased activation in many vascular tissues, including the eye and kidney, in the diabetic state. RBX exerts its inhibition on the cPKC family, and more specifically has affinity for PKCβI and PKCβII over PKCα and other PKC isoforms *(63)*. In addition, in a specific dose range, it demonstrates selective inhibition of PKC over other kinases such as calcium-calmodulin and src-tyrosine kinases *(63)*.

When given orally to diabetic rats, RBX increases retinal blood flow, and improves glomerular filtration rates and albumin excretion *(64)*. It has also been shown to attenuate the microvascular flow disturbances caused by leukocyte adhesion *(65)*. Further studies using intravitreal administration of RBX in diabetic rats showed decreased PKC activation and increased retinal blood flow *(37)*. RBX also suppresses VEGF-mediated retinal vascular permeability in vivo *(62)* and prevents retinal neovascularization development in a pig model of ischemic retinal disease *(66)*. A recent study demonstrated that RBX was well tolerated by diabetic patients in doses up to 16 mg twice daily for 28 days. At these doses, it decreased diabetes-induced retinal circulation time abnormalities without any significant safety issues *(67)*. Subsequent phase 3 studies demonstrated that 32 mg of oral RBX given once daily over 3 years significantly reduced the rate of sustained moderate visual loss *(68)*. In addition, initial macular laser treatment was 26% less frequent in patients on RBX compared to placebo ($p = 0.0008$), and macular edema progressed significantly less frequently to within 100 μm of the fovea *(68)*. To date, 11 clinical trials of this drug have been completed or are currently recruiting that evaluate RBX's additional effects on endothelial dysfunction, peripheral neuropathy, and nephropathy in diabetic patients *(69)*. Clinical trials involving RBX are discussed in further detail in Chap. 18.

CONCLUSIONS

Diabetic complications involving the eye, kidney, heart, and nerve all involve activation of the DAG-PKC pathway. Hyperglycemia increases the activity of this pathway, either directly or indirectly via oxidants and glycated products. PKC inhibition has been shown to ameliorate many of hyperglycemia's adverse effects on the vasculature, including changes in retinal blood flow, thickening of basement membrane and extracellular matrix, and increases in vascular permeability and angiogenesis. Given the presence of multiple PKC isoforms each with specific triggers and actions, the need for targeted therapy is crucial to prevent complications. RBX preferentially inhibits the PKCβ isoform and is well tolerated by diabetic patients. However, it is very likely that the activation of other PKC isoforms also causes significant retinal pathologies and will have to be inhibited in order to stop the progression of diabetic retinopathy.

REFERENCES

1. Diabetes Control and Complications Trial Research Group. Progression of retinopathy with intensive versus conventional treatment in the Diabetes Control and Complications Trial. Ophthalmology 1995;102:647–661.
2. Koya D, King GL. Protein kinase C activation and the development of diabetic complications. Diabetes 1998;47:859–866.
3. Way KJ, Chou E, King GL. Identification of PKC-isoform-specific biological actions using pharmacological approaches. Trends Pharmacol Sci 2000;21:181–187.
4. Nishizuka Y. Intracellular signaling by hydrolysis of phospholipids and activation of protein kinase C. Science 1992;258:607–614.
5. Hofmann J. The potential for isoenzyme-selective modulation of protein kinase C. Faseb J 1997;11:649–669.
6. Kanashiro CA, Khalil RA. Signal transduction by protein kinase C in mammalian cells. Clin Exp Pharmacol Physiol 1998;25:85.
7. Liu WS, Heckman CA. The sevenfold way of PKC regulation. Cell Signal 1998;10:529–542.
8. Mellor H, Parker PJ. The extended protein kinase C superfamily. Biochem J 1998;332:281–292.
9. Newton AC. Regulation of protein kinase C. Curr Opin Cell Biol 1997;9:161–167.
10. Nishizuka Y. Intracellular signaling by hydrolysis of phospholipids and activation of protein kinase C. Science 1992;258:607–614.
11. Nishizuka Y. Protein kinase C and lipid signaling for sustained cellular responses. FASEB 1995;9: 484–496.
12. Liscovitch M, Cantley LC. Lipid second messengers. Cell 1994;77:329–334.
13. Inoguchi T, Battan R, Handler E, et al. Preferential elevation of protein kinase C isoform beta II and diacylglycerol levels in the aorta and heart of diabetic rats: differential reversibility to glycemic control by islet cell transplantation. Proc Natl Acad Sci U S A 1992;89:11059–11063.
14. Shiba T, Inoguchi T, Sportsman JR, et al. Correlation of diacylglcerol level and protein kinase C activity in rat retina to retinal circulation. Am J Physiol 1993;265:E783-E793.
15. Inoguchi T, Xia P, Kunisaki M, et al. Insulin's effect on protein kinase C and diacylglycerol inducted by diabetes and glucose in vascular tissues. Am J Physiol 1994;267:E369-E379.
16. Kunisaki M, Bursell SE, Umeda F, et al. Normalization of diacylglycerol-protein kinase C activation by vitamin E in aorta of diabetic rats and cultured rat smooth muscle cells exposed to elevated glucose levels. Diabetes 1994;43:1372–1377.
17. Park JY, Takahara N, Gabriele A, et al. Induction of endothelin-1 expression by glucose: an effect of protein kinase C activation. Diabetes 2000;49:1239–1248.
18. Igarashi M, Wakasaki H, Takahara N, Ishii H, Jiang Z, Yamauchi T, et al. Glucose or diabetes activates p38 mitogen-activated protein kinase via different pathways. J Clin Invest 1999; 103:185–195.
19. Kang N, Alexander G, Park JK, Maasch C, Buchwalow I, Luft FC et al. Differential expression of protein kinase C isoforms in streptozotocin-induced diabetic rats. Kidney Int 1999; 56:1737–1750.
20. Koya D, Lee IK, Ishii H, Kanoh H, King GL. Prevention of glomerular dysfunction in diabetic rats by treatment with d-alphatocopherol. J Am Soc Nephrol 1997; 8:426–435.
21. Babazono T, Kapor-Drezgic J, Dlugosz JA, Whiteside C. Altered expression and subcellular localization of diacylglycerol-sensitive protein kinase C isoforms in diabetic rat glomerular cells. Diabetes 1998; 47:668–676.
22. Kikkawa R, Haneda M, Uzu T, Koya D, Sugimoto T, Shigeta Y. Translocation of protein kinase C alpha and zeta in rat glomerular mesangial cells cultured under high glucose conditions. Diabetologia 1994; 37:838–841.
23. Ganz MB, Seftel A. Glucose-induced changes in protein kinase C and nitric oxide are prevented by vitamin E. Am J Physiol Endocrinol Metab 2000; 278:E146-E152.
24. Giles TD, Ouyang J, Kerut EK, Given MB, Allen GE, McIlwain EF et al. Changes in protein kinase C in early cardiomyopathy and in gracilis muscle in the BB/Wor diabetic rat. Am J Physiol 1998; 274:H295-H307.
25. Malhotra A, Reich D, Nakouzi A, Sanghi V, Geenen DL, Buttrick PM. Experimental diabetes is associated with functional activation of protein kinase Cepsilon and phosphorylation of troponin I in the heart, which are prevented by angiotensin II receptor blockade. Circ Res 1997; 81:1027–1033.

26. Borghini I, Ania-Lahuerta A, Regazzi R, Ferrari G, Gjinovci A, Wollheim CB et al. Alpha, beta I, beta II, delta, and epsilon protein kinase C isoforms and compound activity in the sciatic nerve of normal and diabetic rats. J Neurochem 1994; 62:686–696.
27. Ishii H, Koya D, King GL. Protein kinase C activation and its role in the development of vascular complications in diabetes mellitus. J Mol Med 1998;76:21–31.
28. Nishizuka Y. The molecular heterogeneity of protein kinase C and its implications for cellular regulation. Nature 1998;334:661–665.
29. Nishizuka Y. The family of protein kinase C for signal transduction. JAMA 1989;262:1826–1833.
30. Yokota T, Ma RC, Park JY, et al. Role of protein kinase C on the expression of platelet-derived growth factor and endothelin-1 in the retina of diabetic rats and cultured retinal capillary pericytes. Diabetes 2003;52:838–45.
31. Bursell SE, Clermont AC, Kinsley BT, et al. Retinal blood flow changes in patients with insulin-dependent diabetes mellitus and no diabetic retonopathy. Invest Ophthalmol Vis Sci 1996;37:886–887.
32. Feke GT, Buzney SM, Ogasawara H, et al. Retinal circulatory abnormalities in type 1 diabetes. Invest Ophthalmol Vis Sci 1994;35:2968–2975.
33. Takagi C, King GL, Clermont AC, et al. Reversal of abnormal retinal hemodynamics in diabetic rats by acarbose, an alpha-glucosidase inhibitor. Curr Eye Res 1995;14:741–749.
34. Small KW, Stefansson E, Hatchell DL. Retinal blood flow in normal and diabetic dogs. Invest Ophthalmol Vis Sci 1987;28:672–675.
35. Konno S, Feke GT, Yoshida A, et al. Retinal blood flow changes in type I diabetes. A long-term follow-up study. Ophthalmol Vis Sci 1996;37:1140–1148.
36. Clermont AC, Aiello LP, Mori F, et al. Vascular endothelial growth factor and severity of nonproliferative diabetic retinopathy mediate retinal hemodynamics in vivo: a potential role for vascular endothelial growth factor in the progression of nonproliferative diabetic retinopathy. Am J Ophthalmol 1997;124:433–446.
37. Bursell SE, Takagi C, Clermont AC, et al. Specific retinal diacylglycerol and protein kinase C beta isoform modulation mimics abnormal retinal hemodynamics in diabetic rats. Invest Ophthalmol Vis Sci 1997;38:2711–2720.
38. Deng D, Evans T, Mukerjee K, et al. Diabetes-induced vascular dysfunction in the retina: role of endothelins. Diabetologia 1999;42:1228–1234.
39. Takagi C, Bursell SE, Lin YW, et al. Regulation of retinal hemodynamics in diabetic rats by increased expression and action of endothelin-1. Invest Ophthalmol Vis Sci 1996;37:2504–2518.
40. Chakravarthy U, Hayes RG, Stitt AW, et al. Constitutive nitric oxide synthase expression in retinal vascular endothelial cells is suppressed by high glucose and advanced glycation and end products. Diabetes 1998;47:945–952.
41. Abiko T, Abiko A, Clermont AC, et al. Characterization of retinal leukostasis and hemodynamics in insulin resistance and diabetes. Diabetes 2003;52:829–837.
42. Williamson JR, Kilo C. Extracellular matrix changes in diabetes mellitus. In: Comparative pathobiology of major age-related diseases, edited by Scarpelli DG, Migahi G (Liss, New York, 1984), pp. 269–288.
43. Meier M, King GL. Protein kinase C activation and its pharmacological inhibition in vascular disease. Vascular Med 2000;5:173–185.
44. Bruneval P, Foidart JM, Nochy D, et al. Glomerular matrix proteins in nodular glomerulosclerosis in association with light chain deposition disease and diabetes mellitus. Hum Pathol 1985;16: 477–484.
45. Scheinman JI, Fish AJ, Matas AJ, et al. The immunohistopathology of glomerular antigens. II. The glomerlar basement membrane, actomyosis, and fibroblast surface antigens in normal, diseased, and transplanted human kidneys. Am J Pathol 1978;90:71–88.
46. Wolf G, Sharma K, Chen Y, et al. High glucose-induced proliferation in mesangial cells is reversed by autocrine TGF-beta. Kidney Int 1992;42:647–656.
47. Moussad EE, Brigstock DR. Connective tissue growth factor: what's in a name? Mol Genet Metab 2000;71:276–292.
48. Murphy M, Godson C, Cannon S, et al. Suppression subtractive hybridization identifies high glucose levels as a stimulus for expression of connective tissue growth factor and other genes in hman mesangial cells. J Biol Chem 1999;274:5830–5834.

49. Riser BL, Denichilo M, Cortes P, et al. Regulation of connective tissue growth factor activity in cultured rat mesangial cells and its expression n experimental diabetic glomerulosclerosis. J Am Soc Nephrol 2000;11:25–38.
50. Messina JL, Standaert ML, Ishizuka T, et al. Role of protein kinase C in insulin's regulation of c-fos transcription. J Biol Chem 1992;267:9223–9228.
51. Chiu R, Boyle WJ, Meek J, et al. The c-Fos protein interacts with c-Jun/AP-1 to simulate transcription o f AP-1 responsive genes. Cell 1988;54:541–552.
52. Franza BR Jr, Raushcer F, Jd Josephs SF, et al. The Fos complex and Fos-related antigens recognize sequence elements that contain AP-1 binding sites. Science 1988;239:1150–1153.
53. Zhang J, Wang L, Petrin J, et al. Characterization of site-specific mutants altered at protein kinase C beta 1 isozyme autophosphorylation sites.Proc Natl Acad Sci U S A 1993;90:6130–6134.
54. Williamson JR, Chang K, Tilton RG, et al. Increased vascular permeability in spontaneously diabetic BB/W rats and in rats with mild versus severe streptozocin-induced diabetes. Prevention by aldose reductase inhibitors and castration. Diabetes 1987;36:813–821.
55. Lynch JJ, Ferro TJ, Blumenstock FA, et al. Increased endothelial albumin permeability mediated by protein kinase C activation. J Clin Invest 1990;85:1991–1998.
56. Oliver JA. Adenylate cyclase and protein kinase C mediate opposite actions on endothelial junctions. J Cell Physiol 1990;145:536–542.
57. Stasek JE Jr, Patterson CE, Garcia JG. Protein kinase C phosphorylates caldesmon77 and vimentin and enhances albumin permeability across cultured bovine pulmonary artery endothelial cell monolayers. J Cell Physiol 1992;153:62–75.
58. Turner CE, Pavalko FM, Burridge K. The role of phosphorylation and limited proteolytic cleavage of talin and vinculin in the disruption of focal adhesion integrity. J Biol Chem 1989;264:11938–11944.
59. Werth DK, Niedel JE, Pastan I, et al. A cytoskeletal substrate of protein kinase C. J Biol Chem 1983;258:11423–11426.
60. Aiello LP, Avery RL, Arrig PG, et al. Vascular endothelial growth factor in ocular fluid of patients with diabetic retinopathy and other retinal disorders. N Engl J Med 1994;331:1480–1487.
61. Xia P, Aiello LP, Ishii H, et al. Characterization of vascular endothelial growth factor's effect on the activation of protein kinase C, its isoforms, and endothelial cell growth. J Clin Invest 1996;98:2018–2026.
62. Aiello LP, Bursell SE, Clermont A, et al. Vascular endothelial growth factor-induced retinal permeability is mediated by protein kinase C in vivo and suppressed by an orally effective beta-isoform-selective inhibitor. Diabetes 1997;46:1473–1480.
63. Jirousek MR, Gillig JR, Gonzalez CM, et al. (S)-13-[(dimethylamino)methyl]-10,11,14,15-tetrahydro-4,9:16,21-dimetheno-1H,13H-dibenzo[e,k]pyrrolo[3,4-h][1,4,13]oxadiazacyclohexadecene-1,3(2H)-dione (LY-333531) and related analogues: isozyme selective inhibitors of protein kinase C beta. J Med Chem 1996;39:2664–2671.
64. Ishii H, Jirousek MR, Koya D, et al. Amelioration of vascular dysfunctions in diabetic rats by an oral PKC β inhibitor. Science 1996;272:728–731.
65. Nonaka A, Kiryu J, Tsujikawa A, et al. PKC-eta inhibitor (LY 333531) attenuates leukocyte entrapment in retinal microcirculation of diabetic rats. Invest Ophthalmol Vis Sci 2000;41:2707–2706.
66. Danis RP, Bingaman DP, Jirousek M, et al. Inhibition of intraocular neovascularization cuased by retinal ischemia in pigs by PKCbeta inhibition with LY 333531. Invest Ophthalmol Vis Sci 1998;39:17–179.
67. Aiello LP, Clermont A, Arora V, et al. Inhibition of PKC β by oral administration of ruboxistaurin is well tolerated and ameliorates diabetes-induced retinal hemodynamic abnormalities in patients. Invest Ophthalmol Vis Sci 2006;47:86–92.
68. PKC-DRS2 Group, Aiello LP, Davis MD, Girach A, Kles KA, Milton RC, Sheetz MJ, Vignati L, Zhi XE. Effect of ruboxistaurin on visual loss in patients with diabetic retinopathy. Ophthalmology 2006;113:2221–2230.
69. Trials involving ruboxistaurin. At ClinicalTrials.gov: A service of the U.S. National Institutes of Health. http://clinicaltrials.gov/ct2/results?intr=%22Ruboxistaurin%22&show_flds=Y&flds=Xabehimn (Accessed on Nov 11, 2007)

9 Oxidative Stress in Diabetic Retinopathy

Ruth B. Caldwell, Azza E.B. El-Remessy, and Robert W. Caldwell

CONTENTS

ABSTRACT

An association between oxidative stress and the development of diabetes complications has been recognized for over 20 years. Increased production of reactive oxygen species has been strongly implicated in the pathogenesis of diabetic retinopathy. However, in spite of overwhelming evidence supporting the damaging consequences of oxidative stress and its established role in experimental models of diabetes, the results of large-scale clinical trials with classic antioxidants have failed to show any benefit for diabetic patients. The disappointing results of antioxidant trials in patients underline the importance of identifying the specific sites and sources of oxidative stress in the tissues of diabetic patients. This chapter summarizes the current perspective on how diabetes induces oxidative stress in the retina, how diabetes-induced oxidative stress may lead to the development of diabetic retinopathy and reviews strategies for treatment or prevention of diabetic retinopathy by reducing oxidative stress.

Key Words: Diabetic retinopathy; oxidative stress; reactive oxygen species; antioxidants; inflammation; cytokines.

From: *Contemporary Diabetes*: *Diabetic Retinopathy*
Edited by: E. Duh © Humana Press, Totowa, NJ

INTRODUCTION

As has been explained in earlier chapters, development of diabetic retinopathy follows a pattern similar to that seen with ischemic retinopathy, beginning with a period of vascular dysfunction and breakdown of the blood-retinal barrier, which may be followed by active proliferation of new vessels in the retina and vitreous (for review, see *(1, 2)*). Large-scale clinical trials have demonstrated that hyperglycemia is the primary pathogenic factor in the development of diabetic complications, including diabetic retinopathy *(3, 4)*. While the specific mechanisms by which elevated blood glucose causes tissue injury in the diabetic retina are not fully understood, studies in animal models as well as in clinical specimens have shown that diabetic retinopathy is associated with increases in inflammatory mediators, including VEGF, TNFα, IL-6, IL-1β, and MCP-1 *(5–10)*. This results in increased endothelial cell expression of adhesion molecules, such as ICAM-1 and PECAM, and with leukocyte accumulation and attachment to the retinal blood vessels (leukostasis) *(11)*. Leukostasis is thought to contribute to increases in vascular permeability and subsequent neovascularization. During retinopathy, leukocytes become activated *(12)* and are thought to influence retinal edema, ischemia, and angiogenesis *(13)*. Macrophages are also important participants in the inflammatory process *(14)* and have been implicated in retinal neovascularization in models of ischemic retinopathy *(15, 16)*. Microglial cells (resident macrophages) are also activated during diabetes *(7, 17)*. Activated monocytes, neutrophils, and microglial cells are all important sources of oxidative stress.

The association between oxidative stress and the progression of diabetes and its complications has been recognized for over 20 years *(18)*. Increased production of reactive oxygen species (ROS) has been strongly implicated in the pathogenesis of diabetic retinopathy (for review, see *(2, 19)*). However, in spite of overwhelming evidence supporting the damaging consequences of oxidative stress and its established role in experimental models of diabetes, the results of large-scale clinical trials with classic antioxidants have failed to show any benefit for diabetic patients (for review, see *(20)*). The disappointing results of antioxidant trials in patients underline the importance of identifying the specific sites and sources of oxidative stress in the tissues of diabetic patients. In this chapter we will summarize the current perspective on how diabetes induces oxidative stress in the retina, how diabetes-induced oxidative stress may lead to the development of diabetic retinopathy and consider therapeutic approaches for preventing the onset and progression of the retinal complications of diabetes.

SOURCES OF OXIDATIVE STRESS IN THE DIABETIC RETINA

Overview

The term "oxidative stress" refers to the condition in which there is a serious imbalance between the production of oxidants (including both reactive oxygen species (ROS) and reactive nitrogen species (RNS)), and antioxidant defense, leading to potential tissue damage (for review, see *(21)*). Prominent members of the ROS group are superoxide, hydroxyl radical, and peroxy radical. Key members of the RNS group are nitric oxide, peroxynitrite, and their derivatives. Oxidative reactions are essential for mechanisms of host defense mediated by neutrophils, macrophages, and other cells of the immune system. However, when oxidants are overproduced they cause tissue injury and cell death. In normal conditions, antioxidants are present in tissues to neutralize free radicals and prevent excessive oxidative stress *(22, 23)*. Antioxidants have been variably defined as substances that, when present at low concentrations compared to those of an oxidizable substrate, significantly delay or inhibit oxidation of the substrate *(24)* or as a metabolic intermediate, i.e., a substrate that protects biological tissues from free-radical damage and is able to be recycled or regenerated by biological reductants *(25)*. A variety of compounds (flavonoids, uric acid, bilirubin, albumin, vitamin E, vitamin C, α-lipoic acid, and glutathione) and various enzymes (catalase, superoxide dismutase, glutathione peroxidase) have been described as antioxidants.

Formation of ROS is increased in diabetes/hyperglycemia, and is directly related to the vascular dysfunction and complications of diabetes. Several initiating events and sources of ROS in diabetes have been described and include disruption of the mitochondrial electron transport chain, formation of advanced glycation end (AGE) products, auto-oxidation of glucose, flux through the aldose reductase/polyol pathway, uncoupling of NOS, and activation of PKC and NAD(P)H oxidase *(26, 27)*. Overproduction of superoxide can lead to scavenging of NO, reducing its bioavailability and to production of peroxynitrite and other reactive species, with subsequent vascular dysfunction and pathology *(28)*. The primary source of ROS is considered to be overproduction of superoxide anion by the mitochondrial electron transport chain which then initiates superoxide production by other sources *(27)*. However, it is quite likely that several sources of superoxide production are activated by hyperglycemia and that the activities of these sources are connected and increased through a series of positive feedback relationships (Fig. 1). The contributing events and ROS sources will be discussed, some only briefly as they are the subjects of other chapters in this book.

Mitochondrial Electron Transport Chain (ETC)

Hyperglycemia can disrupt normal mitochondrial function and substantially increase superoxide production. This action appears to occur through the increased hyperglycemia-derived electron donors mostly from the citric acid cycle – NADH and $FADH_2$ – which increase electron flow through the ETC complexes as well as the efflux of protons from the mitochondrial matrix across the inner mitochondrial membrane by complexes I, III, and IV. This leads to a substantial increase in mitochondrial membrane potential and the preferential inhibition of electron flow through complex III. This inhibition disrupts normal ETC electron flow and promotes the leak of electrons leading to formation of superoxide *(29)*. The increase in superoxide formation leads to oxidative damage of mitochondrial and cellular lipids, proteins, and nucleic acids which contribute heavily to the pathology of hyperglycemic/diabetic state. These damaging events are amplified by the fact that free-radical defense mechanisms such as superoxide dismutase, catalase, glutathione peroxidase, and levels of the intracellular antioxidant GSH are also substantially compromised during diabetes (for review, see *(19)*). The key role of mitochondrial ROS formation in diabetes-induced oxidative damage in the retina has been demonstrated by recent studies using transgenic mice that overexpress mitochondrial SOD. These experiments showed that overexpressing mitochondrial SOD protects the retina from diabetes-induced oxidative stress *(30)*. Moreover, studies using the same

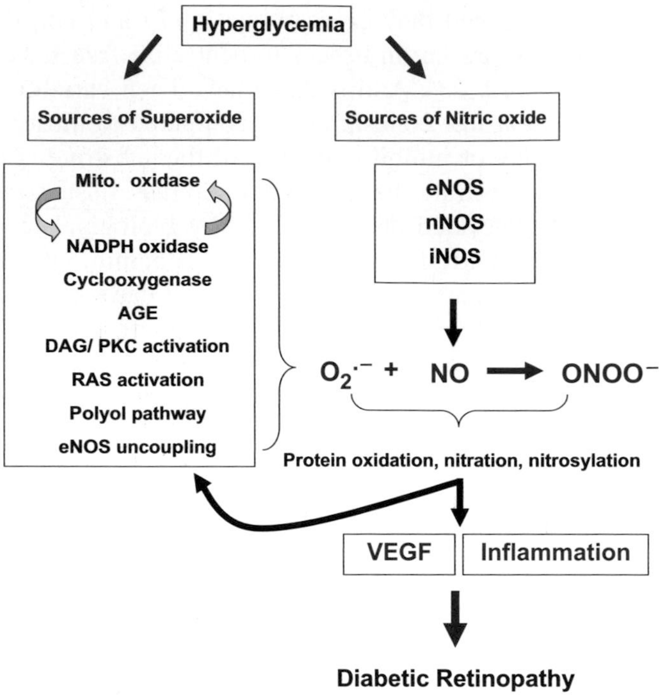

Fig. 1. Sources of ROS and RNS in the diabetic retina.

mice confirmed that retinal mitochondria undergo oxidative damage in diabetes and that complex III is a source of increased superoxide formation. Most importantly, the retinas of these mice were protected from diabetes-induced capillary degeneration, indicating the key role of mitochondrial ROS formation in this pathological process *(31)*.

Advanced Glycation End (AGE) Product Formation

Hyperglycemia is the initiating event in formation of AGEs as gluco-carbonyl adducts with amino acids (such as lysine) and can involve auto-oxidation of glucose to glyoxal. Besides being able to crosslink a number of proteins and alter their physical properties, AGEs interact with a specific receptor, RAGE to activate PKC-δ and subsequently NADPH oxidase *(32)*. AGEs appear to activate NADPH oxidase in neural cells through activation of PKC-δ *(33)*. Studies in patients, animals, and tissue culture models have clearly demonstrated the role of AGE formation in the complications of diabetes *(34,35)*.

Cyclo-oxygenase (COX)

Expression of the inducible form of COX, COX-2 rises markedly with diabetes, high glucose, and oxidant stress *(36, 37)*. This greater COX-2 expression causes an increased rate of conversion of prostaglandin G_2 to prostaglandin H_2, which increases ROS formation through the functionally linked peroxidase activity of COX-2. This results in exacerbation of oxidative stress *(38)*. COX-2 inhibition has been noted to protect against diabetic neuropathy in STZ-diabetic mice *(39)*. Treatment with aspirin or other nonsteroidal anti-inflammatory inhibitors of COX-1, COX-2, and prostaglandin synthesis has been shown to prevent signs of vascular lesions in the retinas of diabetic animals *(40, 41)*, suggesting that this pathway could be important in the development of diabetic retinopathy.

Flux Through Aldose Reductase (AR) Pathway

AR is the first step in the polyol pathway. In hyperglycemia conditions, AR reduces glucose to sorbitol and consumes NADPH. Since regeneration of the antioxidant-reduced glutathione requires NADPH, the active AR pathway can increase levels of ROS. Conversion of sorbitol to fructose requires reduction of NAD^+ to NADH, leading to higher levels of oxidized triose phosphates, precursors of AGEs and of diacylglycerol (DAG) through α-glycerol-3-phosphate. Thus, activities through the AGE and PKC pathways are enhanced. The potential role of the AR pathway in the development of diabetic retinopathy is supported by studies in experimental animal models and endothelial cells treated with high glucose *(42, 43)*.

Activation of Protein Kinase C (PKC)

PKC has many isoforms which are activated by diacylglycerol (DAG). De novo synthesis of DAG comes largely from glycolytic intermediates and stepwise acylation of glycerol-3-phosphate. All the classic and novel PKC isoforms are activated by DAG, but primarily the ß and α isoforms appear to be involved in diabetes *(44)*. Studies have shown increased levels of DAG in vascular tissue of diabetic subjects *(45)* as well as elevated DAG levels in cultured vascular cells exposed to high glucose. Hyperglycemia can also indirectly activate PKC through activation of AGE receptors and polyol pathway products. DAG can also be synthesized through the phospholipase pathways activated by growth factors, cytokines, and hormones, such as angiotensin II, which are elevated in diabetes *(46–48)*. PKC can also be activated by peroxynitrite, superoxide, and high amounts of NO *(49)*.

Endothelial NO Synthase (eNOS)

Uncoupled NOS can be a source of superoxide production. When the cellular supply of its substrate, L-arginine or the required co-factor tetrahydrobiopterin is limited, NOS becomes uncoupled and utilizes molecular oxygen as a principal substrate, producing superoxide instead of NO *(50–52)*. Superoxide can combine rapidly with NO to form peroxynitrite or other oxidants *(53)*. L-Arginine can be limited by several means. A state of imbalance between L-arg availability and NOS activity can occur when cellular transport of L-arginine is inhibited, as with oxidative stress associated with cardiovascular disease. Conditions of prolonged and elevated NOS activity *(54, 55)*, reduced recycling of L-citrulline back to L-arginine *(56)*, and/or elevated catabolism of L-arginine by arginase *(57–59)* can also reduce L-arginine availability to NOS. Diabetes has been shown to reduce cellular transport of L-arginine and enhance vascular and hepatic arginase activity *(60)*.

Derby Hospitals NHS Foundation
Trust
Library and Knowledge Service

Formation of peroxynitrite and superoxide can also cause NOS uncoupling due to oxidation of tetrahydrobiopterin, leading to further formation of superoxide. It has also been reported that hydrogen peroxide, a byproduct of superoxide, can itself stimulate eNOS activity *(61)*. This may result in a positive feedback loop, stimulating further increases in superoxide production. Further evidence of ROS involvement in eNOS uncoupling and vascular dysfunction has been provided by experiments showing that native LDL enhances superoxide formation in blood vessels and that this effect can be reversed by acute treatment with supplemental L-arginine *(62)*. Additionally, blood vessels dysfunctional because of oxidized LDL exposure regain their ability to vasodilate in response to serotonin or acetylcholine upon treatment with L-arginine *(63, 64)*. Thus, supplemental L-arginine treatment may ameliorate vascular injury by limiting superoxide formation. However, a number of studies in animals and humans have found no benefit or worsening of adverse outcomes when administration of supplemental L-arginine is prolonged *(65, 66)*. These negative outcomes may be related to the action of L-arginine in increasing arginase activity *(67)*. A study with rabbits showed that chronic administration of L-arginine for 3 days caused decreased NO production in response to acetylcholine which was associated with increased arginase activity in both liver and aorta. In contrast, chronic treatment with L-citrulline for the same period was beneficial in supporting NO production *(68)*. L-Citrulline, a byproduct in the formation of NO, is recycled back to L-arginine, contributing to sustained L-arginine supply for NOS activity *(69)*. L-Citrulline is also an allosteric inhibitor of arginase *(70)*. Therefore, L-citrulline may suppress arginase activity.

Certain eNOS polymorphisms in humans have been associated with severe diabetic retinopathy *(71)*. The eNOS4b/b polymorphism, which increases NOS expression and activity, is associated with severe diabetic retinopathy. In contrast, persons with the eNOS4a/a homozygous deletion in which NOS expression and activity are reduced have absent or background diabetic retinopathy *(72)*. It is possible that those with a high eNOS expression phenotype are more prone to eNOS uncoupling when L-arginine availability and BH4 levels are reduced. An uncoupled highly expressed and activated enzyme would produce higher levels of peroxynitrite through a combination of superoxide and NO, leading to increased VEGF levels *(73)*, a major feature of diabetic retinopathy.

Inducible NOS (iNOS)

Excessive NOS activity and peroxynitrite formation may also be involved in vascular and cellular injury associated with diabetic retinopathy. Peroxynitrite can modify protein and lipid structure via multiple mechanisms *(74)*. These include nitration of tyrosine residues or thiol oxidation, which can alter cell signaling events, and DNA strand breakage, which leads to activation of the nuclear enzyme poly-ADP-ribose polymerase (PARP). Studies showing that diabetes-induced activation of PARP, leukostasis, and formation of acellular capillaries in the retina are all accompanied by increases in the nitration of tyrosine residues of retinal proteins imply a role for peroxynitrite in diabetic retinopathy *(75)*. These effects are blocked in mice deficient in inducible NOS, suggesting that the activity of this enzyme has a critical role in the development of diabetic retinopathy. The potential role of peroxynitrite and protein tyrosine nitration in retinopathy is further supported by studies showing that knocking out eNOS prevents vaso-obliteration in the mouse model of ischemic retinopathy *(76)* and by data showing that treatment with aminoguanidine, which inhibits inducible NOS (iNOS) and reduces AGE, also inhibits the development of microvascular lesions of diabetic retinopathy in animals *(77–79)*.

In contrast with the constitutive isoforms of NOS (eNOS and nNOS), the activity of iNOS is regulated primarily at the transcriptional level. NO formation by iNOS is independent of agonist stimulation and does not require a rise in intracellular calcium. iNOS is expressed in macrophages, microglia, glial cells, neurons, and vascular cells of the retina and can play multiple roles in inflammatory response. During inflammation, iNOS is upregulated by multiple stimuli, for example cytokines such as IL-1β activate NFκB, which upregulates the transcription of iNOS. In macrophages, monocytes, and other cells the induction of iNOS and the presence of L-arginine are sufficient to initiate the generation of NO. Kinetics of NO production by iNOS differs greatly from the production by eNOS or nNOS in that iNOS produces very large, toxic amounts of NO in a sustained manner, whereas the constitutive NOS isoforms produce NO within seconds and its activities are direct and short acting.

There are multiple intracellular mechanisms through which NO may act as a proinflammatory mediator (for review, see *(80)*). When it is produced by activated macrophages, NO kills microorganisms and nitrosylates macromolecules. Large amounts of "inflammatory NO" from myeloid cells are usually generated side by side with large amounts of superoxide anion. As explained these two can form peroxynitrite which mediates cytotoxic effects of NO, such as DNA damage, LDL oxidation, isoprostane formation, tyrosine nitration, and modification of enzyme activity.

The role of iNOS in diabetic retinopathy has been supported by numerous experiments showing beneficial effects of iNOS inhibitors in blocking signs of diabetic retinopathy (for review, see *(81)*). Moreover, recent studies with mice have shown that iNOS deletion prevents the development of vascular lesions and blocks the loss of neuronal cells in the diabetic retina *(75)*. While the results of these experiments are promising, it is important to remember that NO made by iNOS is of benefit to host defense reactions by contributing to microbial killing. The exact role of iNOS-derived NO in diabetic retinopathy awaits further elucidation and evaluation

NADPH Oxidase

NADPH oxidase is considered to be a major source of ROS in diabetes. Recently, the NOX family of NADPH oxidases has emerged as a major source of ROS induction *(82)*. Studies have shown that both the mitochondria and the NADPH oxidase are involved in the sustained accumulation of ROS in a serum-withdrawal model of cell death *(83)*. Importantly, it was found that the mitochondria and the NADPH oxidase do not act independently but rather function in a cooperative manner to extend the production of ROS. Data showing increased activity of NADPH oxidase in diabetic patients and animals and in high glucose-treated endothelial cells *(84–87)* suggest that NADPH oxidase is an important source of hyperglycemia-induced ROS formation. Recent studies indicate that superoxide production by NADPH oxidase has a primary role in VEGF expression and vitreoretinal neovascularization in a mouse model for ischemic retinopathy

(88A). Studies of cultured retinal endothelial cells have implicated activity of NADPH oxidase in high glucose-mediated increases in VEGF expression. Moreover, increased expression of the NADPH oxidase catalytic subunit NOX2 (previously known as gp91phox) is correlated with early signs of diabetic retinopathy, including increases in ROS and VEGF, leukostasis, and breakdown of the blood-retinal barrier *(89)*. Furthermore, in vitro studies show that inhibiting NADPH oxidase blocks the effects of high glucose in stimulating VEGF expression.

The generation of ROS through activation of NADPH oxidase in neutrophils is a well-known process with various means of regulation, including phosphorylation, GTPase activation, and protein–protein interactions (for review, see *(90)*). Neutrophil NOX consists of a heterodimer with a large catalytic subunit, NOX2, and a small subunit, p22phox. Enzyme activation is controlled by recruitment of the regulatory proteins p40phox, p47phox, and p67phox. Assembly of the complex is initiated upon phosphorylation of p47phox *(91)*. The p67phox subunit mediates direct binding of the complex with activated Rac *(92)*. Rac initiates the electron transfer reaction that produces superoxide. Several isoforms of Rac proteins exist, including Rac1, Rac1b, Rac2, and Rac3. Rac1 is widely expressed and is likely the main Rac GTPase for NADPH oxidase activation in nonhematopoietic cells, including vascular endothelial cells. Rac2 is expressed in hematopoietic cells only and is the most relevant isoform for activation of neutrophil NADPH. Rac1 and Rac2 proteins are 92% homologous and show great overlap in their biological effects. However, mice deficient in Rac2 show defects in neutrophil function and NADPH oxidase activity that are not rescued by the remaining fraction of Rac1 (for review, see *(90)*).

The Rac1–ROS signaling pathway has been strongly implicated in vascular disease. Studies of murine models of diabetes and endothelial cells treated with high glucose have shown enhanced Rac1 activity. Moreover, inhibition of Rac1 by a dominant negative mutant of Rac1 protected against oxidative stress and vascular dysfunction induced by diabetes in mice *(93)*. Current literature suggests that the most relevant NOX isoforms in endothelial cells are NOX1 and NOX2. NOX1 is expressed at higher levels than NOX2 in normal endothelial cells *(94, 95)*. However, studies have shown that NOX2 is upregulated in the diabetic retina and in high glucose-treated retinal vascular endothelial cells *(89)*. Moreover, diabetes-induced leukostasis and hyperpermeability are blocked in NOX2-deficient mice *(88B)*. These results are consistent with previous studies implicating NOX2 expression in ischemia-reperfusion injury in the brain *(96)*. Thus, it is likely that NOX2 activity has a key role in diabetes and hyperglycemia-induced vascular injury. It should be noted that endothelial cells also express high levels of Nox4 (indeed, greater than Nox2 levels). The function of NOX4 is not yet understood, but it has been suggested that NOX4 may contribute to the basal levels of superoxide formation in unstimulated cells *(97)*.

ANTIOXIDANTS IN DIABETIC RETINOPATHY

Overview

The retina has several defense mechanisms to minimize oxidative stress. These include nonenzyme systems such as α-tocopherol, glutathione, and vitamins A, C, and E. Enzyme systems, such as superoxide dismutase, catalase, glutathione reductase, and glutathione peroxidase, help to maintain the intracellular concentration of glutathione and NADPH necessary for the optimal function of cellular antioxidant defense mechanisms. Other antioxidants include α-lipoic acid, mixed carotenoids, coenzyme Q10, several bioflavonoids, antioxidant minerals (copper, zinc, manganese, selenium), and the cofactors (folic acid, vitamins B1, B2, B6, B12) (for review, see *(98, 99)*). Comparison of antioxidant enzyme activities in retina and retinal microvessels showed that enzyme activities are much higher in the retina than in isolated retinal vascular tissue *(100)*. The higher activity is required to protect the retinal neurons and particularly rod outer segments from oxidative stress due to their high content of polyunsaturated fatty acids, high oxygen consumption, and light exposure. The same study showed that retinal microvascular endothelial cells have substantially less antioxidant activity compared to aortic endothelial cells. This may account for the unique vulnerability of retinal capillaries to oxidative stress under diabetic conditions. Several studies have demonstrated that diabetes-induced increases in lipid peroxidation are paralleled by decreases in antioxidant defense levels. Studies in diabetic patients and experimental animals have shown that antioxidant defense enzymes such as SOD, glutathione reductase, glutathione peroxidase, and catalase are diminished in the retina (for review, see *(19)*). A clinical study found that serum levels of ascorbic acid, a scavenger of free radicals, are significantly decreased in patients with type I or type II diabetes compared to nondiabetic controls *(101)*. These findings suggest that diabetics have diminished antioxidant defense and are more vulnerable to oxidative damage.

Glutathione (GSH)

Reduced GSH is a major component of the intracellular defense system. It functions as a direct free-radical scavenger and as a cosubstrate for glutathione peroxidase (GPx). GSH acts as a free-radical scavenger by trapping ROS that otherwise would react with cellular thiol groups (for review, see *(102)*). This process is accomplished through enzyme-catalyzed reactions in which GSH peroxidases (GPx) use GSH in the reduction of peroxides. GPx metabolizes hydrogen peroxide to water by using reduced GSH as a hydrogen donor. GSH reductase (GRx) functions to regenerate GSH from GSH disulfide. This GSH enzyme system protects the retina from toxic effects of ROS and helps maintain normal cellular redox potential.

The retina has a very active system for maintaining GSH in its reduced form *(103)*. Normal GSH levels are maintained by a balance between its synthesis and utilization by the GSH redox cycle, and alteration of either or both of these processes can result in abnormal GSH levels (for review, see *(104)*). Decreases in retinal GSH levels have been found to be associated with increased concentrations of oxidized GSH in diabetic rats and mice *(30, 105–107)*. Decreased GSH concentrations have also been observed in vitreous and blood samples of patients with diabetic retinopathy as compared with nondiabetic controls *(108, 109)*. In addition, a study of pericytes from human retinas found that GRx mRNA is decreased, whereas GPx mRNA is increased in diabetic patients as compared with controls *(110)*. On the other hand, studies with rats have suggested that GRx activity is reduced in diabetic retinas *(111)*. Further investigation is needed to determine the reasons for these apparent contradictions.

Superoxide Dismutase (SOD)

The SODs are ubiquitous components of cellular antioxidant systems and effectively protect retinal tissue against free-radical oxidation of membrane phospholipids. Different isoforms of SOD are located at different sites within the cell. CuZn-SOD is located in both the cytoplasm and the nucleus. In contrast MnSOD is found only in the mitochondria, but can be released into the extracellular space (for review, see *(99)*). The SODs act as a major defense system against the cytotoxic effects of superoxide radicals by catalyzing the conversion of superoxide anion to oxygen and hydrogen peroxide. The activity and the expression of SOD are downregulated in the retinas of diabetic or galactosemic rats *(79, 112)*. It has also been shown that diabetes causes decreases in CuZn-SOD mRNA in human pericytes but that levels of MnSOD mRNA were not affected *(110)*. Studies in diabetic rats have shown that therapies that inhibit the development of retinopathy, including aminoguanidine and antioxidants, also prevent diabetes-induced decreases in retinal SOD levels and normalize SOD activity (for review, see *(19)*). Furthermore, treatment with SOD mimetics and overexpression of MnSOD protect the retina from diabetes-induced oxidative stress and prevent glucose-induced mitochondrial dysfunction and apoptosis of retinal capillary cells *(30, 31, 113)*.

Catalase

Catalase catalyzes the conversion of hydrogen peroxide to water and oxygen and thus protects against hydrogen peroxide-mediated oxidative damage. The enzyme also has peroxidase activity and reacts with organic peroxides and hydrogen donors to form water and organic alcohols. It is located mainly in cellular peroxisomes and to some extent in the cytosol. The enzyme is especially important in conditions where content of GSH is limited or when activity of GPx in diminished. The effects of diabetes on catalase activity in the retina are somewhat contradictory. Studies have shown modest increases in catalase activity in the diabetic rat retina *(112)*, whereas activity in the diabetic mouse retina is apparently decreased *(114)*.

EFFECTS OF OXIDATIVE STRESS IN THE DIABETIC RETINA

Overview

Recent studies have identified ROS as key second messengers in multiple signaling pathways that initiate diverse biological responses (for review, see *(115, 116)*). First, ROS can modify the activity of redox-sensitive protein kinases (such as members of the MAPK family, Akt, PKC, PKD, and JAK (Janus kinase)) either indirectly via inactivation of tyrosine phosphatases or in some cases by direct activation. Second, ROS can alter the activity of redox-sensitive transcription factors such as AP-1 (activator protein 1), NF-κB (nuclear factor κB), HIF-1 (hypoxia-inducible factor 1), and STAT (signal transducer and activator of transcription). This latter effect can occur directly or secondary to altered activity of upstream kinases. Third, ROS can modulate the activity of redox-sensitive molecules such as thioredoxin. Fourth, ROS can directly affect the function of enzymes, receptors, or ion channels. Finally, ROS-mediated production of inflammatory cytokines such as TNF-α may in turn increase NADPH oxidase activity and expression, thereby completing the vicious circle of inflammation *(117)*.

Growth Factors and Cytokines

Increases in oxidative stress have been linked to increased production of VEGF upon high glucose treatment in vitro and in the diabetic retina *(84, 118–121)*. The mechanisms by which oxidative stress contributes to VEGF overexpression are not fully understood. However, inhibiting NOS or scavenging peroxynitrite has been shown to prevent signs of diabetic retinopathy in rats *(73, 105)*, suggesting that formation of reactive nitrogen species plays a role in the pathology. Studies using tissue culture models suggest that high glucose-induced peroxynitrite formation increases VEGF expression by a mechanism involving the activation of STAT3 *(122, 123)*. Studies have shown that constitutive activation of STAT3 is correlated with increased rates of VEGF expression and angiogenesis *(124–128)*. Because VEGF stimulation of retinal microvascular endothelial cells can induce its own expression via the activation of STAT3 *(123, 129)*, it appears likely that the effects of diabetes in causing pathological overgrowth of the retinal microvasculature are due in part to VEGF's actions in triggering its autocrine expression. VEGF autocrine production in the microvascular endothelium has been described in hypoxia, brain tumors, when the cell-to-cell junctions are disrupted or during in vitro angiogenesis induced by AGE products *(127, 130)*.

PEDF is a noninhibitory member of the serpin superfamily. It was first discovered as a neurotrophic factor, but it is now known to function as an endogenous inhibitor of angiogenesis and a blocker of VEGF-induced permeability *(131–134)*. VEGF and PEDF appear to have a reciprocal relationship in the eyes of patients with proliferative diabetic retinopathy in that levels of VEGF are increased whereas levels of PEDF are decreased *(135)*. The protective role of PEDF in preventing retinopathy has been supported by studies showing that intravitreal injection of PEDF significantly reduces vascular hyperpermeability in models of diabetes and oxygen-induced retinopathy. The permeability-blocking effect was correlated with decreased levels of retinal inflammatory factors, including VEGF, VEGF receptor-2, MCP-1, TNF-α, and ICAM-1 *(136)*. In cultured retinal capillary endothelial cells, PEDF significantly decreased TNF-α and ICAM-1 expression induced by hypoxia. These protective actions of PEDF may involve an antioxidant function in that PEDF has been shown to protect cultured retinal pericytes from AGE-induced injury through its antioxidative properties *(137)*. It has also been shown to block angiotensin II signaling and to inhibit TNF-alpha-induced IL-6 expression in endothelial cells by suppressing NADPH oxidase-mediated ROS generation *(138, 139)*. PEDF was also found to inhibit AGE-induced retinal vascular hyperpermeability by blocking ROS-mediated expression of VEGF *(140)* and to block ROS-induced apoptosis and dysfunction of cultured retinal pericytes *(141)*. Further evidence supporting an antioxidant action of PEDF comes from studies of ocular fluids from patients with proliferative diabetic retinopathy which showed that levels of PEDF are positively correlated with total antioxidant capacity *(142, 143)*.

Diabetic retinopathy exhibits signs of chronic inflammatory disease *(144)*. As has been explained in the section on sources of ROS, iNOS expression is increased in retinas of diabetic patients and experimental animal models, and inhibiting iNOS or knocking out the iNOS gene protects against diabetic retinopathy *(75, 81)*. Production of large amounts of NO and ROS can trigger a variety of inflammatory reactions. Extracellular release of superoxide, produced in leukocytes as a respiratory burst, is an important mechanism of pathogen killing and also leads to endothelial damage resulting in increased vascular permeability as well as cell death. Intracellular production of NO and ROS also can promote the release of other mediators of inflammation. ROS can increase chemokine and cytokine expression, which can increase adhesion molecule expression on both the endothelium and the inflammatory cells, thus affecting inflammatory cell recruitment to the sites of vascular damage. Recent studies in animal and tissue culture models indicate that diabetes- or high glucose-induced increases in expression of VEGF and ICAM-1 as well as retinal leukostasis and breakdown of the blood-retinal barrier depend critically on the activity of NADPH oxidase in triggering the activation of STAT3 *(89, 122)*. The role of NADPH oxidase in diabetes-induced retinal vascular inflammation has been confirmed by studies showing that diabetes or high glucose increase NADPH oxidase expression in the vascular wall and that inhibition of NADPH oxidase or deletion of its catalytic subunit NOX2 reduces signs of vascular inflammation in the diabetic retina *(88)*.

Cytoxicity

Studies in clinical specimens and animal models have shown that retinal capillary cells undergo accelerated apoptosis prior to the appearance of clinical signs of diabetic retinopathy *(79, 145)*. Experimental diabetes or treatment of endothelial cells or pericytes with high glucose has been shown to result in increased levels of oxidative stress and activation of caspase 3 and NF-κB, suggesting a causal relationship between oxidative stress and vascular injury (for review, see *(19)*). Studies showing that overexpression of mitochondrial SOD reduces oxidative stress, protects the retina from diabetes-induced abnormalities in the mitochondria, and prevents vascular pathology strongly support the role of mitochondrial-derived ROS in diabetic vascular injury *(31)*.

Nearly 50 years ago, Bloodworth proposed that diabetic retinopathy is not just a disease of the vasculature but a multifactorial disease involving the retinal neurons and glia *(146)*. Early histopathologic studies noted the loss of neurons in patients with diabetic retinopathy. Since then, studies using electroretinography, dark adaptation, contrast sensitivity, and color vision tests have conclusively demonstrated that neuroretinal function is compromised before the onset of vascular lesions in humans (for review, see *(147, 148)*). While extensive research effort has been focused on defining the vascular pathology in the diabetic retina, neurodegenerative changes also occur. These include increased apoptosis of ganglion cells; glial cell reactivity, microglial activation, and altered glutamate metabolism. The metabolic factors that lead to this neuronal cell death have been suggested to include loss of insulin-mediated trophic support *(149–151)* and/or injury due to accumulation of excess hexosamines *(152)*, tumor necrosis factor-alpha *(7, 153)*, or glutamate (for review, see *(147)*). Studies showing that treatments that target formation of ROS exert neuroprotective effects suggest that diabetes-induced oxidative stress also has a key role in the pathogenesis of the neuronal degeneration *(154–155)*.

Müller cells undergo reactive gliosis following acute retinal injury or chronic neuronal stress *(156)*. Gliosis is characterized by glial cell proliferation, changes in cell shape due to alterations in intermediate filament production (GFAP), and secretion of NO and VEGF (for review, see *(157)*). The progression of gliosis in diabetic retina has been correlated with increases in ROS/RNS formation *(158–161)* as well as with increased levels of inflammatory mediators *(162, 163)*.

VEGF's function as an endothelial cell survival factor is well established *(164)*. However, VEGF also appears to have a role in promoting neuronal cell survival. Genetic studies in mice with a deletion of the hypoxia response element in the VEGF gene promoter have shown that mice with reduced VEGF levels develop adult-onset motor neuron degeneration similar to that seen in patients with amyotrophic lateral sclerosis *(165)*. VEGF has also been found to reduce neuronal injury in stroke *(165)*. The mechanism(s) of these effects are not yet clear, but may involve both a direct action on neural cells that express VEGFR1 and 2 as well as an indirect action in promoting angiogenesis and reducing tissue ischemia. In the developing retina VEGFR-1 and -2 are expressed specifically in Muller glial cells. Studies in the developing retina showed that inhibiting the activity of VEGFR1 and 2 in the avascular regions of the developing neural retina results in a loss of cells in the inner retinal layers, suggesting that retinal neurons and/or glial cells may be VEGF dependent *(166)*.

Paradoxically, even though levels of VEGF and VEGFR2 are increased in the diabetic retina, VEGF's prosurvival function is compromised in that endothelial cells, neurons, and glial cells undergo apoptosis *(145, 147, 164, 167)*. These observations suggest that VEGF prosurvival signaling is altered by the diabetic state. VEGF activation of VEGFR2 transduces prosurvival signals via the PI3-kinase/Akt signaling pathway *(168)*. However, VEGF also activates p38 MAP kinase, which is a known modulator of proapoptotic signals in endothelial cells *(169)*. Blockade of VEGF-mediated activation of PI3 kinase or Akt signaling can lead to increases in apoptosis by enhancing the activation of p38 MAP kinase *(170)*. Studies in retinal endothelial cells have shown a similar phenomenon of accelerated apoptosis even in the presence of exogenous VEGF when cells are exposed to high glucose or oxidative stress *(171, 172)*. This proapoptotic effect is associated with activation of p38 MAP kinase, inhibition of Akt-kinase, and tyrosine nitration of the regulatory subunit of PI3 kinase p85 *(171)*. Given that p85 is a known target for peroxynitrite-induced nitration on tyrosine which blocks its interaction with the PI3 kinase catalytic subunit p110 *(173)*, these data suggest that peroxynitrite can alter cell survival responses mediated by PI3-kinase. More work is needed to determine whether this mechanism also plays a role in ROS-mediated impairment of neuronal and glial cell survival function.

THERAPEUTIC STRATEGIES FOR REDUCING OXIDATIVE STRESS

Overview

As has been explained in the section "Antioxidants in Diabetic Retinopathy," formation of ROS is increased in diabetes and is directly related to the complications of diabetes. A number of treatments that reduce levels of oxidative stress have also shown promise in reducing signs of diabetic retinopathy in experimental models (Fig. 2). Therapies with potential actions in reducing ROS will be discussed in this section, some only briefly as they are the subjects of other chapters in this book.

Antioxidants

The causal role of oxidants in diabetic retinopathy is well established, and antioxidant therapy has shown great promise when tested in tissue culture and experimental animal models. However, antioxidant agents that scavenge formed oxidants have not

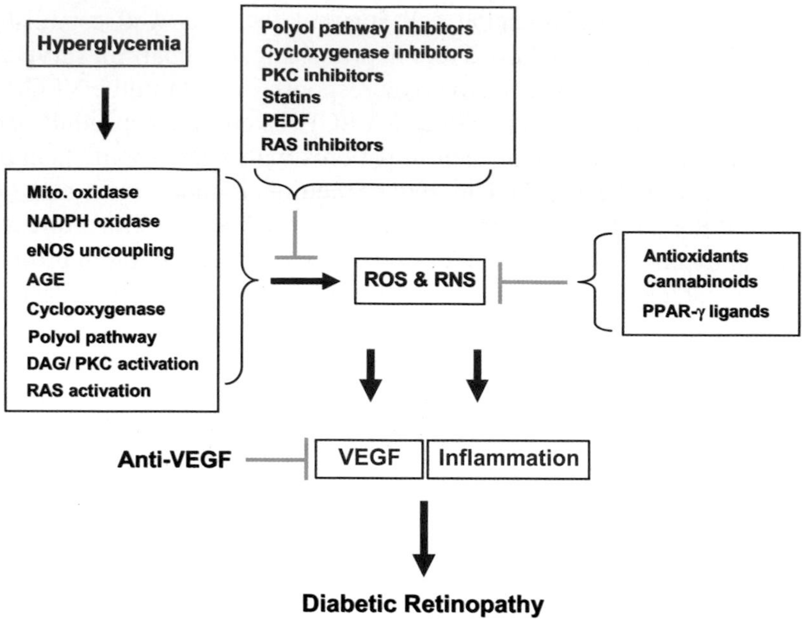

Fig. 2. Therapeutic strategies for reducing ROS and RNS in the diabetic retina.

proven to be very effective clinically. Treatment with vitamin E (α-tocopherol) for 4 months raised retinal blood flow in patients with type I diabetes and mild or no retinopathy *(174)*, but other large studies failed to show a beneficial effect. Chronic treatment with vitamin E also failed to decrease cardiovascular events in a large study with a high percentage of diabetic patients *(20)*. A major limitation of treatment with vitamin E or other antioxidants is that these therapies scavenge already-formed oxidants, but do not prevent their formation.

PKC Inhibitors

As has been noted, PKC has been clearly established as both a source and a target of reactive oxygen species in diabetic retinopathy. Clinical trials testing the efficacy of the PKC-beta inhibitor ruboxistaurin have supported the hypothesis that PKC activation, especially the β isoform, plays an important role in the development of diabetic macular edema (for review, see *(45)*). However, while ruboxistaurin treatment was found to improve visual acuity in patients with diabetic macular edema, clinical trials showed that it did not reduce or reverse the progression of diabetic macular edema or prevent the development of proliferative diabetic retinopathy *(175)*.

Inhibitors of the Renin-Angiotensin System

Studies in animal and tissue culture models have implicated the renin-angiotensin system (RAS) in the development and progression of retinal vascular diseases, including diabetic retinopathy. Angiotensin II (Ang II) is the main mediator of the RAS and has been shown to activate PKC. Ang II induces vascular injury through several mechanisms, including ROS formation and inflammation. Several small studies of patients with type I or type II diabetes have shown beneficial effects of inhibiting the RAS in reducing the risk of diabetic retinopathy. A larger trial in patients with type I diabetes showed that treatment with an angiotensin-converting enzyme (ACE) inhibitor reduced the risk for progression of retinopathy. Another study in patients with type II diabetes found that treatment with an ACE inhibitor reduced the need for laser photocoagulation treatment. However, questions remain as to the effect of blood pressure control on development and progression of microvascular complications in the retina. A large clinical trial is in progress to determine whether blockade of the RAS with an Ang II-receptor blocker can prevent the incidence and progression of retinopathy in normotensive or mildly hypertensive diabetic patients (for review, see *(176, 177)*).

Inhibitors of the Polyol Pathway

As has been discussed in the section "Sources of Oxidative Stress in the Diabetic Retina," the importance of the aldose reductase (AR) polyol pathway in the development of diabetic retinopathy has been strongly supported by studies in experimental animals and endothelial cells treated with high glucose *(42, 43)*, However, clinical studies using AR inhibitors in patients have failed to show a beneficial effect in preventing diabetic retinopathy (for review, see *(178)*).

HMG-CoA Reductase Inhibitors (Statins)

Increases in serum lipid levels are positively correlated with visual impairment due to macular edema and formation of hard exudates in the retinas of diabetic patients *(179)*. The lipid-lowering agents statins have been shown to reduce the risk of cardiovascular events in diabetic patients *(180, 181)*. Recent studies have shown that statins possess remarkable vasoprotective effects in a variety of diseases, including diabetes *(182–184)*. These protective effects are exerted mainly on the microvasculature, are independent of their cholesterol-lowering properties, and appear to be the result of both anti-inflammatory and antioxidant functions *(185)*. The efficacy of statin therapy for diabetic retinopathy has not been fully studied, but several small trials in patients with macular edema have found positive effects on hard exudates, clinically significant macular edema, and simple diabetic retinopathy *(186–188)*.

PEDF

As has been discussed in the section "Effects of Oxidative Stress in the Diabetic Retina," PEDF has been shown to have prominent antioxidant function in various in vitro model systems. Studies showing that retinal and choroidal neovascularization as well as ischemia-induced neurotoxicity and proliferative neovascularization can be inhibited by intraocular gene transfer of PEDF *(189–192)* suggest that a strategy for enhancing the expression and function of this protein could be effective in treating diabetic retinopathy. A phase I trial investigating the effect of a single intraocular injection of an adenoviral vector-expressing human PEDF in patients with advanced choroidal neovascularization due to age-related macular degeneration has been completed with promising results *(193)*. Further study is needed to determine the efficacy of PEDF in preventing diabetic retinopathy.

Cannabinoids

Recent studies indicate that cannabinoids may also be useful in reducing oxidative stress. Cannabinoids have a variety of potentially beneficial properties including anti-inflammatory *(194)* and antioxidant actions *(195)*. Several synthetic, nonpsychoactive cannabinoids have shown promising results in the reducing oxidative stress, suppressing inflammation, and inhibiting neurotoxicity in conditions of central nervous system injury. Phase 3 clinical trials have demonstrated the efficacy and safety of dexanabinol in the treatment of traumatic brain injury due to its abilities to antagonize N-methyl-D-aspartate receptors, scavenge reactive oxygen species, and suppress inflammation *(196)*. Another synthetic, nonpsychoactive compound, cannabidiol (CBD), has been found to block neuronal damage resulting from cerebral ischemia *(197)*. CBD has recently been approved for the treatment of inflammation, pain, and spasticity in patients with multiple sclerosis. A recent study demonstrated potent antioxidant and anti-inflammatory effects of CBD where it blocked the effects of high glucose in increasing mitochondrial superoxide generation, NF-kappa B activation, nitrotyrosine formation, upregulation of iNOS and adhesion molecules ICAM-1 and VCAM-1, transendothelial migration of monocytes, and monocyte-endothelial adhesion in human coronary endothelial cells *(198)*. CBD has also been shown to have potent neuroprotective actions in the retina *(199)*. Studies showing that CBD also prevents diabetes-induced neurotoxicity and preserves blood-retinal barrier function in experimental diabetes suggest that it could also be useful in the treatment of diabetic retinopathy *(155)*.

Cyclo-oxygenase-2 (COX-2) Inhibitors

As has been outlined in the section "Antioxidants in Diabetic Retinopathy," COX-2 expression is increased during diabetes *(37)* and elevated COX-2 increases ROS formation *(38)*. COX-2 inhibition has been noted to protect against diabetic neuropathy in animals *(39)*. High doses of aspirin, a nonselective inhibitor of both COX-1 and-2, have been reported to prevent some signs of diabetic retinopathy in diabetic patients and experimental animals *(78, 200, 201)*. However, other clinical trials showed that treatment with high-dose aspirin did not prevent the development of high-risk proliferative retinopathy and did not reduce the risk of visual loss, nor did it increase the risk of vitreous hemorrhage *(202)*. Clinical trials are in progress to evaluate the effectiveness of celecoxib on proliferative diabetic retinopathy *(179)*. Unfortunately, chronic use of selective COX-2 inhibitors has been associated with increased risks of adverse cardiovascular events *(203)*.

Peroxisome Proliferator-Activated Receptor γ Ligands

Thiazolidinediones and glitazones are insulin-sensitizer agents that bind to and activate the nuclear receptor peroxisome proliferator-activated receptor γ (PPARγ). Although these drugs are used primarily for lowering blood glucose levels, studies have shown that they are also effective in reducing arterial inflammation and oxidative stress (for review, see *(204)*). The ability of PPARγ ligands to improve endothelial dysfunction by reducing oxidative stress has prompted the initiation of clinical trials designed to investigate their effects on cardiovascular disease in diabetes. A large clinical trial with pioglitazone showed a beneficial effect in reducing all-cause mortality, nonfatal myocardial infarction, and stroke in patients with type 2 diabetes and pre-existing cardiovascular disease *(205)*. However, this positive outcome was also accompanied adverse findings, including increases in the incidence of edema not attributable to heart failure and increases in heart failure. Moreover, the frequency of each of these adverse outcomes was greater than the reduction in incidence of cardiovascular events by the drug treatment. Furthermore, pioglitazone also caused greater increases in body weight than with other antihyperglycemic therapies, including insulin. Studies in which diabetic rats were treated with rosiglitazone have shown blockade of early signs of diabetic retinopathy *(206)*. However the efficacy of PPARγ ligands in improving diabetic retinopathy in patients has not yet been determined.

REFERENCES

1. Frank RN. Diabetic retinopathy. N Engl J Med 2004;350(1):48–58.
2. Caldwell RB, Bartoli M, Behzadian MA, et al. Vascular endothelial growth factor and diabetic retinopathy: Role of oxidative stress. Curr Drug Targets 2005;6(4):511–24.
3. Effect of intensive blood-glucose control with metformin on complications in overweight patients with type 2 diabetes (ukpds 34). Uk prospective diabetes study (ukpds) group. Lancet 1998;352(9131): 854–65.
4. The effect of intensive treatment of diabetes on the development and progression of long-term complications in insulin-dependent diabetes mellitus. The diabetes control and complications trial research group. N Engl J Med 1993;329(14):977–86.
5. Mitamura Y, Takeuchi S, Matsuda A, Tagawa Y, Mizue Y, Nishihira J. Monocyte chemotactic protein-1 in the vitreous of patients with proliferative diabetic retinopathy. Ophthalmologica 2001;215(6):415–8.
6. Hernandez C, Segura RM, Fonollosa A, Carrasco E, Francisco G, Simo R. Interleukin-8, monocyte chemoattractant protein-1 and il-10 in the vitreous fluid of patients with proliferative diabetic retinopathy. Diabet Med 2005;22(6):719–22.
7. Krady JK, Basu A, Allen CM, et al. Minocycline reduces proinflammatory cytokine expression, microglial activation, and caspase-3 activation in a rodent model of diabetic retinopathy. Diabetes 2005;54(5):1559–65.
8. Antonetti DA, Barber AJ, Khin S, Lieth E, Tarbell JM, Gardner TW. Vascular permeability in experimental diabetes is associated with reduced endothelial occludin content: Vascular endothelial growth factor decreases occludin in retinal endothelial cells. Penn state retina research group. Diabetes 1998;47(12):1953–9.
9. Starita C, Patel M, Katz B, Adamis AP. Vascular endothelial growth factor and the potential therapeutic use of pegaptanib (macugen) in diabetic retinopathy. Dev Ophthalmol 2007;39:122–48.
10. Meleth AD, Agron E, Chan CC, et al. Serum inflammatory markers in diabetic retinopathy. Invest Ophthalmol Vis Sci 2005;46(11):4295–301.
11. Joussen AM, Poulaki V, Le ML, et al. A central role for inflammation in the pathogenesis of diabetic retinopathy. Faseb J 2004;18(12):1450–2.
12. Miyamoto K, Hiroshiba N, Tsujikawa A, Ogura Y. In vivo demonstration of increased leukocyte entrapment in retinal microcirculation of diabetic rats. Invest Ophthalmol Vis Sci 1998;39(11):2190–4.
13. Ishida S, Yamashiro K, Usui T, et al. [significance of leukocytes in the regulation of retinal edema, ischemia, and angiogenesis]. Nippon Ganka Gakkai Zasshi 2004;108(4):193–201.

14. Furuta T, Saito T, Ootaka T, et al. The role of macrophages in diabetic glomerulosclerosis. Am J Kidney Dis 1993;21(5):480–5.
15. Yoshida S, Yoshida A, Ishibashi T, Elner SG, Elner VM. Role of mcp-1 and mip-1alpha in retinal neovascularization during postischemic inflammation in a mouse model of retinal neovascularization. J Leukoc Biol 2003;73(1):137–44.
16. Ishida S, Usui T, Yamashiro K, et al. Vegf164-mediated inflammation is required for pathological, but not physiological, ischemia-induced retinal neovascularization. J Exp Med 2003;198(3):483–9.
17. Rungger-Brandle E, Dosso AA, Leuenberger PM. Glial reactivity, an early feature of diabetic retinopathy. Invest Ophthalmol Vis Sci 2000;41(7):1971–80.
18. Giugliano D, Ceriello A, Paolisso G. Oxidative stress and diabetic vascular complications. Diabetes Care 1996;19(3):257–67.
19. Kowluru RA, Chan PS. Oxidative stress and diabetic retinopathy. Exp Diabetes Res 2007;2007:43603.
20. Pennathur S, Heinecke JW. Mechanisms for oxidative stress in diabetic cardiovascular disease. Antioxid Redox Signal 2007;9(7):955–69.
21. Rosen P, Nawroth PP, King G, Moller W, Tritschler HJ, Packer L. The role of oxidative stress in the onset and progression of diabetes and its complications: A summary of a congress series sponsored by unesco-mcbn, the american diabetes association and the german diabetes society. Diabetes Metab Res Rev 2001;17(3):189–212.
22. Halliwell B. Antioxidants in human health and disease. Annu Rev Nutr 1996;16:33–50.
23. Sies H. Oxidative stress: From basic research to clinical application. Am J Med 1991;91(3C):31S-8S.
24. Halliwell B. Antioxidant characterization. Methodology and mechanism. Biochem Pharmacol 1995;49(10):1341–8.
25. Packer L, Tritschler HJ. Alpha-lipoic acid: The metabolic antioxidant. Free Radic Biol Med 1996;20(4):625–6.
26. Nishikawa T, Edelstein D, Brownlee M. The missing link: A single unifying mechanism for diabetic complications. Kidney Int Suppl 2000;77:S26–30.
27. Brownlee M. Biochemistry and molecular cell biology of diabetic complications. Nature 2001;414(6865):813–20.
28. Yung LM, Leung FP, Yao X, Chen ZY, Huang Y. Reactive oxygen species in vascular wall. Cardiovasc Hematol Disord Drug Targets 2006;6(1):1–19.
29. Paradies G, Petrosillo G, Pistolese M, Ruggiero FM. Reactive oxygen species generated by the mitochondrial respiratory chain affect the complex iii activity via cardiolipin peroxidation in beef-heart submitochondrial particles. Mitochondrion 2001;1(2):151–9.
30. Kowluru RA, Kowluru V, Xiong Y, Ho YS. Overexpression of mitochondrial superoxide dismutase in mice protects the retina from diabetes-induced oxidative stress. Free Radic Biol Med 2006; 41(8):1191–6.
31. Kanwar M, Chan PS, Kern TS, Kowluru RA. Oxidative damage in the retinal mitochondria of diabetic mice: Possible protection by superoxide dismutase. Invest Ophthalmol Vis Sci 2007;48(8):3805–11.
32. Li L, Renier G. Activation of nicotinamide adenine dinucleotide phosphate (reduced form) oxidase by advanced glycation end products links oxidative stress to altered retinal vascular endothelial growth factor expression. Metabolism 2006;55(11):1516–23.
33. Nitti M, Furfaro AL, Traverso N, et al. Pkc delta and nadph oxidase in age-induced neuronal death. Neurosci Lett 2007;416(3):261–5.
34. Goldin A, Beckman JA, Schmidt AM, Creager MA. Advanced glycation end products: Sparking the development of diabetic vascular injury. Circulation 2006;114(6):597–605.
35. Yan SF, Barile GR, D'Agati V, Du Yan S, Ramasamy R, Schmidt AM. The biology of rage and its ligands: Uncovering mechanisms at the heart of diabetes and its complications. Curr Diab Rep 2007;7(2):146–53.
36. Cosentino F, Eto M, De Paolis P, et al. High glucose causes upregulation of cyclooxygenase-2 and alters prostanoid profile in human endothelial cells: Role of protein kinase c and reactive oxygen species. Circulation 2003;107(7):1017–23.
37. Li J, Chen YJ, Quilley J. Effect of tempol on renal cyclooxygenase expression and activity in experimental diabetes in the rat. J Pharmacol Exp Ther 2005;314(2):818–24.
38. Pop-Busui R, Sima A, Stevens M. Diabetic neuropathy and oxidative stress. Diabetes Metab Res Rev 2006;22(4):257–73.

39. Kellogg AP, Pop-Busui R. Peripheral nerve dysfunction in experimental diabetes is mediated by cyclooxygenase-2 and oxidative stress. Antioxid Redox Signal 2005;7(11–12):1521–9.
40. Zheng L, Howell SJ, Hatala DA, Huang K, Kern TS. Salicylate-based anti-inflammatory drugs inhibit the early lesion of diabetic retinopathy. Diabetes 2007;56(2):337–45.
41. Kern TS, Miller CM, Du Y, et al. Topical administration of nepafenac inhibits diabetes-induced retinal microvascular disease and underlying abnormalities of retinal metabolism and physiology. Diabetes 2007;56(2):373–9.
42. Sun W, Oates PJ, Coutcher JB, Gerhardinger C, Lorenzi M. A selective aldose reductase inhibitor of a new structural class prevents or reverses early retinal abnormalities in experimental diabetic retinopathy. Diabetes 2006;55(10):2757–62.
43. El-Remessy AB, Abou-Mohamed G, Caldwell RW, Caldwell RB. High glucose-induced tyrosine nitration in endothelial cells: Role of enos uncoupling and aldose reductase activation. Invest Ophthalmol Vis Sci 2003;44(7):3135–43.
44. Koya D, Jirousek MR, Lin YW, Ishii H, Kuboki K, King GL. Characterization of protein kinase c beta isoform activation on the gene expression of transforming growth factor-beta, extracellular matrix components, and prostanoids in the glomeruli of diabetic rats. J Clin Invest 1997;100(1):115–26.
45. Das Evcimen N, King GL. The role of protein kinase c activation and the vascular complications of diabetes. Pharmacol Res 2007;55(6):498–510.
46. Zhang L, Ma J, Gu Y, Lin S. Effects of blocking the renin-angiotensin system on expression and translocation of protein kinase c isoforms in the kidney of diabetic rats. Nephron Exp Nephrol 2006;104(3):e103–11.
47. Malhotra A, Kang BP, Cheung S, Opawumi D, Meggs LG. Angiotensin ii promotes glucose-induced activation of cardiac protein kinase c isozymes and phosphorylation of troponin i. Diabetes 2001;50(8):1918–26.
48. Wilkinson-Berka JL. Angiotensin and diabetic retinopathy. Int J Biochem Cell Biol 2006;38(5–6):752–65.
49. Abou-Mohamed G, Johnson JA, Jin L, et al. Roles of superoxide, peroxynitrite, and protein kinase c in the development of tolerance to nitroglycerin. J Pharmacol Exp Ther 2004;308(1):289–99. Epub 2003 Oct 16.
50. Heinzel B, John M, Klatt P, Bohme E, Mayer B. Ca2+/calmodulin-dependent formation of hydrogen peroxide by brain nitric oxide synthase. Biochem J 1992;281 (Pt 3):627–30.
51. Mayer B, John M, Heinzel B, et al. Brain nitric oxide synthase is a biopterin- and flavin-containing multi-functional oxido-reductase. FEBS Lett 1991;288(1–2):187–91.
52. Presta A, Liu J, Sessa WC, Stuehr DJ. Substrate binding and calmodulin binding to endothelial nitric oxide synthase coregulate its enzymatic activity. Nitric Oxide 1997;1(1):74–87.
53. Stamler JS, Jaraki O, Osborne J, et al. Nitric oxide circulates in mammalian plasma primarily as an s-nitroso adduct of serum albumin. Proc Natl Acad Sci U S A 1992;89(16):7674–7.
54. Drexler H, Hayoz D, Munzel T, et al. Endothelial function in chronic congestive heart failure. Am J Cardiol 1992;69(19):1596–601.
55. Rector TS, Bank AJ, Mullen KA, et al. Randomized, double-blind, placebo-controlled study of supplemental oral l-arginine in patients with heart failure. Circulation 1996;93(12):2135–41.
56. Graier WF, Posch K, Wascher TC, Kostner GM. Role of superoxide anions in changes of endothelial vasoactive response during acute hyperglycemia. Horm Metab Res 1997;29(12):622–6.
57. Mayhan WG, Rubinstein I. Acetylcholine induces vasoconstriction in the microcirculation of cardiomyopathic hamsters: Reversal by l-arginine. Biochem Biophys Res Commun 1992;184(3):1372–7.
58. Gold ME, Wood KS, Byrns RE, Buga GM, Ignarro LJ. L-arginine-dependent vascular smooth muscle relaxation and cgmp formation. Am J Physiol 1990;259(6 Pt 2):H1813–21.
59. Parker JO, Parker JD, Caldwell RW, Farrel B, Kaesemeyer WH. The effect of supplemental l-arginine on tolerance development during continuous transdermal nitroglycerin therapy. J Am Coll Card 2002;39(7):1199–203.
60. Romero MJ, Platt DH, Tawfik HE, El-Remessy AB, Bartoli M, Labazi M, Caldwell RB, Caldwell RW. Diabetes-induced coronary dysfunction involves increased arginase activity. Circ Res 2008; 102(1):95–102
61. Shimizu S, Nomoto M, Naito S, Yamamoto T, Momose K. Stimulation of nitric oxide synthase during oxidative endothelial cell injury. Biochem Pharmacol 1998;55(1):77–83.

62. Pritchard KA, Jr., Groszek L, Smalley DM, et al. Native low-density lipoprotein increases endothelial cell nitric oxide synthase generation of superoxide anion. Circ Res 1995;77(3):510–8.
63. Tanner FC, Noll G, Boulanger CM, Luscher TF. Oxidized low density lipoproteins inhibit relaxations of porcine coronary arteries. Role of scavenger receptor and endothelium-derived nitric oxide. Circulation 1991;83(6):2012–20.
64. Jay MT, Chirico S, Siow RC, et al. Modulation of vascular tone by low density lipoproteins: Effects on L-arginine transport and nitric oxide synthesis. Exp Physiol 1997;82(2):349–60.
65. Jeremy RW, McCarron H, Sullivan D. Effects of dietary L-arginine on atherosclerosis and endothelium-dependent vasodilatation in the hypercholesterolemic rabbit. Response according to treatment duration, anatomic site, and sex. Circulation 1996;94(3):498–506.
66. Schulman SP, Becker LC, Kass DA, et al. L-arginine therapy in acute myocardial infarction: The vascular interaction with age in myocardial infarction (vintage mi) randomized clinical trial. Jama 2006;295(1):58–64.
67. Morris SM, Jr. Regulation of enzymes of urea and arginine synthesis. Annu Rev Nutr 1992;12:81–101.
68. Socha HM, Romero MJ, Caldwell RB, Caldwell RW. Oral citrulline administration enhances no-dependent vasodilation. FASEB (Exp Biol) 2006:Abs 703.4.
69. Romero MJ, Platt DH., Caldwell, R.B., Caldwell, R.W. Therapeutic use of citrulline in cardiovascular disease.. Cardiovasc Drug Rev 2006;24(3–4):189–295.
70. Shearer JD, Richards JR, Mills CD, Caldwell MD. Differential regulation of macrophage arginine metabolism: A proposed role in wound healing. Am J Physiol 1997;272(2 Pt 1):E181–90.
71. Taverna MJ, Elgrably F, Selmi H, Selam JL, Slama G. The t-786c and c774t endothelial nitric oxide synthase gene polymorphisms independently affect the onset pattern of severe diabetic retinopathy. Nitric Oxide 2005;13(1):88–92.
72. Taverna MJ, Sola A, Guyot-Argenton C, et al. Enos4 polymorphism of the endothelial nitric oxide synthase predicts risk for severe diabetic retinopathy. Diabet Med 2002;19(3):240–5.
73. El-Remessy AB, Behzadian MA, Abou-Mohamed G, Franklin T, Caldwell RW, Caldwell RB. Experimental diabetes causes breakdown of the blood-retina barrier by a mechanism involving tyrosine nitration and increases in expression of vascular endothelial growth factor and urokinase plasminogen activator receptor. Am J Pathol 2003;162(6):1995–2004.
74. Pacher P, Beckman JS, Liaudet L. Nitric oxide and peroxynitrite in health and disease. Physiol Rev 2007;87(1):315–424.
75. Zheng L, Du Y, Miller C, et al. Critical role of inducible nitric oxide synthase in degeneration of retinal capillaries in mice with streptozotocin-induced diabetes. Diabetologia 2007;50(9):1987–96.
76. Brooks SE, Gu X, Samuel S, et al. Reduced severity of oxygen-induced retinopathy in enos-deficient mice. Invest Ophthalmol Vis Sci 2001;42(1):222–8.
77. Hammes HP, Martin S, Federlin K, Geisen K, Brownlee M. Aminoguanidine treatment inhibits the development of experimental diabetic retinopathy. Proc Natl Acad Sci U S A 1991;88(24): 11555–8.
78. Kern TS, Engerman RL. Pharmacological inhibition of diabetic retinopathy: Aminoguanidine and aspirin. Diabetes 2001;50(7):1636–42.
79. Kern TS, Tang J, Mizutani M, et al. Response of capillary cell death to aminoguanidine predicts the development of retinopathy: Comparison of diabetes and galactosemia. Invest Ophthalmol Vis Sci 2000;41(12):3972–8.
80. Guzik TJ, Korbut R, Adamek-Guzik T. Nitric oxide and superoxide in inflammation and immune regulation. J Physiol Pharmacol 2003;54(4):469–87.
81. Toda N, Nakanishi-Toda M. Nitric oxide: Ocular blood flow, glaucoma, and diabetic retinopathy. Prog Retin Eye Res 2007;26(3):205–38.
82. Lambeth JD. Nox enzymes and the biology of reactive oxygen. Nat Rev Immunol 2004;4(3):181–9.
83. Lee SB, Bae IH, Bae YS, Um HD. Link between mitochondria and nadph oxidase 1 isozyme for the sustained production of reactive oxygen species and cell death. J Biol Chem 2006;281(47):36228–35.
84. Ellis EA, Guberski DL, Somogyi-Mann M, Grant MB. Increased h2o2, vascular endothelial growth factor and receptors in the retina of the bbz/wor diabetic rat. Free Radic Biol Med 2000;28(1):91–101.
85. Inoguchi T, Sonta T, Tsubouchi H, et al. Protein kinase c-dependent increase in reactive oxygen species (ros) production in vascular tissues of diabetes: Role of vascular nad(p)h oxidase. J Am Soc Nephrol 2003;14(8 Suppl 3):S227–32.

86. Sonta T, Inoguchi T, Tsubouchi H, et al. Evidence for contribution of vascular nad(p)h oxidase to increased oxidative stress in animal models of diabetes and obesity. Free Radic Biol Med 2004;37(1):115–23.
87. Griendling KK, Sorescu D, Ushio-Fukai M. nad(p)h oxidase: Role in cardiovascular biology and disease. Circ Res 2000;86(5):494–501.
88A. Al-Shabrawey M, Bartoli M, El-Remessy AB, et al. Inhibition of nad(p)h oxidase activity blocks vascular endothelial growth factor overexpression and neovascularization during ischemic retinopathy. Am J Pathol 2005;167(2):599–607.
88B. Al-Shabrawey M, Rojas M, Sanders T et al., Role of NADPH oxidase in retinal vascular inflammation. Invest Ophthalmol Vis Sci 2008;49(7):3239-3244.
89. Al-Shabrawey M, Bartoli M, El-Remessy AB, et al. Signs of diabetic. Role of NADPH oxidase and STAT3 in statin-mediated protection against diabetic retinopathy. Invest Ophthalmol Vis Sci 2008;49(7)3231–3238.
90. Hordijk PL. Regulation of nadph oxidases: The role of rac proteins. Circ Res 2006;98(4):453–62.
91. Heyworth PG, Curnutte JT, Nauseef WM, et al. Neutrophil nicotinamide adenine dinucleotide phosphate oxidase assembly. Translocation of p47-phox and p67-phox requires interaction between p47-phox and cytochrome b558. J Clin Invest 1991;87(1):352–6.
92. Koga H, Terasawa H, Nunoi H, Takeshige K, Inagaki F, Sumimoto H. Tetratricopeptide repeat (tpr) motifs of p67(phox) participate in interaction with the small gtpase rac and activation of the phagocyte nadph oxidase. J Biol Chem 1999;274(35):25051–60.
93. Vecchione C, Aretini A, Marino G, et al. Selective rac-1 inhibition protects from diabetes-induced vascular injury. Circ Res 2006;98(2):218–25.
94. Sorescu D, Somers MJ, Lassegue B, Grant S, Harrison DG, Griendling KK. Electron spin resonance characterization of the nad(p)h oxidase in vascular smooth muscle cells. Free Radic Biol Med 2001;30(6):603–12.
95. Van Buul JD, Fernandez-Borja M, Anthony EC, Hordijk PL. Expression and localization of nox2 and nox4 in primary human endothelial cells. Antioxid Redox Signal 2005;7(3–4):308–17.
96. Green SP, Cairns B, Rae J, et al. Induction of gp91-phox, a component of the phagocyte nadph oxidase, in microglial cells during central nervous system inflammation. J Cereb Blood Flow Metab 2001;21(4):374–84.
97. Ago T, Kitazono T, Ooboshi H, et al. Nox4 as the major catalytic component of an endothelial nad(p)h oxidase. Circulation 2004;109(2):227–33.
98. Jain SK. Superoxide dismutase overexpression and cellular oxidative damage in diabetes. A commentary on "Overexpression of mitochondrial superoxide dismutase in mice protects the retina from diabetes-induced oxidative stress". Free Radic Biol Med 2006;41(8):1187–90.
99. Maritim AC, Sanders RA, Watkins JB, 3rd. Diabetes, oxidative stress, and antioxidants: A review. J Biochem Mol Toxicol 2003;17(1):24–38.
100. Paget C, Lecomte M, Ruggiero D, Wiernsperger N, Lagarde M. Modification of enzymatic antioxidants in retinal microvascular cells by glucose or advanced glycation end products. Free Radic Biol Med 1998;25(1):121–9.
101. Jennings PE, Jones AF, Florkowski CM, Lunec J, Barnett AH. Increased diene conjugates in diabetic subjects with microangiopathy. Diabet Med 1987;4(5):452–6.
102. Ghezzi P. Regulation of protein function by glutathionylation. Free Radic Res 2005;39(6):573–80.
103. Winkler BS, Giblin FJ. Glutathione oxidation in retina: Effects on biochemical and electrical activities. Exp Eye Res 1983;36(2):287–97.
104. Meister A. Glutathione metabolism and its selective modification. J Biol Chem 1988;263(33):17205–8.
105. Kowluru RA, Engerman RL, Kern TS. Abnormalities of retinal metabolism in diabetes or experimental galactosemia viii. Prevention by aminoguanidine. Curr Eye Res 2000;21:814–9.
106. Kern TS, Kowluru RA, Engerman RL. Abnormalities of retinal metabolism in diabetes or galactosemia: Atpases and glutathione. Invest Ophthalmol Vis Sci 1994;35(7):2962–7.
107. Muriach M, Bosch-Morell F, Alexander G, et al. Lutein effect on retina and hippocampus of diabetic mice. Free Radic Biol Med 2006;41(6):979–84.
108. Sampathkumar R, Balasubramanyam M, Tara C, Rema M, Mohan V. Association of hypoglutathionemia with reduced Na+/K+ atpase activity in type 2 diabetes and microangiopathy. Mol Cell Biochem 2006;282(1–2):169–76.

109. Cicik E, Tekin H, Akar S, et al. Interleukin-8, nitric oxide and glutathione status in proliferative vitreoretinopathy and proliferative diabetic retinopathy. Ophthalmic Res 2003;35(5):251–5.
110. Li W, Yanoff M, Jian B, He Z. Altered mrna levels of antioxidant enzymes in pre-apoptotic pericytes from human diabetic retinas. Cell Mol Biol (Noisy-le-grand) 1999;45(1):59–66.
111. Obrosova IG, Fathallah L, Greene DA. Early changes in lipid peroxidation and antioxidative defense in diabetic rat retina: Effect of dl-alpha-lipoic acid. Eur J Pharmacol 2000;398(1):139–46.
112. Kowluru RA, Kern TS, Engerman RL. Abnormalities of retinal metabolism in diabetes or experimental galactosemia. IV. Antioxidant defense system. Free Radic Biol Med 1997;22(4):587–92.
113. Du Y, Miller CM, Kern TS. Hyperglycemia increases mitochondrial superoxide in retina and retinal cells. Free Radic Biol Med 2003;35(11):1491–9.
114. Obrosova IG, Drel VR, Kumagai AK, Szabo C, Pacher P, Stevens MJ. Early diabetes-induced biochemical changes in the retina: Comparison of rat and mouse models. Diabetologia 2006;49(10):2525–33.
115. Bubici C, Papa S, Dean K, Franzoso G. Mutual cross-talk between reactive oxygen species and nuclear factor-kappa b: Molecular basis and biological significance. Oncogene 2006;25(51):6731–48.
116. Dworakowski R, Anilkumar N, Zhang M, Shah AM. Redox signalling involving nadph oxidase-derived reactive oxygen species. Biochem Soc Trans 2006;34(Pt 5):960–4.
117. Gauss KA, Nelson-Overton LK, Siemsen DW, Gao Y, Deleo FR, Quinn MT. Role of nf-{kappa}b in transcriptional regulation of the phagocyte nadph oxidase by tumor necrosis factor-{alpha}. J Leukoc Biol 2007.
118. Ellis EA, Grant MB, Murray FT, et al. Increased nadh oxidase activity in the retina of the bbz/wor diabetic rat. Free Radic Biol Med 1998;24(1):111–20.
119. Kuroki M, Voest EE, Amano S, et al. Reactive oxygen intermediates increase vascular endothelial growth factor expression in vitro and in vivo. J Clin Invest 1996;98(7):1667–75.
120. Obrosova IG, Minchenko AG, Marinescu V, et al. Antioxidants attenuate early up regulation of retinal vascular endothelial growth factor in streptozotocin-diabetic rats. Diabetologia 2001;44(9):1102–10.
121. El-Remessy A, Behzadian MA, Abou-Mohamed G, Franklin T, Caldwell RW, Caldwell RB. Peroxynitrite increases vascular permeability in experimental diabetes by a mechanism involving increased expression of vegf and urokinase plasminogen activator receptor (upar). Am J Pathol 2003;162:1995–2004.
122. Bartoli M, Lemtalsi T, Platt DH, El-Remessy AB, Caldwell RB. Diabetes induces activation of stat3 via nad(p)h oxidase-dependent induction of src kinase. Submitted.
123. Platt DH, Bartoli M, El-Remessy AB, et al. Peroxynitrite increases vegf expression in vascular endothelial cells via stat3. Free Radic Biol Med 2005;39(10):1353–61.
124. Funamoto M, Fujio Y, Kunisada K, et al. Signal transducer and activator of transcription 3 is required for glycoprotein 130-mediated induction of vascular endothelial growth factor in cardiac myocytes. J Biol Chem 2000;275(14):10561–6.
125. Niu G, Wright KL, Huang M, et al. Constitutive stat3 activity up-regulates vegf expression and tumor angiogenesis. Oncogene 2002;21(13):2000–8.
126. Osugi T, Oshima Y, Fujio Y, et al. Cardiac-specific activation of signal transducer and activator of transcription 3 promotes vascular formation in the heart. J Biol Chem 2002;277(8):6676–81.
127. Schaefer LK, Ren Z, Fuller GN, Schaefer TS. Constitutive activation of stat3alpha in brain tumors: Localization to tumor endothelial cells and activation by the endothelial tyrosine kinase receptor (vegfr-2). Oncogene 2002;21(13):2058–65.
128. Valdembri D, Serini G, Vacca A, Ribatti D, Bussolino F. In vivo activation of jak2/stat-3 pathway during angiogenesis induced by gm-csf. Faseb J 2002;16(2):225–7.
129. Bartoli M, Platt D, Lemtalsi T, et al. Vegf differentially activates stat3 in microvascular endothelial cells. Faseb J 2003;17(11):1562–4. Epub 2003 Jun 17.
130. Yamagishi S, Yonekura H, Yamamoto Y, et al. Advanced glycation end products-driven angiogenesis in vitro. Induction of the growth and tube formation of human microvascular endothelial cells through autocrine vascular endothelial growth factor. J Biol Chem 1997;272(13):8723–30.
131. Tombran-Tink J, Barnstable CJ. Pedf: A multifaceted neurotrophic factor. Nat Rev Neurosci 2003;4(8):628–36.
132. Barnstable CJ, Tombran-Tink J. Neuroprotective and antiangiogenic actions of pedf in the eye: Molecular targets and therapeutic potential. Prog Retin Eye Res 2004;23(5):561–77.

133. Stellmach V, Crawford SE, Zhou W, Bouck N. Prevention of ischemia-induced retinopathy by the natural ocular antiangiogenic agent pigment epithelium-derived factor. Proc Natl Acad Sci U S A 2001;98(5):2593–7. Epub 001 Jan 23.
134. Liu H, Ren JG, Cooper WL, Hawkins CE, Cowan MR, Tong PY. Identification of the antivasopermeability effect of pigment epithelium-derived factor and its active site. Proc Natl Acad Sci U S A 2004;101(17):6605–10. Epub 2004 Apr 19.
135. Gao G, Li Y, Zhang D, Gee S, Crosson C, Ma J. Unbalanced expression of vegf and pedf in ischemia-induced retinal neovascularization. FEBS Lett 2001;489(2–3):270–6.
136. Zhang SX, Wang JJ, Gao G, Shao C, Mott R, Ma JX. Pigment epithelium-derived factor (PEDF) is an endogenous antiinflammatory factor. Faseb J 2006;20(2):323–5.
137. Yamagishi S, Inagaki Y, Amano S, Okamoto T, Takeuchi M, Makita Z. Pigment epithelium-derived factor protects cultured retinal pericytes from advanced glycation end product-induced injury through its antioxidative properties. Biochem Biophys Res Commun 2002;296(4):877–82.
138. Yamagishi S, Nakamura K, Ueda S, Kato S, Imaizumi T. Pigment epithelium-derived factor (PEDF) blocks angiotensin ii signaling in endothelial cells via suppression of nadph oxidase: A novel anti-oxidative mechanism of PEDF. Cell Tissue Res 2005;320(3):437–45.
139. Yamagishi S, Inagaki Y, Nakamura K, et al. Pigment epithelium-derived factor inhibits tnf-alpha-induced interleukin-6 expression in endothelial cells by suppressing nadph oxidase-mediated reactive oxygen species generation. J Mol Cell Cardiol 2004;37(2):497–506.
140. Yamagishi S, Nakamura K, Matsui T, et al. Pigment epithelium-derived factor inhibits advanced glycation end product-induced retinal vascular hyperpermeability by blocking reactive oxygen species-mediated vascular endothelial growth factor expression. J Biol Chem 2006;281(29):20213–20.
141. Amano S, Yamagishi S, Inagaki Y, et al. Pigment epithelium-derived factor inhibits oxidative stress-induced apoptosis and dysfunction of cultured retinal pericytes. Microvasc Res 2005;69(1–2):45–55.
142. Yokoi M, Yamagishi S, Saito A, et al. Positive association of pigment epithelium-derived factor with total antioxidant capacity in the vitreous fluid of patients with proliferative diabetic retinopathy. Br J Ophthalmol 2007;91(7):885–7.
143. Yoshida Y, Yamagishi SI, Matsui T, et al. Positive correlation of pigment epithelium-derived factor (PEDF) and total anti-oxidant capacity in aqueous humor of patients with uveitis and proliferative diabetic retinopathy. Br J Ophthalmol 2007.
144. Joussen AM, Murata T, Tsujikawa A, Kirchhof B, Bursell SE, Adamis AP. Leukocyte-mediated endothelial cell injury and death in the diabetic retina. Am J Pathol 2001;158(1):147–52.
145. Mizutani M, Kern TS, Lorenzi M. Accelerated death of retinal microvascular cells in human and experimental diabetic retinopathy. J Clin Invest 1996;97(12):2883–90.
146. Bloodworth JM, Jr. Diabetic retinopathy. Diabetes 1962;11:1–22.
147. Barber AJ. A new view of diabetic retinopathy: A neurodegenerative disease of the eye. Prog Neuropsychopharmacol Biol Psychiatry 2003;27(2):283–90.
148. Antonetti DA, Barber AJ, Bronson SK, et al. Diabetic retinopathy: Seeing beyond glucose-induced microvascular disease. Diabetes 2006;55(9):2401–11.
149. Barber AJ, Lieth E, Khin SA, Antonetti DA, Buchanan AG, Gardner TW. Neural apoptosis in the retina during experimental and human diabetes. Early onset and effect of insulin. J Clin Invest 1998;102(4):783–91.
150. Barber AJ, Nakamura M, Wolpert EB, et al. Insulin rescues retinal neurons from apoptosis by a phosphatidylinositol 3-kinase/akt-mediated mechanism that reduces the activation of caspase-3. J Biol Chem 2001;276(35):32814–21.
151. Yu XR, Jia GR, Gao GD, Wang SH, Han Y, Cao W. Neuroprotection of insulin against oxidative stress-induced apoptosis in cultured retinal neurons: Involvement of phosphoinositide 3-kinase/akt signal pathway. Acta Biochim Biophys Sin (Shanghai) 2006;38(4):241–8.
152. Nakamura M, Barber AJ, Antonetti DA, et al. Excessive hexosamines block the neuroprotective effect of insulin and induce apoptosis in retinal neurons. J Biol Chem 2001;276(47):43748–55.
153. El-Remessy AB, Al-Shabrawey M, Khalifa Y, Tsai NT, Caldwell RB, Liou GI. Neuroprotective and blood-retinal barrier-preserving effects of cannabidiol in experimental diabetes. Am J Pathol 2006;168(1):235–44.
154. Maher P, Hanneken A. Flavonoids protect retinal ganglion cells from oxidative stress-induced death. Invest Ophthalmol Vis Sci 2005;46(12):4796–803.

155. Ali TK, Matragoon S, Pillai BA, Liou GI, El-Remessy AB. Peroxynitrite mediates retinal neurodegeneration by inhibiting nerve growth factor survival signaling in experimental and human diabetes. Diabetes 2008;57(4):889-898.
156. Dyer MA, Cepko CL. Control of muller glial cell proliferation and activation following retinal injury. Nat Neurosci 2000;3(9):873–80.
157. Bringmann A, Pannicke T, Grosche J, et al. Muller cells in the healthy and diseased retina. Prog Retin Eye Res 2006;25(4):397–424.
158. Goureau O, Regnier-Ricard F, Courtois Y. Requirement for nitric oxide in retinal neuronal cell death induced by activated muller glial cells. J Neurochem 1999;72(6):2506–15.
159. Asnaghi V, Gerhardinger C, Hoehn T, Adeboje A, Lorenzi M. A role for the polyol pathway in the early neuroretinal apoptosis and glial changes induced by diabetes in the rat. Diabetes 2003;52(2):506–11.
160. Baydas G, Tuzcu M, Yasar A, Baydas B. Early changes in glial reactivity and lipid peroxidation in diabetic rat retina: Effects of melatonin. Acta Diabetol 2004;41(3):123–8.
161. Du Y, Sarthy VP, Kern TS. Interaction between no and cox pathways in retinal cells exposed to elevated glucose and retina of diabetic rats. Am J Physiol Regul Integr Comp Physiol 2004;287(4):R735–41.
162. Gerhardinger C, Costa MB, Coulombe MC, Toth I, Hoehn T, Grosu P. Expression of acute-phase response proteins in retinal muller cells in diabetes. Invest Ophthalmol Vis Sci 2005;46(1):349–57.
163. Shelton MD, Kern TS, Mieyal JJ. Glutaredoxin regulates nuclear factor kappa-b and intercellular adhesion molecule in muller cells: Model of diabetic retinopathy. J Biol Chem 2007;282(17):12467–74.
164. Duh E, Aiello LP. Vascular endothelial growth factor and diabetes: The agonist versus antagonist paradox. Diabetes 1999;48(10):1899–906.
165. Storkebaum E, Carmeliet P. vegf: A critical player in neurodegeneration. J Clin Invest 2004;113(1): 14–8.
166. Robinson GS, Ju M, Shih SC, et al. Nonvascular role for vegf: Vegfr-1, 2 activity is critical for neural retinal development. Faseb J 2001;15(7):1215–7.
167. Martin PM, Roon P, Van Ells TK, Ganapathy V, Smith SB. Death of retinal neurons in streptozotocin-induced diabetic mice. Invest Ophthalmol Vis Sci 2004;45(9):3330–6.
168. Gerber HP, McMurtrey A, Kowalski J, et al. Vascular endothelial growth factor regulates endothelial cell survival through the phosphatidylinositol 3″-kinase/akt signal transduction pathway. Requirement for flk-1/kdr activation. J Biol Chem 1998;273(46):30336–43.
169. Rousseau S, Houle F, Landry J, Huot J. P38 map kinase activation by vascular endothelial growth factor mediates actin reorganization and cell migration in human endothelial cells. Oncogene 1997;15(18):2169–77.
170. Gratton JP, Morales-Ruiz M, Kureishi Y, Fulton D, Walsh K, Sessa WC. Akt down-regulation of p38 signaling provides a novel mechanism of vascular endothelial growth factor-mediated cytoprotection in endothelial cells. J Biol Chem 2001;276(32):30359–65.
171. el-Remessy AB, Bartoli M, Platt DH, Fulton D, Caldwell RB. Oxidative stress inactivates vegf survival signaling in retinal endothelial cells via pi 3-kinase tyrosine nitration. J Cell Sci 2005;118 (Pt 1):243–52.
172. Gu X, El-Remessy AB, Brooks SE, Al-Shabrawey M, Tsai NT, Caldwell RB. Hyperoxia induces retinal vascular endothelial cell apoptosis through formation of peroxynitrite. Am J Physiol Cell Physiol 2003;285(3):C546–54.
173. Hellberg CB, Boggs SE, Lapetina EG. Phosphatidylinositol 3-kinase is a target for protein tyrosine nitration. Biochem Biophys Res Commun 1998;252(2):313–7.
174. Bursell SE, Clermont AC, Aiello LP, et al. High-dose vitamin E supplementation normalizes retinal blood flow and creatinine clearance in patients with type 1 diabetes. Diabetes Care 1999;22(8): 1245–51.
175. Aiello LP, Clermont A, Arora V, Davis MD, Sheetz MJ, Bursell SE. Inhibition of pkc beta by oral administration of ruboxistaurin is well tolerated and ameliorates diabetes-induced retinal hemodynamic abnormalities in patients. Invest Ophthalmol Vis Sci 2006;47(1):86–92.
176. Clermont A, Bursell SE, Feener EP. Role of the angiotensin ii type 1 receptor in the pathogenesis of diabetic retinopathy: Effects of blood pressure control and beyond. J Hypertens Suppl 2006;24(1):S73–80.
177. Sjolie AK. Prospects for angiotensin receptor blockers in diabetic retinopathy. Diabetes Res Clin Pract 2007;76 (1 Suppl):S31–9.

178. Oates PJ, Mylari BL. Aldose reductase inhibitors: Therapeutic implications for diabetic complications. Expert Opin Investig Drugs 1999;8(12):2095–119.
179. Comer GM, Ciulla TA. Pharmacotherapy for diabetic retinopathy. Curr Opin Ophthalmol 2004;15(6):508–18.
180. Collins R, Armitage J, Parish S, Sleigh P, Peto R. Mrc/bhf heart protection study of cholesterol-lowering with simvastatin in 5963 people with diabetes: A randomised placebo-controlled trial. Lancet 2003;361(9374):2005–16.
181. Colhoun HM, Betteridge DJ, Durrington PN, et al. Primary prevention of cardiovascular disease with atorvastatin in type 2 diabetes in the collaborative atorvastatin diabetes study (cards): Multicentre randomised placebo-controlled trial. Lancet 2004;364(9435):685–96.
182. Danesh FR, Kanwar YS. Modulatory effects of hmg-coa reductase inhibitors in diabetic microangiopathy. Faseb J 2004;18(7):805–15.
183. Tawfik HE, El-Remessy AB, Matragoon S, Ma G, Caldwell RB, Caldwell RW. Simvastatin improves diabetes-induced coronary endothelial dysfunction. J Pharmacol Exp Ther 2006;373(6):415–427.
184. Miyahara S, Kiryu J, Yamashiro K, et al. Simvastatin inhibits leukocyte accumulation and vascular permeability in the retinas of rats with streptozotocin-induced diabetes. Am J Pathol 2004;164(5):1697–706.
185. Bonetti PO, Lerman LO, Napoli C, Lerman A. Statin effects beyond lipid lowering–are they clinically relevant? Eur Heart J 2003;24(3):225–48.
186. Baghdasarian SB, Jneid H, Hoogwerf BJ. Association of dyslipidemia and effects of statins on nonmacrovascular diseases. Clin Ther 2004;26(3):337–51.
187. Gupta A, Gupta V, Thapar S, Bhansali A. Lipid-lowering drug atorvastatin as an adjunct in the management of diabetic macular edema. Am J Ophthalmol 2004;137(4):675–82.
188. Sen K, Misra A, Kumar A, Pandey RM. Simvastatin retards progression of retinopathy in diabetic patients with hypercholesterolemia. Diabetes Res Clin Pract 2002;56(1):1–11.
189. Duh EJ, Yang HS, Suzuma I, et al. Pigment epithelium-derived factor suppresses ischemia-induced retinal neovascularization and vegf-induced migration and growth. Invest Ophthalmol Vis Sci 2002;43(3):821–9.
190. Mori K, Gehlbach P, Ando A, McVey D, Wei L, Campochiaro PA. Regression of ocular neovascularization in response to increased expression of pigment epithelium-derived factor. Invest Ophthalmol Vis Sci 2002;43(7):2428–34.
191. Mori K, Gehlbach P, Yamamoto S, et al. Aav-mediated gene transfer of pigment epithelium-derived factor inhibits choroidal neovascularization. Invest Ophthalmol Vis Sci 2002;43(6):1994–2000.
192. Takita H, Yoneya S, Gehlbach PL, Duh EJ, Wei LL, Mori K. Retinal neuroprotection against ischemic injury mediated by intraocular gene transfer of pigment epithelium-derived factor. Invest Ophthalmol Vis Sci 2003;44(10):4497–504.
193. Campochiaro PA, Nguyen QD, Shah SM, et al. Adenoviral vector-delivered pigment epithelium-derived factor for neovascular age-related macular degeneration: Results of a phase i clinical trial. Hum Gene Ther 2006;17(2):167–76.
194. Buckley NE, McCoy KL, Mezey E, et al. Immunomodulation by cannabinoids is absent in mice deficient for the cannabinoid cb(2) receptor. Eur J Pharmacol 2000;396(2–3):141–9.
195. Hampson AJ, Grimaldi M, Lolic M, Wink D, Rosenthal R, Axelrod J. Neuroprotective antioxidants from marijuana. Ann NY Acad Sci 2000;899(1):274–82.
196. Maas AI, Murray G, Henney H, 3rd, et al. Efficacy and safety of dexanabinol in severe traumatic brain injury: Results of a phase iii randomised, placebo-controlled, clinical trial. Lancet Neurol 2006;5(1):38–45.
197. Braida D, Pegorini S, Arcidiacono MV, Consalez GG, Croci L, Sala M. Post-ischemic treatment with cannabidiol prevents electroencephalographic flattening, hyperlocomotion and neuronal injury in gerbils. Neurosci Lett 2003;346(1–2):61–4.
198. Rajesh M, Mukhopadhyay P, Batkai S, et al. Cannabidiol attenuates high glucose-induced endothelial cell inflammatory response and barrier disruption. Am J Physiol Heart Circ Physiol 2007;293(1):H610–9.
199. El-Remessy AB, Khalil IE, Matragoon S, et al. Neuroprotective effect of (-)delta9-tetrahydrocannabinol and cannabidiol in n-methyl-d-aspartate-induced retinal neurotoxicity: Involvement of peroxynitrite. Am J Pathol 2003;163(5):1997–2008.
200. Powell ED, Field RA. Studies on salicylates and complement in diabetes. Diabetes 1966;15(10):730–3.

201. Effect of aspirin alone and aspirin plus dipyridamole in early diabetic retinopathy. A multicenter randomized controlled clinical trial. The damad study group. Diabetes 1989;38(4):491–8.
202. Effects of aspirin treatment on diabetic retinopathy. Etdrs report number 8. Early treatment diabetic retinopathy study research group. Ophthalmology 1991;98(5 Suppl):757–65.
203. Fitzgerald GA. Coxibs and cardiovascular disease. N Engl J Med 2004;351(17):1709–11.
204. Ceriello A. Controlling oxidative stress as a novel molecular approach to protecting the vascular wall in diabetes. Curr Opin Lipidol 2006;17(5):510–8.
205. Dormandy JA, Charbonnel B, Eckland DJ, et al. Secondary prevention of macrovascular events in patients with type 2 diabetes in the proactive study (prospective pioglitazone clinical trial in macrovascular events): A randomised controlled trial. Lancet 2005;366(9493):1279–89.
206. Muranaka K, Yanagi Y, Tamaki Y, et al. Effects of peroxisome proliferator-activated receptor gamma and its ligand on blood-retinal barrier in a streptozotocin-induced diabetic model. Invest Ophthalmol Vis Sci 2006;47(10):4547–52.

B

Pathophysiological Process in Diabeitc Retinopathy

10 Pericyte Loss in the Diabetic Retina

*Frederick Pfister, Yuxi Feng,
and Hans-Peter Hammes*

CONTENTS

ABSTRACT

Retinal pericytes are enigmatic cells. The lack of a panpericyte marker and the diversity of possible origins suggest that there is not one pericyte population in a given organ. The important functions of pericytes related to the specific demands of the retina are the control of endothelial survival and growth, and the tightness of the blood retinal barrier. Pericyte loss is a common early phenomenon of all diabetic mammalians. An important molecular contribution to pericyte functionality comes from the angiopoietin-Tie system that is involved in the maturation of the developing vascular network as well as in its destabilization and angiogenesis. Hyperglycemia induces upregulation of angiopoietin-2 which inhibits the pericyte-recruiting function of Ang-1 suggesting a novel, active, mechanism in pericyte loss, rather than a passive intoxication by glycolytic intermediates. Post-translational modification involving intracellular methylglyoxal-type AGEs and enzymatic modification of transcription factors are involved in glucose-induced transcription changes of Ang-2. Metabolic signal blockers as well as catalytic antioxidants prevent Ang-2 upregulation as well as diabetic pericyte loss in vivo.

Key Words: Pericytes; Endothelial cells; Müller cells; Angiopoietins; Diabetes; Methylglyoxal.

From: *Contemporary Diabetes*: *Diabetic Retinopathy*
Edited by: E. Duh © Humana Press, Totowa, NJ

INTRODUCTION

Promoted by the observation that they are selectively lost in early diabetic retinopathy, pericytes have attracted the interest of researchers from many disciplines. Still, pericytes are enigmatic cells. Neither their origin, nor their normal function has been fully delineated, and the biological meaning and the causes and consequences of their loss in the diabetic retina are still under investigation. It is useful to review current knowledge about the cellular crosstalk between vascular cells, before adding a further level of complexity by addressing the cellular crosstalk between vascular and neuroglial cells *(1, 2)* Pericytes are functionally codependent on endothelial cell, and each cell type provides its counterpart with growth factors and contact-dependent signals that influence survival and/or proliferation *(3)*. Diabetic pericyte loss may represent one of the prominent examples in which the survival impact of pericytes is critically lost for endothelial cells.

Origin and Differentiation

Resident retinal pericytes derive from mesodermal and from neural crest origin during development *(4)*. The relative contribution of common embryonic stem cell precursor which may incorporate into vessels under the influence of pericyte-recruiting factors such as PDGF-B remains unclear *(5)*. During postnatal vascular repair conditions, and during angiogenesis, endothelial cell transdifferentiation into pericytes has been suggested *(6)*. Recently, evidence for a bone marrow origin of mural cells supporting adult angiogenesis has been presented *(7)*. Whether endothelial precursor cells from nondiabetic origin can integrate into diabetic retinal capillaries and replace functional pericytes is also unclear *(8)*.

Pericytes are able to transdifferentiate into other cell types. For example, in the rat brain, phagocytic pericytes assume microglia cell functions *(9)*. The conversion of pericytes to tissue macrophages has been observed, suggesting an active contribution to a variety of clearance and defense functions *(10)*. In the brain, a transitional cell phenotype of pericytes compatible with a fibroblast morphology and localization, but with a surface expression pattern of a pericyte (see later) has been reported. In particular, pericytes can differentiate into vSMC and fibroblasts, and the reverse transformation of vSMC and fibroblasts into pericytes is possible *(10–15)*. In vitro observations suggest further transdifferential potential into adipogenic, chondrogenic, and osteogenic cells *(16, 17)*, reflecting the heterogeneity of pericyte populations in general.

Morphology and Distribution

Pericytes are regular components of capillaries in almost all human tissues and organs *(10)*. In contrast to arteries and arterioles, where the coverage consists of single or multilayers of vascular smooth muscle cells (vSMC), the capillary system is exclusively covered by individual pericytes. It has been suggested that vSMC and pericytes represent phenotypic variations of a continuous cell lineage, because of morphological similarities and the expression of common markers such as smooth muscle actin and desmin *(3)*. In the capillary system, pericytes are readily identifiable by the protuberant position within the capillary basement membrane and the shape *(18, 19)* (Fig. 1). They

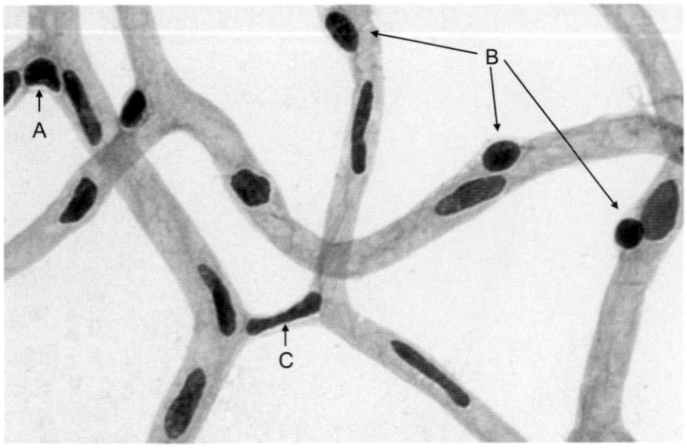

Fig. 1. Retinal vessels isolated from a nondiabetic rat retina by enzymatic digestion with a pepsin/trypsin combination. "A" denotes a type of pericyte at the branching site of capillaries (approx. 20% of all pericytes in a normal rat retina); "B" indicates three different phenotypes of pericytes in longitudinal orientation of capillaries; "C" indicates a pericyte stretched between two capillary branches. PAS staining, original magnification 600x.

sometimes extend cytoplasmatic processes, varying in length, arrangement, and form in the different capillary beds, suggesting mobility *(20)*. Pericytes in the retina are completely embedded within the capillary basement membrane *(21)*, surrounding the endothelial cells which form the capillary tube ("intramural pericytes").

The density of pericyte coverage of capillaries varies from organ to organ. The highest relative ratio of pericytes to endothelial cells is found in the retinal microvasculature (1:1), followed by brain capillaries (5:1–3:1), skeletal muscle capillaries (5:1), and the cardiac muscle capillaries (10:1) (Fig. 2) *(22)*. One explanation for the exclusively high pericyte coverage of capillaries in the retina is the function of blood vessels in this specialized organ. On one hand, blood supply to the retina is among the highest within the body, as determined by perfusion/organ weight. On the other hand, the need for vessel tightness is particularly high, as any extra fluid deposition would interfere with proper retinal function. The greater the number of pericytes covering the endothelial cell tube, the better the barrier function *(23)*. This explains why capillaries of the brain and the retina show the highest relative frequency of pericytes to endothelial cells. Another relation is noteworthy, i.e., that tissues with the slowest endothelial cell turnover show the largest pericyte coverage *(24, 25)*. Both common notions suggest that primary pericyte functions in the retina relate to the maintenance of the blood-retinal barrier and support of endothelial cell survival.

Cellular Crosstalk

The unique position of pericytes next to the endothelial monolayer predicts a direct interaction. This unique position within the common basement membrane and the proximity to perivascular cells renders the pericyte a privileged candidate for cellular crosstalk under physiological and pathological conditions. Pericytes communicate with their

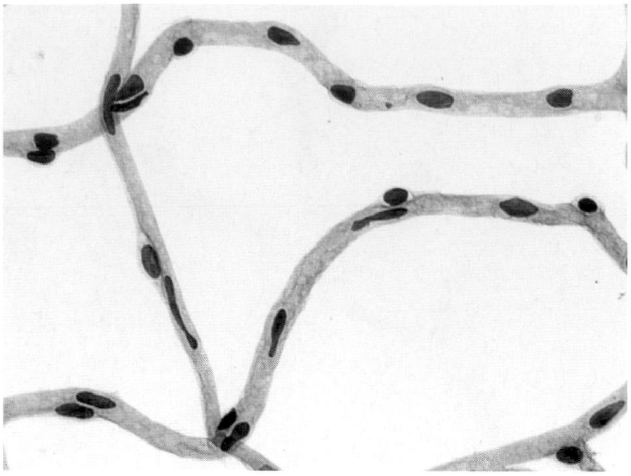

Fig. 2. Retinal digestion preparation of a nondiabetic rat retina. Note the approx. 1:1 ratio of pericytes and endothelial cells. PAS staining, original magnification 400x.

neighboring endothelial cells via various adhesive structures, such as gap junctions, tight junctions, adhesion plaques, and so-called peg and pocket contacts *(26, 27)*. These communications are the basis for the variety of direct or indirect consequences of pericytes on endothelial survival and proliferation.

Gap junctions between endothelial cells and pericytes are membranous channels directly connecting the cytoplasms of both cell types. These junctions are involved in the exchange of nucleotides and small molecules between pericytes and endothelial cells *(28)*. Major components of gap junctions are the connexins of which Cx-37,-42, and -57 have been identified in the eye. Gap junctions provide a substantial role in controlling endothelial cell proliferation during physiological angiogenesis *(29, 30)*. Tight junctions are membrane proteins which interconnect endothelial cells and pericytes. Pericytes are frequently located adjacent to or over tight endothelial junctions, supporting a direct barrier-promoting role. These contacts form a diffusion barrier that controls paracellular fluid transport through the capillary wall. By this, the number of pericytes determines the number of tight junction proteins. Importantly, membrane protein families of tight junctions are the claudins and the occludins. Cell culture experiments demonstrated that pericytes induce occludin production of brain endothelial cells. Occludin expression is induced by the pericyte-derived Angiopoietin-1. In brain microvessels, the induction of occludin expression enhances the tightness of tight junctions. Further studies suggested that the attenuation or inhibition of the angiopoietin-1/Tie-2 signaling leads to dysfunction of blood brain barrier in disease *(31)*. These data exemplify the importance of pericytes for the maintenance of endothelial barrier function. Another variant of cell contact between pericytes and endothelial cell is the adhesion plaque which is rich in fibronectin depositions. These cell contacts anchor the pericyte to the endothelium during the transfer of contractile forces such as during contraction or during propagation of shear stress *(20, 32–34)*.

Identification

The phenotypic nature of pericytes was largely disclosed by transmission and scanning electron microscopy. However, due to the morphological similarities of rodent retinal capillary endothelial cells and pericytes, markers allowing for the distinction of retinal capillary cells were crucial for quantitative analysis.

There is still no "pan pericyte marker" due to the versatility of pericytes, even in one organ such as the retina *(27)*. Common markers of pericytes are smooth muscle actin (SMA), desmin, the proteoglycan NG2, and the platelet-derived growth factor-receptor beta (PDGFR-beta). The aminopeptidase N, the identification of the expression of XlacZ gene in pericytes (and vSMC), and the regulator of G-signaling 5 (RGS5) are also used for identification *(14, 35–44)*. By comparing cDNA microarrays of mouse brain of PDGF-B knockout with wildtype embryos, several downregulated genes were expressed in brain capillary pericytes of wildtype tissue, such as the ATP-sensitive potassium channel complex (Kir 6.1), the sulfonylurea receptor 2 (SUR2) and the delta homolog 1 (DLK1) *(45)*.

The XlacZ4 mouse is widely used as a model to study the role of pericytes and SMC because it expresses a reporter gene under control of a pericyte/SMC-specific promoter. However, according to our analysis, approximately 55–65% of retinal pericytes express the XlacZ4 and the expression is context dependent. Common to all markers mentioned is that they fail to recognize all pericytes at all stages *(26)*.

FUNCTION

Contractility

Pericytes are the capillary counterparts to SMC on arterioles and arteries *(44, 46)*. One remarkable feature that pericytes have in common with SMC is their contractile phenotype. Pericytes contain both smooth muscle and nonsmooth muscle isoforms of actin and myosin, however, with an uneven distribution within the pericyte population *(39)*. The differential expression of SMA in pericytes may reflect the continuum from SMC of arteries and arterioles to pericytes of true capillaries and may correlate with the physical forces that pericytes are exposed to. The same pericytes are immunolabeled with smooth muscle tropomyosin and cGK suggestive of a contractile function *(37, 47, 48)*. Meanwhile, several factors are identified that regulate pericytes contractility. While alpha 2-adrenergic agonists, cholinergic agonists, histamine, serotonin, angiotensin II, and endothelin-1 lead to vasoconstriction, beta-2 adrenergic agonists, NO, and atrial natriuretic peptide lead to a dilatation of the pericyte-covered capillaries *(34)*. As demonstrated in in vivo studies, pericytes in brain and retinal capillaries constrict in response to electrical stimulation, superperfusion with ATP and noradrenalin. These data provide firm evidence that pericyte control capillary blood flow in response to local modulation by vasoactive mechanisms *(49)*. However, whether the hyperglycemic milieu or the loss of pericytes has an impact on contractility, in particular when basement membrane components have changed under hyperglycaemic conditions, awaits further clarification.

Role in Vessel Formation and Stabilization

The function of pericytes that has been most intensively studied is their role in endothelial proliferation and angiogenesis. Studies also highlighted the importance of pericytes for vessel maturation in embryonic development, in vascular remodeling, and in guidance of sprouting angiogenesis *(50–54)*. Endothelial cells alone can initiate, but not complete vessel formation. After the primary network of vessels has formed during vasculogenesis, maturation of the primitive network ensues. During this process, pericytes are recruited to the forming vasculature. Important molecular pathways, involved in pericyte recruitment during embryonic vessel maturation, are platelet-derived growth factor-beta (PDGF-B) and its receptor (PDGFR-B), transforming growth factor-beta (TGF-β) and its receptor and the angiopoietin/Tie-2 system (Ang/Tie-2). While the PDGF/PDGF-receptor system is crucial for pericyte migration and proliferation during vascular maturation, the angiopoietin/Tie-2 system is essential for subsequent vessel stabilization, and TGF-β is involved in the interaction of vascular cells with extracellular matrix (ECM) and ECM production and further mural cell differentiation. Inhibition of pericyte recruitment to capillaries by interfering with the recruitment leads to abnormal remodeling of developing vessels, a process that is reversed by administration of endothelial survival factors *(55)*. During this angiogenic remodeling the initial vascular network is also modified through both pruning and vessel enlargement *(56, 57)*.

In sprouting angiogenesis, pericytes are actively involved *(56)*. Under the influence of VEGF, endothelial cells start to evade from their resident site toward a VEGF gradient *(58)*. Endothelial cell proliferation and migration of sprouting tip cells include the degradation and losing of ECM and is dependent on tip cell guidance *(59)*. In this process, pericytes are recruited to vessels by the platelet-derived growth factor PDGF-B/PDGFR-B system *(60)*, but other factors such as sphingosine-1-phosphate-1 (S1P-1) and the angiopoietins are also involved *(61)*. For the completion of vessel maturation, active TGF-ß signaling via the ALK-1 and Smad5 pathway is needed *(62)*.

Vessels are resistant to hyperoxic vasoregression when covered with pericytes. This led to the concept of the "window of plasticity" determined by pericyte recruitment lagging behind endothelial sprouting *(63)*. By the use of complementary phase-specific pericyte markers outlined earlier, it was shown that pericytes play an active role in physiological and pathological angiogenesis, as they are frequently found near, at or even in front of the tips of endothelial sprouts *(14, 27, 64)*. When remodeling ceases, pericytes contribute to the stabilization of vessels by the production of collagen and ECM proteins, such as fibronectin, laminin, and glycosaminglycans to the basal lamina *(33, 65–68)*. Once the entire vascular system has formed, the major function of pericytes becomes the maintenance of a functional vascular network by their ability to control endothelial cell proliferation and vascular tone and by making endothelial cells refractory to shifts in oxygen tension and growth factor levels *(69–72)*. Another paracrine signaling pathway implicated in vessel stabilization is the angiopoietin/Tie-2 system. Angiopoietins (Ang-1 and Ang-2) signal via the tyrosine kinase receptor Tie-2. Pericytes are a predominant source of Ang-1 *(54, 73)*. Ang-1 in endothelial cells is believed to maintain vessel integrity by its ability to stabilize nascent vessels and to promote tightness of vessel barrier function, presumably by facilitating communication between ECs and pericytes *(31)*.

LOSS IN DIABETIC RETINOPATHY

Given the complex cell-cell crosstalk outlined earlier, and the high numbers of pericytes covering retinal capillaries, the observation that pericytes are lost in a diabetic retina predicts profound consequences for the integrity of the affected tissue.

Important insight into the cellular changes that underlie diabetic retinopathy dates back to the early 1960s. Kuwabara and Cogan developed a method that allowed for the direct inspection of the affected retina liberated from neuroglial tissues due to differential susceptibility against trypsin digestion. As a result of their work and that of others presented later, they identified pericyte loss as one of the earliest changes in the diabetic retina *(18)*, though not truly specific for the diabetic retina. However, the time course of pericyte loss in humans and the degree remain unclear.

Thus, although the specificity and the primacy of pericyte loss in the human diabetic retina are not verified, the pericyte biology outlined earlier, and the clear evidence of pericyte abolition suggests an important impact in the evolution of diabetic retinopathy.

As appropriate human original material is unavailable, data on the degree and the time course of pericyte function mostly derive from animal models as widespread as from mice to monkeys.

With the following paragraphs summarizing data on different animal species with regard to early diabetic lesions in the retina, it becomes clear that pericyte loss in diabetes is a universal event, not restricted to specific conditions or species. Therefore, it is unlikely that humans are an exception from the rule.

Animal models of diabetic retinopathy were either spontaneously diabetic caused by genetic or inbreed alterations, or diabetes was induced by chemicals such as streptozotocin. In addition, dietary modifications were used to imitate diabetic hyperhexosemia with sufficient duration to assess retinal vascular changes such as pericyte loss. Mice with modified expressions of genes involved in pericyte behavior during developmental angiogenesis were also proposed as retinopathy models.

The unequivocal identification of pericytes succeeds in retinal digest preparations. Modifications of the original protocol for digestion not only improved the completeness of the resulting vessel network, but also allowed for advanced analytical methods, in particular, when the fixation procedure was modified, or enzymatic isolation of the vasculature was omitted. One important requirement of the morphological distinction between endothelial cells and pericytes, which is more difficult in rodents than in primates or humans (only exception: Chinese hamster), is the staining. Using differential staining techniques, a selective labeling of pericytes improved the completeness of pericyte identification *(74)*.

Rats

Rats are the most commonly used models of experimental diabetic retinopathy. Permanent hyperglycemia is usually achieved by chemical induction with streptozotocin (STZ). The type of diabetes resembles more type 1 than type 2 with severe hyperglycemia and moderate hypoinsulinemia. In this model, pericyte loss is reproducible, depending on the strain used *(75)*. Sprague-Dawley rats which are often used for studies in experimental diabetic nephropathy develop pericyte loss later than Lewis or Wistar rats. Brown Norway or Fisher rats, sometimes used in short-term gene expression experiments, have not been fully characterized for diabetic pericyte loss and other relevant retinal lesions so that their usefulness remains unclear.

STZ-diabetic Lewis and Wistar rats generally show a 30–50% reduction of pericyte numbers after 6–9 months of diabetes *(74, 76–78)*. Specifically, in STZ-diabetic Wistar rats a pericyte dropout over 30% has been reported after 30 weeks of experimental hyperglycemia *(77)*. In STZ-diabetic Wistar rats supplemented with sucrose the loss was even more pronounced *(79)*.

There are spontaneous diabetic rat models which resemble type 1 diabetes more closely because of their pathogenesis. The insulin-dependent diabetic BB Wistar rat and the spontaneous diabetic SDT rat, both develop typical retinal lesions including pericyte loss, due to hyperglycemia. In the diabetic BB Wistar rats, signs of degenerating pericytes and a decreased pericyte/endothelial cell ratio were observed after 8–11 months. In diabetic spontaneous diabetic Torii rat, the loss of pericytes and the formation of acellular capillaries have been described in the majority of the observed eyes (80%) *(80, 81)*. The quantity of pericyte loss would be of particular interest as these animals develop intraretinal neovascularizations. In nondiabetic models mice with a conditional depletion of PDGF-B this only happens if pericyte coverage drops below 50% *(82)*.

Rat models of type 2 diabetes show similar morphological characteristics suggesting that pericyte loss and other changes characteristic for retinopathy are caused by hyperglycemia-mediated mechanisms *(83–85)*. As in other animal models, the addition of sucrose to the diet in genetically obese fatty fa/fa rats resulted in a pronounced decrease in pericytes and signs of pericyte degeneration *(84)*.

Mice

Mice are cheap to house and easy to breed, but they were less favored than rats as models of diabetic retinopathy. With the widespread use of genetically manipulated mice, their use, in particular in combination with chronic hyperglycemia, has become popular, although their retinopathic phenotype is considered less severe and the identification of pericytes more difficult than rats. Furthermore, some mouse strains are unsuitable as models, because of the lack of a deep capillary network, in which hyperglycemia-induced lesions occur first. Retinae of some strains inherited tend to degenerate imposing a potential analytical bias between hyperglycemic and degenerative cell loss. In turn, mice are better to study, because of the availability of molecular tools such as antibodies for specific characterization.

Like in rats, diabetes induction in mice is performed by injection of STZ and ensuing hyperglycemia persists. Studies in C57BL6 mice revealed that retinal capillaries show a significant loss of pericyte beginning 6 months after STZ-diabetes induction, which continued to increase through the 18 months examined *(86)*.

A transgenic mouse model of diabetes is the spontaneous diabetic Ins2Akita mouse. A point mutation in the insulin 2 gene results in misfolding and accumulation of the maturing insulin in beta cells of the pancreas. Subsequent hypoinsulinemia leads to spontaneous hyperglycemia with a rapid onset 4–5 weeks after birth. Male Ins2Akita mice remain constant on glucose levels over 500 mg ml^{-1} during life, while females have lower blood glucose and HbA1c levels. After 6 months of experimental hyperglycemia Ins2Akita males develop morphological characteristics of diabetic retinopathy, including the loss of pericytes of approximately 15% *(87, 125)*.

Diabetic db/db mice as a model for type 2 diabetes show a more than 25% decrease in pericyte density after 15 months of disease duration *(88)*. Pericyte dropout may start earlier in the course of diabetes, but systematic studies on the time course are not available (Pfister, Sauerhöfer, Möller, and Hammes, unpublished). The somewhat milder overall phenotype of retinal changes in mice may result from a higher antioxidative defense capacity as suggested recently *(89)*.

Chinese Hamster

Another rodent model of diabetic retinopathy is the Chinese spontaneous diabetic hamster. In this species, two different levels of hyperglycemia are achieved by breeding, one with mild hyperglycemia (blood glucose between 6 and 15 mmol L^{-1}), the other one with severe hyperglycemia (blood glucose between 25 and 30 mmol L^{-1}) over a period of 12 months. Our own studies revealed a comparable early dropout of pericytes of both the mild and the severe diabetic group (approximately 25% after 3 months), and a maximum loss of pericytes in the severely diabetic group of 57% after 12 months. Despite the extended pericyte dropout, these animals do not develop microaneuryms. Therefore, the proposed link between pericyte loss and a local weakening of the capillary wall as a cause for microaneuryms formation is questionable *(90)*.

Dog

Pericyte-deficient capillaries and the presence of pericyte ghosts in diabetic dogs have been reported in this model *(91–94)*. As researchers working with dogs use quantitation of pericyte ghosts, but not quantitative retinal morphometry, information on the real degree of pericyte loss is not available (the method of counting pericyte ghosts cannot detect ghosts above and below capillaries and can therefore miss up to 50% of the actual deficit).

As hyperglycemia affects the retina as a whole, Engerman and Kern, using dogs, asked whether pericyte loss was uniformly distributed throughout the retina as expected. Indeed, by dividing the retina into four quadrants, they identified equal numbers of pericytes throughout the retina. However, the numbers of acellular capillaries were preponderant in the upper temporal quadrant which led the authors to speculate that pericyte loss and acellular capillaries occur by different mechanisms. Like in rats, a qualitative loss of smooth muscle cells was also found in dogs, extending the concept of a loss of mural cells also to smooth muscle cells *(95)*.

Apart from these experimental animals, pericyte loss has been observed in diabetic monkeys, however, without precise data about onset or degree *(96, 97)*.

Animal Models Mimicking Retinal Pericyte Loss

As noted earlier, the PDGF-B/ß-receptor and the Ang/Tie-2 system are important in the recruitment of pericytes to the retinal vasculature. Mice with modifications of these factors are suitable to understand the vascular consequences of pericyte deficiencies. Other factors like VEGF and IGF-1 can play a critical role in the survival of retinal vessels and in the pathogenesis of proliferative diabetic retinopathy.

PDGF-B-PDGF-SSR

Genetic ablation of PDGF-B has major effects on the brain microvasculature. Studies using PDGF-B deficient mouse embryos demonstrated a complete lack of microvascular pericytes and the development of numerous capillary microaneurysms that ruptured at birth, when blood pressure increases. Endothelial cells of sprouting capillaries in the mutant mice appeared to be unable to attract PDGFR-b-positive pericyte progenitor cells *(98)*. Hemorrhages are also prevalent in mice with a deletion of the cognate receptor PDGFR-b, and in mice in which the proper recruitment of pericytes was abolished by an antagonistic mAb against PDGFR-beta. The perinatal death of these animals precluded retinal studies. However, as some of the lesions in vessels of affected mice were reminiscent of early retinal lesions in diabetes, heterozygous PDGF-B mice were used to study the retinal vasculature. The retinae showed a 28% reduction in the number of pericytes compared to wildtype littermates and an increase in acellular capillaries during adulthood, implying that pericytes have survival-promoting functions for established retinal capillary. This concept was supported by the findings that pericyte dropout in PDGF-B deficient mice was further aggravated when chronic hyperglycemia was superimposed *(99)*.

Since the perinatal lethality of homozygous PDGF-B mice precluded vascular studies of the retina, mice with an endothelium-restricted ablation of PDGF-B were created to study pericyte recruitment, vasoregression, and proliferation. The level of pericyte coverage was determined in different areas of the brain and in the retina. It was observed that pericyte loss up to 50% was accompanied by vasoregression in the retina, whereas pericyte deficits exceeding 50% induced retinal vasoproliferations mimicking proliferative diabetic retinopathy. Thus, there is an obvious discrepancy between hyperglycemia-induced pericyte loss > 50% and a genetically induced loss.

Angiopoietin-Tie

The Angiopoietin-Tie family consists of several members of ligands (Ang-1–4) and of receptor tyrosine kinases (Tie-1/2). While Ang-1–4 act via ligation to Tie-2, no active ligand for Tie-1 has been unequivocally identified. Tie-2 has been identified on cells important for vascular cell survival and angiogenesis, including pericytes *(54)*].

The interaction of Ang-1 with Tie-2 is crucial for the timely and coordinated recruitment of pericytes to the developing vascular system. The concept that angiopoietin-1 acting via the receptor tyrosine kinase Tie-2 determines endothelial cell survival, sprouting, vessel remodeling, and stabilization though the recruitment of pericytes still hold true for retinal vessels. The activity of Tie-2 is differentially regulated as the natural antagonist of Ang-1, angiopoietin-2 (Ang-2) inhibits the phosphorylation of Tie-2, induced by Ang-1. Ang-2 cooperates with VEGF to induce angiogenesis, while Ang-2 in absence of VEGF induces capillary regression *(100)*. To assess the pathogenetic role of the angiopoietin-Tie system in diabetic pericyte loss, the expression of Ang-1 and -2 was studied in a diabetic rat model, in which the onset of pericyte dropout is exactly known. It was found that Ang-2 is 37-fold upregulated prior to the onset of pericyte dropout. Injection of recombinant Ang-2 into the vitreous of nondiabetic rats reproduced pericyte dropout within days, and the 25% pericyte loss of diabetic C56BL6/J mice after 6 months of diabetes was abolished in a diabetic mouse with a 50% reduction of Ang-2 gene dose *(101)*. Constitutive overexpression of Ang-2 in photoreceptor cells induces reduced pericyte coverage in the deep capillary layers of the retina *(102)*. Diabetes aggravates the pericyte deficiency and promotes acellular capillaries over time, similarly to the changes in PDGF-B+/– mice. These data suggest that hyperglycemic regulation of angiopoietin-2 plays a crucial role in the survival of pericytes in the diabetic retina and the subsequent development of pathology. This notion leads to the question of the regulation of growth factors such as angiopoietin-2 by glucose and its intracellular metabolites. This will be addressed later.

VEGF-VEGFR2

VEGF is a major determinant of retinal vascular development and responses to injury. The murine *VEGF* gene is alternatively transcribed to yield the VEGF120, VEGF164, and VEGF188 isoforms, which differ in their potential to bind to heparan sulfate. While the VEGF164 mouse yielded regular pericyte-recruiting patterns in all vascular beds, the VEGF120 mouse had major defects in pericyte recruitment to capillaries and arterioles, but not to venules. As signs of impaired vessel maturation and patency, extravasations of red blood cells were also observed. Endothelial cells provide pericyte-recruiting factors like PDGF-B, and VEGF120 mice had lower PDGF-B expression suggesting that the defect was secondary to the endothelial defect. Endothelial cells of larger vessels express VEGF-R1, but the affinity of VEGF120 to this receptor is lower than other VEGF isoforms. It is thus unclear whether this axis contributes significantly to pericyte recruitment to capillaries in the retina. The 188 isoform of VEGF did not yield a defect in pericyte recruitment to capillaries. In essence, VEGF may play a significant role in pericyte recruitment, but the specific and predominant mechanism working in the eye, and in particular in the capillary network, may be difficult to dissect *(103)*.

IGF-1/IGF-R

The growth hormone-IGF-1-IGF-1 receptor system has been involved in the pathogenesis of proliferative diabetic retinopathy since the early days when pituitary ablation was the only feasible approach. However, the question of a possible involvement in incipient changes was only addressed recently by Ruberte et al. They used a mouse overexpressing IGF-1 in several organs, including the retina. The transgene was found in the outer nuclear layer and in photoreceptors. After 2 months of paracrine IGF-1 exposure, quantitative retinal morphometry in retinal digest preparations revealed an almost 50% reduction of pericyte numbers, while the numbers of endothelial cells remained unexpectedly unchanged. Of note, acellular capillaries were more numerous already at this early time point. In analogy to cells exposed to high glucose in the presence of low IGF-1 the authors claimed a cooperative effect of glucose and IGF-1 on the observed ocular alterations *(104)*.

MECHANISMS OF LOSS

The underlying causes and mechanisms of early pericyte dropout in diabetic retinopathy remain still unclear. It is possible that pericyte loss is a result of passive processes, such as degeneration and apoptosis. For example, STZ-diabetic Wistar rats showed a 2.65 fold increase in the numbers of TUNEL positive cells (including pericytes) in retinae after 11 months of hyperglycemia *(105)*. Pericyte death was also present in retinal vessels of diabetic patients suggesting its relevance in clinical disease *(106)*.

Biochemical Pathways

Aldose Reductase

The selective damage of pericytes by chronic hyperglycemia may be explained by altered biochemical pathways which have been implicated in the pathogenesis of microvascular damage, so that pericyte loss may be the consequence of hyperglycemic toxicity. The four biochemical pathways that have been discussed over years to be involved in the pathogenesis of diabetic complications are i. increased activity of the polyol-pathway, ii. activation of PKC isoforms by de novo synthesis of diacylglycerol, iii. increased flux through the hexosamine pathway and iiii. supply of glycolytic intermediates for the formation of AGEs. The first pathway to be studied in this regard was the aldose reductase pathway, as immunological evidence had suggested the selective presence of aldose reductase in pericytes *(107)*. When glucose levels in cells are low, the enzyme aldose reductase functions by detoxifying aldehydes to inactive alcohols. When glucose levels in cells rise in diabetes, the enzyme starts to reduce glucose to sorbitol, and this process consumes the cofactor NADPH. Since NADPH is an essential cofactor for the regeneration of an important intracellular antioxidant, reduced glutathione, its depletion may induce a significant impact on cellular defense against oxidative stress. According to novel findings, the expression and the activity of aldose reductase are increased in bovine retinal pericytes in vitro when cultured in high glucose *(108)*, and are accompanied by elevated intracellular sorbitol levels. Whether this leads to increased pericyte death and is amenable to pharmacological inhibition has not yet been demonstrated. Overall, in line with the notion that the absolute levels of aldose reductase in the retina may be too low to contribute significantly to retinopathy development, the majority of experimental, and one large clinical trial failed to establish this pathway as playing a major role.

Age Formation

Chronic hyperglycemia-induced formation of reactive oxygen species and AGEs, which accumulate in pericytes in vivo *(109)*, might be able to initiate pericyte degeneration. Injection of exogenous AGE into nondiabetic animals resulted in a selective uptake in pericytes *(110)*. In principle, repeated injection of high doses of AGE-modified rat serum can induce selective pericyte loss in normal rats after 2 weeks *(111)*. Moreover, endogenous AGEs can form and accumulate in pericytes *(112)*. While the ingestions of exogenous AGEs is consistent with the propensity of phagocytosis of pericytes, the formation of endogenous AGEs in pericytes is inconsistent with the prior finding that pericytes and SMCs are able to downregulate glucose uptake to protect themselves from hyperglycemic damage *(113)*. It is thus speculated that pericytes take up AGEs from the circulation or from the direct vicinity suggesting a clearing function under specific conditions. Since the tissue load with AGEs changes over time in diabetes, the role of pericytes as AGE-removing cell compartment becomes increasingly relevant. However, the time course of AGE accumulation in pericytes (occurring over several months) is inconsistent with the time course of pericyte loss (starting after approximately 8 weeks of diabetes with a plateau after 6 months in diabetic animals), suggesting that AGEs may not be causally involved in incipient pericyte loss.

Modification of LDL

Another piece of evidence suggests that pericytes may be injured by toxic plasma proteins which predominantly form in the diabetic milieu. Pericytes are differentially susceptible to damage by modified LDL in vitro *(114)*. As in vivo correlate, the combination of elevated glucose and lipids in ApoE–/– db/db mice led to an almost doubling of pericyte ghosts after 6 months of exposure. The majority of genes upregulated in human pericytes exposed to modifications of LDL such as oxidized-glycated LDL belong to the families of signal transduction, enzymes, and lipid metabolism *(115)*. One interesting gene regulated by exposure of pericytes to modified lipids is TIMP-3, which controls vessel stability and maturation in vitro *(116)*. Exposure of cultured human retinal pericytes to glycated-oxidized LDL repressed TIMP-3 expression by 2.41 fold vs. pericytes exposed to unmodified LDL. Given the close cell-cell communication based on physical contacts between endothelial cells and pericytes, it is conceivable that the MMP-TIMP system can play a significant role in execution of vascular stabilization by pericytes, and to the respective alteration in diabetes *(117)*. Although a clear clinical benefit of lipid-lowering treatment for diabetic retinopathy has not been demonstrated *(118, 119)*, the preclinical data and evidence from associative studies suggest an association between lipoprotein profiles and the severity of retinopathy at least in type 1 diabetes *(120)*. It must be kept in mind that lipid-lowering drugs can have an independent effect on pericyte survival. For instance, it was recently reported that statins, in particular simvastatin, a potent HMG-CoA reductase inhibitor, can selectively induce pericyte apoptosis in vitro.

Loss Through Active Elimination

Alternative to early pericyte loss in diabetic retinopathy being the result of hyperglycemic injury, a different concept was proposed. It is possible that pericyte loss is an active process involving migration of pericytes away from the capillaries, driven by the Angiopoietin-Tie system. As described, gain of function experiments in nondiabetic animals revealed the induction of pericyte dropout in the vicinity of the Ang-2 overexpressing site. Superimposition of diabetes aggravated the most important vascular readout, i.e., the formation of acellular capillaries. Loss of function studies in the presence of diabetes yielded the prevention of pericyte dropout and the reduction of acellular capillary formation. Ang-2 is expressed in three cell types of the retina, i.e., the endothelial cell, the Müller cells, and the horizontal cells. In situ hybridization of diabetic retinae with Ang-2 yielded the expression particularly in Müller cells. However, the regulation of Ang-2 in chronic hyperglycemia has not been understood until recently.

For a better understanding, a short summary of the biochemical state of the art is given.

As mentioned, four pathways have been investigated over many years to explain how diabetes can affect diabetic vascular target cells: the sorbitol pathway, the hexosamine pathway, and the protein kinase C pathway, and increased production of AGEs. Recently, these seemingly independent biochemical pathways have been linked by the findings that one single mechanism, hyperglycemia-induced mitochondrial overproduction of reactive oxygen species, is the underlying cause, which, mediated through the enzyme poly-ADP-ribose polymerase, blocks activities of the critical glycolytic enzyme glyceraldehyde-3-phosphate dehydrogenase *(121, 122)*. In normal cells, glucose is metabolized through glycolysis and the tricarbon cycle to generate electron donors for the mitochondrial respiratory chain. Here, energy (ATP) is generated in a precisely regulated way. In hyperglycemic cells, increased flux through glycolysis and the TCA cycle generates a voltage gradient of electrons surpassing a certain threshold which is then blocked inside complex III of the mitochondrial electron transport chain. From complex III, the surplus of electrons is purported to coenzyme Q together with molecular oxygen producing superoxide. The mitochondrial form of superoxide dismutase detoxifies this radical via hydrogen peroxide to water in the presence of oxygen. The link between the four biochemical pathways, and the mitochondrial overproduction of ROS was made, when it became evident that an important change in hyperglycemic cells and in experimental animals was the reduced activity of the glycolytic enzyme glyceraldehyde-3-phosphate dehydrogenase. When examining for biochemical modifications of the enzyme, it was observed that hyperglycemia-induced superoxides caused polymers of ADP ribose to attach and reduce enzyme activity. These changes were prevented with the inhibition of superoxide generation, and with the inhibition of the nuclear enzyme poly-ADP-ribose polymerase using a specific PARP inhibitor. The latter is activated upon DNA strand brakes known to form in hyperglycemic cells. Reduced GAPDH activity induced by PARP activation activates the biochemical pathways by increasing intermediates such as diacyl-glycerol (PKC pathway), glyceraldehyde-3-phosphate (AGE pathway), fructose-6-phosphate (hexosamine pathway), and intracellular glucose (sorbitol pathway). Thus, hyperglycemia links to biochemical pathway abnormalities via a common denominator, mitochondrial overproduction of reactive oxygen species. Methyglyoxal is the most important intracellular AGE precursor. Methylglyoxal-induced hydroimidazolones are the predominant modifications of intracellular proteins. They react with amino groups of arginine in intracellular proteins to form AGEs, which are detoxified by the glyoxalase system *(123)*.

Methylglyoxal has been recently implicated in the mechanism of how high glucose regulates gene expression. It was found that increased glucose flux in renal microvascular endothelial cells caused increased modification of the corepressor mSin3A by methylglyoxal resulting in recruitment of the enzyme O-GlcNAc transferase to an mSin3A-Sp3 complex. Subsequently, Sp3 modification by O-linked N-acetylglucosamine decreased its binding to a glucose-responsive GC box in the Ang-2 promoter and the activation of Ang-2 transcription (Fig. 3) *(124)*. The same mechanism was operative in retinal Müller cells consistent with in vivo data from retinae of diabetic rats and mice. These data are consistent with the novel hypothesis, i.e., that pericyte loss is actively induced by glial cell overexpression Ang-2 in response to high glucose.

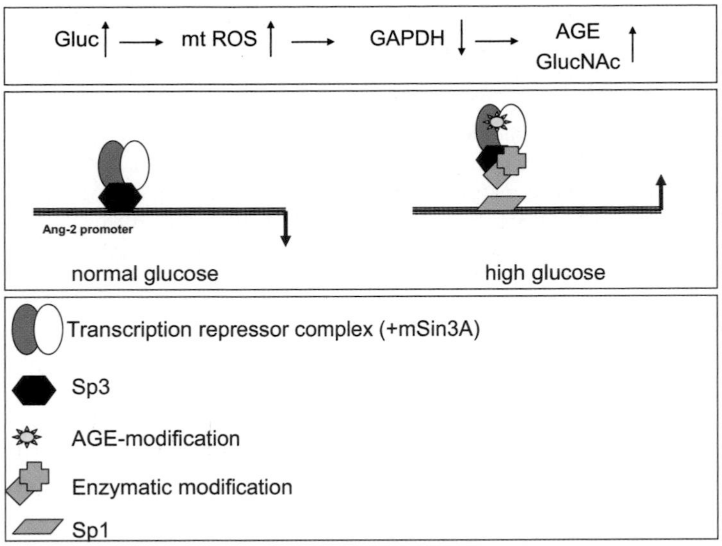

Fig. 3. Schematic representation of transcriptional Ang2 derepression in hyperglycaemic endothelial (and Müller) cells. High glucose induces cellular changes resulting in increased AGE formation which modifies the transcriptional corepressor mSin3A. Subsequent modifications involving GlucNAc of the transcription factor Sp3 lead to binding of Sp1 causing Ang2 expression (124).

From the unifying hypothesis, two classes of compounds have been proposed to alleviate hyperglycemic damage: metabolic signal blockers and catalytic antioxidants.

Among the first class of compounds are specific PARP inhibitors, among the second are catalytic antioxidants. Animal experiments using PARP inhibitors, and the catalytic antioxidant dexlipotam consistently showed a reduction of diabetes-induced increased Ang-2 expression and an inhibition of pericyte dropout *(77)*.

SUMMARY

Since the observation that pericyte loss is an early morphological change in the natural history of diabetic retinopathy, substantial progress has been made over the years in the understanding of the factors and mechanisms involved. The central change causing pericyte loss is chronic elevation of glucose with subsequent generation of reactive oxygen species. The molecular scenery encompasses post-translational modification of corepressor and transcription factors finally resulting in altered expression of genes crucially involved in the cellular crosstalk of the retinal vasculature. These changes are amenable to therapeutic interventions.

REFERENCES

1. Antonetti, D.A., et al., Diabetic retinopathy: seeing beyond glucose-induced microvascular disease. Diabetes, 2006. 55(9): p. 2401–11.
2. West, H., W.D.Richardson, and M. Fruttiger, Stabilization of the retinal vascular network by reciprocal feedback between blood vessels and astrocytes. Development, 2005. 132(8): p. 1855–62.
3. Sims, D.E., Diversity within pericytes. Clin Exp Pharmacol Physiol, 2000. 27(10): p. 842–6.

4. Etchevers, H.C., et al., The cephalic neural crest provides pericytes and smooth muscle cells to all blood vessels of the face and forebrain. Development, 2001. 128(7): p. 1059–68.
5. Yamashita, J., et al., Flk1-positive cells derived from embryonic stem cells serve as vascular progenitors. Nature, 2000. 408(6808): p. 92–6.
6. DeRuiter, M.C., et al., Embryonic endothelial cells transdifferentiate into mesenchymal cells expressing smooth muscle actins in vivo and in vitro. Circ Res, 1997. 80(4): p. 444–51.
7. Rajantie, I., et al., Adult bone marrow-derived cells recruited during angiogenesis comprise precursors for periendothelial vascular mural cells. Blood, 2004. 104(7): p. 2084–6.
8. Caballero, S., et al., Ischemic vascular damage can be repaired by healthy, but not diabetic, endothelial progenitor cells. Diabetes, 2007. 56(4): p. 960–7.
9. van Deurs, B., Observations on the blood-brain barrier in hypertensive rats, with particular reference to phagocytic pericytes. J Ultrastruct Res, 1976. 56(1): p. 65–77.
10. Thomas, W.E., Brain macrophages: on the role of pericytes and perivascular cells. Brain Res Brain Res Rev, 1999. 31(1): p. 42–57.
11. Hirschi, K.K., S.A. Rohovsky, and P.A. D'Amore, PDGF, TGF-beta, and heterotypic cell-cell interactions mediate endothelial cell-induced recruitment of 10T1/2 cells and their differentiation to a smooth muscle fate. J Cell Biol, 1998. 141(3): p. 805–14.
12. Nicosia, R.F., and S. Villaschi, Rat aortic smooth muscle cells become pericytes during angiogenesis in vitro. Lab Invest, 1995. 73(5): p. 658–66.
13. Villaschi, S., R.F. Nicosia, and M.R. Smith, Isolation of a morphologically and functionally distinct smooth muscle cell type from the intimal aspect of the normal rat aorta. Evidence for smooth muscle cell heterogeneity. In Vitro Cell Dev Biol Anim, 1994. 30A(9): p. 589–95.
14. Nehls, V., K. Denzer, and D. Drenckhahn, Pericyte involvement in capillary sprouting during angiogenesis in situ. Cell Tissue Res, 1992. 270(3): p. 469–74.
15. Sundberg, C., et al., Pericytes as collagen-producing cells in excessive dermal scarring. Lab Invest, 1996. 74(2): p. 452–66.
16. Farrington-Rock, C., et al., Chondrogenic and adipogenic potential of microvascular pericytes. Circulation, 2004. 110(15): p. 2226–32.
17. Schor, A.M., et al., Pericytes derived from the retinal microvasculature undergo calcification in vitro. J Cell Sci, 1990. 97 (Pt 3): p. 449–61.
18. Cogan, D.G., D. Toussaint, and T. Kuwabara, Retinal vascular patterns. IV. Diabetic retinopathy. Arch Ophthalmol, 1961. 66: p. 366–78.
19. Kuwabara, T., and D.G. Cogan, Retinal vascular patterns. VI. Mural cells of the retinal capillaries. Arch Ophthalmol, 1963. 69: p. 492–502.
20. Allt, G. and J.G. Lawrenson, Pericytes: cell biology and pathology. Cells Tissues Organs, 2001. 169(1): p. 1–11.
21. Sims, D.E., The pericyte–a review. Tissue Cell, 1986. 18(2): p. 153–74.
22. Sims, D.E., Recent advances in pericyte biology–implications for health and disease. Can J Cardiol, 1991. 7(10): p. 431–43.
23. Shepro, D. and N.M. Morel, Pericyte physiology. Faseb J, 1993. 7(11): p. 1031–8.
24. Tilton, R.G., et al., Pericyte degeneration and acellular capillaries are increased in the feet of human diabetic patients. Diabetologia, 1985. 28(12): p. 895–900.
25. Wakui, S., et al., Transforming growth factor-beta and urokinase plasminogen activator presents at endothelial cell-pericyte interdigitation in human granulation tissue. Microvasc Res, 1997. 54(3): p. 262–9.
26. Armulik, A., A. Abramsson, and C.Betsholtz, Endothelial/Pericyte Interactions. Circ Res, 2005. 97(6): p. 512–23.
27. Gerhardt, H. and C. Betsholtz, Endothelial-pericyte interactions in angiogenesis. Cell Tissue Res, 2003. 314(1): p. 15–23.
28. Larson, D.M., M.P. Carson, and C.C. Haudenschild, Junctional transfer of small molecules in cultured bovine brain microvascular endothelial cells and pericytes. Microvasc Res, 1987. 34(2): p. 184–99.
29. Crocker, D.J., T.M. Murad, and J.C.Geer, Role of the pericyte in wound healing: an ultrastructural study. Exp Mol Pathol, 1970. 13(1): p. 51–65.
30. Fujimoto, K., Pericyte-endothelial gap junctions in developing rat cerebral capillaries: a fine structural study. Anat Rec, 1995. 242(4): p. 562–5.

31. Hori, S., et al., A pericyte-derived angiopoietin-1 multimeric complex induces occludin gene expression in brain capillary endothelial cells through Tie-2 activation in vitro. J Neurochem, 2004. 89(2): p. 503–13.
32. Courtoy, P.J. , and J. Boyles, Fibronectin in the microvasculature: localization in the pericyte-endothelial interstitium. J Ultrastruct Res, 1983. 83(3): p. 258–73.
33. Hirschi, K.K. and P.A. D'Amore, Pericytes in the microvasculature. Cardiovasc Res, 1996. 32(4): p. 687–98.
34. Rucker, H.K., H.J. Wynder, and W.E. Thomas, Cellular mechanisms of CNS pericytes. Brain Res Bull, 2000. 51(5): p. 363–69.
35. Bondjers, C., et al., Transcription profiling of platelet-derived growth factor-B-deficient mouse embryos identifies RGS5 as a novel marker for pericytes and vascular smooth muscle cells. Am J Pathol, 2003. 162(3): p. 721–9.
36. Cho, H., et al., Pericyte-specific expression of Rgs5: implications for PDGF and EDG receptor signaling during vascular maturation. Faseb J, 2003. 17(3): p. 440–2.
37. Joyce, N.C., et al., cGMP-dependent protein kinase is present in high concentrations in contractile cells of the kidney vasculature. J Cyclic Nucleotide Protein Phosphor Res, 1986. 11(3): p. 191–8.
38. Lindahl, P., et al., Pericyte loss and microaneurysm formation in PDGF-B-deficient mice. Science, 1997. 277(5323): p. 242–5.
39. Nehls, V. and D. Drenckhahn, Heterogeneity of microvascular pericytes for smooth muscle type alpha-actin. J Cell Biol, 1991. 113(1): p. 147–54.
40. Ozerdem, U., et al., NG2 proteoglycan is expressed exclusively by mural cells during vascular morphogenesis. Dev Dyn, 2001. 222(2): p. 218–27.
41. Piva, T.J., D.R. Krause, and K.O. Ellem, UVC activation of the HeLa cell membrane "TGF alpha ase," a metalloenzyme. J Cell Biochem, 1997. 64(3): p. 353–68.
42. Ruiter, D.J., et al., Angiogenesis in wound healing and tumor metastasis. Behring Inst Mitt, 1993(92): p. 258–72.
43. Tidhar, A., et al., A novel transgenic marker for migrating limb muscle precursors and for vascular smooth muscle cells. Dev Dyn, 2001. 220(1): p. 60–73.
44. Song, S., et al., PDGFRbeta + perivascular progenitor cells in tumours regulate pericyte differentiation and vascular survival. Nat Cell Biol, 2005. 7(9): p. 870–9.
45. Bondjers, C., et al., Microarray analysis of blood microvessels from PDGF-B and PDGF-R{beta} mutant mice identifies novel markers for brain pericytes. FASEB J., 2006. 20(10): p. 1703–5.
46. Bergers, G. and S. Song, The role of pericytes in blood-vessel formation and maintenance. Neuro-oncol, 2005. 7(4): p. 452–64.
47. Joyce, N.C., M.F. Haire, and G.E. Palade, Contractile proteins in pericytes. II. Immunocytochemical evidence for the presence of two isomyosins in graded concentrations. J Cell Biol, 1985. 100(5): p. 1387–95.
48. Joyce, N.C., M.F. Haire, and G.E. Palade, Contractile proteins in pericytes. I. Immunoperoxidase localization of tropomyosin. J. Cell Biol, 1985. 100(5): p. 1379–86.
49. Peppiatt, C.M., et al., Bidirectional control of CNS capillary diameter by pericytes. Nature, 2006. 443(7112): p. 700–4.
50. Bauer, H.C., M. Steiner, and H. Bauer, Embryonic development of the CNS microvasculature in the mouse: new insights into the structural mechanisms of early angiogenesis. Exs, 1992. 61: p. 64–8.
51. Gerhardt, H., H. Wolburg, and C. Redies, N-cadherin mediates pericytic-endothelial interaction during brain angiogenesis in the chicken. Dev Dyn, 2000. 218(3): p. 472–9.
52. Egginton, S., et al., The role of pericytes in controlling angiogenesis in vivo. Adv Exp Med Biol, 2000. 476: p. 81–99.
53. Balabanov, R. and P. Dore-Duffy, Role of the CNS microvascular pericyte in the blood-brain barrier. J Neurosci Res, 1998. 53(6): p. 637–44.
54. Wakui, S., et al., Localization of Ang-1, -2, Tie-2, and VEGF expression at endothelial-pericyte interdigitation in rat angiogenesis. Lab Invest, 2006. 86(11): p. 1172–84.
55. Uemura, A., et al., Recombinant angiopoietin-1 restores higher-order architecture of growing blood vessels in mice in the absence of mural cells. J Clin Invest, 2002. 110(11): p. 1619–28.
56. Carmeliet, P., Mechanisms of angiogenesis and arteriogenesis. Nat Med, 2000. 6(4): p. 389–95.

57. Yancopoulos, G.D., et al., Vascular-specific growth factors and blood vessel formation. Nature, 2000. 407(6801): p. 242–8.
58. Gerhardt, H., et al., VEGF guides angiogenic sprouting utilizing endothelial tip cell filopodia. J Cell Biol, 2003. 161(6): p. 1163–77.
59. Anderson, C.R., A.M. Ponce, and R.J. Price, Immunohistochemical identification of an extracellular matrix scaffold that microguides capillary sprouting in vivo. J Histochem Cytochem, 2004. 52(8): p. 1063–72.
60. Betsholtz, C., Insight into the physiological functions of PDGF through genetic studies in mice. Cytokine Growth Factor Rev, 2004. 15(4): p. 215–28.
61. Jain, R.K., Molecular regulation of vessel maturation. Nat Med, 2003. 9(6): p. 685–93.
62. Weinstein, M., X. Yang, and C. Deng, Functions of mammalian Smad genes as revealed by targeted gene disruption in mice. Cytokine Growth Factor Rev, 2000. 11(1–2): p. 49–58.
63. Benjamin, L.E., I. Hemo, and E. Keshet, A plasticity window for blood vessel remodelling is defined by pericyte coverage of the preformed endothelial network and is regulated by PDGF-B and VEGF. Development, 1998. 125(9): p. 1591–8.
64. Ozerdem, U. and W.B. Stallcup, Early contribution of pericytes to angiogenic sprouting and tube formation. Angiogenesis, 2003. 6(3): p. 241–9.
65. Cohen, M.P., R.N. Frank, and A.A. Khalifa, Collagen production by cultured retinal capillary pericytes. Invest Ophthalmol Vis Sci, 1980. 19(1): p. 90–4.
66. Weibel, E.R., On pericytes, particularly their existence on lung capillaries. Microvasc Res, 1974. 8(2): p. 218–35.
67. Schor, A.M., et al., Differentiation of pericytes in culture is accompanied by changes in the extracellular matrix. In Vitro Cell Dev Biol, 1991. 27A(8): p. 651–9.
68. Kennedy, A., R.N. Frank, and M.A. Mancini, In vitro production of glycosaminoglycans by retinal microvessel cells and lens epithelium. Invest. Ophthalmol. Vis. Sci., 1986. 27(5): p. 746–54.
69. Folkman, J. and P.A. D'Amore, Blood Vessel Formation: what is its molecular basis? Cell, 1996. 87(7): p. 1153–55.
70. Lindahl, P., et al., Endothelial-perivascular cell signaling in vascular development: lessons from knockout mice. Curr Opin Lipidol, 1998. 9(5): p. 407–11.
71. Orlidge, A. and P.A. D'Amore, Inhibition of capillary endothelial cell growth by pericytes and smooth muscle cells. J Cell Biol, 1987. 105(3): p. 1455–62.
72. Korff, T., et al., Blood vessel maturation in a 3-dimensional spheroidal coculture model: direct contact with smooth muscle cells regulates endothelial cell quiescence and abrogates VEGF responsiveness. Faseb J, 2001. 15(2): p. 447–57.
73. Sundberg, C., et al., Stable expression of angiopoietin-1 and other markers by cultured pericytes: phenotypic similarities to a subpopulation of cells in maturing vessels during later stages of angiogenesis in vivo. Lab Invest, 2002. 82(4): p. 387–401.
74. Hammes, H.P., et al., Aminoguanidine does not inhibit the initial phase of experimental diabetic retinopathy in rats. Diabetologia, 1995. 38(3): p. 269–73.
75. Kern, T.S., M.C. Tang J, and Du Y. , Differences among rat strains in the rate Eof development of early stages of diabetic retinopathy. Diabetes, 2006. 55 (S1)(A53).
76. Hoffmann, J., et al., Tenilsetam prevents early diabetic retinopathy without correcting pericyte loss. Thromb Haemost, 2006. 95(4): p. 689–95.
77. Lin, J., et al., Effect of R-(+)-alpha-lipoic acid on experimental diabetic retinopathy. Diabetologia, 2006. 49(5): p. 1089–96.
78. Robison, W.G., Jr., et al., Degenerated intramural pericytes ('ghost cells') in the retinal capillaries of diabetic rats. Curr Eye Res, 1991. 10(4): p. 339–50.
79. Papachristodoulou, D., H. Heath, and S.S. Kang, The development of retinopathy in sucrose-fed and streptozotocin-diabetic rats. Diabetologia, 1976. 12(4): p. 367–74.
80. Sima, A.A.F., R. Garcia-Salinas, and P.K. Basu, The BB Wistar rat: an experimental model for the study of diabetic retinopathy. Metabolism, 1983. 32(7, Supplement 1): p. 136–40.
81. Kakehashi, A., Y. Saito, K. Mori, N. Sugi, R. Ono, H. Yamagami, M. Shinohara, H. Tamemoto, S.E. Ishikawa, M. Kawakami, and Y. Kanazawa. Characteristics of diabetic retinopathy in SDR rats. Diabetes Metab Res Rev. 2006. Nov-Dec; 22(6):455–61.

82. Enge, M., et al., Endothelium-specific platelet-derived growth factor-B ablation mimics diabetic retinopathy. Embo J, 2002. 21(16): p. 4307–16.
83. Agardh, C.D., et al., Altered endothelial/pericyte ratio in Goto-Kakizaki rat retina. J Diabetes Complicat, 1997. 11(3): p. 158–62.
84. Dosso, A., et al., Ocular complications in the old and glucose-intolerant genetically obese (fa/fa) rat. Diabetologia, 1990. 33(3): p. 137–44.
85. Kim, S.H., et al., Morphologic studies of the retina in a new diabetic model; SHR/N:Mcc-cp rat. Yonsei Med J, 1998. 39(5): p. 453–62.
86. Feit-Leichman, R.A., et al., Vascular damage in a mouse model of diabetic retinopathy: relation to neuronal and glial changes. Invest Ophthalmol Vis Sci, 2005. 46(11): p. 4281–7.
87. Barber, A.J., et al., The Ins2Akita Mouse as a Model of Early Retinal Complications in Diabetes. Invest Ophthalmol Vis Sci, 2005. 46(6): p. 2210–18.
88. Midena, E., et al., Studies on the retina of the diabetic db/db mouse. I. Endothelial cell-pericyte ratio. Ophthalmic Res, 1989. 21(2): p. 106–11.
89. Obrosova, I.G., et al., Early diabetes-induced biochemical changes in the retina: comparison of rat and mouse models. Diabetologia, 2006. 49(10): p. 2525–33.
90. Hammes, H.P., et al., The relationship of glycaemic level to advanced glycation end-product (AGE) accumulation and retinal pathology in the spontaneous diabetic hamster. Diabetologia, 1998. 41(2): p. 165–70.
91. Engerman, R.L. and T.S. Kern, Experimental galactosemia produces diabetic-like retinopathy. Diabetes, 1984. 33(1): p. 97–100.
92. Engerman, R.L. and T.S. Kern, Retinopathy in galactosemic dogs continues to progress after cessation of galactosemia. Arch Ophthalmol, 1995. 113(3): p. 355–8.
93. Engerman, R.L. and J.W. Kramer, Dogs with induced or spontaneous diabetes as models for the study of human diabetes mellitus. Diabetes, 1982. 31(Suppl 1 Pt 2): p. 26–9.
94. Kern, T.S. and R.L. Engerman, Vascular lesions in diabetes are distributed non-uniformly within the retina. Exp Eye Res, 1995. 60(5): p. 545–9.
95. Gardiner, T.A., et al., Selective loss of vascular smooth muscle cells in the retinal microcirculation of diabetic dogs. Br J Ophthalmol, 1994. 78(1): p. 54–60.
96. Kim, S.Y., et al., Retinopathy in Monkeys with Spontaneous Type 2 Diabetes. Invest Ophthalmol Vis Sci, 2004. 45(12): p. 4543–53.
97. Buchi, E.R., A. Kurosawa, and M.O. Tso, Retinopathy in diabetic hypertensive monkeys: a pathologic study. Graefes Arch Clin Exp Ophthalmol, 1996. 234(6): p. 388–98.
98. Lindahl, P., et al., Pericyte loss and microaneurysm formation in PDGF-B-deficient mice. Science, 1997. 277(5323): p. 242–5.
99. Hammes, H.P., et al., Pericytes and the pathogenesis of diabetic retinopathy. Diabetes, 2002. 51(10): p. 3107–12.
100. Asahara, T., et al., Tie2 Receptor Ligands, Angiopoietin-1 and Angiopoietin-2, Modulate VEGF-Induced Postnatal Neovascularization. Circ Res, 1998. 83(3): p. 233–40.
101. Hammes, H.P., et al., Angiopoietin-2 causes pericyte dropout in the normal retina: evidence for involvement in diabetic retinopathy. Diabetes, 2004. 53(4): p. 1104–10.
102. Feng, Y., et al., Impaired pericyte recruitment and abnormal retinal angiogenesis as a result of angiopoietin-2 overexpression. Thromb Haemost, 2007. 97(1): p. 99–108.
103. Stalmans, I., et al., Arteriolar and venular patterning in retinas of mice selectively expressing VEGF isoforms. J Clin Invest, 2002. 109(3): p. 327–36.
104. Ruberte, J., et al., Increased ocular levels of IGF-1 in transgenic mice lead to diabetes-like eye disease. J Clin Invest, 2004. 113(8): p. 1149–57.
105. Kowluru, R.A. and S. Odenbach, Effect of long-term administration of alpha-lipoic acid on retinal capillary cell death and the development of retinopathy in diabetic rats. Diabetes, 2004. 53(12): p. 3233–8.
106. Mizutani, M., T.S. Kern, and M. Lorenzi, Accelerated death of retinal microvascular cells in human and experimental diabetic retinopathy. J Clin Invest, 1996. 97(12): p. 2883–90.
107. Akagi, Y., et al., Aldose reductase localization in human retinal mural cells. Invest Ophthalmol Vis Sci, 1983. 24(11): p. 1516–19.

108. Berrone, E., et al., Regulation of intracellular glucose and polyol pathway by thiamine and benfotiamine in vascular cells cultured in high glucose. J Biol Chem, 2006. 281(14): p. 9307–13.
109. Yamagishi, S., et al., Advanced glycation endproducts accelerate calcification in microvascular pericytes. Biochem Biophys Res Commun, 1999. 258(2): p. 353–7.
110. Stitt, A.W., et al., Advanced glycation end products (AGEs) co-localize with AGE receptors in the retinal vasculature of diabetic and of AGE-infused rats. Am J Pathol, 1997. 150(2): p. 523–31.
111. Xu, X., et al., Exogenous advanced glycosylation end products induce diabetes-like vascular dysfunction in normal rats: a factor in diabetic retinopathy. Graefes Arch Clin Exp Ophthalmol, 2003. 241(1): p. 56–62.
112. Yamagishi, S.-I., et al., Advanced Glycation Endproducts Accelerate Calcification in Microvascular Pericytes. Biochem Biophys Res Commun, 1999. 258(2): p. 353–7.
113. Kaiser, N., et al., Differential regulation of glucose transport and transporters by glucose in vascular endothelial and smooth muscle cells. Diabetes, 1993. 42(1): p. 80–9.
114. Lyons, T.J., et al., Aminoguanidine and the Effects of Modified LDL on Cultured Retinal Capillary Cells. Invest Ophthalmol Vis Sci, 2000. 41(5): p. 1176–80.
115. Song, W., et al., Effects of oxidized and glycated ldl on gene expression in human retinal capillary pericytes. Invest Ophthalmol Vis Sci, 2005. 46(8): p. 2974–82.
116. Davis, G.E. and W.B. Saunders, Molecular balance of capillary tube formation versus regression in wound repair: role of matrix metalloproteinases and their inhibitors. J Investig Dermatol Symp Proc, 2006. 11(1): p. 44–56.
117. Barth, J.L., et al., Oxidised, glycated LDL selectively influences tissue inhibitor of metalloproteinase-3 gene expression and protein production in human retinal capillary pericytes. Diabetologia, 2007. 50(10): p. 2200–8.
118. Keech, A., R.J. Simes, P. Barter, J. Best, R. Scott, M.R. Taskinen, P. Forder, A. Pillai, T. Davis, P. Glasziou, P. Drury, Y.A. Kesäniemi, D. Sullivan, D. Hunt, P. Colman, M. d'Emden, M. Whiting, C. Ehnholm, and M. Laakso. FIELD study investigators. Effects of long-term fenofibrate therapy on cardiovascular events in 9795 people with type 2 diabetes mellitus (the FIELD study): randomised controlled trial. Lancet. 2005 Nov 26;366(9500): 1849–61.
119. Colhoun, H.M., et al., Primary prevention of cardiovascular disease with atorvastatin in type 2 diabetes in the Collaborative Atorvastatin Diabetes Study (CARDS): multicentre randomised placebo-controlled trial. The Lancet. 364(9435): p. 685–96.
120. Lyons, T.J., et al., Diabetic retinopathy and serum lipoprotein subclasses in the DCCT/EDIC cohort. Invest Ophthalmol Vis Sci, 2004. 45(3): p. 910–8.
121. Brownlee, M., Biochemistry and molecular cell biology of diabetic complications. Nature, 2001. 414(6865): p. 813–20.
122. Hammes, H.-P., Pathophysiological mechanisms of diabetic angiopathy. J Diabetes Complicat, 2003. 17(2, Supplement 1): p. 16–19.
123. Abordo, E.A., H.S. Minhas, and P.J. Thornalley, Accumulation of [alpha]-oxoaldehydes during oxidative stress: a role in cytotoxicity. Biochem Pharmacol, 1999. 58(4): p. 641–48.
124. Yao, D., et al., High glucose increases angiopoietin-2 transcription in microvascular endothelial cells through methylglyoxal modification of mSin3A. J Biol Chem, 2007. 282(42): p. 31038–45.
125. Pfister, F., Y. Feng, F. Vom Hagen, S. Hoffmann, G. Molema, J.L. Hillebrands, M. Shani, U. Deutsch, H.P. Hammes. Pericyte migration: A novel mechanism of pericyte loss in experimental diabetic retinopathy. Diabetes. 2008 Jun 16. [Epub ahed of print]

11 Capillary Dropout in Diabetic Retinopathy

Renu A. Kowluru and Pooi-See Chan

Contents

Abstract

Capillary dropout is a critical process in diabetic retinopathy, resulting in ischemia, release of angiogenic growth factors, and sight-threatening retinal neovascularization.

It is essential to gain a greater understanding of this process in order to develop improved treatments for diabetic retinopathy. This chapter will review the organization, structure, and cellular composition of retinal capillaries. The histopathologic and clinical manifestations of capillary dropout in diabetic retinopathy will be discussed. Methods for detecting capillary dropout and experimental models for studying this phenomenon will be presented. Potential mechanisms for capillary dropout as well as contributory biochemical pathways will be discussed. Finally, the clinical consequences of capillary dropout will be summarized, highlighting the critical importance of this process in the pathophysiology of diabetic retinopathy.

From: *Contemporary Diabetes: Diabetic Retinopathy*
Edited by: E. Duh © Humana Press, Totowa, NJ

Key Words: Diabetic retinopathy, Capillary dropout, Acellular capillaries, Endothelial cell, Apoptosis

DIABETIC RETINOPATHY

Retinopathy, one of the major microvascular complications of diabetes, is the leading cause of blindness throughout the world in the 20–74 year age group. Its effects on the quality of life and loss of productivity for patients and their families are a leading socioeconomic burden on the community. Diabetic retinopathy is a slowly progressing lifelong disease that is exacerbated by high blood pressure, puberty, or pregnancy *(1, 2)*. It affects both type I and type II diabetic patients. With the incidence of type II diabetes increasing worldwide and the age of onset decreasing dramatically, retinopathy is becoming a major global concern.

Retinopathy is a multifactorial complication of diabetes, and sustained hyperglycemia is considered a major cause of slow and cumulative damage to the small blood vessels in the retina *(3, 4)*. The major determinants for the progression of diabetic retinopathy are duration of diabetes and the degree of glycemic control maintained over the years *(5)*. During the initial stages, background retinopathy, small blood vessels may begin to bleed and leak fluid into the surrounding retinal tissue, but the disease remains asymptomatic. As retinal blood vessels continue to get damaged, portions of the retinal microcirculation begin to close down causing the retina to become ischemic. Capillary dropout is a critical process in diabetic retinopathy, resulting in ischemia, release of angiogenic growth factors, and sight-threatening retinal neovascularization *(6)*. As a result, it is necessary to gain a greater understanding of this process in order to develop improved treatments for diabetic retinopathy.

ORGANIZATION, STRUCTURE, COMPOSITION, AND FUNCTION OF RETINAL CAPILLARIES

In order to appreciate how capillaries are damaged in the retina, it is imperative that we have a better understanding of the organization and structure of this delicate but complex tissue. The retina has four major types of cells: vascular (pericytes and endothelial cells), macroglial cells (Muller cells and astrocytes), neurons (photoreceptors, bipolar cells, amacrine and ganglion cells), and microglia (which act as phagocytes). The retinal vessels are highly organized and have three layers of microvessels: a superficial layer in the ganglion cell layer, an intermediate layer in the inner plexiform layer, and a deep layer in the outer plexiform layer (Fig. 1) *(7)*. In humans, the retinal vessels occupy the inner half of the neural retina. The retinal vasculature is separated from the surrounding neural components by the cytoplasm of Muller cells and glial cells. Blood vessels extend outward from the optic disc in all directions spreading their network across the retina, stopping short of the periphery, and also sparing the fovea. Although the arrangement of retinal vessels is unique for each human, the larger blood vessels, in general, occupy the innermost portion of the retina while smaller blood vessels, the capillaries, are found between the nerve fiber and inner nuclear layers *(8)*. The diameter of the capillary network varies in different parts of the retina; the outer mesh ranges from 15 to 130 μm while the superficial network averages about 65 μm *(9)*. The

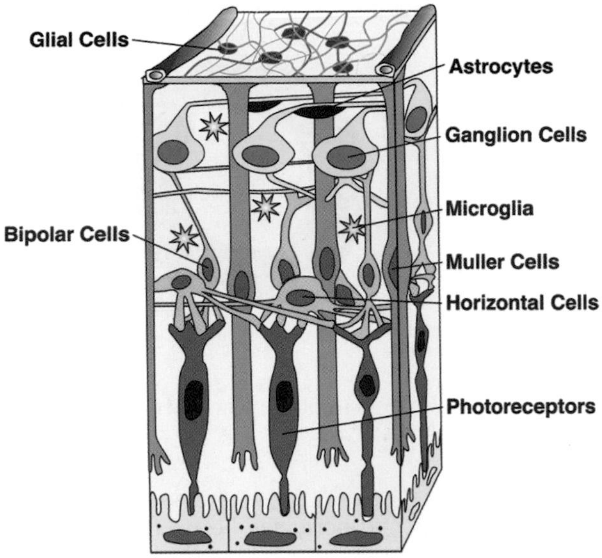

Fig. 1. Organization and structure of retina showing different cell types. The highly organized retinal vessels have three layers of microvessels: a superficial layer in the ganglion cell layer, an intermediate layer in the inner plexiform layer, and a deep layer in the outer plexiform layer. The retinal vasculature is separated from the surrounding neural components by the cytoplasm of Muller cells and glial cells.

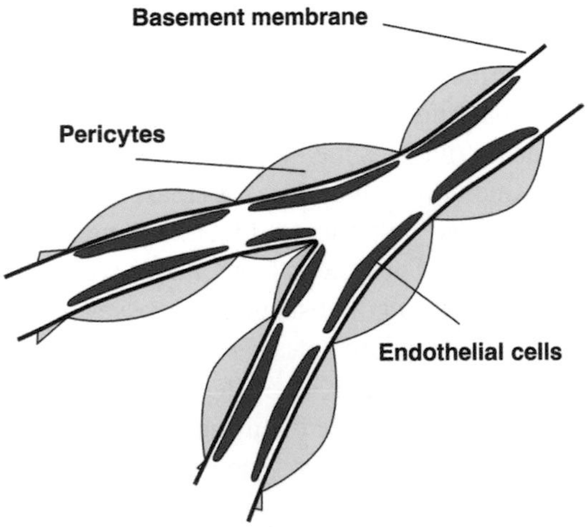

Fig. 2. Retinal capillary structure showing the organization of capillary cells on the basement membrane.

retinal capillary wall is lined by a single layer of endothelial cells encompassed by a basement membrane and surrounded by pericytes (Fig. 2) *(10)*.

The basement membrane, a connective tissue sheath, surrounds the capillaries. It is a definite membrane with a fibrillar structure and has uniform thickness. The retinal capillary basement membrane is mainly composed of collagen types IV and V, laminin and heparan sulfate proteoglycan core protein *(11)*. Its function is to structurally support the endothelial cells and pericytes and also to anchor retinal vessels to adjacent tissues.

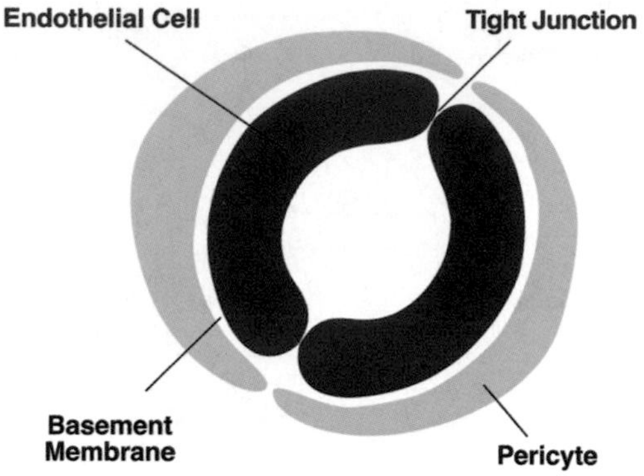

Fig. 3. Cross section of a capillary demonstrating tight junctions in between endothelial cells and coverage by pericytes.

The vascular endothelial cells and pericytes lie on the basement membrane (Fig. 3). Endothelial cells are the predominant cells initially but 3 months after birth, pericytes are observed on the microvessels *(12)*. Fusion of membranes between endothelial cells forms the tight junctional complexes *(7, 13)*. These junctions are largely responsible for the blood–retinal barrier that impedes the outward passage of circulating proteins *(14)*. The integrity of the blood–retinal barrier is essential for normal visual function, and the disruption of this barrier is seen in diabetic retinopathy and other ocular diseases. Under normal conditions, the vascular endothelium also acts as a barrier to the trafficking of leukocytes into the retina. The blood–retinal barrier serves as a selective partition between the retina and the blood circulation enabling the retina to regulate its environment in response to varying metabolic demands. In diabetes the blood–retinal barrier breaks down and permeability to larger molecules, including albumin, is increased *(15)*.

The endothelium is surrounded by pericytes that exchange paracrine signals through a shared basement membrane *(16)*. These cells have nuclei which often appear to protrude from the capillary wall, and have long and slender processes which envelop the wall and overlap neighboring cells *(17)*. They are spaced regularly along the retinal capillary and are in direct contact with endothelial cells. Pericytes are not present on the newly formed capillary beds, but are seen only within the maturing vascular network *(7)*. Pericytes provide structural support, help in contraction and regulate the endothelial cells. Contractility of pericytes confers the ability to regulate retinal vascular tone and blood flow *(18)*.

PATHOLOGY AND CLINICAL MANIFESTATION OF CAPILLARY DROPOUT IN DIABETIC RETINOPATHY

Capillaries function to provide nutrients (glucose, fatty acids, and amino acids) to the retina and to metabolically exchange respiratory gases, and also to remove waste products from the retina in order to maintain retinal homeostasis *(19)*. This fundamental role of the capillaries requires proper functioning of the components of the capillaries. Capillary dropout is characterized by the loss of capillary components that results ultimately in the degeneration or obliteration of capillaries.

In the early stage or background retinopathy, the selective loss of pericytes from the retinal capillaries is consistently shown to occur before any histopathological signs can

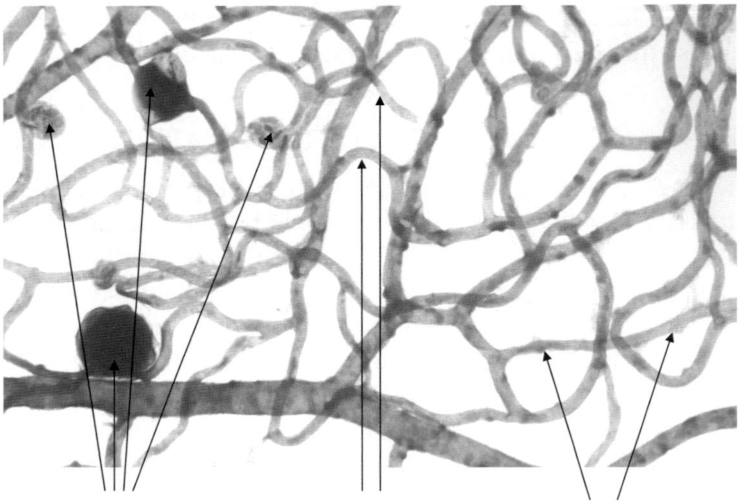

Fig. 4. A trypsin-digest preparation from a patient with diabetic retinopathy showing acellular capillaries that are defined as basement membrane tubes lacking cell nuclei and maintaining at least one-fourth the normal capillary caliber over their length. Pericyte ghosts are the vacant spaces in the capillary basement membrane, formerly occupied by an intramural pericyte nucleus that has degenerated. Capillary microaneurysms of various diameters are clearly seen in this preparation.

be seen. Loss of pericytes that provide support and help in contractility of the capillaries is followed by the loss of endothelial cells. Diabetic patients and animals characteristically demonstrate early pericyte and endothelial cell loss followed by the development of acellular capillaries and microaneurysms (Fig. 4) *(20–22)*.

During the initial stages in background retinopathy, small blood vessels may begin to bleed and leak fluid into the surrounding retinal tissue, but the disease remains asymptomatic. The initial clinical signs a patient presents are microaneurysms and intra-retinal hemorrhages. The frequency and the severity can vary in patients and over 80% patients with diabetes for about 20 years end up showing some of these signs. With progression of the disease, the number and size of intraretinal hemorrhages increases and microcirculatory abnormalities, including leakiness of vessels, are observed by fluorescein angiography. As retinal blood vessels become damaged, peripheral portions of the retinal microcirculation progressively close down. Histopathologic analysis of retinas from diabetic individuals indicates that capillary closure tends to occur on the arterial side of the circulation, often in association with microaneurysms *(23)*. Although this closure initially develops in isolated capillaries, it can eventually extend to groups of capillaries and eventually progress centripetally to involve arterioles *(24)*. Capillary drop-out most commonly involves the mid-peripheral retina, although the central retina is also often involved *(25)*.

Capillary dropout causes the retina to become ischemic, and this signals the release of growth factors leading to the growth of new abnormal blood vessels (neovascularization). New vessels can be intraretinal or can extend into the vitreous cavity of the eye. In addition, they can form within the stroma of the iris and involve the drainage system of the anterior chamber angle of the eye. These new vessels can hemorrhage into the vitreous, resulting in visual loss; in addition, the fibrous tissue accompanying new vessels can cause traction on the retina leading to retinal detachment *(26, 27)*.

METHODS TO MEASURE AND DETECT CAPILLARY DROPOUT

Histological assessment of capillary dropout can be performed in trypsin-digested retina preparations. Capillaries in retinal trypsin digests are stained with periodic acid Schiff-hematoxylin. Acellular capillaries are identified as capillary-sized vessel tubes having no nuclei anywhere along their length (presumably from degeneration of endothelial cells), leaving only a basement membrane tube (Fig. 4). Pericyte ghosts are detected as spaces or pockets in the capillary basement membrane from which pericytes have disappeared *(28)*.

Clinically, the signs of diabetic retinopathy are routinely evaluated by ophthalmologists using fundus examination and photography. Fluorescein angiography helps show physicohemodynamic processes, and has allowed us to understand abnormalities of the capillary bed, including microaneurysms, dilated capillaries, capillary closure and abnormal permeability of the retinal vasculature *(29)*. It can detect microaneurysms and other capillary changes with much greater sensitivity than routine ophthalmoscopy, including leaking vessels, capillary closure and even small new vessels *(30)*. Further, fluorescein angiography has the capability to elucidate detailed microstructural vascular alterations that can escape fundus examination. Microaneurysms that appear as dots on fundus photograph are brightly fluorescent in fluorescein angiography *(31, 32)*. Hemorrhages appear as areas of blocked fluorescence, while hard exudates usually show minimal blocking of fluorescence on fluorescein angiography. Cotton wool spots, which represent areas of ischemic infarction within the nerve fiber layer, appear as fluffy white lesions on fundus examination, and as an area of retinal haziness with blockage of underlying background fluorescence on angiography. Capillary closure is indicated on fluorescein angiography as black patches interrupting the normal capillary pattern (Figs. 5 and 6) *(33)*.

There appears to be a good correlation between the results obtained from fluorescein angiography and trypsin-digested retinal vessels. Comparison of fluorescein angiography of an individual with a trypsin-digested retina preparation a few months afterward demonstrated that areas of capillary nonperfusion correspond to acellular capillary beds *(34)*. In addition, India ink injection preparations fail to fill acellular capillaries, further suggesting their nonfunctional nature *(35)*. These observations support the correspondence between acellular capillaries and capillary dropout.

MODELS TO STUDY RETINAL CAPILLARY DROPOUT IN DIABETES

In order to understand the mechanism of capillary dropout in diabetic retinopathy, suitable models (in vivo and in vitro) are vital. Various animal models have been used to investigate diabetes-induced capillary dropout in the retina. Animal models present an advantage because these models can be used to screen potential therapies for their ability to inhibit the development of retinopathy. In addition, these models have allowed dissection and isolation of various factors associated with the pathogenesis of diabetic retinopathy, and is helping the development of effective strategies to address the problem. For the

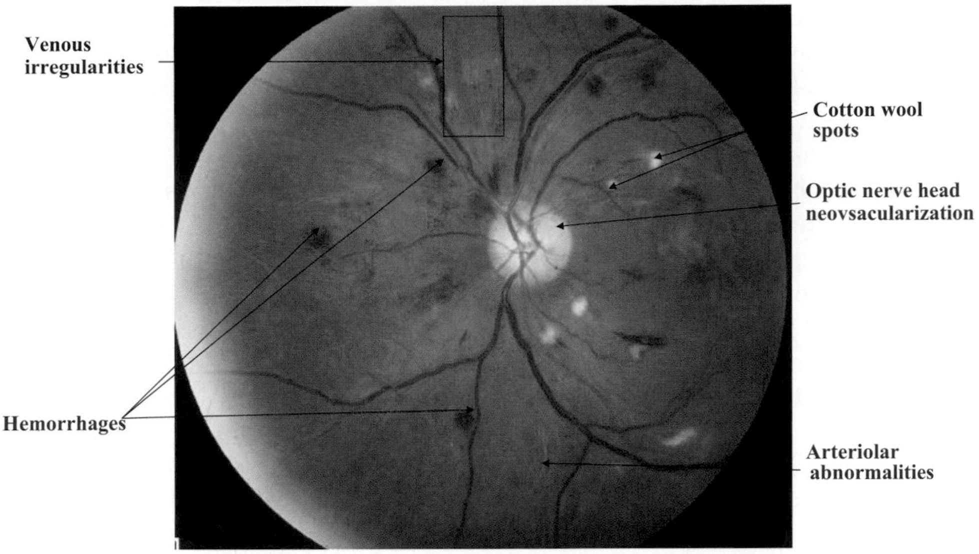

Fig. 5. Fundus photograph of a patient with proliferative diabetic retinopathy showing blot hemorrhages, cotton wool spots, and neovascularization. *Marked areas* of arteriolar abnormalities and venous irregularities suggest very poor blood supply to those areas.

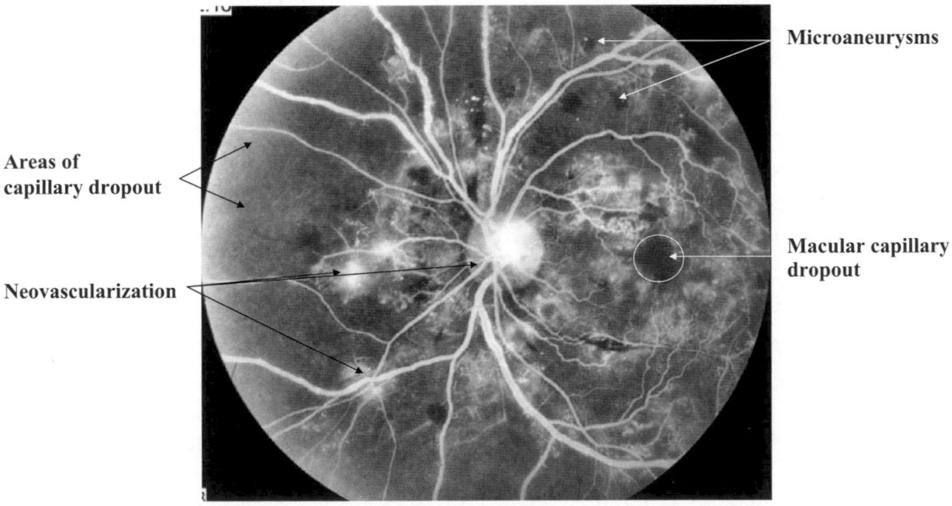

Fig. 6. Angiogram of the same eye (Fig. 5) showing areas of capillary dropout including macular capillary drop out.

most part, data obtained from an animal model can be related to the clinical situation, but this is mainly dependent on the extent to which the clinical pathology can be reliably and successfully duplicated in the animal models. A cautious approach should be used when experimental findings in these models are extrapolated to human conditions. Large animals, such as monkeys, dogs and cats that are chemically made diabetic have been used to understand the pathogenesis of diabetic retinopathy. Monkeys made diabetic by streptozotocin or spontaneously diabetic monkeys have shown capillary cell loss and other significant features of human diabetic retinopathy *(36)*. Pancreatectomized or spontaneously diabetic cats have demonstrated local ischemia and tissue hypoxia in the retina *(37)*, and an acidification of the inner retina that is associated with capillary dropout *(38)*. Diabetic dogs have demonstrated degenerative capillaries, and other histopathology characteristic of retinopathy in diabetic patients *(39, 40)*.

Rodent models (rats and mice), chemically made diabetic with streptozotocin or alloxan, are routinely employed to investigate the development of diabetic retinopathy. Mice present an advantage because they can be genetically manipulated to identify the genes responsible for capillary degeneration *(40–43)*. Capillary dropout and other early histopathological signs of diabetic retinopathy can be observed in rodents at much shorter duration (8–12 months) of diabetes compared to dogs (3–5 years). In addition, the smaller size of the animal provides an advantage in that multiple pathways and therapies can be evaluated using a large number of rodents. Further details about animal models to investigate capillary dropout and other pathology are compiled by Dr. Kern in Chap. 5.

In vitro studies using isolated retinal capillary cells (endothelial cells and pericytes) have helped elucidate the mechanism of capillary dropout in diabetes. These models are useful because the specific gene of interest can be overexpressed or silenced, and the cells can be exposed to specific activators or inhibitors of the pathway of interest without much difficulty *(44–47)*. However, the results should be used with caution because the culture conditions can greatly modify the cells and the in vivo model where multiple diabetes-induced biochemical, physiological, structural, and functional alterations that could work in synergy to contribute to capillary dropout cannot be duplicated.

POTENTIAL MECHANISMS FOR CAPILLARY DROPOUT

At least two mechanisms are thought to contribute to capillary occlusion and obliteration in diabetes: death/apoptosis of capillary cells and vascular occlusion by white blood cells or platelets. In addition, it is quite possible that there could be an interplay between these mechanisms, since capillary cell apoptosis could create an environment favorable for microthrombosis and leukocyte adhesion to endothelial cells, and vice versa.

Capillary Cell Apoptosis

Programmed cell death, commonly termed "apoptosis," may be an important mechanism that contributes to capillary dropout *(22)*. Retinal microvascular cells (pericytes and endothelial cells) and neuronal cells are lost selectively via apoptosis before other histopathology is detectable *(48–50)*, and it is possible that this apoptosis over time contributes to capillary degeneration in DR. In diabetic patients, retinal capillary cells are reported to perish by accelerated cell death *(22)*, and this phenomenon is replicated in animal models of diabetic retinopathy. Apoptosis of retinal microvascular cells in diabetic or galactose-fed rodents can be detected as early as 5–6 months after induction of diabetes, and acellular capillaries and pericyte ghosts are seen after 10–12 months of diabetes *(22, 51–53)*.

The loss of retinal capillary pericytes is considered the earliest morphologic lesion observed in diabetic retinopathy *(54, 55)*. Pericytes with almost no replicative capacity in the adult organism fail to renew *(56)*. This loss of retinal pericytes leaves pockets in the basement membrane, commonly termed as "pericyte ghosts." Apoptotic capillary cells observed in the retina at any given duration of diabetes are very limited in number *(22, 57, 58)*, but this may well be sufficient to result in significant pericyte loss (and appearance of pericyte ghosts) over time. The histopathology of diabetic retinopathy develops over decades in humans and more than 1 year in rats, but apoptosis is a rapidly consummated phenomenon, and apoptotic cells are detectable for only a few hours *(59)*. Thus, accelerated apoptosis could account for the pericyte loss and formation of ghosts in diabetic retinopathy. Although pericyte loss is correlated with acellular capillaries during diabetic microangiopathy *(60–62)*, the specific contribution of pericyte loss to capillary dropout in the pathogenesis of diabetic retinopathy remains unclear. However, studies demonstrating a co-survival relationship of pericytes and endothelial cells in developing and adult vasculature *(63)* suggest that pericytes might have a role in supporting endothelial cell survival. The mean ratio of perictye nuclei to endothelial cell nuclei is 1:1 in normal retinal capillaries, but this ratio decreases to 1:4 (and later 1:10) in diabetic retinopathy *(63, 64)*. Since pericytes are endothelial-supporting cells and they regulate endothelial cells intricately, the loss of pericytes could have negative consequences on endothelial cell survival (for further discussion, see Chap. 10).

Endothelial cells are considered a little less susceptible to damage in diabetes than pericytes *(65)*, and their ability to replicate and replace neighboring cells, though at a very slow rate, could contribute to this *(56, 64)*. Although endothelial cells are capable of making up the deficit for a finite period of time, it is likely that with exposure to the diabetic milieu over time, the replicative capacity of the endothelial cells is exhausted, as occurs in all somatic cells which reach their Hayflick limit *(66, 67)*. In response to cell death in DR, the endothelium maintains a higher than normal rate of cell division over time, and this would be predicted to overextend its replicative capacity. Indeed, it has been suggested that exposure to the diabetic environment could induce a senescent phenotype in endothelial cells so that the normal Hayflick limit is not attainable *(63)*. The precise contribution of endothelial cell apoptosis to capillary dropout remains to be determined. However, it is noteworthy that the ability of a therapy to reduce retinal capillary cell apoptosis in diabetes was predictive of its ability to inhibit retinal capillary degeneration *(50)*. This suggests that apoptosis is an important contributor to capillary dropout in DR. Finally, it is important to note that apoptosis might not be the sole form of cell death in DR, as necrosis has been suggested as well *(68)*.

Proinflammatory Changes/Leukostasis

Diabetes precipitates several molecular and functional abnormalities in the retina suggesting that proinflammatory pathways are a critical contributor in the development of diabetic retinopathy *(69)*. Abnormalities characteristic of inflammation are observed in diabetic retinas and retinal capillary cells cultured in high glucose conditions. These include elevations in proinflammatory cytokines, prostaglandins, nitric oxide (NO), the nuclear transcription factor (NF)-*k*B, and adhesion molecules coupled with up-regulation of leukostasis. These proinflammatory processes could contribute to capillary dropout in diabetic retinopathy by increasing leukostasis and/or via increasing apoptosis of capillary cells *(68, 70–73)*.

The levels of several proinflammatory cytokines including interleukin (IL)-1β, tumor necrosis factor (TNF)-α, IL-6, and IL-8 are increased in the vitreous of patients with proliferative diabetic retinopathy and in retinas from diabetic rodents *(70, 71, 74–76)*. Inflammation is one of the processes implicated in the apoptosis of retinal cells *(68, 71, 77)*, and TNF-α is considered as an important mediator of apoptosis of retinal endothelial cells in diabetes *(78)*.

The eicosanoid prostaglandin E_2 (PGE_2) together with the inducible enzyme that catalyzes its formation, cyclooxygenase-2 (COX-2), are elevated in the retina of diabetic rats *(72, 79–83)*. Besides regulating the levels of vascular endothelial growth factor (VEGF) and retinal vascular permeability during diabetes *(82)*, COX-2 also mediates leukostasis and acellular capillary formation in the retinal microvasculature of diabetic rats *(72, 81)*.

Nitric oxide is an important mediator of inflammation. Its formation is catalyzed by nitric oxide synthases. Inducible nitric oxide synthase (iNOS), in particular, has been reported to contribute to cytotoxicity in some cell types. The expression of iNOS and the levels of NO and peroxynitrite (a product of the reaction between superoxide and NO) are elevated in the retina of diabetic patients and rats *(50, 83–89)*. Diabetic mice that have their iNOS gene knocked out exhibited a significant decrease in retinal capillary degeneration *(90)*.

NF-*k*B, a transcription factor that regulates many genes participating in the inflammatory process and apoptosis, is considered to be a major inducer of most of the proinflammatory proteins including IL-1β, TNF-α, COX-2, iNOS, intercellular adhesion molecule-1 (ICAM-1), and vascular cell adhesion molecule-1 (VCAM-1) *(91)*. NF-*k*B is activated in the retina and retinal capillaries in diabetic conditions *(92–95)*, and it has been implicated in promoting the apoptosis of retinal capillary cells and the formation of acellular capillaries *(92)*. Inhibition of NF-*k*B activation is associated with a reduction in pericyte loss and degeneration of retinal capillaries in diabetic animals *(85, 93, 96)*.

Adhesion molecules including ICAM-1 and VCAM-1 are also up-regulated in the vitreous and serum of patients with diabetic retinopathy *(97–99)*. ICAM-1 and CD18 are considered particularly important in the development of diabetic retinopathy and are suggested to exert their effects via activation of leukostasis *(100, 101)*.

Increased leukostasis has been demonstrated to play an important role in the pathogenesis of diabetic retinopathy *(68, 69, 81, 95, 102–104)*. Leukocytes become less deformable and more activated in diabetes and may be involved in retinal capillary nonperfusion, vascular leakage and endothelial cell damage *(105)*. Acridine orange leukocyte fluorography and fluorescein angiography studies have shown trapped leukocytes directly associated with areas of capillary occlusion and nonperfusion in the diabetic retinal microcirculation *(105, 106)*. Interestingly, with subsequent disappearance of leukocytes, some capillaries remained nonperfused. A detailed discussion of leukostasis and its contribution to capillary dropout in diabetic retinopathy is provided in Chap. 13.

Microthrombosis/Platelet Aggregation

Accumulation of platelets has been observed in the retinal vasculature of diabetic subjects, and these platelet microthrombi were spatially associated with apoptotic endothelial cells *(107)*. Studies have shown that advanced glycation end products (AGEs) inhibit prostacyclin production and induce plasminogen activator inhibitor-1 in microvascular endothelial cells suggesting that AGEs have the ability to cause platelet aggregation and fibrin stabilization, resulting in a predisposition to thrombogenesis

(108, 109). Capillary occlusion by platelet and fibrin thrombi has also been observed in the retina of diabetic rats *(110, 111)*. This suggests that microthrombosis could also contribute to retinal capillary occlusion in DR.

DIABETES-INDUCED BIOCHEMICAL PATHWAYS PROMOTING CAPILLARY DROPOUT

Many metabolic abnormalities that are manifested by elevated glucose, including increased oxidative stress, advanced glycation end product formation, and polyol pathway activation have been implicated in capillary dropout in diabetic retinopathy, but the relative contribution of these biochemical and molecular sequelae of hyperglycemia remains unclear. Chronic hyperglycemia favors glycation reactions, and nonenzymatic glycation can lead to alterations in function and activity of both intracellular and extracellular proteins *(112)*. AGEs can be formed intracellularly and extracellularly in the retina. AGEs increase oxidative and nitrative stress in retinal vascular cells and initiate a sequence of events leading to retinal capillary cell apoptosis via activation of NF-*k*B *(112, 113)*. Treatment of diabetic mice with soluble RAGE, which inhibits interaction of AGEs with AGE receptors, significantly blocked leukostasis as well as blood–retinal barrier breakdown. In addition, diabetes-induced leukostasis and blood–retinal barrier breakdown were significantly augmented in mice transgenic for RAGE, a specific receptor for AGEs *(73)*.

These observations suggest that AGEs could have a significant role in capillary dropout. Additional studies are warranted to confirm the role of AGEs in capillary dropout in diabetic patients.

Oxidative stress is increased in diabetes, and is considered to be a key regulator in the development of diabetic complications *(85, 114, 115)*. Oxidative stress is closely linked to apoptosis in a variety of cell types *(116)*, and reactive oxygen species (ROS) are postulated as causal link between elevated glucose and the other metabolic abnormalities important in the development of diabetic complications *(117)*. As long as glucose levels remain elevated in the retina, the vicious cycle of ROS continues. Antioxidant supplementation in rats or overexpression of mitochondrial manganese superoxide dismutase (MnSOD) in mice inhibit diabetes-induced apoptosis of capillary cells and formation of degenerated capillaries in the retina *(58, 85, 118)*. Increased oxidative stress is observed in retinal capillary cells as well as in other nonvascular retinal cells, including Muller cells and photoreceptors in high glucose conditions *(85, 115, 116)*. Antioxidants and overexpression of MnSOD prevent glucose-induced apoptosis of capillary cells. However, the mechanisms by which oxidative stress contribute to capillary dropout still remain to be elucidated.

CONSEQUENCES OF CAPILLARY DROPOUT

Macular Ischemia

Capillary dropout can lead to the loss of vision in several ways, due to macular ischemia, macular edema, or retinal neovascularization leading to vitreous hemorrhage and tractional retinal detachment. Capillary dropout can result in macular ischemia, a cause of vision loss in nonproliferative diabetic retinopathy. In one study, an enlarged foveal avascular zone was found even in diabetic patients with no retinopathy, compared with healthy subjects *(119)*. But these changes are not reflected in visual acuity loss until the foveal avascular zone is significantly enlarged *(120, 121)*. Measurement of contrast sensitivity has been proposed to be a good visual functional measurement that reflects early changes in retinal circulation and thus may be useful for quantifying disease progression before visual acuity progresses *(122)*.

Neovascularization

Capillary nonperfusion resulting from capillary dropout can subsequently stimulate proliferative retinopathy. Ischemic/hypoxic retina from capillary nonperfusion produces angiogenic growth factors that stimulate the formation of new blood vessels in the retina. These new vessels develop in the retina and at the optic nerve head and later push forward through the internal limiting membrane, and adhere to the posterior surface of the vitreous. These new vessels are very fragile, and as a consequence can break easily leading to vitreous hemorrhage. In addition, the fibrous tissue accompanying these new vessels can produce traction on the retina leading to retinal detachment.

Macular Edema

Capillary dropout has long been known to lead to retinal hypoxia and autoregulatory dilatation of arterioles *(123)* which produces an increase in capillary hydrostatic pressure that could lead to edema *(124)*. With time, blood vessels start leaking into the center of the retina, resulting in the swelling of macula. Impairment of the blood–retinal barrier further complicates the problem. Retinal hypoxia resulting from capillary dropout might lead to an increase in VEGF, known to play an important role in inducing retinal vascular permeability (see Chap. 14). Thus, significant zones of capillary dropout of the foveal capillary network in preproliferative and proliferative diabetic retinopathy are associated with severe forms of diabetic maculopathy with significant edema *(125)*.

THERAPEUTIC APPROACHES TO PREVENT/RETARD CAPILLARY DROPOUT IN DIABETES

It is now widely accepted that good metabolic control is the most effective medical treatment to slow the development and progression of diabetic retinopathy in both type I and type II diabetes.

The Diabetes Control and Complications Trial (DCCT), Epidemiology of Diabetes Interventions and Complications Trial (EDIC), and the United Kingdom Prospective Diabetes Study (UKPDS) have clearly demonstrated that tight blood glucose control reduces, but does not eliminate, the risk of diabetic retinopathy development and progression. The DCCT and the follow-up EDIC studies have shown that instituting good glycemic control in diabetic patients does not have immediate benefits on retinopathy progression. In addition, the benefits of good control persist beyond the period of tight glycemic control *(4, 126)*. This “metabolic memory” phenomenon already becomes important early in the course of diabetes, and tight glycemic control initiated prior to the onset of overt pathology has the most profound long-term impact. Therefore, early intervention with intensive glucose control is critical for preventing the long-term complications of retinopathy. However, good glycemic control, for most patients, is difficult to achieve and maintain for a long duration. This requires modification of behavior and dedication by the patient and loved ones. It also increases the risk of hypoglycemic seizure and possible weight gain *(127)*, thus leaving the patient and physician to strive for the best possible, sensible glycemic control. Consequently, there is a need for additional therapeutic approaches to prevent or delay retinopathy.

Significant research advances have been made regarding the mechanisms of capillary dropout in diabetic retinopathy. These will likely serve as the foundation for clinical studies in the coming years. Therapeutic targeting of specific important mechanisms for capillary dropout could lead to valuable additional treatments to prevent or delay capillary dropout and reduce vision loss in diabetic patients.

ACKNOWLEDGMENTS

Authors would like to thank Dr. T. S. Kern and Dr. R. N. Frank for providing the patient pictures included in this chapter and Mamta Kanwar for technical help. The studies from our laboratory reported here were supported in part by research grants from the National Institutes of Health, the Juvenile Diabetes Foundation International, and by a departmental unrestricted grant from Research to Prevent Blindness.

REFERENCES

1. Klein R, Klein BEK, Jensen SC, Moss SE. The relation of socioeconomics factors to the incidence of proliferative diabetic retinopathy and loss of vision. *Ophthalmology* 101, 68–76 (1994)
2. Chew EY. Epidemiology of diabetic retinopathy. *Hosp Med* 64, 396–399 (2003)
3. Engerman RL, Kern TS. Hyperglycemia as a cause of diabetic retinopathy. *Metabolism* 35(Suppl. 1), 20–23 (1986)
4. Diabetes Control and Complications Trial Research Group. The effect of intensive treatment of diabetes on the development of long-term complications in insulin-dependent diabetes mellitus. *N Engl J Med* 329, 977–986 (1993)
5. Porta M, Bandello F. Diabetic retinopathy: A clinical update. *Diabetologia* 45, 1617–1634 (2002)
6. Davis MD, Norton EWD, Myers FL. *The Airlie House Classification of Diabetic Retinopathy*, Washington, DC, 1969
7. Provis JM. Development of the primate retinal vasculature. *Prog Retin Eye Res* 20, 799–821 (2001)
8. Chan-Ling TL, Halasz P, Stone J. Development of retinal vasculature in the cat: Processes and mechanisms. *Curr Eye Res* 9, 459–478 (1990)
9. Michaelson IC. Vascular morphogenesis in the retina of the cat. *J Anat* 82, 167–174 (1948)
10. Antonelli-Orlidge A, Smith SR, D'Amore PA. Influence of pericytes on capillary endothelial cell growth. *Am Rev Respir Dis* 140, 1129–1131 (1989)
11. Das A, Frank RN, Zhang NL, Samadini E. Increases in collagen type IV and laminin in galactose-induced retinal capillary basement membrane thickening-prevention by an aldose reductase inhibitor. *Exp Eye Res* 50, 269–280 (1990)
12. Shakib M, De Oliveira LF, Henkind P. Development of retinal vessels. II. Earliest stages of vessel formation. *Invest Ophthalmol Vis Sci* 7, 689–700 (1968)
13. Shakib M, Cunha-Vaz JG. Studies on the permeability of the blood–retinal barrier. IV. Junctional complexes of the retinal vessels and their role in the permeability of the blood-retinal barrier. *Exp Eye Res* 5, 229–234 (1966)

14. Gardner TW, Antonetti DA, Barber AJ, Lieth E, Tarbell JA. The molecular structure and function of the inner blood–retinal barrier. *Documenta Ophthalmologica* 97, 3–4 (1999)
15. Cunha-Vaz J, Faria de Abreu JR, Campos AJ. Early breakdown of the blood-retinal barrier in diabetes. *Br J Ophthalmol* 59, 649–656 (1975)
16. Kuwabara T, Cogan DG. Retinal vascular patterns. VI. Mural cells of retinal capillaries. *Arch Ophthalmol* 69, 492–502 (1963)
17. Hogan MJ, Feeney L. The ultrastructure of the retinal vessels. II. The small vessels. *J Ultrastruc Res* 49, 29–46 (1963)
18. Haefliger IO, Zschauer A, Anderson DR. Relaxation of retinal pericyte contractile tone through the nitric oxide-cyclic guanosine monophosphate pathway. *Invest Ophthalmol Vis Sci* 35, 991–997 (1994)
19. Hosoya K, Tomi M. Advances in the cell biology of transport via the inner blood–retinal barrier: Establishment of cell lines and transport functions. *Biol Pharm Bull* 28, 1–8 (2005)
20. Bresnick GH, Davis MD, Myers FL, de Venecia G. Clinicopathologic correlations in diabetic retinopathy. II. Clinical and histologic appearances of retinal capillary microaneurysms. *Arch Ophthalmol* 95, 1215–1220 (1977)
21. Engerman RL. Pathogenesis of diabetic retinopathy. *Diabetes* 38, 1203–1206 (1989)
22. Mizutani M, Kern TS, Lorenzi M. Accelerated death of retinal microvascular cells in human and experimental diabetic retinopathy. *J Clin Invest* 97, 2883–2890 (1996)
23. Ashton N. Arteriolar involvement in diabetic retinopathy. *Br J Ophthal* 37, 282–292 (1953)
24. Engerman RL, Kern TS. Retinopathy in animal models of diabetes. *Diabetes/Metabolism Rev* 11, 109–120 (1995)
25. Niki T, Muraoka K, Shimizu K. Distribution of capillary nonperfusion in early-stage diabetic retinopathy. *Ophthalmology* 91, 1431–1439 (1984)
26. Frank RN. *Diabetic Retinopathy*, Elsevier, Amsterdam, 1995
27. Frank RN. Diabetic Retinopathy. *N Engl J Med* 350, 48–58 (2004)
28. Engerman RL. Animal models of diabetic retinopathy. *Trans Am Acad Ophthalmol Otolaryngol* 81, 710–715 (1976)
29. Kohner EM, Dollery CT, Paterson JW, Oakley NW. Arterial fluorescein studies in diabetic retinopathy. *Diabetes* 16, 1–10 (1967)
30. Novotny HR, Alvis DL. A method of photographing fluorescence in circulating blood in the human retina. *Circulation* 24, 82–86 (1961)
31. Wessing A. Fluorescein appearance of the abnormal fundus. In: Meyer-Schwickerath G, ed. *Fluorescein Angiography of the Retina*, Mosby, Stuttgart, 1969, pp. 53–175
32. Schalnus R, Ohrloff C. The blood–ocular barrier in type I diabetes without diabetic retinopathy: Permeability measurements using fluorophotometry. *Ophthalmic Res* 27, 116–123 (1995)
33. Laatikainen L. The fluorescein angiography revolution: A breakthrough with sustained impact. *Acta Ophthalmologica Scandinavica* 82, 381–392 (2004)
34. Kohner EM, Henkind P. Correlation of fluorescein angiogram and retinal digest in diabetic retinopathy. *Am J Ophthalmol* 69, 403–414 (1970)
35. Ashton N. Studies of the retinal capillaries in relation to diabetic and other retinopathies. *Br J Ophthalmol* 47, 521–538 (1963)
36. Büchi RR, Kurosawa A, Tso MO. Retinopathy in diabetic hypertensive monkeys: A pathologic study. *Graefes Arch Clin Exp Ophthalmol* 234, 388–398 (1996)
37. Linsenmeier RA, Braun RD, McRipley MA, Padnick LB, Ahmed J, Hatchell DL, McLeod DS, Lutty GA. Retinal hypoxia in long-term diabetic cats. *Invest Ophthalmol Vis Sci* 39, 1647–1657 (1998)
38. Budzynski E, Wangsa-Wirawan N, Padnick-Silver L, Hatchell D, Linsenmeier R. Intraretinal pH in diabetic cats. *Curr Eye Res* 30, 229–240 (2005)
39. Engerman RL, Kramer JW. Dogs with induced or spontaneous diabetes as models for the study of human diabetes. *Diabetes* 31(Suppl. 1), 26–29 (1982)
40. Kern TS, Kowluru R, Engerman RL. Dog and rat models of diabetic retinopathy. In: Shafrir E, ed. *Lessons from Animal Diabetes*, Smith-Gordon, London, 1996, pp. 395–408
41. Kern TS, Engerman RL. Comparison of retinal lesions in alloxan-diabetic rats and galactose-fed rats. *Curr Eye Res* 13, 863–867 (1994)

42. Kern TS, Kowluru R, Engerman RL. Questions raised by study of experimental diabetic retinopathy. In: Kaneko SBaT, ed. *Diabetes 1994; Proceedings of the 15th International Diabetes Federation Congress*, Excerpta Medica, Kobe, Japan, 1995, pp. 331–334
43. Kern TS, Engerman RE. Animal model of human disease: A mouse model of diabetic retinopathy. *Comp Pathol Bull* 39, 3–6 (1997)
44. Beltramo E, Berrone E, Giunti S, Gruden G, Perin PC, Porta M. Effects of mechanical stress and high glucose on pericyte proliferation, apoptosis and contractile phenotype. *Exp Eye Res* 83, 989–994 (2006)
45. Kowluru RA, Kowluru V, Ho YS, Xiong Y. Overexpression of mitochondrial superoxide dismutase in mice protects the retina from diabetes-induced oxidative stress. *Free Rad Biol Med* 41, 1191–1196 (2006)
46. Kowluru RA, Kowluru A, Kanwar M. Small molecular weight G-protein, H-Ras, and retinal endothelial cell apoptosis in diabetes. *Mol Cell Biochem* 296, 69–76 (2007)
47. Miller AG, Smith DG, Bhat M, Nagaraj RH. Glyoxalase I is critical for human retinal capillary pericyte survival under hyperglycemic conditions. *J Biol Chem* 281, 11864–11871 (2006)
48. Mizutani M, Gerhardinger C, Lorenzi M. Muller cell changes in human diabetic retinopathy. *Diabetes* 47, 455–459 (1998)
49. Barber AJ, Lieth E, Khin SA, Antonetti DA, Buchanan AG, Gardner TW. Neural apoptosis in the retina during experimental and human diabetes. Early onset and effect of insulin. *J Clin Invest* 102, 783–791 (1998)
50. Kern TS, Tang J, Mizutani M, Kowluru R, Nagraj R, Lorenzi M. Response of capillary cell death to aminoguanidine predicts the development of retinopathy: Comparison of diabetes and galactosemia. *Invest Ophthalmol Vis Sci* 41, 3972–3978 (2000)
51. Barber AJ, Antonetti DA, Kern TS, Reiter CE, Soans RS, Krady JK, Levison SW, Gardner TW, Bronson SK. The Ins2Akita mouse as a model of early retinal complications in diabetes. *Invest Ophthalmol Vis Sci* 46, 2210–2218 (2005)
52. Barile GR, Pachydaki SI, Tari SR, Lee SE, Donmoyer CM, Ma W, Rong LL, Buciarelli LG, Wendt T, Hörig H, Hudson BI, Qu W, Weinberg AD, Yan SF, Schmidt AM. The RAGE axis in early diabetic retinopathy. *Invest Ophthalmol Vis Sci* 46, 2916–2924 (2005)
53. Feit-Leichman RA, Kinouchi R, Takeda M, Fan Z, Mohr S, Kern TS, Chen DF. Vascular damage in a mouse model of diabetic retinopathy: Relation to neuronal and glial changes. *Invest Ophthal Vis Sci* 46, 4281–4287 (2005)
54. Kuwabara T, Cogan DG. Retinal vascular patterns. VII. Acellular change. *Invest Ophthalmol Vis Sci* 4, 1049–1064 (1965)
55. Kador PF, Akagi Y, Terubayashi H, Wyman M, Kinoshita JH. Prevention of pericyte ghost formation in retinal capillaries of galactose-fed dogs by aldose reductase inhibitors. *Arch Ophthalmol* 106, 1099–1102 (1988)
56. Engerman RL, Pfaffenbach D, Davis MD. Cell turnover of capillaries. *Lab Invest* 17, 738–743 (1967)
57. Kowluru RA, Koppolu P. Diabetes-induced activation of caspase-3 in retina: Effect of antioxidant therapy. *Free Radic Res* 36, 993–999 (2002)
58. Kowluru RA, Odenbach S. Effect of long-term administration of alpha lipoic acid on retinal capillary cell death and the development of retinopathy in diabetic rats. *Diabetes* 53, 3233–3238 (2004)
59. Raff MC, Barres BA, Burne JF, Coles HS, Ishizaki Y, Jacobson MD. Programmed cell death and the control of cell survival: Lessons from the nervous system. *Science* 262, 695–700 (1993)
60. Cogan DG, Toussaint D, Kuwabara T. Retinal vascular patterns. IV. Diabetic retinopathy. *Arch Ophthalmol* 66, 366–378 (1961)
61. Dodge AB, D'Amore PA. Cell–cell interactions in diabetic angiopathy. *Diabetes Care* 15, 1168–1180 (1992)
62. Murata M, Ohta N, Fujisawa S, Tsai JY, Sato S, Akagi Y, Takahashi Y, Neuenschwander H, Kador PF. Selective pericyte degeneration in the retinal capillaries of galactose-fed dogs results from apoptosis linked to aldose reductase-catalyzed galactitol accumulation. *J Diabetes Complicat* 16, 363–370 (2002)
63. Gardiner TA, Archer DB, Curtis TM, Stitt AW. Arteriolar involvement in the microvascular lesions of diabetic retinopathy: Implications for pathogenesis. *Microcirculation* 14, 25–38 (2007)

64. Sharma AK, Gardiner TA, Archer DB. A morphologic and autoradiographic study of cell death and regeneration in the retinal microvasculature of normal and diabetic rats. *Am J Ophthalmol* 100, 51–60 (1985)
65. Hammes HP, Lin J, Bretzel RG, Brownlee M, Breier G. Upregulation of the vascular endothelial growth factor/vascular endothelial growth factor receptor sysytem in experimental background diabetic retinopathy of the rats. *Diabetes* 47, 401–406 (1998)
66. Hayflick L. The limited in vitro lifetime of human diploid cell strains. *Exp Cell Res* 37, 614–636 (1965)
67. Linskens MH, Harley CB, West MD, Campisi J, Hayflick L. Replicative senescence and cell death. *Science* 267, 17 (1995)
68. Joussen AM, Murata T, Tsujikawa A, Kirchhof B, Bursell SE, Adamis AP. Leukocyte-mediated endothelial cell injury and death in the diabetic retina. *Am J Pathol* 158, 147–152 (2001)
69. Joussen AM, Poulaki V, Le ML, Koizumi K, Esser C, Janicki H, Schraermeyer U, Kociok N, Fauser S, Kirchhof B, Kern TS, Adamis AP. A central role for inflammation in the pathogenesis of diabetic retinopathy. *FASEB J* 18, 1450–1452 (2004)
70. Kowluru RA, Odenbach S. Role of interleukin-1beta in the pathogenesis of diabetic retinopathy. *Br J Ophthalmol* 88, 1343–1347 (2004)
71. Kowluru RA, Odenbach S. Role of interleukin-1beta in the development of retinopathy in rats: Effect of antioxidants. *Invest Ophthalmol Vis Sci* 45, 4161–4166 (2004)
72. Kern TS, Miller CM, Du Y, Zheng L, Mohr S, Ball SL, Kim M, Jamison JA, Bingaman DP. Topical administration of nepafenac inhibits diabetes-induced retinal microvascular disease and underlying abnormalities of retinal metabolism and physiology. *Diabetes* 56, 373–379 (2007)
73. Kaji Y, Usui T, Ishida S, Yamashiro K, Moore TC, Moore J, Yamamoto Y, Yamamoto H, Adamis AP. Inhibition of diabetic leukostasis and blood–retinal barrier breakdown with a soluble form of a receptor for advanced glycation end products. *Invest Ophthalmol Vis Sci* 48, 858–865 (2007)
74. Carmo A, Cunha-Vaz JG, Carvalho AP, Lopes MC. L-arginine transport in retinas from streptozotocin diabetic rats: Correlation with the level of IL-1 beta and NO synthase activity. *Vision Res* 39, 3817–3823 (1999)
75. Yuuki T, Kanda T, Kimura Y, Kotajima N, Tamura J, Kobayashi I, Kishi S. Inflammatory cytokines in vitreous fluid and serum of patients with diabetic vitreoretinopathy. *J Diabetes Complicat* 15, 257–259 (2001)
76. Zheng L, Gong B, Hatala DA, Kern TS. Retinal ischemia and reperfusion causes capillary degeneration: Similarities to diabetes. *Invest Ophthalmol Vis Sci* 48, 361–367 (2007)
77. Joussen AM, Poulaki V, Mitsiades N, Cai WY, Suzuma I, Pak J, Ju ST, Rook SL, Esser P, Mitsiades CS, Kirchhof B, Adamis AP, Aiello LP. Suppression of Fas-FasL-induced endothelial cell apoptosis prevents diabetic blood–retinal barrier breakdown in a model of streptozotocin-induced diabetes. *FASEB J* 17, 76–78 (2003)
78. Kociok N, Radetzky S, Krohne TU, Gavranic C, Joussen AM. Pathological but not physiological retinal neovascularization is altered in TNF-Rp55-receptor-deficient mice. *Invest Ophthalmol Vis Sci* 47, 5057–5065 (2006)
79. Naveh-Floman N, Weissman C, Belkin M. Arachidonic acid metabolism by retinas of rats with streptozotocin-induced diabetes. *Curr Eye Res* 3, 1135–1139 (1984)
80. Johnson EI, Dunlop ME, Larkins RG. Increased vasodilatory prostaglandin production in the diabetic rat retinal vasculature. *Curr Eye Res* 18, 79–82 (1999)
81. Joussen AM, Poulaki V, Mitsiades N, Kirchhof B, Koizumi K, Dohmen S, Adamis AP. Nonsteroidal anti-inflammatory drugs prevent early diabetic retinopathy via TNF-alpha suppression. *FASEB J* 16, 438–440 (2002)
82. Ayalasomayajula SP, Kompella UB. Celecoxib, a selective cyclooxygenase-2 inhibitor, inhibits retinal vascular endothelial growth factor expression and vascular leakage in a streptozotocin-induced diabetic rat model. *Eur J Pharmacol* 458, 283–289 (2003)
83. Du Y, Sarthy VP, Kern TS. Interaction between NO and COX pathways in retinal cells exposed to elevated glucose and retina of diabetic rats. *Am J Physiol Regul Integr Comp Physiol* 287, R734–R741 (2004)
84. Kowluru RA, Engerman RL, Kern TS. Abnormalities of retinal metabolism in diabetes or experimental galactosemia VIII. Prevention by aminoguanidine. *Curr Eye Res* 21, 814–819 (2000)

85. Kowluru RA, Tang J, Kern TS. Abnormalities of retinal metabolism in diabetes and experimental galactosemia. VII. Effect of long-term administration of antioxidants on the development of retinopathy. *Diabetes* 50, 1938–1942 (2001)
86. Abu El-Asrar AM, Desmet S, Meersschaert A, Dralands L, Missotten L, Geboes K. Expression of the inducible isoform of nitric oxide synthase in the retinas of human subjects with diabetes mellitus. *Am J Ophthalmol* 132, 551–556 (2001)
87. Du Y, Smith MA, Miller CM, Kern TS. Diabetes-induced nitrative stress in the retina, and correction by aminoguanidine. *J Neurochem* 80, 771–779 (2002)
88. Kowluru RA. Effect of re-institution of good glycemic control on retinal oxidative stress and nitrative stress in diabetic rats. *Diabetes* 52, 818–823 (2003)
89. Kowluru RA, Kanwar M, Kennedy A. Metabolic memory phenomenon and accumulation of peroxynitrite in retinal capillaries. *Exp Diabetes Res* 2007, 1–7 (2007)
90. Zheng L, Du Y, Miller C, Gubitosi-Klug RA, Kern TS, Ball S, Berkowitz BA. Critical role of inducible nitric oxide synthase in degeneration of retinal capillaries in mice with streptozotocin-induced diabetes. *Diabetologia* 50, 1987–1996 (2007)
91. Lee JI, Burckart GJ. Nuclear factor kappa B: Important transcription factor and therapeutic target. *J Clin Pharmacol* 38, 981–993 (1998)
92. Romeo G, Liu WH, Asnaghi V, Kern TS, Lorenzi M. Activation of nuclear factor-kappaB induced by diabetes and high glucose regulates a proapoptotic program in retinal pericytes. *Diabetes* 51, 2241–2248 (2002)
93. Kowluru RA, Koppolu P, Chakrabarti S, Chen S. Diabetes-induced activation of nuclear transcriptional factor in the retina, and its inhibition by antioxidants. *Free Radic Res* 37, 1169–1180 (2003)
94. Kowluru RA, Chakrabarti S, Chen S. Re-Institution of good metabolic control in diabetic rats on the activation of caspase-3 and nuclear transcriptional factor (NF-kB) in the retina. *Acta Diabetologica* 44, 194–199 (2004)
95. Zheng L, Szabo C, Kern TS. Poly(ADP-ribose) polymerase is involved in the development of diabetic retinopathy via regulation of nuclear factor-kappaB. *Diabetes* 53, 2960–2967 (2004)
96. Zheng L, Howell SJ, Hatala DA, Huang K, Kern TS. Salicylate-based anti-inflammatory drugs inhibit the early lesion of diabetic retinopathy. *Diabetes* 56, 337–345 (2007)
97. Barile GR, Chang SS, Park LS, et al. Soluble cellular adhesion molecules in proliferative vitreoretinopathy and proliferative diabetic retinopathy. *Curr Eye Res* 19, 219–227 (1999)
98. Matsumoto K, Sera Y, Ueki Y, Inukai G, Niiro E, Miyake S. Comparison of serum concentrations of soluble adhesion molecules in diabetic microangiopathy and macroangiopathy. *Diabet Med* 19, 822–826 (2002)
99. van Hecke MV, Dekker JM, Nijpels G, Moll AC, Heine RJ, Bouter LM, Polak BC, Stehouwer CD. Inflammation and endothelial dysfunction are associated with retinopathy: The Hoorn Study. *Diabetologia* 48, 1300–1306 (2005)
100. Osborn L. Leukocyte adhesion to endothelium in inflammation. *Cell* 62, 3–6 (1990)
101. Matsuoka M, Ogata N, Minamino K, Matsumura M. Leukostasis and pigment epithelium-derived factor in rat models of diabetic retinopathy. *Mol Vis* 13, 1058–1065 (2007)
102. Schröder S, Palinski W, Schmid-Schönbein GW. Activated monocytes and granulocytes, capillary nonperfusion, and neovascularization in diabetic retinopathy. *Am J Pathol* 139, 81–100 (1991)
103. Miyamoto K, Khosrof S, Busell SE, Rohan R, Murata T, Clermont AC, Aiello LP, Ogura Y, Adamis AP. Prevention of leukostasis and vascular leakage in streptozotocin-induced diabetic retinopathy via intercellular adhesion molecule-1 inhibition. *Proc Natl Acad Sci USA* 96, 10836–10841 (1999)
104. Moore TC, Moore JE, Kaji Y, Frizzell N, Usui T, Poulaki V, Campbell IL, Stitt AW, Gardiner TA, Archer DB, Adamis AP. The role of advanced glycation end products in retinal microvascular leukostasis. *Invest Ophthalmol Vis Sci* 44, 4457–4464 (2003)
105. Miyamoto K, Ogura Y. Pathogenetic potential of leukocytes in diabetic retinopathy. *Sem in Ophthalmol* 14, 233–239 (1999)
106. Hossain P. Scanning laser ophthalmoscopy and fundus fluorescent leucocyte angiography. *Br J Ophthalmol* 83, 1250–1253 (1999)
107. Boeri D, Maiello M, Lorenzi M. Increased prevalence of microthromboses in retinal capillaries of diabetic individuals. *Diabetes* 50, 1432–1439 (2001)

108. Yamagishi S, Yamamoto Y, Harada S, Hsu CC, Yamamoto H. Advanced glycosylation end products stimulate the growth but inhibit the prostacyclin-producing ability of endothelial cells through interactions with their receptors. *FEBS Lett* 384, 103–106 (1996)
109. Yamagishi S, Fujimori H, Yonekura H, Yamamoto Y, Yamamoto H. Advanced glycation endproducts inhibit prostacyclin production and induce plasminogen activator inhibitor-1 in human microvascular endothelial cells. *Diabetologia* 41, 1435–1441 (1998)
110. Ishibashi T, Tanaka K, Taniguchi Y. Platelet aggregation and coagulation in the pathogenesis of diabetic retinopathy in rats. *Diabetes* 30, 601–605 (1981)
111. Sima AAF, Chakrabarti S, Garcia-Salinas R, Basu PK. The BB-rat: An authentic model of human diabetic retinopathy. *Curr Eye Res* 4, 1087–1092 (1985)
112. Stitt AW. The role of advanced glycation in the pathogenesis of diabetic retinopathy. *Exp Mol Pathol* 75, 95–108 (2003)
113. Kowluru RA. Effect of advanced glycation end products on accelerated apoptosis of retinal capillary cells under in vitro conditions. *Life Sci* 76, 1051–1060 (2005)
114. Baynes JW, Thrope SR. Role of oxidative stress in diabetic complications: A new perspective on an old paradigm. *Diabetes* 48, 1–9 (1999)
115. Du XL, Edelstein D, Rossetti L, Fantus IG, Goldberg H, Ziyadeh F, Wu J, Brownlee M. Hyperglycemia-induced mitochondrial superoxide overproduction activates the hexosamine pathway and induces plasminogen activator inhibitor-1 expression by increasing Sp1 glycosylation. *Proc Natl Acad Sci* 97, 12222–12226 (2000)
116. Baumgartner-Parzer SM, Wagner L, Pettermann M, Grillari J, Gessl A, Waldhausl W. High-glucose-triggered apoptosis in cultured endothelial cells. *Diabetes* 44, 1323–1327 (1995)
117. Brownlee M. The pathobiology of diabetic complications: A unifying mechanism. *Diabetes* 54, 1615–1625 (2005)
118. Kanwar M, Chan PS, Kern TS, Kowluru RA. Oxidative damage in the retinal mtochondria of diabetic mice: Possible protection by superoxide dismutase. *Invest Ophthalmol Vis Sci* 48, 3805–3811 (2007)
119. Arend O, Wolf S, Harris A, Reim M. The relationship of macular microcirculation to visual acuity in diabetic patients. *Arch Ophthalmol* 113, 610–614 (1995)
120. Bresnick GH, Condit R, Syrjala S, Palta M, Groo A, Korth K. Abnormalities of the foveal avascular zone in diabetic retinopathy. *Arch Ophthalmol* 102, 1286–1293 (1984)
121. Arend O, Wolf S, Jung F, Bertram B, Pöstgens H, Toonen H, Reim M. Retinal microcirculation in patients with diabetes mellitus: Dynamic and morphological analysis of perifoveal capillary network. *Br J Ophthalmol* 75, 514–518 (1991)
122. Arend O, Remky A, Evans D, Stüber R, Harris A. Contrast sensitivity loss is coupled with capillary dropout in patients with diabetes. *Invest Ophthalmol Vis Sci* 38, 1819–1824 (1997)
123. Hickman JB, Frayser R. Studies of the retinal circulation in man: Observations on vessel diameter, arteriovenous oxygen difference, and mean circulation time. *Circulation* 33, 302–316 (1966)
124. Kristinsson JK, Gottfredsdóttir MS, Stefánsson E. Retinal vessel dilatation and elongation precedes diabetic macular oedema. *Br J Ophthalmol* 81, 274–278 (1997)
125. Golubovic-Arsovska M. Correlation of diabetic maculopathy and level of diabetic retinopathy. *Prilozi* 27, 139–150 (2006)
126. Diabetes Control and Complications Trial/Epidemiology of Diabetes Interventions and Complications Research Group. Effect of intensive therapy on the microvascular complications of type 1 diabetes mellitus. *JAMA* 287, 2563–2569 (2002)
127. Diabetes Control and Complications Trial Research Group. Hypoglycemia in the diabetes control and complications trial. *Diabetes* 46, 271–286 (1997)

12 Neuroglial Dysfunction in Diabetic Retinopathy

Heather D. VanGuilder, Thomas W. Gardner, and Alistair J. Barber

CONTENTS

ABSTRACT

Diabetic retinopathy is a vision-threatening disease that impacts many, if not all the different types of cells in the retina. This chapter reviews evidence that the dysfunction of the neuroglial cells of the retina contributes to the pathology of diabetic retinopathy. The basic histology of the neurons and glial cells of the retina is summarized, along with a discussion of the functions of these different cell types, and how they operate collectively to mediate vision. Then the effect of diabetes on retinal function is summarized, along with a discussion of how neurodegeneration, glial dysfunction, and neuroinflammation each may play a part in loss of vision. Finally, the history of research on neuroglial dysfunction in diabetic retinopathy is summarized in order to appreciate the evolution of the notion that vision loss is mediated through abnormalities in neuroglial cells.

From: *Contemporary Diabetes: Diabetic Retinopathy*
Edited by: E. Duh © Humana Press, Totowa, NJ

Key Words: Retina; Neuron; Retinal ganglion cell; Microglia; Macroglia; Astrocyte; Müller cell; Neurodegeneration; Visual function; Electroretinogram.

THE RETINA IS A MULTICELLULAR PHOTON SENSOR AND PHOTOMULTIPLIER

The retina is a unique component of the central nervous system (CNS), containing a variety of neurons and glial cells. This elegant and complex structure converts visual stimuli into chemical and electrical signals that are transmitted to the brain via the optic nerve. Clinicians and neuroscientists view the retina from distinct perspectives, and both disciplines provide instructive lessons about retinal composition and function. Clinicians view the fundus of the retina as the sum of the visible structures – retinal blood vessels, pigment epithelium, choroid and, to some extent, the vitreous humor. By contrast, neuroscientists concentrate on the cellular organization that is largely invisible to clinicians. This brief overview of retinal structure and function emphasizes the critical role of the invisible neurosensory retina in normal vision, to illustrate how these characteristics may predispose it to compromise the metabolic stresses of diabetes. These relationships are essential to the interpretation of the clinical features of diabetic retinopathy and the processes that disrupt vision.

The cellular anatomy of the mammalian retina was revealed in great detail by Ramón y Cajal more than 100 years ago, when he defined the neuronal subclasses as well as the Müller cells and astrocytes, using Golgi silver staining methods. He recognized the laminar structure of the retina and the fact that neurons comprise the majority of retinal cells. This structure, highly conserved throughout vertebrate evolution from fish to humans, is comprised of three layers of neurons and two layers of synapses, which are minute structures that facilitate interneuronal communication through the release of, and response to, chemical transmitter substances *(1)*.

The neurons are categorized as follows:

First-order: photoreceptors, which produce a neurochemical response to photons

Second-order: bipolar, horizontal, and amacrine ("without axons") cells, which conduct and regulate signals from photoreceptors

Third-order: ganglion cells, which collect and integrate information from second-order neurons that are organized into opposing on/off receptive fields and transmit electrical impulses via axons which terminate primarily in the lateral geniculate body of the thalamus.

THE NEURONS OF THE RETINA

The histological configuration of the retina implies that communication between neurons can be broken down into at least three distinct stages. Retinal neurons are organized in three layers separated by two plexuses of densely packed synaptic connections that enable different types of neurons to communicate with each other. The two layers of synapses (plexiform layers) mediate signal transduction from the photoreceptors (first-order neurons) through bipolar interneurons (second-order neurons) to the ganglion cells (third-order neurons). The axons of the retinal ganglion cells cofasciculate to form the optic nerve, which transmits integrated visual signals to be interpreted by the occipital cortex.

Photoreceptors are organized with their cell bodies (inner segments) in the outer nuclear layer and the stacked discs (outer segments), which contain photon-detecting photopigments, (rhodopsin and opsins), in the photoreceptor layer, with a thin cilium connecting the two layers. Photoreceptors number approximately 126 million in young adult human retinas, a factor of 10 more than the ganglion cells *(2)*, thus reflecting the high degree of signal integration within the retina. Photoreceptors synapse with rod ON (light-stimulated) bipolar cells and cone photoreceptors synapse with ON and OFF (light-inhibited) bipolar cells. The ON and OFF bipolar cells synapse, in turn, with ON and OFF ganglion cells, respectively (Fig. 1). In this manner, second-order neurons integrate signals from groups of adjacent photoreceptors, and in concert with third-order neurons, ganglion cells, provide the center-surround receptive fields that lead to the ability to detect contrast and motion *(3)*.

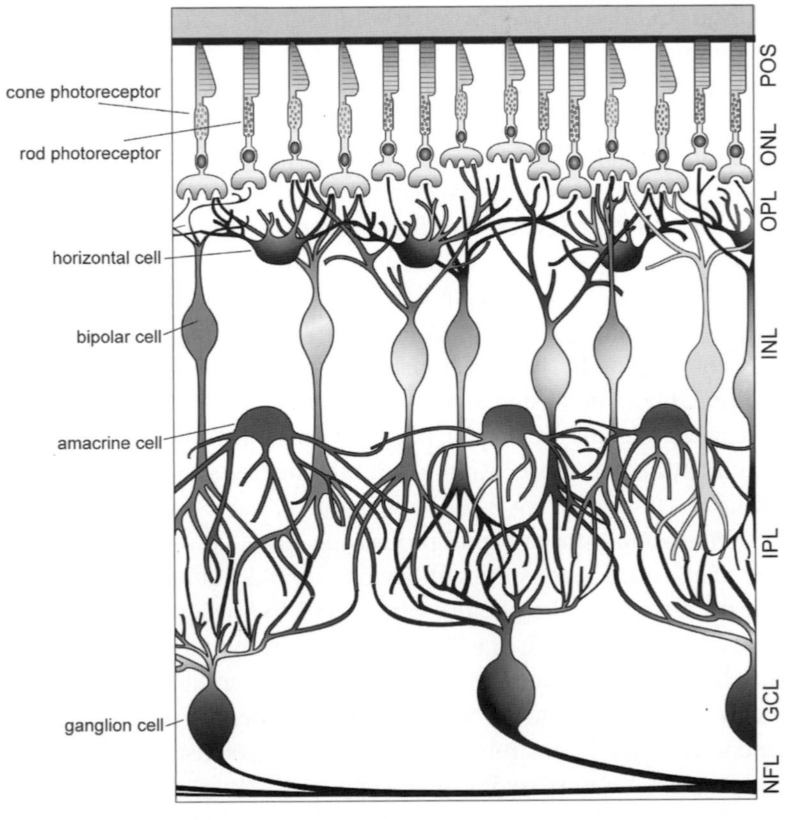

Fig. 1. Organization of retinal neurons. Neurons of the retina are organized into three distinct layers of cell bodies (nuclear layers), separated by two layers of densely packed synapses (plexiform layers). Light passes through the entire retina to the photoreceptors, which transduce visual signals into chemical signals that are transmitted vertically through bipolar cells to the ganglion cells. These signals are modulated by two stages of horizontal signal processing mediated by the horizontal and amacrine cells. *POS* photoreceptor outer segments; *ONL* outer nuclear layer; *OPL* outer plexiform layer; *INL* inner nuclear layer; *IPL* inner plexiform layer; *GCL* ganglion cell layer; *NFL* nerve fiber layer.

The photoreceptors absorb photons of light and begin a cascade of signal transduction. Rod photoreceptors are extremely sensitive to light, and maintain vision in low illumination (scotopic conditions), while cone photoreceptors mediate color vision in bright light (photopic conditions), and afford a high degree of visual acuity. The primate retina contains a fovea, which has a high concentration of cone photoreceptors to augment acuity. Signals are transmitted from photoreceptors by synaptic connections in the outer plexiform layer to bipolar cells and horizontal cells. Horizontal cells provide modulatory input to photoreceptor terminals, and also perform pan-retinal signal averaging through a network of inter-horizontal gap junctions to refine visual information. Bipolar cells, subtypes of which selectively connect with rod or cone photoreceptors, transmit signals from the photoreceptors to the ganglion cells, while amacrine cells refine both bipolar and ganglion cell output. Together, these vertical and lateral interactions allow the retina to function over a wide dynamic range.

Synaptic communication in the retina is mediated by a variety of neurotransmitters. Photoreceptors and bipolar cells release the excitatory neurotransmitter, glutamate, while horizontal and amacrine cells release the inhibitory neurotransmitter, gamma-aminobutyric acid (GABA). In addition, neurotransmitters, including dopamine, acetylcholine, and norepinephrine, are also involved in neurotransmission. Glutamate and GABA, however, are the predominant signaling molecules and contribute to synaptic communication among almost all retinal neurons. These substances act on neurons to generate an intraneuronal electrical potential that subsequently results in the release of chemical neurotransmitters from the receiving cell, enabling transduction of visual information through multiple types of retinal neurons. In the complex signal processing pathway of the retina, the outer plexiform layer (OPL) contains connections between photoreceptors, horizontal cells, and bipolar cells, while the inner plexiform layer (IPL) comprises connections between the bipolar, amacrine, and ganglion cells. Each plexiform layer achieves one step in the vertical transmission of visual signals through the retina, as well as additional horizontal signal modification mediated by horizontal and amacrine cells, which sharpen signals by emphasizing pertinent information, while minimizing interference and extraneous noise. Although a high degree of redundancy may preserve basic neurotransmission in many pathological states, each neuronal subtype fulfills a specific and fundamental role in signal processing that is critical to various aspects of normal vision. The functional aspects of various retinal neurons, such as the constitutively active dark current of the photoreceptors and the necessity for ganglion cells to maintain large, complex dendritic branches, impose a tremendous metabolic requirement that the limited retinal vasculature and retinal pigment epithelium must meet without interfering with the phototransduction by the photoreceptor outer segments. To meet this requirement, retinal neurons rely heavily on effective vascular and supporting glial cell function for waste removal and trophic support *(4–8)*.

THE GLIAL CELLS OF THE RETINA

The glial cells of the retina form three main populations: astrocytes, Müller cells, and microglia (Fig. 2). Astrocytes originate in the optic nerve and migrate into the maturing retina to form a monolayer apposed to the inner limiting membrane, where they interact with neurons and vascular cells *(7, 9)*, and contribute to the maintenance of the inner

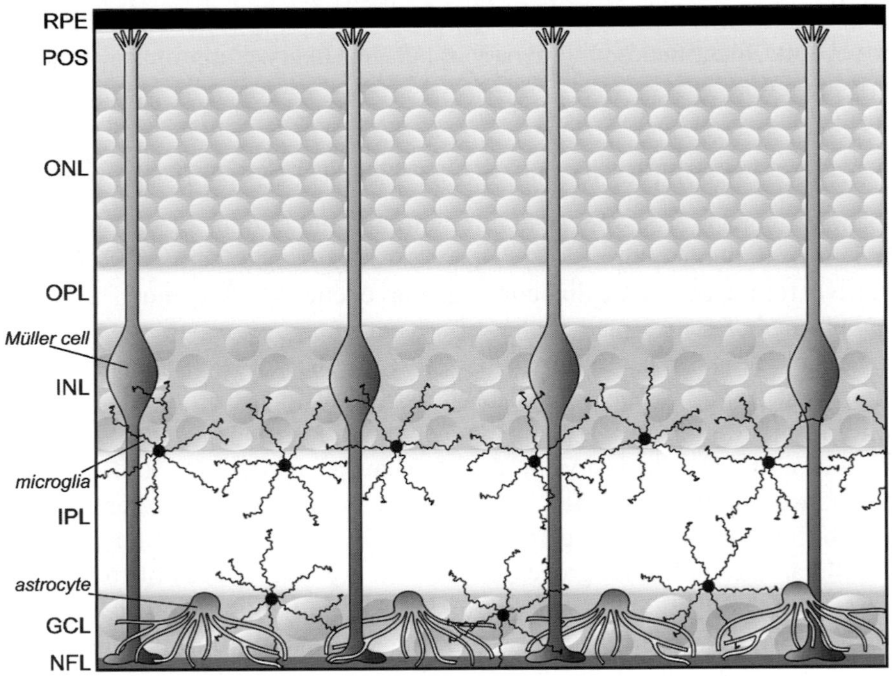

Fig. 2. Localization of retinal glia. Glial cells are differentially distributed throughout the neural retina. Müller cells are large radial glia that span the entire thickness of the retina, with endfeet contacting the inner limiting membrane and microvilli projecting through the outer limiting membrane to the subretinal space. Astrocytes are located primarily in the inner retina along the nerve fiber layer, where they appose the inner limiting membrane. Microglia reside in the inner retina, typically in the inner plexiform layer/ganglion cell layer and inner plexiform layer/inner nuclear layer interfaces.

part of the blood–retina barrier *(10)*. Müller cells are unique radial glia cells that closely interact with retinal neurons, providing nutritional support and regulating neuronal microenvironments by removing GABA and glutamate from synapses *(6)*. Microglia are monocyte-derived cells with immunological functions in the immuno-privileged CNS. As such, microglial activation is implicated in retinal immune responses that often contribute to neurodegeneration and inflammation. These cells produce inflammatory cytokines, but also provide neuroprotective substances that aid in the support of neuronal and vascular cells *(11)*. Together, these three types of glial cells support and influence neuronal and vascular function. Healthy functioning of glial and vascular cells is required to provide nutrients, waste disposal and trophic support to the neural retina, but it is the neurons and glia themselves that induce and maintain the vascular phenotype optimal for their own survival. Gross pathological abnormalities have been identified in retinal vasculature with diabetes, including pericyte ghosts, acellular capillaries, leukostasis, and tight junction breakdown, all of which have the potential to contribute to vascular leakage and nonperfusion *(12–14)*. These events may induce glial-cell changes, such as astrocyte and Müller-cell reactivity and microglial activation, which can further exacerbate vascular dysfunction through the release of cytokines and vascular endothelial growth factor (VEGF) *(15–24)*. These changes may alter retinal neurons in ways that are not yet fully identified and understood, but that likely compromise the functional output of the retina.

DIABETES REDUCES RETINAL FUNCTION

Diabetic retinopathy is associated with multifactorial deficits of vision *(25–28)* and impaired electroretinographic (ERG) responses *(29–34)*. Although the development of proliferative retinopathy and diabetic macular edema are the most severe vision-threatening characteristics of diabetic retinopathy *(35)*, even patients without clinically detectable retinal vasculopathy can experience subtle vision impairment *(36, 37)*. Psychophysical testing is one method of assessing distinct aspects of patients' visual function and monitoring vision changes over time, even when patients are not consciously aware of impaired vision. It also provides an opportunity to determine when diabetes-induced deficits of vision, which range from mild impairment to blindness *(38)*, first become apparent at a perceptive level. In diabetic retinopathy, many pathological cellular and molecular processes occur in the early stages of the disease, and may inflict subtle changes on retinal function before retinopathy is anatomically evident. Routine clinical evaluation of patients' sensory capacity has the potential to expose deficits of vision that individuals may be unaware of in daily life. Several clinical studies have described a loss of visual function in diabetic patients in the very early stages of diabetes, and often in the absence of classically recognized symptoms of diabetic retinopathy *(32, 39)*. These deficits include decreased hue discrimination and contrast sensitivity, delayed dark adaptation, abnormal visual fields, and decreased visual acuity *(28, 37, 40–42)*. Spatial resolution and/or contrast sensitivity are two of the most commonly studied aspects of vision consistently altered by diabetes. Early reports suggest a high frequency of declining contrast sensitivity that is more strongly correlated with disease duration that with lack of metabolic control *(26)*. A similar study detected significant visual dysfunction in 60% of patients with background retinopathy, but also in nearly 40% of patients with no detectable signs of vascular disease *(43)*. Defects in color perception have also been reported in patients with minimal or no retinopathy, and involve both blue–yellow and red–green discrimination *(26, 43)*. More recent research consistent with these findings has reported loss of color and contrast sensitivity in patients after a short duration of diabetes, and with no discernable signs of retinopathy, by fundus examination or fluorescein angiography, demonstrating a generalized loss of central vision and hue discrimination, as well as significant decreases in both static and dynamic spatial resolution *(25, 44)*. Together, these changes suggest a broad impairment of retinal neuronal function.

The electroretinogram (ERG) is used to assess the electrophysiological response of the retina to various visual stimuli, and potentially provides a physiological basis for the loss of function observed in psychophysical studies. The ERG wave represents the characteristic sequence of neuronal activation that forms this response, reflecting the duration and amplitude of functional output throughout the retina. The a-wave, an initial negative deflection of the ERG signal, represents photoreceptor hyperpolarization resulting from the cessation of the photocurrent that flows continuously in the absence of light. The second major component of the ERG is the positive b-wave, which is thought to originate from depolarization of rod–bipolar neurons and Müller glia. A series of small wavelets, termed oscillatory potentials (OPs), contribute to the ascending edge of the b-wave, and are attributed partially to amacrine cell activity. The OPs and the b-wave reflect the inner-retina function, and exhibit abnormalities in the form of decreased response amplitudes and delayed peak-times in patients with diabetes, even with good glycemic control and no detectable vascular lesions *(29, 33, 34, 37, 45, 46)*. These data suggest that diabetes affects multiple neuronal subtypes throughout the retina, including photoreceptors, bipolar cells, and amacrine cells, while more advanced ERG techniques reveal similar abnormalities in ganglion-cell responses. ERG deficits may contribute to loss of visual sensitivity in patients with diabetes, which ranges from mild to severe, and which includes reductions in overall acuity, dark adaptation, scotopic vision, contrast and contour sensitivity, and hue discrimination *(25, 27, 42–44, 47)*.

Ganglion-cell function can be measured more specifically with the multifocal pattern ERG, which uses a complex stimulus pattern rather than a flash of light *(30)*. In patients with diabetes but without overt vascular complications, ganglion-cell responses to medium- and large-grated stimuli have been reported to be reduced *(31)*, and delayed in the macular region *(30, 33)*. Less frequently, defects in photoreceptor response are reported in similar patient cohorts exhibiting impaired activation of the blue-cone system and increased a-wave latency *(45, 47, 48)* although other studies report no functional changes in the outer retina *(34, 37)*. These data provide a physiological basis for decreased performance in psychophysical testing, and implicate diabetes in the disruption of the functional output of the various neurons and synaptic connections that mediate normal vision. In addition, this sensitive technique often detects the abnormal responses of retinal neurons in the absence of vascular lesions. A number of researchers suggest that ganglion-cell electrophysiology shows promise as a supplemental diagnostic tool usable in patients with subclinical diabetic retinopathy, correlating the underlying electrophysiological impairment with loss of vision *(49–51)*, and currently the predictive capacity of the multifocal ERG is being investigated as a potential early diagnostic tool *(52)*.

The application of ERG studies to experimental rodent models of diabetes has yielded data similar to those obtained from clinical studies, demonstrating retinal dysfunction in the first few weeks of diabetes. In these animals, OP amplitudes are consistently depressed and delayed throughout the first 12 weeks of diabetes *(53–55)*, with abnormalities detected after only 2 days of hyperglycemia in one recent study *(56)*. Additional work has demonstrated reductions in b-wave amplitude after 2–4 weeks of diabetes *(57, 58)*. Interestingly, several studies report electrophysiological changes in the a-wave of diabetic rodents *(53, 56, 57)*, while photoreceptor response is more variable in patients with diabetes. A degree of variability exists in rodents particularly due to differences in retinal pigmentation, sex, and strain. Despite discrepancies in reported amplitude and latency measures, however, these studies are in general agreement that diabetes compromises the functional integrity of the neural retina, resulting in both inner- and outer-retinal dysfunction. The pairing of psychophysical and ERG data suggests a broad dysfunction of retinal neurons, involving both rod and cone photoreceptors, bipolar cells, amacrine cells, and ganglion cells. ERG abnormalities in rodents, as in humans, develop in the early stages of diabetes when the retina appears anatomically normal *(54, 57)*. Rodent models of diabetes provide clinically relevant ERG data with the added benefit of enabling investigation into potential mechanisms contributing to retinal dysfunction.

DIABETES INDUCES NEURODEGENERATION IN THE RETINA

It has long been suggested that diabetic retinopathy involves a neurodegenerative component *(59)*. In the 1960s, both Wolter and Bloodworth identified degenerating or "pyknotic" neurons in postmortem retinas from human donors with diabetes *(60, 61)*. Since then, several studies have investigated the effects of diabetes on retinal neurons, with the recognition that at some level, these elements must contribute to visual impairment in diabetic retinopathy, and may explain the electrophysiological abnormalities in humans and rodents with diabetes. Perhaps the most basic observation has been that elements of the retina, distinct from the vasculature, undergo apoptosis in experimental diabetes. An early study demonstrated retinal-cell apoptosis in rats after a short period of diabetes *(62, 63)*. Work elaborating on this finding established that diabetes significantly increased retinal apoptosis, detected by TUNEL, resulting in a significant reduction in cell counts in STZ-diabetic rats *(64)*. Since then, this finding has been confirmed in multiple rodent models of diabetes including the streptozotocin (STZ) rat, the STZ mouse, and the spontaneously diabetic $Ins2^{Akita}$ mouse *(17, 65, 66)*. Additional studies have demonstrated degeneration and cell loss in multiple types of retinal neurons in both the inner and outer nuclear layers, including photoreceptors *(57, 67)*, dopaminergic and cholinergic amacrine cells *(65)*, and bipolar cells *(19, 68–70)*. Consistent with the theory that diabetes induces neuroretinal apoptosis, proapoptotic molecules, including activated caspase-3 have been detected in retinas from humans and rodents with diabetes *(17, 21, 65, 66, 71, 72)*.

In addition to cell loss, morphometric analysis has identified significant thinning of the retina after varying durations of diabetes. The thickness of the inner and outer nuclear layers is reduced after 10 weeks of diabetes in mice and 24 weeks of diabetes in rats *(64, 66, 67)*, suggesting a chronic depletion of neurons. Further, diabetes is associated with decreased nerve- fiber diameter and degeneration of the nerve fiber layer, which is likely due to a loss of ganglion cells or ganglion cell axons *(73–75)*. Diabetes is associated with atrophy of retinal axons in humans *(76, 77)*, and the processes of retinal neurons, including nerve terminals, ganglion cell dendrites, centrifugal axons, and horizontal cell axons appear dystrophic in diabetic rodents *(57, 67, 78, 79)*. One of the most consistent findings in retinas of diabetic rodents is a decreased thickness of the IPL, which contain synaptic connections between bipolar, amacrine, and ganglion cells. In a seminal publication, Barber et al. (1998) reported a 22% reduction in thickness of the IPL after 7.5 months in STZ-diabetes in rats *(64)*. Subsequent work elaborating this finding reported a 9.9% decrease in the thickness of the IPL after 1 month of diabetes in STZ-diabetic Sprague-Dawley rats, and a 15% decrease after 1 month of STZ-diabetes in Brown-Norway rats *(57)*. More recently, a third study reported a 10% decrease in inner plexiform thickness of STZ-diabetic Sprague-Dawley rats after 6 months of diabetes *(67)*. Although one study using STZ-diabetic mice did not observe inner plexiform thinning in the first 8 weeks of diabetes *(66)*, characterization of the spontaneously diabetic $Ins2^{Akita}$ mouse revealed that after 22 weeks of hyperglycemia, the IPL was reduced by 16.7 and 27% in the central and peripheral retina, respectively *(17)*. Although the timing and severity of decreased thickness of the IPL varied in these reports, overall the data clearly demonstrate that diabetes induces a generalized neurodegeneration of the retina. While the changes summarized here are well-characterized, work to determine the molecular mechanisms leading to neuronal dysfunction and apoptosis is far from complete.

Reports of anomalous biochemical composition of retinal neurons indicate that the pathological processes which impact retinal function begin early in diabetes. One study suggested that diabetes upregulates whole-retina neuronal nitric oxide synthase (NOS), which was accompanied by an increase in the number of NOS-containing bipolar cells *(69)*. In contrast, a study using a shorter duration of diabetes reported an early depletion of NOS-positive neurons that was sustained through later time points *(80)*. Consistent with this finding, a recent study found a decrease in NOS-immunoreactive amacrine cells and a redistribution of nitric oxide precursors after a short period of diabetes *(81)*. Tyrosine hydroxylase protein content is also reduced in dopaminergic amacrine cells concomitant with an overall decrease in brain-derived neurotrophic factor *(82)*. Glutamate receptors and calcium-binding proteins are upregulated in the inner and OPL, as well as in ganglion, bipolar, and amacrine cells of one-month STZ-diabetic rats *(83)*. Additional work also indicates that diabetes alters the retinal expression of neuronal transcription factors, ion channels, and GABA receptors *(84)*. These studies reveal that several aspects of neuronal biochemistry are altered by diabetes.

Despite the potential that synaptic degeneration and impaired neurotransmission are likely contributing components of diabetes-induced retinal dysfunction and visual impairment, little is known concerning the effects of diabetes on retinal synapses. Several reports and comprehensive reviews, however, propose impaired synaptic transmission as a potential mechanism underlying functional deficits evidenced by abnormal ERG responses *(83)*. Alterations in visual function precede the emergence of clinical diabetic retinopathy in humans, and significant depletion of retinal neurons and the development of vascular lesions, which often do not appear until 3–6 months in rodent models of diabetes *(16)*. This implies that subcellular changes in retinal neurons may play a role in early retinal dysfunction in a manner similar to the pathological changes in cells of the vasculature that are apparent soon after the onset of diabetes *(15, 18, 22, 68, 85, 86)*.

DIABETES ALTERS THE FUNCTION OF GLIAL CELLS IN THE RETINA

Pathological changes in retinal glial cells occur with diabetes and likely impair their functions in neuronal and vascular support, which include providing nutritional support to neurons, processing glutamate and other neurotransmitters released from the synaptic cleft, and maintaining the blood–retina barrier. Diabetes disrupts retinal glutamate metabolism, a process particular to Müller cells in the mammalian retina. Early work demonstrated a 45% reduction in the conversion of glutamate to glutamine in rat retina after 3 months of STZ diabetes, which was accompanied by a 1.6-fold increase in total retinal glutamate *(87)*. Glutamate also increases in the vitreous of patients with proliferative diabetic retinopathy *(88)*. While the de novo synthesis of amino acids is unchanged, glutamate oxidation is significantly reduced in rat retina by diabetes.

Further, the activity and content of the enzyme that converts glutamate to glutamine, glutamine synthetase, are significantly decreased in retinas from diabetic rats *(89)*. These data indicate an early failure of the Müller-cell glutamate metabolism, in which both the transamination of glutamate to alpha ketoglutarate and the amination of glutamate to glutamine are significantly impaired after a short period of experimental diabetes. Similar findings have been obtained from studies of cultured Müller cells isolated from retinas of control and diabetic rats. In these cells, the activity of the electrogenic glutamate transporter was dysfunctional after 4 weeks of diabetes, and was reduced by 67% after 13 weeks *(90)*. More recently, it was demonstrated that a short period of diabetes increases immunoreactivity to D-aspartate, a nonmetabolisable substrate for the GLAST glutamate/aspartate transporter,in retinal Müller cells, and that these cells undergo gliosis in the early stages of diabetes *(91)*.

In the healthy retina, glial fibrillary acidic protein (GFAP) is largely restricted to astrocytes, where it provides structural integrity and stability to the cytoskeleton of glial filaments *(92)*. In diabetes, GFAP expression is reduced in astrocytes but is significantly induced, in Muller cells indicative of gliosis. Early studies demonstrated this phenomenon using rodent models of diabetes, including the streptozotocin (STZ)-induced diabetic rat and the spontaneously diabetic BB/Wor rat, and demonstrated a fivefold increase in Müller-cell GFAP expression, concomitant with a decrease in astrocyte GFAP expression, that occurred progressively from 1 to 4 months of hyperglycemia *(15, 87)*. Additional work has confirmed this finding, demonstrating upregulated Muller cell GFAP content after short periods of diabetes ranging from 6 to 12 weeks *(18, 62, 79, 93, 94)*, as well as after chronic hyperglycemia in rodents *(19)*, in conjunction with decreased astrocytic GFAP. This finding has been confirmed in human retinal tissue from patients with approximately 10 years of diabetes, which demonstrates increased GFAP expression in Müller cells distributed throughout the entire retina, as well as whole-retina increases in GFAP content *(95)*. The GFAP expression by Müller glia has been similarly reported to increase with disruption of the retinal pigment epithelium and the blood–retina–barrier, as well as in response to neuronal loss *(96)*. Although the specific function of GFAP in retinal Müller cells remains to be fully identified, this protein is implicated in the stability of Müller-cell processes and the inner limiting membrane *(97)*. The drastic redistribution of GFAP in retina after short durations of diabetes likely indicates the progression of retinal gliosis in response to the disease *(98)*.

Increased production of VEGF by retinal glia is another consequence of diabetes *(99)*. The VEGF induction is not only implicated in the aberrant growth and increased permeability of retinal blood vessels that contribute to the classic vascular symptoms of diabetic retinopathy *(100)*, but also functions as a trophic factor for multiple types of retinal cells *(101, 102)*. The VEGF mRNA and protein are expressed by neurons and Müller glia in mammalian and human retina *(103)*, which has been attributed to the role of these cells in influencing maintenance of the blood–retina barrier. Growing evidence supports the role of retinal neurons and glia in increased VEGF production in both humans and rodents with diabetes *(99, 104, 105)*. In retinas from human donors with proliferative and nonproliferative diabetic retinopathy that exhibit increased Müller-cell GFAP expression, VEGF and its inducible angiogenic cofactor and inducible NOS have been reported to increase in Müller glia *(106, 107)*. Studies of diabetic-rat retina have demonstrated similar effects, with increased VEGF protein and mRNA occurring predominantly in the Müller cells *(108)*. Due to the close interaction of Müller cells with neuronal and vascular cells in the retina, these pathological abnormalities likely contribute to diabetes-induced retinal dysfunction.

Retinal microglial are also impacted by diabetes, although further study is required to clarify the causes and effects of microglial activation in diabetic retinopathy. Microglia become hypertrophic in rat retina after 1 month of diabetes, and the number of reactive microglia is significantly increased in the OPL after 4 months, while increases in the outer nuclear and photoreceptor layers occur after 14 months *(19)*. Diabetes upregulates inflammatory cytokines, such as TNF alpha, which activate microglia and induce the production of cytotoxins that may lead to retinal cell death. The activation of microglia after 4 weeks of diabetes, prior to neuronal death, was recently reported to occur in discrete regions of the rodent retina, and likely indicates localized inflammatory responses to diabetic insults on retinal cell populations *(21)*.

NEUROINFLAMMATION IN DIABETIC RETINOPATHY

The pathological alterations in retinal neurons and glial cells in diabetes generally remain below the threshold of detection by ophthalmoscopy. Ophthalmologists have therefore focused on the details of the vascular lesions such as number of microaneurysms, area of macular thickening, quadrants of venous beading or hemorrhages, or degree of neovascularization, to classify and stage diabetic retinopathy. A broader perspective of fundus changes that include increased retinal blood flow and permeability, tissue edema, gliosis, macrophage infiltration and leukostasis, tissue damage (including neuronal apoptosis), and attempts at repair (such as neovascularization) are pathophysiological features that can be considered components of chronic retinal inflammation.

The nature of this chronic activation of the defense mechanisms within the retina, as well as the systemic immune-cell response to inflammatory markers on the vasculature, are still under intense investigation, but clearly includes the release of numerous peptide growth factors *(109)*, activation of the complement pathway *(110)*, increased expression of Fas ligand *(111)*, activation of microglial cells *(19)*, and macrophage infiltration *(112)*. Adaptive inflammation is a normal, highly conserved physiologic response to any type of tissue injury including viral infection, traumas or tumors, and constitutes an attempt to heal the injury and maintain tissue viability. For example, increased expression of interleukins, VEGF or recruitment of macrophages may be designed to remove damaged cells and help maintain the viability of their surviving neighbors. This inflammatory response is turned off when the initial insult subsides. However, when the injury persists, the response continues unabated, and the deleterious effects of proinflammatory cytokine- and immune-cell activation may outweigh the benefits. Consideration of the dual roles of the retinal immune response in diabetes is important because, though the targeted inhibition of proinflammatory molecules may provide beneficial effects in the short term, chronic administration may impair the integrity of existing vascular or neuronal cells required for normal retinal function.

HISTORICAL PERSPECTIVE ON DIABETIC RETINOPATHY

The first description of diabetic retinopathy by von Graefe in 1856 *(113)* discussed the presence of yellow liquid exudates and red hemorrhages in the retina of a patient with diabetes. Over the ensuing 150 years, clinicians have focused on the visually detectable appearance of pigmented red lesions in the retina as the primary feature of diabetic retinopathy. This approach is analogous to the finding of pigment clumping as the primary feature of retinitis pigmentosa, whereas modern molecular and genetic studies have confirmed that primary defects reside in the photoreceptors, and pigmentary migration is a secondary hyperplastic response to photoreceptor cell death. There is a long history of anatomical and electrophysiological evidence for alterations in the neurosensory retina as a prominent consequence of diabetes. In 1961 and 1962, Wolter *(60)* and Bloodworth *(61)* emphasized the loss of retinal neurons in areas remote from vascular changes as a prominent feature in histopathological studies of postmortem human eyes. Their studies were followed by Simonsen's discovery in 1969 *(114)* that patients with diabetic retinopathy had impaired ERG responses. Simonsen's observations were extended by Bresnick, who found that the b-wave amplitudes, implicit times, and OPs were reduced in patients with diabetic retinopathy. In fact, the ERG changes proved to be better predictors of progression from severe nonproliferative to high-risk proliferative retinopathy than the vascular changes revealed by fundus photographs *(115, 116)*. In 1986, Bresnick *(59)* proposed that diabetic retinopathy be viewed as a neurosensory disorder. His proposal was supported by numerous reports of impaired contrast sensitivity *(42, 117)*, dark adaptation *(40, 118)* and color vision *(119, 120)* in patients with varying degrees of retinopathy. In 1997, Ghirlanda *(121)* proposed that the initial impact of diabetes on the retina involves the neurosensory retina, and that microvascular abnormalities maybe a secondary development.

During the late 1990s, several reports showing specific cellular defects in the neurosensory retina in human eyes and animal models of diabetes began to provide a mechanistic basis for the functional alterations that had been long observed. These studies included evidence of Müller- cell activation in human eyes *(95)*, abnormal glutamate metabolism *(87, 89)*, microglial cell activation *(18, 19)* and neuronal apoptosis *(63, 64, 66)*. Taken together, these data conclusively demonstrated that diabetes exerts a major impact on the neuroglial parenchyma of the retina. Thus, the term "microvascular disease" fails to adequately describe diabetic retinopathy. We propose that it should be replaced by a more comprehensive understanding of diabetic retinopathy as functional and structural alterations in the retina due to diabetes.

The question arises as to why nearly half a century transpired before the neurovascular concept of diabetic retinopathy began to gain acceptance. Clinical fluorescein angiography was introduced in 1960 *(122)*, and the classic studies of vascular lesions in trypsin-digested retinas were published in 1961 *(123)*. These studies emphasized the same features in the retina observed clinically; that is, microaneurysms, hemorrhages, nonperfused capillaries and neovascularization. During the 1970s and early 1980s, efforts were appropriately applied to treat vision-threatening stages of diabetic retinopathy such as macular edema and proliferative retinopathy. The positive outcomes of the Diabetic Retinopathy Study and Early Treatment Diabetic Retinopathy Study provided promise that lasers and vitrectomy would contain the problem of diabetic retinopathy. In spite of its effectiveness in preventing legal blindness, however, patients and ophthalmologists realized that laser photocoagulation reduced the risk of vision loss only by about 50%, and successfully treated patients often had unsatisfactory vision for seeing fine details and colors, or driving at night. Moreover, numerous clinical trials of potential pharmacotherapeutic compounds have failed to arrest the development or progression of vision loss in patients, so there may now be more willingness to consider broader alternative approaches to the treatment of diabetic retinopathy. As of late 2007, no drug which targets retinal blood vessels has been approved for clinical use by the Food and Drug Administration. VEGF inhibitors are under investigation for diabetic macular edema and proliferative diabetic retinopathy *(23, 124)*, and while the results of early-stage studies are promising, the long-term effects of blocking VEGF are uncertain. In addition to its role in vascular permeability and neovascularization, VEGF signaling also provides trophic support for neurons *(125–127)* as well as vascular cells, so prolonged interruption of VEGF action may not only reduce macular edema and vascularization but also compromise the viability of the retinal cells required for vision.

Recent research using rodent models of diabetes has identified a number of compounds with potential antiinflammatory and neuroprotective properties. Growth factors, including nerve growth factor (NGF), insulin-like growth factor (IGF-1) and brain derived neurotrophic factor (BDNF), have been demonstrated to prevent diabetes-related neuroretinal cell death in STZ rats *(62, 70, 82)*. In 2005, Krady et al. demonstrated the efficacy of minocycline, a semisynthetic tetracycline, as an inhibitor of retinal inflammation, microglial activation and caspase-3 activation in STZ-diabetic rats *(21)*. The prostaglandin F2alpha analogue, latanoprost, is another neuroprotective agent reported to decrease both the number of activated caspase-3-immunoreactive cells, and the number of TUNEL-positive cells in STZ rat retina, indicating its effectiveness in the suppression of diabetes-induced apoptosis *(128)*. Cannabidiol, a nonpsychotropic cannabinoid, also possesses neuroprotective and antiinflammatory properties, and is capable of reducing oxidative stress, inflammation, and neurotoxicity in STZ-diabetic rat retina *(68)*. These encouraging findings suggest that retinal neurodegeneration and inflammation, two potentially vision-threatening complications of diabetes, can be diminished in rodent models of diabetes. Further work is required, however, to investigate existing and novel compounds in preclinical testing before clinical trials on targeted pharmacotherapies can be initiated.

NEUROGLIAL DYSFUNCTION IN DIABETIC RETINOPATHY.

The spectrum, interrelationships, and significance of changes in retinal neuroglial cells in diabetes remain incompletely defined at this point. It is clear, however, that the impact of diabetes on the retina includes impaired outer-retina function (delayed dark adaptation) and inner-retina dysfunction (impaired visual fields, impaired contrast sensitivity, and color vision). Likewise, histopathologic studies reveal evidence of retinal pigment epithelial degeneration, as well as atrophy of the ganglion cell layer, and inner nuclear and plexiform layers. The death of retinal neurons appears to be by apoptosis associated with caspase activation. In keeping with the recognition that neurons and glial cells have a linked function, LaNoue et al. *(89)* observed that retinal conversion of glutamate to glutamine is impaired by diabetes. Thus, glutamate may accumulate in the interstitial fluid, leading to neuronal glutamate excitotoxicity and dysregulation of normal synaptic transmission.

The relationship between neurons and glial cells in the CNS is intimately symbiotic. One class of cells cannot function correctly without the other. The metabolic support provided by Müller cells and astrocytes in the retina is undoubtedly critical to the functional neural output of the retina, and contributes to maintenance of the vasculature.

Dysfunction in one or more of these elements, therefore, will almost certainly result in altered visual function. Future studies of vision loss in diabetes must consider how neurons and glial cells interact with each other and with elements of the vasculature under both normal and diabetic conditions, in order to create a more comprehensive understanding of retinal function and vision loss in diabetes.

REFERENCES

1. Duke-Elder S. The emergence of vision in the animal world. Annals of the Royal College of Surgeons of England 1958;23(1):1–24.
2. Kolb H. How the retina works. Am Sci 2003;91:28–36.
3. Schiller PH, Sandell JH, Maunsell JH. Functions of the ON and OFF channels of the visual system. Nature 1986;322(6082):824–5.
4. Haydon PG, Carmignoto G. Astrocyte control of synaptic transmission and neurovascular coupling. Physiol Rev 2006;86(3):1009–31.
5. Dubois-Dauphin M, Poitry-Yamate C, de Bilbao F, Julliard AK, Jourdan F, Donati G. Early postnatal Muller cell death leads to retinal but not optic nerve degeneration in NSE-Hu-Bcl-2 transgenic mice. Neuroscience 2000;95(1):9–21.
6. Newman E, Reichenbach A. The Muller cell: a functional element of the retina. Trends Neurosci 1996;19(8):307–12.
7. Newman EA. Glial modulation of synaptic transmission in the retina. Glia 2004;47(3):268–74.
8. Antonetti DA, Barber AJ, Bronson SK, et al. Diabetic retinopathy: seeing beyond glucose-induced microvascular disease. Diabetes 2006;55(9):2401–11.
9. Schnitzer J. Retinal astrocytes: their restriction to vascularized parts of the mammalian retina. Neurosci Lett 1987;78(1):29–34.
10. Gardner TW, Lieth E, Khin SA, et al. Astrocytes increase barrier properties and ZO-1 expression in retinal vascular endothelial cells. Invest Ophthalmol Vis Sci 1997;38(11):2423–7.
11. Xu H, Chen M, Mayer EJ, Forrester JV, Dick AD. Turnover of resident retinal microglia in the normal adult mouse. Glia 2007;55(11):1189–98.
12. Arevalo JF, Fromow-Guerra J, Quiroz-Mercado H, et al. Primary intravitreal bevacizumab (Avastin) for diabetic macular edema: results from the Pan-American Collaborative Retina Study Group at 6-month follow-up. Ophthalmology 2007;114(4):743–50.
13. Lobo CL, Bernardes RC, Figueira JP, de Abreu JR, Cunha-Vaz JG. Three-year follow-up study of blood-retinal barrier and retinal thickness alterations in patients with type 2 diabetes mellitus and mild nonproliferative diabetic retinopathy. Arch Ophthalmol 2004;122(2):211–7.
14. Kern TS, Engerman RL. A mouse model of diabetic retinopathy. Arch Ophthalmol 1996;114(8):986–90.
15. Barber AJ, Antonetti DA, Gardner TW. Altered expression of retinal occludin and glial fibrillary acidic protein in experimental diabetes. The Penn State Retina Research Group. Invest Ophthalmol Vis Sci 2000;41(11):3561–8.
16. Feit-Leichman RA, Kinouchi R, Takeda M, et al. Vascular damage in a mouse model of diabetic retinopathy: relation to neuronal and glial changes. Invest Ophthalmol Vis Sci 2005;46(11):4281–7.
17. Barber AJ, Antonetti DA, Kern TS, et al. The Ins2Akita mouse as a model of early retinal complications in diabetes. Invest Ophthalmol Vis Sci 2005;46(6):2210–8.
18. Rungger-Brandle E, Dosso AA, Leuenberger PM. Glial reactivity, an early feature of diabetic retinopathy. Invest Ophthalmol Vis Sci 2000;41(7):1971–80.
19. Zeng XX, Ng YK, Ling EA. Neuronal and microglial response in the retina of streptozotocin-induced diabetic rats. Vis Neurosci 2000;17(3):463–71.
20. Bek T. Immunohistochemical characterization of retinal glial cell changes in areas of vascular occlusion secondary to diabetic retinopathy. Acta Ophthalmol Scand 1997;75(4):388–92.
21. Krady JK, Basu A, Allen CM, et al. Minocycline reduces proinflammatory cytokine expression, microglial activation, and caspase-3 activation in a rodent model of diabetic retinopathy. Diabetes 2005;54(5):1559–65.

ISBN	Qty	Sales Order
9781934115831	1	F 9917825 1

Customer P/O No	Cust P/O List
72103344	75.50 GBP

Title: Diabetic retinopathy. edited by Elia Duh

Format: C (Cloth/HB)
Author: Duh, Elia
Publisher: Humana ; Springer [distributor]
Fund:
Location:
Loan Type:
Coutts CN: 8364536

Order Specific Instructions

Ship To: UK 73623001 F
DERBY HOSPITALS NHS FOUND
DERBY CITY GENERAL HOSPIT
UTTOXETER ROAD
DERBY
DERBYSHIRE
DE22 3NE

Volume:
Edition:
Year: 2008
Pagination: 480 p.
Size: 26 cm

P00L39A8C
DERBY HOSPITALS NHS FOUNDATION TRUS

Routing
Sorting
Y02K03Y
Covering – BXXXX
Despatch

298289784 UKRWLG40 RC2

COUTTS INFORMATION SERVICES LTD.:

22. Antonetti DA, Barber AJ, Khin S, Lieth E, Tarbell JM, Gardner TW. Vascular permeability in experimental diabetes is associated with reduced endothelial occludin content: vascular endothelial growth factor decreases occludin in retinal endothelial cells. Penn State Retina Research Group. Diabetes 1998;47(12):1953–9.
23. Ng EW, Shima DT, Calias P, Cunningham ET, Jr., Guyer DR, Adamis AP. Pegaptanib, a targeted anti-VEGF aptamer for ocular vascular disease. Nat Rev Drug Discov 2006;5(2):123–32.
24. Amrite AC, Ayalasomayajula SP, Cheruvu NP, Kompella UB. Single periocular injection of celecoxib-PLGA microparticles inhibits diabetes-induced elevations in retinal PGE2, VEGF, and vascular leakage. Invest Ophthalmol Vis Sci 2006;47(3):1149–60.
25. Di Leo MA, Caputo S, Falsini B, et al. Nonselective loss of contrast sensitivity in visual system testing in early type I diabetes. Diabetes Care 1992;15(5):620–5.
26. Hardy KJ, Lipton J, Scase MO, Foster DH, Scarpello JH. Detection of colour vision abnormalities in uncomplicated type 1 diabetic patients with angiographically normal retinas. Br J Ophthalmol 1992;76(8):461–4.
27. Holm K, Larsson J, Lovestam-Adrian M. In diabetic retinopathy, foveal thickness of 300 mum seems to correlate with functionally significant loss of vision. Doc Ophthalmol 2007;114(3):117–24.
28. Hyvarinen L, Laurinen P, Rovamo J. Contrast sensitivity in evaluation of visual impairment due to diabetes. Acta Ophthalmol (Copenh) 1983;61(1):94–101.
29. Bearse MA, Jr., Han Y, Schneck ME, Barez S, Jacobsen C, Adams AJ. Local multifocal oscillatory potential abnormalities in diabetes and early diabetic retinopathy. Invest Ophthalmol Vis Sci 2004;45(9):3259–65.
30. Caputo S, Di Leo MA, Falsini B, et al. Evidence for early impairment of macular function with pattern ERG in type I diabetic patients. Diabetes Care 1990;13(4):412–8.
31. Di Leo MA, Falsini B, Caputo S, Ghirlanda G, Porciatti V, Greco AV. Spatial frequency-selective losses with pattern electroretinogram in type 1 (insulin-dependent) diabetic patients without retinopathy. Diabetologia 1990;33(12):726–30.
32. Fortune B, Schneck ME, Adams AJ. Multifocal electroretinogram delays reveal local retinal dysfunction in early diabetic retinopathy. Invest Ophthalmol Vis Sci 1999;40(11):2638–51.
33. Palmowski AM, Sutter EE, Bearse MA, Jr., Fung W. Mapping of retinal function in diabetic retinopathy using the multifocal electroretinogram. Invest Ophthalmol Vis Sci 1997;38(12):2586–96.
34. Ghirlanda G, Di Leo MA, Caputo S, et al. Detection of inner retina dysfunction by steady-state focal electroretinogram pattern and flicker in early IDDM. Diabetes 1991;40(9):1122–7.
35. Davis MD, Fisher MR, Gangnon RE, et al. Risk factors for high-risk proliferative diabetic retinopathy and severe visual loss: Early Treatment Diabetic Retinopathy Study Report #18. Invest Ophthalmol Vis Sci 1998;39(2):233–52.
36. Han Y, Adams AJ, Bearse MA, Jr., Schneck ME. Multifocal electroretinogram and short-wavelength automated perimetry measures in diabetic eyes with little or no retinopathy. Arch Ophthalmol 2004;122(12):1809–15.
37. Di Leo MA, Caputo S, Falsini B, Porciatti V, Greco AV, Ghirlanda G. Presence and further development of retinal dysfunction after 3-year follow up in IDDM patients without angiographically documented vasculopathy. Diabetologia 1994;37(9):911–6.
38. Sinclair SH. Diabetic retinopathy: the unmet needs for screening and a review of potential solutions. Expert review of medical devices 2006;3(3):301–13.
39. Ewing FM, Deary IJ, Strachan MW, Frier BM. Seeing beyond retinopathy in diabetes: electrophysiological and psychophysical abnormalities and alterations in vision. Endocrine reviews 1998;19(4):462–76.
40. Frost-Larsen K, Larsen HW, Simonsen SE. Value of electroretinography and dark adaptation as prognostic tools in diabetic retinopathy. Dev ophthalmol 1981;2:222–34.
41. Spaide RF, Fisher YL. Intravitreal bevacizumab (Avastin) treatment of proliferative diabetic retinopathy complicated by vitreous hemorrhage. Retina 2006;26(3):275–8.
42. Sokol S, Moskowitz A, Skarf B, Evans R, Molitch M, Senior B. Contrast sensitivity in diabetics with and without background retinopathy. Arch Ophthalmol 1985;103(1):51–4.
43. Trick GL, Burde RM, Gordon MO, Santiago JV, Kilo C. The relationship between hue discrimination and contrast sensitivity deficits in patients with diabetes mellitus. Ophthalmology 1988;95(5):693–8.
44. Dosso AA, Bonvin ER, Morel Y, Golay A, Assal JP, Leuenberger PM. Risk factors associated with contrast sensitivity loss in diabetic patients. Graefes Arch Clin Exp Ophthalmol 1996;234(5):300–5.

Derby Hospitals NHS Foundation Trust
Library and Knowledge Service

45. Liu W, Deng Y. The analysis of electroretinography of diabetes mellitus. Yan Ke Xue Bao 2001;17(3): 173–5, 9.
46. Tzekov R, Arden GB. The electroretinogram in diabetic retinopathy. Survey of ophthalmology 1999;44(1):53–60.
47. Holopigian K, Greenstein VC, Seiple W, Hood DC, Carr RE. Evidence for photoreceptor changes in patients with diabetic retinopathy. Invest Ophthalmol Vis Sci 1997;38(11):2355–65.
48. Mortlock KE, Chiti Z, Drasdo N, Owens DR, North RV. Silent substitution S-cone electroretinogram in subjects with diabetes mellitus. Ophthalmic Physiol Opt 2005;25(5):392–9.
49. Simonsen SE. The value of the oscillatory potential in selecting juvenile diabetics at risk of developing proliferative retinopathy. Acta Ophthalmol (Copenh) 1980;58(6):865–78.
50. Han Y, Schneck ME, Bearse MA, Jr., et al. Formulation and evaluation of a predictive model to identify the sites of future diabetic retinopathy. Invest Ophthalmol Vis Sci 2004;45(11):4106–12.
51. Han Y, Bearse MA, Jr., Schneck ME, Barez S, Jacobsen CH, Adams AJ. Multifocal electro retinogram delays predict sites of subsequent diabetic retinopathy. Invest Ophthalmol Vis Sci 2004;45(3):948–54.
52. Bearse MA, Jr., Adams AJ, Han Y, et al. A multifocal electroretinogram model predicting the development of diabetic retinopathy. Progress in retinal and eye research 2006;25(5):425–48.
53. Hancock HA, Kraft TW. Oscillatory potential analysis and ERGs of normal and diabetic rats. Invest Ophthalmol Vis Sci 2004;45(3):1002–8.
54. Sakai H, Tani Y, Shirasawa E, Shirao Y, Kawasaki K. Development of electroretinographic alterations in streptozotocin-induced diabetes in rats. Ophthalmic Res 1995;27(1):57–63.
55. Yonemura D, Aoki T, Tsuzuki K. Electroretinogram in diabetic retinopathy. Arch Ophthalmol 1962;68:19–24.
56. Phipps JA, Fletcher EL, Vingrys AJ. Paired-flash identification of rod and cone dysfunction in the diabetic rat. Invest Ophthalmol Vis Sci 2004;45(12):4592–600.
57. Aizu Y, Oyanagi K, Hu J, Nakagawa H. Degeneration of retinal neuronal processes and pigment epithelium in the early stage of the streptozotocin-diabetic rats. Neuropathology 2002;22(3):161–70.
58. Li Q, Zemel E, Miller B, Perlman I. Early retinal damage in experimental diabetes: electroretinographical and morphological observations. Exp Eye Res 2002;74(5):615–25.
59. Bresnick GH. Diabetic retinopathy viewed as a neurosensory disorder. Arch Ophthalmol 1986;104(7): 989–90.
60. Wolter JR. Diabetic retinopathy. Am J Ophthalmol 1961;51:1123–41.
61. Bloodworth JM, Jr. Diabetic retinopathy. Diabetes 1962;11:1–22.
62. Hammes HP, Federoff HJ, Brownlee M. Nerve growth factor prevents both neuroretinal programmed cell death and capillary pathology in experimental diabetes. Mol Med 1995;1(5):527–34.
63. Kerrigan LA, Zack DJ, Quigley HA, Smith SD, Pease ME. TUNEL-positive ganglion cells in human primary open-angle glaucoma. Arch Ophthalmol 1997;115(8):1031–5.
64. Barber AJ, Lieth E, Khin SA, Antonetti DA, Buchanan AG, Gardner TW. Neural apoptosis in the retina during experimental and human diabetes. Early onset and effect of insulin. J Clin Invest 1998;102(4):783–91.
65. Gastinger MJ, Singh RS, Barber AJ. Loss of cholinergic and dopaminergic amacrine cells in streptozotocin-diabetic rat and Ins2Akita-diabetic mouse retinas. Invest Ophthalmol Vis Sci 2006;47(7):3143–50.
66. Martin PM, Roon P, Van Ells TK, Ganapathy V, Smith SB. Death of retinal neurons in streptozotocin-induced diabetic mice. Invest Ophthalmol Vis Sci 2004;45(9):3330–6.
67. Park SH, Park JW, Park SJ, et al. Apoptotic death of photoreceptors in the streptozotocin-induced diabetic rat retina. Diabetologia 2003;46(9):1260–8.
68. El-Remessy AB, Al-Shabrawey M, Khalifa Y, Tsai NT, Caldwell RB, Liou GI. Neuroprotective and blood-retinal barrier-preserving effects of cannabidiol in experimental diabetes. Am J Pathol 2006;168(1):235–44.
69. Park JW, Park SJ, Park SH, et al. Up-regulated expression of neuronal nitric oxide synthase in experimental diabetic retina. Neurobiol Dis 2006;21(1):43–9.
70. Seigel GM, Lupien SB, Campbell LM, Ishii DN. Systemic IGF-I treatment inhibits cell death in diabetic rat retina. J Diabetes Complicat 2006;20(3):196–204.
71. Abu-El-Asrar AM, Dralands L, Missotten L, Al-Jadaan IA, Geboes K. Expression of apoptosis markers in the retinas of human subjects with diabetes. Invest Ophthalmol Vis Sci 2004;45(8):2760–6.

72. Mohr S, Xi X, Tang J, Kern TS. Caspase activation in retinas of diabetic and galactosemic mice and diabetic patients. Diabetes 2002;51(4):1172–9.
73. Chihara E, Matsuoka T, Ogura Y, Matsumura M. Retinal nerve fiber layer defect as an early manifestation of diabetic retinopathy. Ophthalmology 1993;100(8):1147–51.
74. Chakrabarti S, Sima AA. The effect of myo-inositol treatment on basement membrane thickening in the BB/W-rat retina. Diabetes Research Clin Pract 1992;16(1):13–7.
75. Scott TM, Foote J, Peat B, Galway G. Vascular and neural changes in the rat optic nerve following induction of diabetes with streptozotocin. J Anat 1986;144:145–52.
76. Sugimoto M, Sasoh M, Ido M, Wakitani Y, Takahashi C, Uji Y. Detection of early diabetic change with optical coherence tomography in type 2 diabetes mellitus patients without retinopathy. Ophthalmologica Journal international d'ophtalmologie International journal of ophthalmology 2005;219(6):379–85.
77. Meyer-Rusenberg B, Pavlidis M, Stupp T, Thanos S. Pathological changes in human retinal ganglion cells associated with diabetic and hypertensive retinopathy. Graefes Arch Clin Exp Ophthalmol 2006;245(7):1009–18.
78. Gastinger MJ, Barber AJ, Khin SA, McRill CS, Gardner TW, Marshak DW. Abnormal centrifugal axons in streptozotocin-diabetic rat retinas. Invest Ophthalmol Vis Sci 2001;42(11):2679–85.
79. Agardh E, Bruun A, Agardh CD. Retinal glial cell immunoreactivity and neuronal cell changes in rats with STZ-induced diabetes. Curr Eye Res 2001;23(4):276–84.
80. Roufail E, Soulis T, Boel E, Cooper ME, Rees S. Depletion of nitric oxide synthase-containing neurons in the diabetic retina: reversal by aminoguanidine. Diabetologia 1998;41(12):1419–25.
81. Goto R, Doi M, Ma N, Semba R, Uji Y. Contribution of nitric oxide-producing cells in normal and diabetic rat retina. Jpn J Ophthalmol 2005;49(5):363–70.
82. Seki M, Tanaka T, Nawa H, et al. Involvement of brain-derived neurotrophic factor in early retinal neuropathy of streptozotocin-induced diabetes in rats: therapeutic potential of brain-derived neurotrophic factor for dopaminergic amacrine cells. Diabetes 2004;53(9):2412–9.
83. Ng YK, Zeng XX, Ling EA. Expression of glutamate receptors and calcium-binding proteins in the retina of streptozotocin-induced diabetic rats. Brain Res 2004;1018(1):66–72.
84. Ramsey DJ, Ripps H, Qian H. Streptozotocin-induced diabetes modulates GABA receptor activity of rat retinal neurons. Exp Eye Res 2007;85(3):413–22.
85. Barber AJ, Antonetti DA. Mapping the blood vessels with paracellular permeability in the retinas of diabetic rats. Invest Ophthalmol Vis Sci 2003;44(12):5410–6.
86. Yokota T, Ma RC, Park JY, et al. Role of protein kinase C on the expression of platelet-derived growth factor and endothelin-1 in the retina of diabetic rats and cultured retinal capillary pericytes. Diabetes 2003;52(3):838–45.
87. Lieth E, Barber AJ, Xu B, et al. Glial reactivity and impaired glutamate metabolism in short-term experimental diabetic retinopathy. Penn State Retina Research Group. Diabetes 1998;47(5):815–20.
88. Ambati J, Chalam KV, Chawla DK, et al. Elevated gamma-aminobutyric acid, glutamate, and vascular endothelial growth factor levels in the vitreous of patients with proliferative diabetic retinopathy. Arch Ophthalmol 1997;115(9):1161–6.
89. Lieth E, LaNoue KF, Antonetti DA, Ratz M. Diabetes reduces glutamate oxidation and glutamine synthesis in the retina. The Penn State Retina Research Group. Exp Eye Res 2000;70(6):723–30.
90. Puro DG. Diabetes-induced dysfunction of retinal Muller cells. Trans Am Ophthalmol Soc 2002;100: 339–52.
91. Ward MM, Jobling AI, Kalloniatis M, Fletcher EL. Glutamate uptake in retinal glial cells during diabetes. Diabetologia 2005;48(2):351–60.
92. Eng LF, Ghirnikar RS, Lee YL. Glial fibrillary acidic protein: GFAP-thirty-one years (1969–2000). Neurochem Res 2000;25(9–10):1439–51.
93. Asnaghi V, Gerhardinger C, Hoehn T, Adeboje A, Lorenzi M. A role for the polyol pathway in the early neuroretinal apoptosis and glial changes induced by diabetes in the rat. Diabetes 2003;52(2):506–11.
94. Li Q, Puro DG. Diabetes-induced dysfunction of the glutamate transporter in retinal Muller cells. Invest Ophthalmol Vis Sci 2002;43(9):3109–16.
95. Mizutani M, Gerhardinger C, Lorenzi M. Muller cell changes in human diabetic retinopathy. Diabetes 1998;47(3):445–9.
96. Sarthy VP. Muller cells in retinal health and disease. Archivos de la Sociedad Espanola de Oftalmologia 2000;75(6):367–8.

97. Lundkvist A, Reichenbach A, Betsholtz C, Carmeliet P, Wolburg H, Pekny M. Under stress, the absence of intermediate filaments from Muller cells in the retina has structural and functional consequences. J Cell Sci 2004;117(Pt 16):3481–8.
98. Fletcher EL, Phipps JA, Ward MM, Puthussery T, Wilkinson-Berka JL. Neuronal and glial cell abnormality as predictors of progression of diabetic retinopathy. Curr pharm Des 2007;13(26):2699–712.
99. Pe'er J, Folberg R, Itin A, Gnessin H, Hemo I, Keshet E. Upregulated expression of vascular endothelial growth factor in proliferative diabetic retinopathy. Br J Ophthalmol 1996;80(3):241–5.
100. Frank RN. Diabetic retinopathy. N Engl J Med 2004;350(1):48–58.
101. Kilic U, Kilic E, Jarve A, et al. Human vascular endothelial growth factor protects axotomized retinal ganglion cells in vivo by activating ERK-1/2 and Akt pathways. J Neurosci 2006;26(48):12439–46.
102. Schlingemann RO. Role of growth factors and the wound healing response in age-related macular degeneration. Graefes Arch Clin Exp Ophthalmol 2004;242(1):91–101.
103. Famiglietti EV, Stopa EG, McGookin ED, Song P, LeBlanc V, Streeten BW. Immunocytochemical localization of vascular endothelial growth factor in neurons and glial cells of human retina. Brain Res 2003;969(1–2):195–204.
104. Hammes HP, Lin J, Bretzel RG, Brownlee M, Breier G. Upregulation of the vascular endothelial growth factor/vascular endothelial growth factor receptor system in experimental background diabetic retinopathy of the rat. Diabetes 1998;47(3):401–6.
105. Hirata C, Nakano K, Nakamura N, et al. Advanced glycation end products induce expression of vascular endothelial growth factor by retinal Muller cells. Biochem Biophys Res Commun 1997;236(3):712–5.
106. Amin RH, Frank RN, Kennedy A, Eliott D, Puklin JE, Abrams GW. Vascular endothelial growth factor is present in glial cells of the retina and optic nerve of human subjects with nonproliferative diabetic retinopathy. Invest Ophthalmol Vis Sci 1997;38(1):36–47.
107. Abu El-Asrar AM, Meersschaert A, Dralands L, Missotten L, Geboes K. Inducible nitric oxide synthase and vascular endothelial growth factor are colocalized in the retinas of human subjects with diabetes. Eye (London, England) 2004;18(3):306–13.
108. Murata T, Nakagawa K, Khalil A, Ishibashi T, Inomata H, Sueishi K. The relation between expression of vascular endothelial growth factor and breakdown of the blood-retinal barrier in diabetic rat retinas. Lab Invest; J Tech Methods Pathol 1996;74(4):819–25.
109. Gariano RF, Gardner TW. Retinal angiogenesis in development and disease. Nature 2005;438(7070): 960–6.
110. Zhang J, Gerhardinger C, Lorenzi M. Early complement activation and decreased levels of glycosylphosphatidylinositol-anchored complement inhibitors in human and experimental diabetic retinopathy. Diabetes 2002;51(12):3499–504.
111. Joussen AM, Poulaki V, Mitsiades N, et al. Suppression of Fas-FasL-induced endothelial cell apoptosis prevents diabetic blood-retinal barrier breakdown in a model of streptozotocin-induced diabetes. Faseb J 2003;17(1):76–8.
112. Cusick M, Chew EY, Chan CC, Kruth HS, Murphy RP, Ferris FL, III. Histopathology and regression of retinal hard exudates in diabetic retinopathy after reduction of elevated serum lipid levels. Ophthalmology 2003;110(11):2126–33.
113. Wolfensberger TJ, Hamilton AM. Diabetic retinopathy–an historical review. Semin Ophthalmol 2001;16(1):2–7.
114. Simonsen SE. ERG in Juvenile Diabetics: a prognostic study. Symposium on the Treatment of Diabetic Retinopathy MF Goldberg and SL Fine, editors Arlington: US Dept of Health, Education and Welfare 681–689 1969.
115. Bresnick GH, Palta M. Oscillatory potential amplitudes. Relation to severity of diabetic retinopathy. Arch Ophthalmol 1987;105(7):929–33.
116. Bresnick GH, Palta M. Predicting progression to severe proliferative diabetic retinopathy. Arch Ophthalmol 1987;105(6):810–4.
117. Della Salla S, Bertoni G, Somazzi L, Stubbe F, Wilkins AJ. Impaired contrast sensitivity in diabetic patients with and without retinopathy: a new technique for rapid assessment. Br J Ophthalmol 1985;69(2):(136–142).
118. Abraham FA, Haimovitz J, Berezin M. The photopic and scotopic visual thresholds in diabetics without diabetic retinopathy. Metab Pediatr Syst Ophthalmol 1988;11(1–2):76–7.

119. Roy MS, Gunkel RD, Podgor MJ. Color vision defects in early diabetic retinopathy. Arch Ophthalmol 1986;104(2):225–8.
120. Daley ML, Watzke RC, Riddle MC. Early loss of blue-sensitive color vision in patients with type I diabetes. Diabetes Care 1987;10(6):777–81.
121. Ghirlanda G, Di Leo MA, Caputo S, Cercone S, Greco AV. From functional to microvascular abnormalities in early diabetic retinopathy. Diabetes/Metab Rev 1997;13(1):15–35.
122. Novotny HR, Alvis DL. A method of photographing fluorescence in circulating blood in the human retina. Circulation 1961;24:82–6.
123. Cogan DG, Toussaint D, Kuwabara T. Retinal vascular patterns. IV. Diabetic retinopathy. Arch Ophthalmol 1961;66:366–78.
124. Qaum T, Xu Q, Joussen AM, et al. VEGF-initiated blood-retinal barrier breakdown in early diabetes. Invest Ophthalmol Vis Sci 2001;42(10):2408–13.
125. Jin KL, Mao XO, Greenberg DA. Vascular endothelial growth factor: direct neuroprotective effect in in vitro ischemia. Proc Natl Acad Sci USA 2000;97(18):10242–7.
126. Storkebaum E, Carmeliet P. VEGF: a critical player in neurodegeneration. J Clin Invest 2004; 113(1):14–8.
127. Nishijima K, Ng YS, Zhong L, et al. Vascular endothelial growth factor-a is a survival factor for retinal neurons and a critical neuroprotectant during the adaptive response to ischemic injury. Am J Pathol 2007.
128. Nakanishi Y, Nakamura M, Mukuno H, Kanamori A, Seigel GM, Negi A. Latanoprost rescues retinal neuro-glial cells from apoptosis by inhibiting caspase-3, which is mediated by p44/p42 mitogen-activated protein kinase. Exp Eye Res 2006;83(5):1108–17.

13 The Role of Inflammation in the Pathophysiology of Diabetic Retinopathy

Lauren E. Swenarchuk, Linda E. Whetter, and Anthony P. Adamis

CONTENTS

ABSTRACT

The inflammatory nature of diabetic retinopathy (DR) was first suggested by the finding that it occurred less frequently among diabetic patients taking salicylates for rheumatoid arthritis. Subsequent work has identified many features that are characteristic of inflammation, including increased blood flow, vascular permeability, and edema, as well as the influx of cells that are associated with inflammatory responses. While DR involves defects in many retinal cell types, the retinal vasculature appears to be the principal locus of the inflammation-linked damage.

From: *Contemporary Diabetes: Diabetic Retinopathy*
Edited by: E. Duh © Humana Press, Totowa, NJ

In experimental studies employing rodent models of diabetes, diabetic retinal vascular leakage, capillary nonperfusion, and endothelial cell damage are temporally and spatially correlated with a low-level leukocyte influx and persistent retinal leukostasis. This leukostasis is mediated by retinal upregulation of intercellular adhesion molecule-1 (ICAM-1), together with an increased expression of its cognate integrin ligands on neutrophils. Subsequently, endothelial cell injury and death result from Fas/FasL-mediated apoptosis.

In response to this injury, the endothelium maintains a sustained high rate of cell division, which is believed to result in exhaustion of its regenerative capacity. This stress is further exacerbated by a diabetes-induced defect in the ability of endothelial precursor cells to repair the damaged vasculature. While the vascular damage is primarily a function of infiltrating leukocytes, DR also is associated with ischemic neovascularization, a process that is amplified by the influx of macrophages.

Numerous cytokines are upregulated in DR, and two of these, vascular endothelial growth factor (VEGF) and tumor necrosis factor-α (TNF-α), are believed to play important roles in the inflammation-linked retinal damage. Upregulation of VEGF causes much of the increase in retinal ICAM-1 and the resultant leukostasis, with the $VEGF_{165}$ isoform being especially important in promoting inflammatory responses. TNF-α also is involved in the upregulation of ICAM-1, and preclinical studies have established that inhibitors of both VEGF and TNF-α are able to reduce the DR-associated pathology.

The concept that DR is a low-grade inflammatory condition has proved useful in the clinic. Inhibitors of VEGF and TNF-α have shown efficacy in reducing the DR-related vision loss while high-dose aspirin has proved effective in reducing the number of DR-associated microaneurysms. There is thus reason for hope that further elucidation of the underlying cellular and molecular mechanisms of DR-associated inflammation will lead to the development of new molecularly targeted therapies and to the rational use of approaches employing more than one therapeutic agent.

Key Words: Bevacizumab; Inflammation; Leukostasis; Pegaptanib; Ranibizumab; Tumor necrosis factor-alpha; Vascular endothelial growth factor.

INTRODUCTION

The concept that diabetic retinopathy (DR) is inflammatory in nature has been under investigation since the 1960s following the results of a study demonstrating a lower incidence of DR in patients treated with salicylates for rheumatoid arthritis *(1)*. Subsequent work has provided further support for this linkage and has identified many characteristic inflammatory features that accompany the progress of DR in patients and in animal models. These include increased blood flow and vascular permeability, edema, infiltration of inflammatory cells such as macrophages, and the development of neovascularization (Table 1) *(2–27)*. Numerous physiologic derangements are believed to act in mediating the linkage between hyperglycemia and retinal damage, including the accumulation of polyols, reactive oxygen intermediates, and advanced glycation end products, in addition to the activation of protein kinase-C (reviewed by Brownlee *(28)*, Sheetz and King *(29)*, and Caldwell et al. *(30)*). These topics are discussed elsewhere in this book, and will be referred to here when they have a bearing on inflammatory processes.

Table 1
Inflammatory features that characterize diabetic retinopathy (adapted from Antonetti et al. *(2)*)

Increased blood flow and vascular permeability *(2)*
Tissue (macular) edema *(2)*
Neovascularization *(2)*
Increased expression of inflammatory mediators *(3–16)*
Accelerated retinal neural *(17)* and microvascular *(18)* cell death
Macrophage infiltration *(8,19)*
Microglial cell activation *(20–22)*
Increased leukocyte adhesion *(23,24)*
Complement activation *(25)*
Fas ligand upregulation *(26)*
Acute-phase response protein expression *(27)*

The retinal abnormalities in DR involve neurons, glial elements, and the retinal microvasculature *(31)*. While some of the earliest detectable defects in DR include alterations in neuronal function *(2, 31)*, for which there is some evidence for an inflammatory contribution *(27, 32)*, most research into inflammatory changes concerns DR-associated damage to the retinal vasculature. As described in accompanying chapters, the processes leading to the DR-associated vasculopathy include leukocyte entrapment, formation of acellular capillaries, capillary dropout, and local hypoxia. The focus of this chapter is on the inflammatory nature of many of the molecular and cellular processes leading to this vascular damage, as well as on the pathologic neovascularization that often accompanies it. Finally, clinical findings validating the role of inflammation in DR are described.

PATHOPHYSIOLOGY OF DIABETIC RETINAL VASCULAR INJURY: THE ROLE OF LEUKOSTASIS

Several lines of correlative preclinical and clinical evidence have demonstrated that DR is associated with increased levels of leukocytes. In a key early clinical study, McLeod et al. *(33)* reported that neutrophil numbers were significantly elevated in the choroidal and retinal vasculature of patients with diabetes mellitus and that this elevation was accompanied by an increased expression of intercellular adhesion molecule-1 (ICAM-1) in both tissues. Subsequently, it was determined that vitreous levels of soluble ICAM-1 were significantly higher in the eyes of diabetic patients compared to nondiabetic controls *(34)*. Macrophages also have been detected in surgically removed membranes *(19)* and vitreous samples of *(8)* patients with proliferative DR. In other studies, the choriocapillaris of eyes from diabetic patients had approximately twice the number of polymorphonuclear leukocytes as in nondiabetic controls, together with an elevated level of nonviable endothelial cells, leading to choriocapillary dropout *(35)*. Increased numbers of polymorphonuclear cells also have been observed in the retinal vasculature of spontaneously diabetic monkeys, again associated with capillary closure *(36)*. Moreover, in an early study with diabetic rats in which the disease was induced by injection with alloxan, retinal populations of monocytes and granulocytes increased severalfold in advanced diabetes mellitus compared to controls *(37)*, while capillary occlusions and endothelial cell damage accompanied these increases.

Whether the leukocyte accumulation was merely an epiphenomenon of a vasculopathy for which a primary cause lay elsewhere, or whether the leukocytes were directly involved in producing the damage could not be elucidated from these correlative studies. Support for a direct causative role for leukocytes in diabetic vasculopathy was derived from the results of further studies with rodent models of diabetes mellitus, including the streptozotocin (STZ)-induced diabetic rat and transgenic mice. In the normal rat, low levels of retinal leukostasis were observed in the retinal vasculature *(38)*, but numbers of adherent leukocytes began to increase within a few days of STZ induction (Fig. 1) *(23, 38)*. The increase did not represent an overt vasculitis but rather a cumulative and persistent elevation of leukocyte numbers (Fig. 2A) coupled with a progressive increase in vascular leakage (Fig. 2B) *(23)*. Some of the static leukocytes were associated with capillary blockage, leading to localized areas of downstream nonperfusion; subsequent disappearance of the leukocytes was accompanied by capillary reperfusion in some instances, but in others, the capillaries remained closed (Fig. 3A–F) *(23)*.

Analysis of the molecular mechanisms underlying these events has revealed a pivotal role for the interaction between ICAM-1 on endothelial cells and its integrin ligands on the leukocytes. Retinal ICAM-1 mRNA expression was increased in the diabetic rats compared to nondiabetic controls (Fig. 4), and this elevation was essential for both the increased leukostasis (Fig. 5A) and the increase in vascular leakage (Fig. 5B); both were significantly reduced by 49 and 86%, respectively, following systemic administration of an anti-ICAM-1 antibody *(23)*. In a follow-up study, neutrophils from diabetic rats had increased surface expression of α integrin subunits CD11a and CD11b and β integrin subunit CD18 (CD11a/CD11b combine with CD18 to form the ligand for ICAM-1); systemic administration of an anti-CD18 antibody decreased retinal leukostasis by 62% *(39)*. A similar elevation of CD18 expression has recently been demonstrated in neutrophils of patients suffering from DR *(40)*.

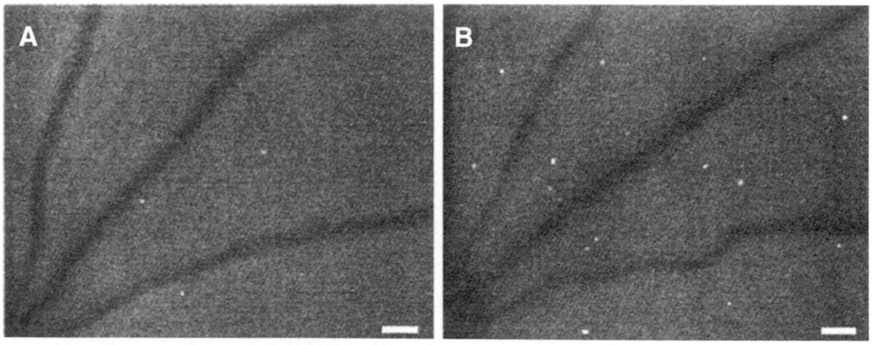

Fig. 1. Diabetes induces retinal leukostasis. Representative retinal leukostasis observed with acridine orange leukocyte fluorography in nondiabetic (**A**) and diabetic (**B**) rats; diabetic rats were analyzed 1 week after induction of diabetes. Scale bars: 100 μm. (Reproduced from Miyamoto et al. 1999 *(23)* with permission from Proc Natl Acad Sci USA. Copyright 1999 National Academy of Sciences, USA).

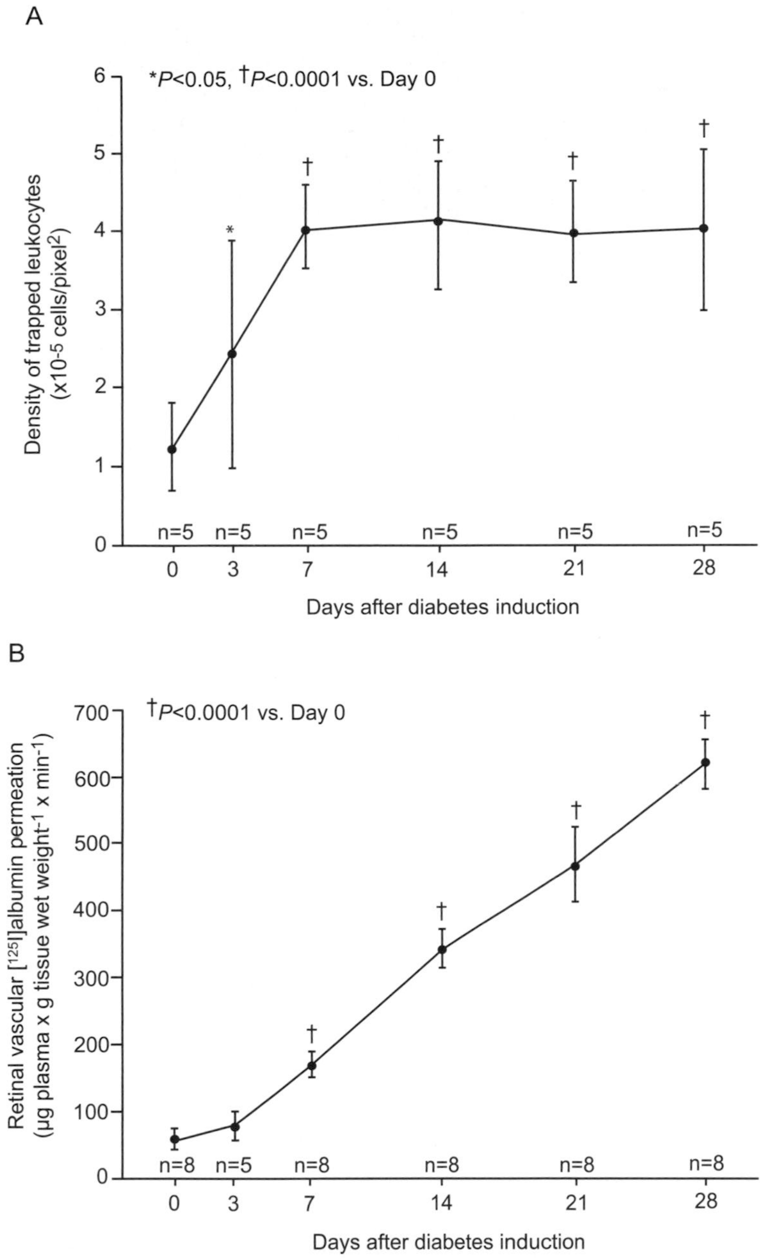

Fig. 2. Retinal leukostasis and vascular leakage are significantly increased over time. (**A**) Leukostasis was serially quantified in nondiabetic rats (Day 0) and in rats with streptozotocin-induced diabetes of varying duration using acridine orange leukocyte fluorography. (**B**) Vascular leakage was quantified at the same time points by evaluating radioactive albumin permeation into retinal tissue. Data represent mean ± standard deviation. (Reproduced from Miyamoto et al. 1999 *(23)* with permission from Proc Natl Acad Sci USA. Copyright 1999 National Academy of Sciences, USA.)

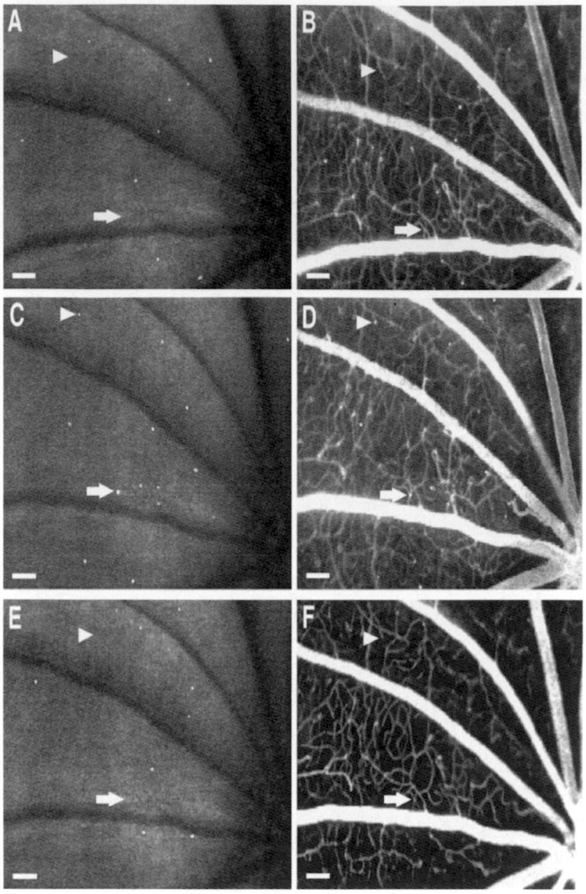

Fig. 3. Leukocytes induce capillary occlusion. Serial studies were completed 1 week (**A**, **B**), 2 weeks (**C**, **D**), and 4 weeks (**E**, **F**) after diabetes induction in rats by using both acridine orange leukocyte fluorography (**A**, **C**, **E**) and fluorescein angiography (**B**, **D**, **F**). The arrows show a patent capillary that is not blocked by a leukocyte (**A**, **B**) that subsequently becomes occluded downstream from a static leukocyte (**C**, **D**), and then subsequently opens up when the leukocyte disappears (**E**, **F**). The arrowheads show a patent capillary not blocked by a leukocyte (**A**, **B**) that becomes occluded downstream from a static leukocyte (**C**, **D**) and then remains closed after the leukocyte has disappeared (**E, F**). Scale bars: 100 μm. (Reproduced from Miyamoto et al. 1999 *(23)* with permission from Proc Natl Acad Sci USA. Copyright 1999 National Academy of Sciences, USA.)

Possible mechanisms linking leukostasis with increased permeability may include a direct action on tight junction disruption *(41, 42)* as well as local upregulation of vascular endothelial growth factor (VEGF), either from the hypoxia induced by nonperfusion or from release by the leukocytes themselves *(43–46)*. A major factor, however, appears to be the concomitant increase in endothelial cell injury and death *(24, 26, 47)*, also reported in an earlier clinical study *(18)*. Prevention of the interaction between leukocytes and the retinal vascular endothelium by the administration of antibodies to CD18 or ICAM-1 resulted in inhibition of leukostasis and endothelial cell apoptosis *(47)*. Similarly, the genetic ablation of CD18 or ICAM-1 resulted in markedly reduced

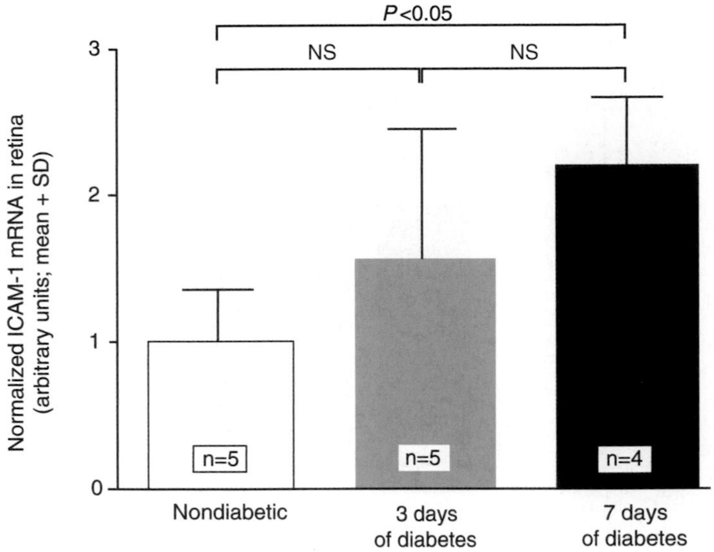

Fig. 4. Retinal intercellular adhesion molecule-1 (ICAM-1) expression is induced in diabetes. Rat retinal ICAM-1 levels after 7 days of diabetes were 2.2-fold higher than in nondiabetic controls ($P < 0.05$). All mRNA levels were normalized to 18S ribosomal RNA (used as a control for quantity of RNA loaded). NS = not significant. (Reproduced from Miyamoto et al. 1999 *(23)* with permission from Proc Natl Acad Sci USA. Copyright 1999 National Academy of Sciences, USA).

leukocyte adhesion, endothelial injury (Fig. 6A), and blood-retinal barrier (BRB) breakdown (Fig. 6B) in animals with chronic diabetes *(24)*.

Additional studies have demonstrated that the vascular damage in the rat STZ-induced diabetes model results from apoptosis mediated by the interaction of Fas and its ligand FasL *(26)*. Induction of diabetes resulted in upregulation of FasL on neutrophils while Fas was upregulated in the retinal vasculature; in addition, neutrophils from diabetic rats, unlike those from control animals, induced endothelial cell apoptosis in vitro. In addition, the systemic administration of an anti-FasL antibody inhibited endothelial cell apoptosis (Fig. 7A) and BRB breakdown (Fig. 7B), although this treatment did not reduce leukocyte adhesion to the diabetic retinal vasculature *(26)*.

There is also evidence supporting a role for platelets in the pathogenesis of DR in that platelet microthrombi have been identified in the retinas of diabetic patients *(48)*. Platelet microthrombi have also been found to accumulate in the retinas of diabetic rats *(49, 50)*. The accumulation of platelet microthrombi occurred within 2 weeks after induction with STZ and contributed actively to inflammation through adhesion molecule upregulation and VEGF and platelet-derived growth-factor release *(50)*. Inhibition of endothelial cell apoptosis with an anti-FasL antibody prevented the accumulation of platelets, suggesting that their accumulation was secondary to endothelial cell damage; when this damage was allowed to proceed in platelet-depleted rats, there was a worsening of the BRB breakdown *(50)*.

It remains to be determined whether the inflammatory phenomena observed in the rodent models are sufficient to account for the slowly developing retinopathy that is characteristic of clinical diabetes. In this connection, it is noteworthy that the course of

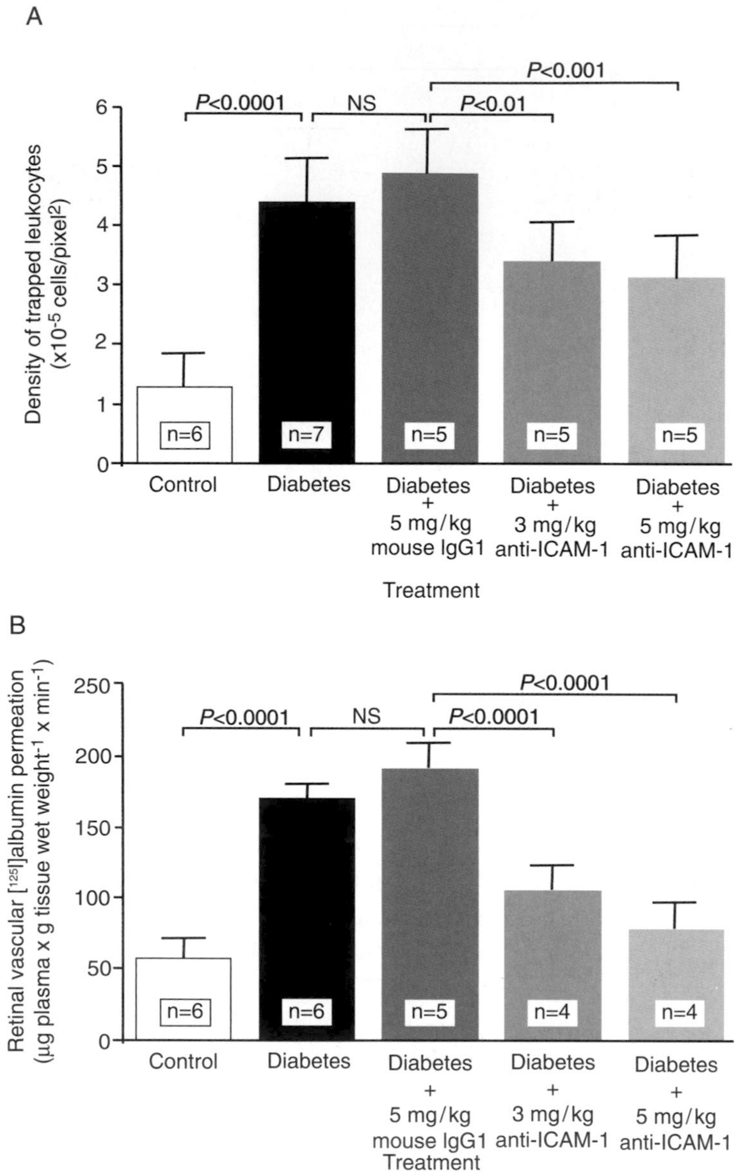

Fig. 5. Diabetes-induced retinal leukostasis and vascular leakage involve intercellular adhesion molecule-1 (ICAM-1). (**A**) The density of trapped leukocytes was significantly increased 1 week after diabetes induction in rats; systemic administration of an ICAM-1 neutralizing antibody ($5\,mg/kg^{-1}$) decreased leukocyte density by 48.5% ($P < 0.001$). (**B**) Similarly, diabetes-induced vascular permeability, as assessed by permeation of radioactive albumin was reduced 85.6% ($P < 0.0001$) with administration of the anti–ICAM-1 antibody. NS = not significant. Data represent mean ± standard deviation. (Reproduced from Miyamoto et al. 1999 *(23)* with permission from Proc Natl Acad Sci USA. Copyright 1999 National Academy of Sciences, USA.)

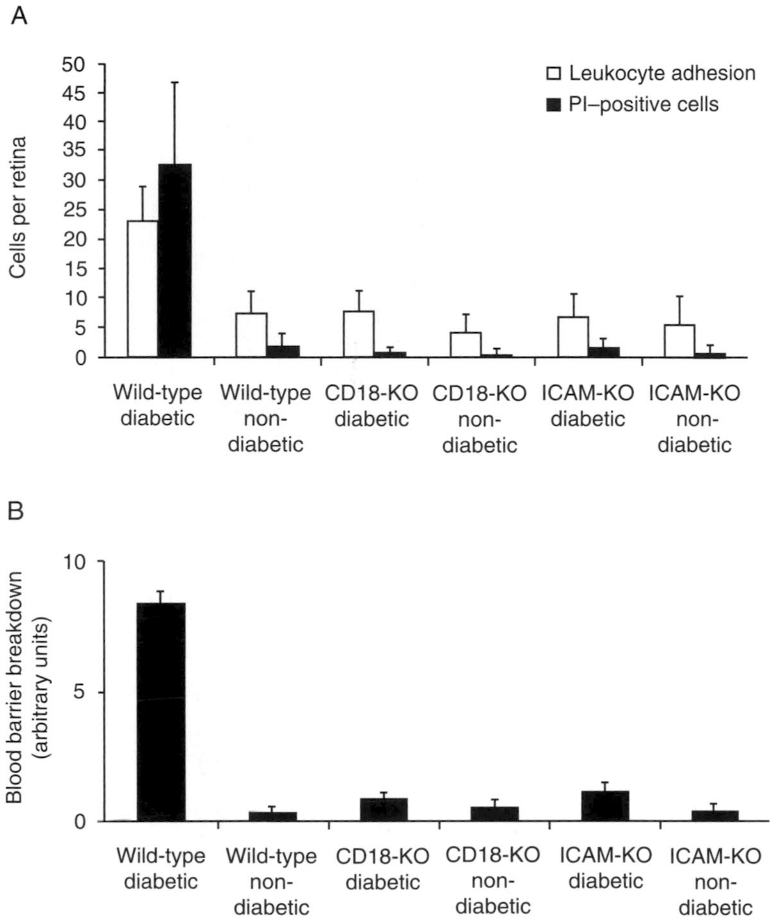

Fig. 6. Genetic ablation of either CD18 or intercellular adhesion molecule-1 (ICAM-1) dramatically reduces leukocyte adhesion, retinal endothelial damage, and blood–retinal barrier (BRB) breakdown in diabetic mice. (**A**) Adherent leukocytes were quantified in the retinal vasculature following in situ labeling with *Concanavalin* A (*open bars*). After 11 months of diabetes, the number of adherent leukocytes in the wild-type mice was 3.7-fold greater than in the age-matched, nondiabetic, wild-type controls ($P < 0.001$). In contrast, the number of adherent leukocytes in both the diabetic CD18 and ICAM-1 knockout (KO) mice did not differ significantly from that of the nondiabetic, wild-type controls or the nondiabetic, CD18, and ICAM-1 KO controls ($P > 0.05$ for all). Endothelial cell injury was assessed with propidium iodide (PI), which labels nonviable cells (*filled bars*). While 11-month diabetic, wild-type mice had a marked increase in PI-positive cells ($P < 0.001$), diabetic CD18, and ICAM-1 KO mice had significantly fewer PI-positive cells than diabetic wild-type mice ($P < 0.001$). Nondiabetic, wild-type mice and the nondiabetic, CD18, and ICAM-1 KO mice also had few PI-positive retinal endothelial cells. (**B**) BRB breakdown was assessed with the use of Evans Blue dye, which binds covalently to albumin. In wild-type mice, long-term diabetes led to a 27.7-fold increase in vascular leakage whereas in both CD18 and ICAM-1 KOs the diabetes-associated increase was much less (1.6- and 2.75-fold, respectively). Data represent mean ± standard deviation. (Reproduced from Joussen et al. 2004 *(24)* with permission from Fedn of Am Societies for Experimental Bio [FASEB] Copyright 2004 by Fedn of Am Societies for Experimental Bio (FASEB).)

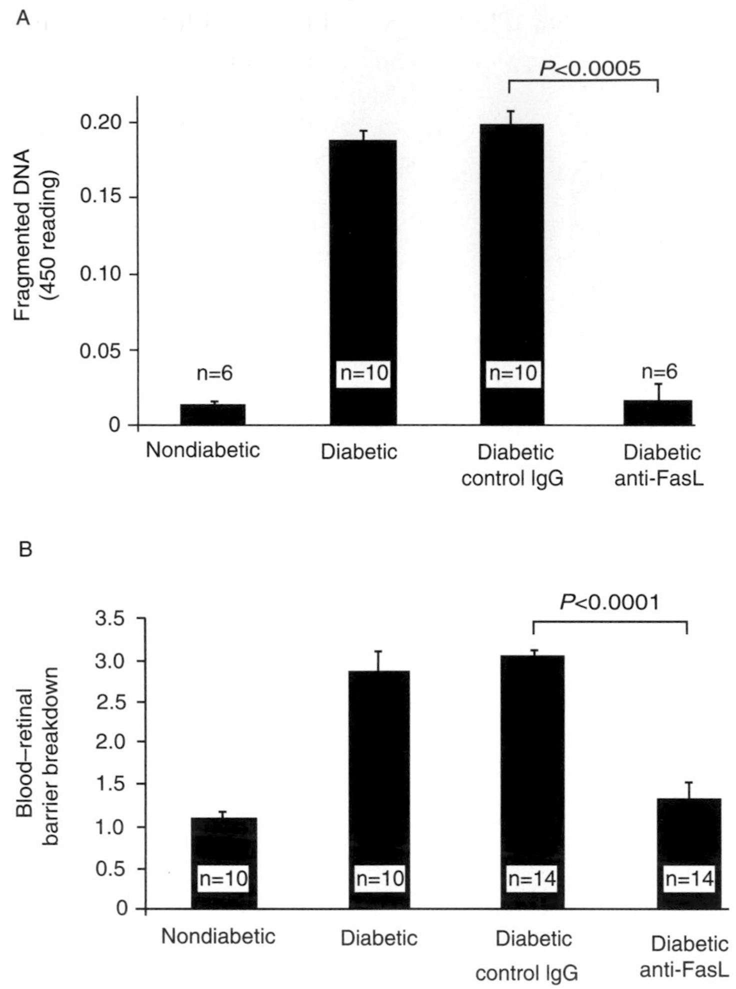

Fig. 7. FasL inhibition suppresses apoptosis and blood–retinal barrier (BRB) breakdown. (**A**) Retinal cell death was quantified 2 weeks after induction of diabetes in rats using a DNA fragmentation enzyme-linked immunosorbant assay 48 h after systemic administration of an anti-FasL antibody or a control antibody. Fragmented retinal DNA levels increased by 13.84 ± 0.41-fold in diabetic animals. Systemic administration of the anti-FasL antibody reduced this to nearly nondiabetic levels (1.22 ± 0.82-fold), whereas no attenuating effect was seen after treatment with a control IgG antibody. (**B**) BRB breakdown was determined by Evans Blue performed 48 h after treatment with the anti-FasL antibody or a control antibody. Retinal permeability in the 2-week diabetic rats increased to 2.6 times the value in nondiabetic animals; treatment with the anti-FasL antibody reduced this to a factor of 1.33. Data represent mean ± standard deviation. (Reproduced from Joussen et al. 2003 *(26)* with permission from Fedn of Am Societies for Experimental Bio [FASEB] Copyright 2003 by Fedn of Am Societies for Experimental Bio (FASEB)).

the DR is accompanied by an enhanced rate of endothelial cell proliferation and death in experimental *(18, 51)* and clinical *(18)* disease, suggesting that the replicative capacity of endothelial cells may eventually become exhausted and lead to capillary dropout *(18)*. Moreover, subsequent studies have also demonstrated that endothelial precursor cells from diabetic patients are impaired in several essential functions, including migration in response to the cytokine stromal-derived factor-1 *(52)*, proliferation, adhesion, and incorporation into vascular structures *(53)*. These deficiencies led to their inability to repair the retinal vascular damage characteristic of diabetes *(54)*.

Thus, it appears that the diabetic retinal vasculature is being subjected to sustained stress, leading to the exhaustion of its inherent capacity for self-repair, conditions that are exacerbated by the reduction in replenishment from bone-marrow-derived endothelial precursor cells. Further work will be required to confirm that aberrant leukocyte adhesion is also responsible for the clinical pathology. One potential approach to testing this hypothesis in the clinic would be the development of agents that interfere with the ICAM-1 interaction that appears to be essential for the excess leukostasis observed in the rodent models.

INFLAMMATORY CELLS PROMOTE AND REGULATE THE DEVELOPMENT OF ISCHEMIC OCULAR NEOVASCULARIZATION

In addition to the damage to the existing retinal vasculature, DR may be accompanied by a proliferative neovascularization. While there is no animal model that accurately reproduces the course of proliferative DR, a retinopathy of prematurity model has been used in a number of studies to investigate the processes that regulate ischemic neovascularization. For these experiments, neonatal rats were raised in the presence of an elevated concentration of oxygen before returning to normal ambient oxygen levels *(55)*. The inflammatory nature of the neovascular response to ischemia was suggested by immunohistochemical evidence demonstrating the presence of monocytes in the pathologic neovascular fronds. Further, neovascularization could be significantly suppressed by the depletion of monocyte lineage cells by intravitreous injection of clodronate liposomes (Figs. 8B,C) *(55)*. In contrast, the physiologic vascularization that occurs during normal retinal development was affected only minimally by this treatment (Figs. 8B,D) *(55)*. This suppression of pathologic neovascularization may reflect a role of infiltrating monocyte lineage cells in amplifying the response to ischemia (Figs. 8E–J) *(55)*. An inherent potential for a positive feedback mechanism exists since VEGF induces activation *(56, 57)* and chemoattraction *(56–58)* of monocyte lineage cells, which in turn express and release it *(59, 60)*, especially in conditions of hypoxia (Fig. 8K) *(55)*. Evidence that monocytes play a role in pathologic angiogenesis has also been reported by other groups that have induced choroidal neovascularization by laser wounding; neovascularization was again suppressed by techniques that inhibited monocyte lineage cell recruitment, including their depletion with clodronate liposomes *(61, 62)* and genetic ablation of C-C chemokine receptor-2, the receptor for monocyte chemoattractant protein-1 *(63)*.

In addition to the evidence implicating monocyte lineage cells in promoting pathologic vascularization, another population of inflammatory cells, T lymphocytes, was also mobilized *(55)*. These cells were involved in the negative regulation of neovascularization, which was demonstrated by studies in which systemic injection of an antibody against CD2, a key adhesion molecule important for T lymphocyte-mediated responses, significantly increased pathologic neovascularization (Fig. 9A–C) *(55)*. Immunocytochemical data demonstrated that these cells were positive for CD8 and CD25 antigens, characteristic of activated cytotoxic T lymphocytes (CTLs) (Fig. 9D–I) *(55)*.

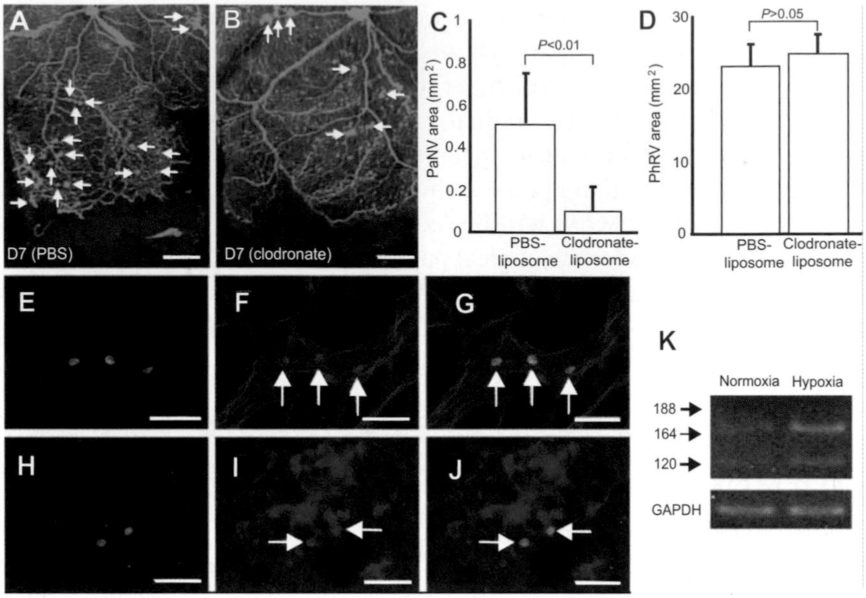

Fig. 8. Monocytes contribute to pathologic retinal neovascularization. To induce an avascular retina, postnatal Day 0 (P0) rats were maintained for 10 days in 80% oxygen and were interrupted daily for 30 min in room air followed by a progressive return to 80% oxygen. On P10, which corresponds to study Day 0 (D0), they were placed in room air for an additional 7 days (D7) to induce retinal neovascularization. Pathologic neovascularization (PaNV) at D7 (*arrows*) was not inhibited when treated with phosphate buffered saline-control liposomes ($n = 8$) (A) but was reduced with clodronate liposomes ($n = 8$) (**B**). The area of PaNV (**C**) was significantly reduced with clodronate liposomes vs. control liposomes ($P < 0.01$), whereas physiologic neovascular area (PhRV) (**D**) was not ($P > 0.05$). Data represent mean ± standard deviation. (**E–J**) Monocyte adhesion was observed just before and during pathologic neovascularization (**H–J**). A fluorescein conjugated anti-CD13 antibody was used to label monocytes (**E, H**). Retinal vasculature and adherent leukocytes were labeled with rhodamine-conjugated *Concanavalin* A (**F, I**). Superposition of the figures identifies the *Concanavalin* A–stained cells as CD13-positive leukocytes (*arrows*) (**G, J**). (**K**) VEGF mRNA levels were markedly increased in response to hypoxia (1% oxygen) when compared to normoxia (21% oxygen) in cultured peripheral blood monocytes from D7 rats with retinopathy. Scale bars: (**A, B**) 0.5 mm and (**E–J**) 50 μm. (Reproduced from Ishida et al. 2003 *(55)* with permission from J Exp Med).

The involvement of T lymphocytes appears to be a mobilization of a physiologic pruning mechanism that is operative during physiologic development of the retinal vasculature during embryogenesis *(64)*. Vascular pruning in physiologic retinal angiogenesis is mediated, at least in part, through T lymphocyte expression of FasL, which induces apoptosis of the endothelial cells *(64)*. To assess whether a similar mechanism might be involved in controlling the pathologic neovascularization, CD-8–positive CTLs were isolated from the blood of rats with retinopathy and cocultured with human microvascular endothelial cells. Compared to CTLs from age-matched control animals, coculture with CTLs from rats with retinopathy led to a marked increase in endothelial cell apoptosis. Most of this increase was eliminated by pretreatment of the CTLs with an antibody to FasL; in contrast, exposure of the CTLs to a control antibody did not

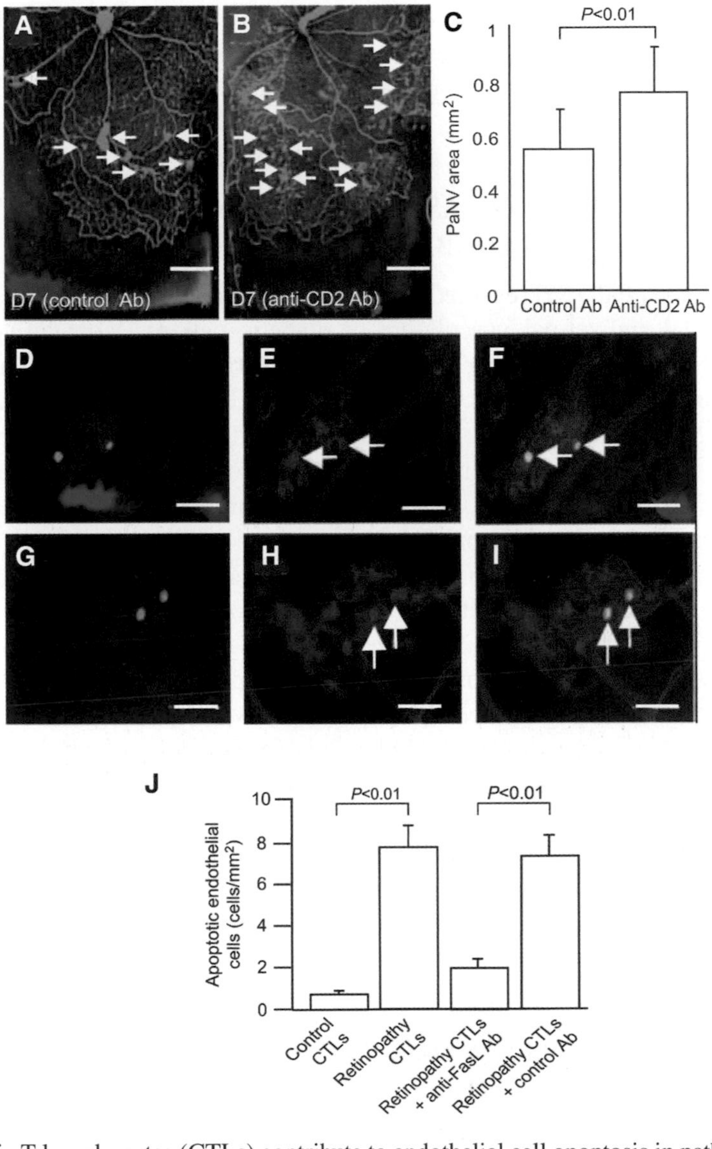

Fig. 9. Cytotoxic T lymphocytes (CTLs) contribute to endothelial cell apoptosis in pathologic retinal neovascularization. (**A**) Pathologic neovascularization in a rat ischemic retinopathy model (see Fig. 8 for description) showed pathologic vascular budding at Day 7 (D7) (*arrows*) with a systemically administered control antibody ($n = 9$), which was increased when treated with an antibody against CD2 (**B**), an adhesion molecule for T lymphocytes ($n = 11$); treatment with the anti-CD2 antibody resulted in a significant increase ($P < 0.01$) in pathologic neovascular (PaNV) area (**C**). Data represent mean ± standard deviation. Adherent leukocytes at the vascular fronds were positive for fluorescein-conjugated antibodies against CD8 (**D**) and CD25 (interleukin-2 (IL-2) receptor; **G**), demonstrating that they were activated CTLs. Superimposition of these images upon those obtained with rhodamine-conjugated *Concanavalin* A (**E, H**), which binds to leukocytes and vascular endothelium, demonstrated that these activated CTLs were binding to the endothelium of the vascular fronds (**F, I**). (**J**) In leukocyte–endothelial cocultures, CTLs isolated from the peripheral blood of rats with retinopathy significantly increased the number of apoptotic endothelial cells vs. CTLs from control rats ($P < 0.01$). An anti-FasL antibody significantly inhibited CTL-mediated apoptosis ($n = 18$–24 in each condition; $P < 0.01$). Data represent mean ± standard deviation. Scale bars: (**A, B**) 0.5 mm and (**D–I**) 50 μm. (Reproduced from Ishida et al. 2003 *(55)* with permission from J Exp Med.)

prevent the increase of endothelial cell death in these cocultures (Fig. 9J) *(55)*. These data are consistent with the hypothesis that CTL-mediated apoptosis of endothelial cells through the Fas/FasL pathway is important in the negative regulation of pathologic neovascularization.

GROWTH FACTORS AS MEDIATORS OF INFLAMMATION IN DIABETIC RETINOPATHY

Since McLeod et al. *(33)* reported that ICAM-1 expression was significantly elevated in the choroidal and retinal vasculature of diabetic patients, correlative studies have established that a variety of other inflammatory response mediators are also elevated in the ocular fluid or retinal tissue. These include VEGF *(3,4)*, interleukin-1β *(5)*, interleukin-6 *(6–8)*, interleukin-8 *(7, 8)*, stromal-derived factor-1 *(9)*, angiotensin II *(10)*, angiopoietin-1 *(11)*, angiopoietin-2 *(11, 12)*, erythropoietin *(13, 14)*, tumor necrosis factor-α (TNF-α) *(5, 15)*, monocyte chemoattractant protein-1 *(16)*, and RANTES (Regulated on Activation, Normal T-cell Expressed and Presumably Secreted) *(16)*. These studies, which focus on one or a few factors, are also being supplemented by more global approaches, including proteomic catalogs from the vitreous of diabetic human eyes *(65, 66)* as well as gene expression studies on Müller cells *(27)* and retinas *(67)* of diabetic rats. Elevations of a wide variety of proteins have been demonstrated in DR; the most recent of these reports has provided evidence that carbonic anhydrase, a heretofore unsuspected candidate, might be a viable molecular target for future therapies *(66)*. Apart from VEGF and TNF-α, however, the evidence for the involvement of the majority of these proteins in DR remains correlative. The remainder of this discussion focuses on the evidence for the involvement of these two cytokines that have been examined in some detail in connection to their roles in DR-related inflammation. As VEGF is also the subject of other chapters in this book, this particular discussion will focus on the evidence for its proinflammatory actions.

VEGF as a Proinflammatory Factor in Diabetic Retinopathy

The involvement of VEGF in DR has been studied more extensively than that of any other single factor. This work has included numerous correlative studies reporting elevated VEGF levels in the vitreous of patients suffering from DR or diabetic macular edema (DME) (reviewed in Starita et al. *(68)*). While the increases in VEGF are likely to reflect a number of processes, it is noteworthy that VEGF is upregulated by several factors that are themselves associated with DR, including reactive oxygen intermediates *(69)*, advanced glycation end products *(70)*, insulin-like growth factor-1 *(71)*, and TNF-α *(72)*. There is now increasing evidence that the actions of VEGF in promoting DR are inflammatory in nature.

Given the particular pathophysiology of DR, several properties of VEGF are especially relevant in its role as a proinflammatory agent. These include its many actions as a promoter of ocular neovascularization *(73)*, its role as the most potent known promoter of vascular permeability *(74)*, its expression by many retinal cell types *(75, 76)*, and its upregulation by hypoxia *(75, 77)*. In early studies, Tolentino et al. *(78)* found that intravitreous injection of VEGF in monkeys led to iris neovascularization, with the development of tortuous, beaded vessels as well as microaneurysms, endothelial cell hyperplasia, and neovascular glaucoma, demonstrating an important role for VEGF in ocular neovascular disease. The remainder of this section concentrates on more recent experiments that have examined the inflammatory nature of VEGF in promoting both the BRB breakdown and the ischemia-mediated neovascularization that are characteristic of DR.

VEGF as a Mediator of Diabetes-associated Retinal Leukostasis and BRB Breakdown

As discussed earlier, DR is associated with a chronic elevation of retinal leukostasis, which has in turn been identified as a major contributor to endothelial cell injury and BRB breakdown. Like the studies examining the roles of ICAM-1 and its cognate integrins in these processes, studies of VEGF have employed the STZ-induced diabetic rat, and they have been further supplemented by experiments examining the effect of intravitreous VEGF in nondiabetic animals.

Within a week of STZ induction, retinal expression of VEGF mRNA was elevated by 3.2-fold with respect to controls (Fig. 10A) *(79)*, together with the concomitant increases in vascular permeability, BRB breakdown *(79)*, and elevated expression of ICAM-1 *(80)* that have been described earlier. These diabetes-induced increases were significantly reduced by the systemic administration of a VEGF receptor fusion protein that blocks the bioactivity of VEGF *(79, 80)*; in fact, STZ-mediated upregulation of ICAM-1 expression was essentially eliminated (Fig. 10B), suggesting that in this model VEGF is responsible for much of the subsequent ICAM-1-mediated leukostasis. In a parallel experiment, intravitreous injection of VEGF in nondiabetic rats also resulted in increased retinal leukocyte adhesion (Fig. 11), together with retinal ICAM-1 upregulation and increased vascular permeability *(81)*. Both retinal vascular permeability (Fig. 12A) and leukocyte accumulation (Fig. 12B) could be inhibited by a systemically administered anti-ICAM-1 antibody *(81)*. Thus, VEGF elevations, whether caused by diabetes or intravitreous injection, led to the development of similar retinal pathologic consequences. Taken together, these data support a model in which diabetes-induced elevations of retinal VEGF lead to upregulation of retinal expression of ICAM-1 and increased leukostasis. As described earlier, the final outcome of these events is leukocyte-mediated vascular damage.

$VEGF_{164/165}$ as a Proinflammatory Cytokine

Data from experiments with rodent models have suggested that only one VEGF isoform $VEGF_{165}$ acts as an especially pathogenic proinflammatory cytokine. These experiments have focused on $VEGF_{164}$ and $VEGF_{120}$ (corresponding to human $VEGF_{165}$ and $VEGF_{121}$, respectively). Experiments comparing intravitreous injection of $VEGF_{164}$ and $VEGF_{120}$ in nondiabetic rats demonstrated that $VEGF_{164}$ was approximately twice as effective in promoting increased retinal ICAM-1 expression, leukocyte adhesion, and BRB breakdown *(82)*. Moreover, in diabetic animals, selective inhibition of $VEGF_{164}$, through intravitreous injection of pegaptanib, an RNA aptamer that binds $VEGF_{164}$ while sparing $VEGF_{120}$, significantly inhibited retinal leukostasis and BRB breakdown. The inhibition of BRB breakdown by pegaptanib was particularly marked in early diabetes (2 weeks

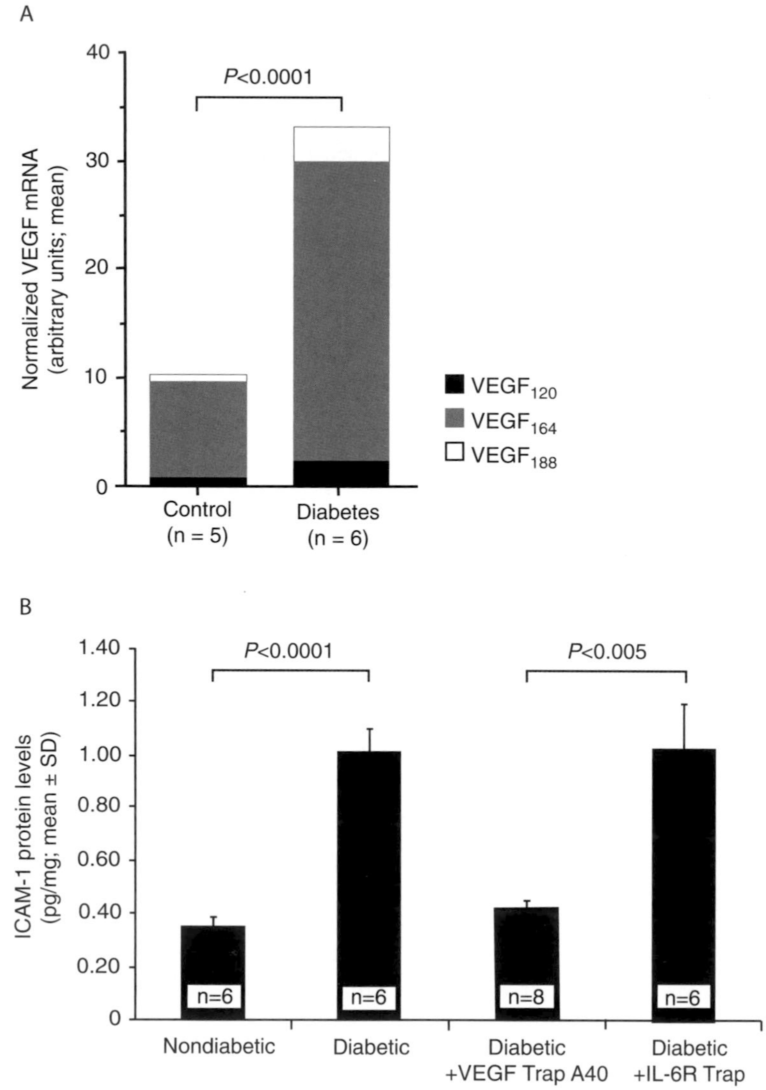

Fig. 10. Increased retinal expression of vascular endothelial growth factor (VEGF) mRNA in early diabetes. (**A**) In 1-week diabetic rats, expression of VEGF mRNA was upregulated approximately 3-fold with respect to control rats ($P < 0.001$); mRNA levels were normalized to 18S ribosomal RNA (used as a control for quantity of RNA loaded). $VEGF_{165}$ was the predominant isoform in both control and diabetic rats. (Copyright 2001 by Investigative Ophthalmology & Visual Science. Reproduced from Qaum et al. 2001 *(79)* with permission from Investigative Ophthalmology & Visual Science) (**B**) Diabetic rats showed a 3-fold increase in intercellular adhesion molecule-1 (ICAM-1) protein levels (from 0.35 + 0.035 pg/mg^{-1} to 1.007 ± 0.09 pg/mg^{-1}; $P < 0.0001$; $n = 6$) when compared to nondiabetic control rats. The ICAM-1 levels were reduced to the levels of the nondiabetic animals (from 1.007 ± 0.09 pg mg^{-1} to 0.42 ± 0.03 pg mg^{-1}; $P < 0.0005$; $n = 8$) on systemic treatment with a VEGF receptor-1/Fc fusion protein (VEGF $TrapA_{40}$) but not interleukin-6 receptor Trap ($n = 6$), a control fusion protein. (Reprinted from Joussen et al. 2002, *(80)* with permission from the American Society for Investigative Pathology).

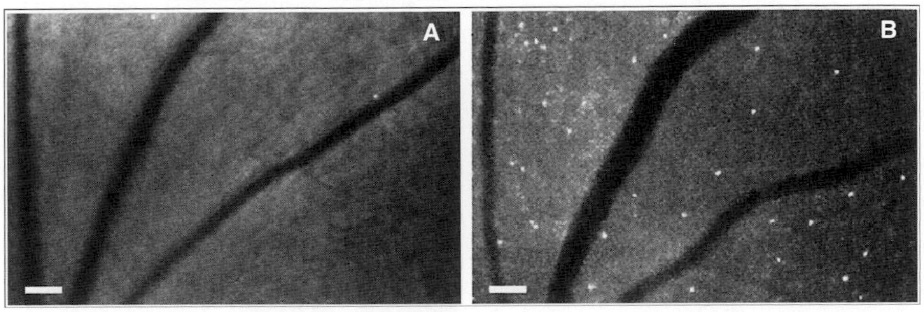

Fig. 11. Vascular endothelial growth factor (VEGF) induces retinal leukostasis. Appearance of a normal rat retina before (**A**) and 48 h after (**B**) intravitreous injection of 50 ng VEGF; retinal leukostasis was assessed by acridine orange leukocyte fluorography. Numerous static leukocytes are visible (*white dots*) as well as vessel dilation and tortuosity. Scale bar: 100 μm. (Reprinted from Miyamoto et al. 2000 *(81)* with permission from the American Society for Investigative Pathology.)

after induction; Fig. 13A), but was still evident in established diabetes at 3 months (Fig. 13B) *(82)*. The suppression effected by intravitreous pegaptanib in these experiments was comparable to that described earlier in the studies with the VEGF receptor fusion protein that binds to all VEGF isoforms *(79, 80)*, suggesting that $VEGF_{164/165}$ is responsible for much of the retinal vasculopathy that results from the diabetes-induced elevation of VEGF.

Additional support for the inflammatory nature of $VEGF_{164/165}$ has come from the retinopathy of prematurity model of ischemic neovascularization in which the expression of $VEGF_{164}$ was markedly enhanced compared to $VEGF_{120}$ *(55)*. Intravitreous injection of pegaptanib or the VEGF receptor fusion protein inhibited leukocyte adhesion by approximately 50%; both also dramatically inhibited pathologic vascularization (Fig. 14A) *(55)*. Unlike the fusion protein, which also inhibited physiologic retinal revascularization, intravitreous pegaptanib spared this process (Fig. 14B) *(55)*. In part, the enhanced pathogenicity of $VEGF_{164/165}$ in the ischemic ocular neovascularization model may reflect the greater potency of $VEGF_{164/165}$ compared to $VEGF_{120/121}$ in acting as a chemoattractant for infiltrating macrophages *(58)*, which are known to amplify pathologic neovascularization, as discussed earlier.

TUMOR NECROSIS FACTOR-α

TNF-α is a key proinflammatory cytokine that has been implicated in several immunological disorders *(83)*. The main cellular source of TNF-α is macrophages *(84)*, although other immune cells such as T lymphocytes *(85)*, neutrophils *(86)*, and a variety of other cell types, including endothelial cells, can synthesize TNF-α as well *(84)*. Stimulation of its cognate receptors by TNF-α can lead to a multitude of cellular responses, including the recruitment of leukocytes and monocytes, induction of apoptosis, stimulation of adhesion molecule expression, and stimulation of synthesis and release of a variety of other cytokines and inflammatory mediators *(84)*. In addition to its actions in mediating specific pathologic features of diabetes, including nephropathy

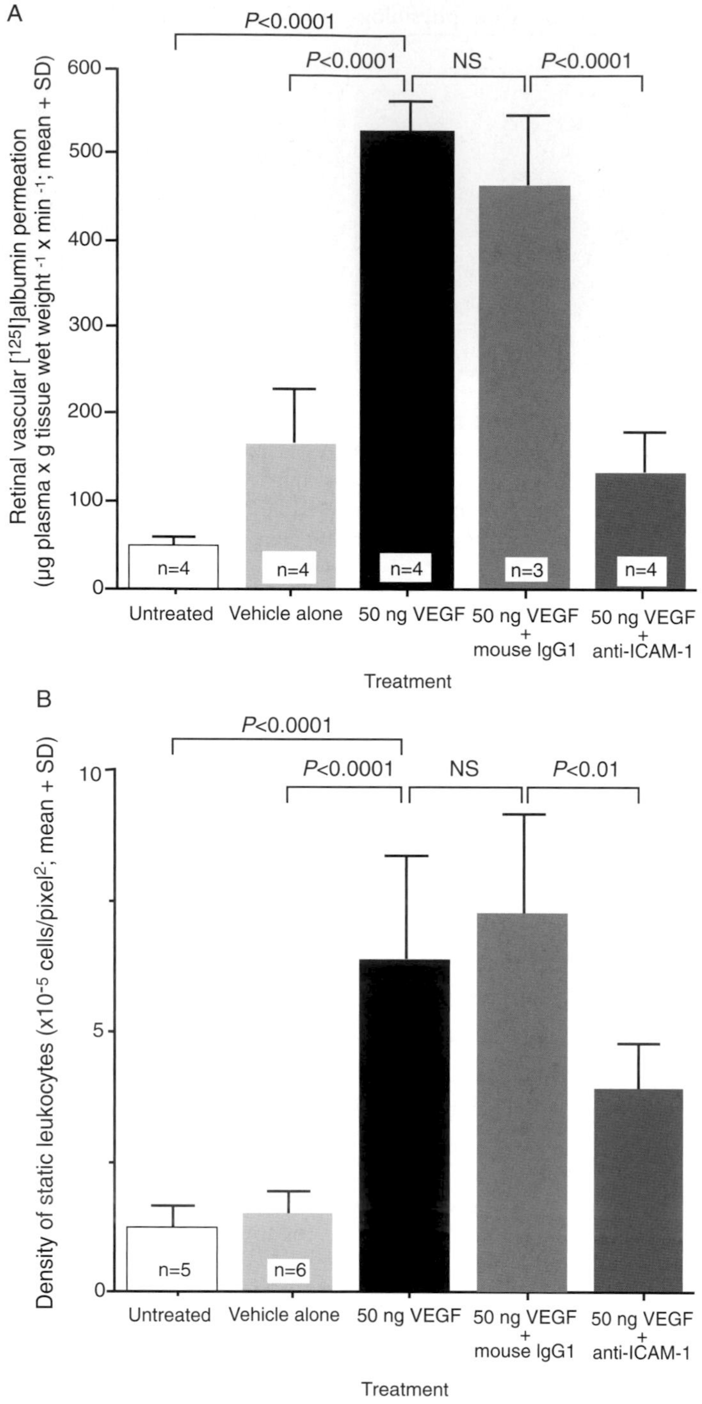

Fig. 12. Effect of anti-intercellular adhesion molecule-1 (ICAM-1) monoclonal antibody on permeability and leukostasis after intravitreous vascular endothelial growth factor (VEGF) injection. Rats receiving intravitreous VEGF had a 3.2-fold increase in vascular permeability (**A**), as measured by assessing radioactive albumin permeation into retinal tissue; systemic administration of an anti–ICAM-1 antibody significantly reduced vascular leakage when compared to a control antibody ($P < 0.0001$). Similar increases in VEGF-mediated leukostasis (**B**) also were blocked with the anti–ICAM-1 antibody. NS = not significant. (Reprinted from Miyamoto et al. 2000 *(81)* with permission from the American Society for Investigative Pathology).

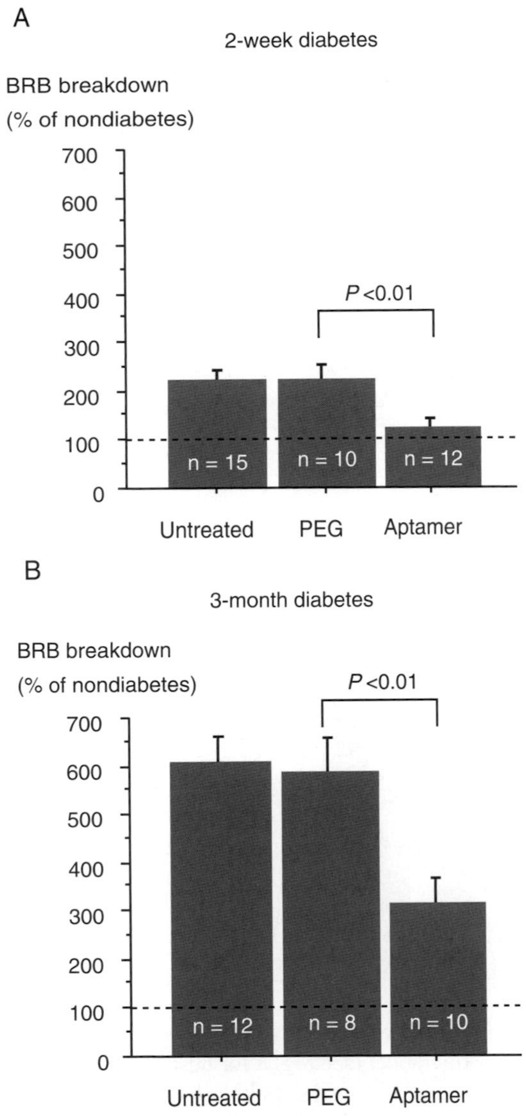

Fig. 13. Pegaptanib, an antivascular endothelial growth factor $(VEGF)_{165}$ aptamer, reduces diabetic blood–retinal barrier (BRB) breakdown. In 2-week diabetic rats (**A**), intravitreous treatment with pegaptanib resulted in an 82.6% reduction of BRB breakdown when compared to polyethylene glycol (PEG) alone ($P < 0.01$). In established diabetes (**B**), there was 55% inhibition of BRB breakdown with pegaptanib ($P < 0.01$). BRB breakdown was assessed by a fluorescein-conjugated dextran method; data represent mean ± standard deviation. (Reproduced from Ishida et al. 2003 *(82)* with permission from Investigative Ophthalmology & Visual Science. Copyright 2003 by Investigative Ophthalmology & Visual Science.)

(84) and retinopathy, TNF-α has also been found to contribute to the induction of pancreatic β-cell apoptosis in mice *(87)* and to insulin resistance in adipose tissue *(88)*.

Evidence supporting a role for TNF-α in DR comes from studies demonstrating elevations of TNF-α in ocular fibrovascular membranes *(15)*, platelets *(89)*, and plasma

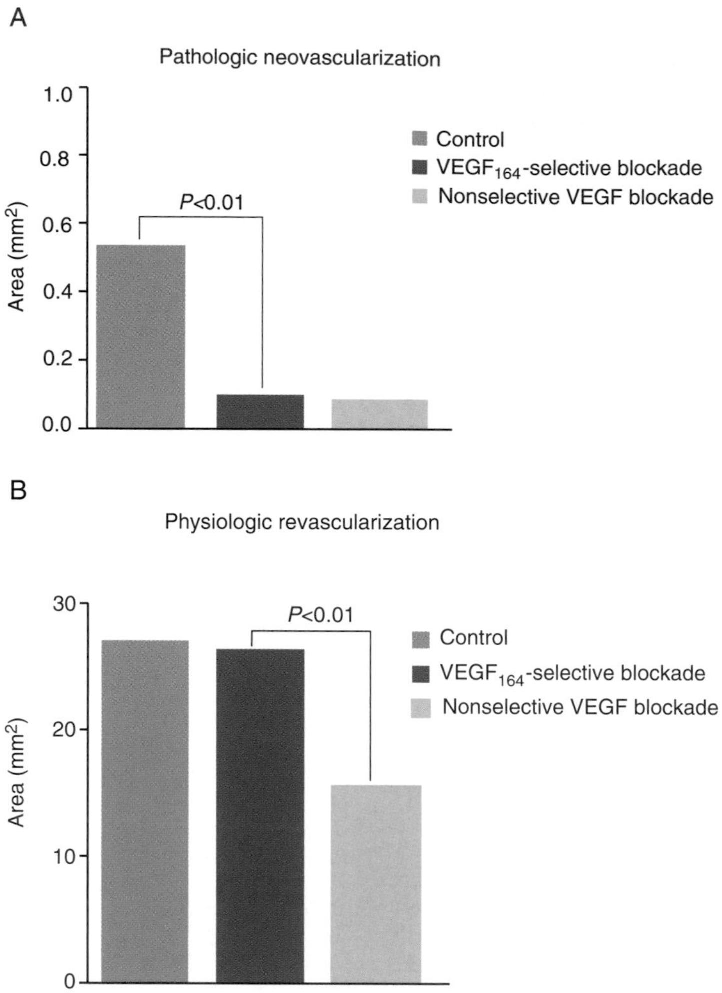

Fig. 14. Antivascular endothelial growth factor (VEGF) blockade inhibits pathologic neovascularization. In a rat ischemic retinopathy model (see Fig. 8 for description), pathologic neovascular budding into the vitreous (**A**) was significantly suppressed either by pegaptanib, an anti-$VEGF_{164}$ aptamer, or a VEGF receptor-1/Fc fusion protein that blocks the activity of all VEGF isoforms. In contrast, the effect of $VEGF_{164}$ inhibition on physiologic revascularization (that occurring in normal developing rat retinas) (**B**) was negligible, but pan-isoform inhibition with the fusion protein led to significant suppression of revascularization. (Reproduced from Ishida et al. 2003 *(55)* with permission from J Exp Med.)

(90) or serum *(5)* of patients with DR. Vitreous elevations in TNF-α in patients with proliferative DR were reported in one study *(5)*, although another study found no difference in the vitreous levels of TNF-α between those with proliferative DR and those with noninflammatory retinopathies *(7)*. A correlation between the expression of a particular TNF-α polymorphism and a susceptibility to DR has also been reported *(91)*.

The direct involvement of TNF-α in the vascular pathology associated with DR was examined by Joussen et al. *(92)* in the STZ-induced diabetic rat. Systemic administration of etanercept, a soluble TNF-α receptor/Fc construct significantly reduced diabetes-induced elevation of ICAM-1 and suppressed leukocyte adhesion and BRB breakdown but did not affect retinal VEGF levels *(92)*. One possible explanation for these findings is that etanercept inhibited TNF-α–mediated upregulation of VEGF receptor-2 expression *(93)*. Another potential mechanism, not exclusive of effects on VEGF receptor-2, involves TNF-α–induced activation of protein kinase C-β2, which in turn has been correlated with increased leukocyte adhesion to endothelial cells *(90)*. Irrespective of the molecular details, these data indicate that the TNF-α–mediated effects on ICAM-1, leukocyte adhesion, and BRB breakdown are independent of VEGF so that combinatorial approaches involving the inactivation of both proteins may hold promise.

STUDIES WITH ANTI-INFLAMMATORY AGENTS LINK DIABETIC RETINOPATHY AND INFLAMMATION

Nonsteroidal Anti-inflammatory Drugs (NSAIDs)

As mentioned earlier, Powell and Field *(1)* first proposed the link between DR and inflammation on the basis of a 1964 retrospective study, in which the incidence of DR appeared to be significantly reduced among diabetic patients suffering from rheumatoid arthritis. The authors suggested that one possibility for the lowered incidence was the high dosing of salicylates taken as anti-inflammatory medications in this cohort. This proposal has since provided the impetus for a number of studies confirming this effect and examining potential underlying cellular and molecular mechanisms. In a 5-year dog study, the daily administration of aspirin at doses of 20 mg/kg^{-1} resulted in a significant reduction in the development of retinal hemorrhages and acellular capillaries *(94)*; this dose is equivalent to 1.4 g per day for a 70-kg patient, which is lower than the usual clinical doses. In the STZ rat model of diabetes, the administration of high-dose aspirin (50 mg/kg^{-1} per day) resulted in a significant suppression of BRB breakdown as well as a reduction in the adhesion of leukocytes to retinal arterioles, venules, and capillaries *(92)*. These reductions were accompanied by a significant inhibition of diabetes-induced retinal expression of ICAM-1 and a decrease in neutrophil expression of the integrin subunits CD11a, CD11b, and CD18. In addition, the upregulation of ICAM-1 expression was inhibited by the administration of meloxicam, an inhibitor of cyclooxygenase-2 (COX-2), although meloxicam did not affect the diabetes-induced integrin expression on neutrophils, nor did aspirin or meloxicam affect the elevated retinal levels of VEGF *(92)*. These results suggest that anti-inflammatory agents might provide additive benefits if combined with targeted anti-VEGF therapies.

In further experiments with the STZ-induced diabetic rat model, periocular injection of celecoxib-poly (lactide-co-glycolide) microparticles, also directed against COX-2, significantly reduced diabetes-induced BRB breakdown and elevations in prostaglandin E_2 and VEGF expression *(95)*. Similar protective effects for the retinal vasculature were reported in STZ-induced rats given daily aspirin doses of 30 mg/kg^{-1}; this treatment did not prevent abnormalities in glial cells or neurons, suggesting that inflammatory changes associated with diabetes are focused on the vasculature *(96)*. However, it was later found that three different salicylate-based drugs (aspirin, sodium salicylate, and sulfasalazine) were all able to inhibit diabetes-induced loss of both capillaries and retinal ganglion cells in rats *(32)*. These effects were accompanied by inhibition of the action of nuclear factor-κB, a transcription factor important in increasing proinflammatory gene transcription, so that upregulation of ICAM-1, vascular cell adhesion molecule, inducible nitrogen oxide synthase, and COX-2 were all inhibited *(32)*. Finally, it was recently reported that the application of nepafenac, a NSAID-prodrug COX-1 and COX-2 inhibitor that reaches the retina when applied topically, was also able to inhibit damage to the retinal vasculature in the diabetic rat *(97)*.

The original proposal by Powell and Field *(1)*, that salicylates could offer therapeutic benefit in DR, was examined in two randomized, controlled trials. Analysis of data from the Early Treatment of Diabetic Retinopathy Study *(98)* determined that relatively low doses of aspirin (650 mg per day) provided no clinical benefit to patients with mild to severe nonproliferative or early proliferative DR. More encouraging results were seen in the Dipyridamole Aspirin Microangiopathy of Diabetes Study *(99)* in which patients with early-stage retinopathy received aspirin at doses of 990 mg per day. There was a significant slowing in the progressive increase in the number of microaneurysms, a surrogate for increased severity of retinopathy, in the aspirin-treated group *(99)*. As described earlier, this area remains under intensive study, with the promise that topically applied drugs in this group may be useful in treating DR *(97)*.

Corticosteroids

Corticosteroids have long been the agents of choice in treating inflammatory disorders, and the synthetic corticosteroid triamcinolone acetonide has been employed in many preclinical and clinical investigations in the treatment of DR and other ocular diseases with an inflammatory component *(100)*. Evidence for the mechanisms underlying the anti-inflammatory effects of triamcinolone in the eye has been derived from preclinical studies on cultured human choroidal endothelial cells where it significantly inhibited the upregulation of ICAM-1 by inflammatory cytokines *(101)*. In addition, triamcinolone also reduced the expression of VEGF in response to hypoxia in cultured retinal pigment epithelium cells *(102)*. These findings have laid the basis for numerous clinical investigations with intravitreous triamcinolone, discussed in detail in Chapter 19 of this book.

Anti-TNF-α Antibody

Direct evidence supporting a role for TNF-α in DR comes from a small case series in which infliximab, an antibody directed against TNF-α, was administered intravenously to four patients with seven eyes affected by DR *(103)*. Within 1 month, improvements in visual acuity and reductions in macular thickness were seen in five of the eyes. Similar improvements were also seen using the same approach to treat age-related macular degeneration *(104)*. These data, while based on very small samples, nonetheless suggest that therapies directed against TNF-α well may prove to be a useful target in treating DR, whether used alone or in combination with agents that inactivate VEGF. Moreover, the recent experience with VEGF-targeted agents suggests that inactivating TNF-α with agents that can be delivered intravitreously may provide greater therapeutic benefit compared to the intravenous administration used heretofore.

Anti-VEGF Agents

Pegaptanib

The preclinical data suggesting that $VEGF_{165}$ was especially pathogenic, and that its inhibition with pegaptanib could reverse BRB breakdown, provided the basis for a proof-of-concept Phase 2 double-masked, multicenter, randomized, controlled trial enrolling 172 patients with DME *(105)*. Patients received intravitreous pegaptanib (0.3 mg, 1 mg, or 3 mg) or sham injections at study entry, Week 6, and Week 12, with additional injections and/or focal photocoagulation given at the investigator's discretion through 30 weeks; final assessments were made 6 weeks later. In this dose-ranging study, no additional benefit was conferred at doses above 0.3 mg. This dose proved significantly superior to sham for all prespecified endpoints (median visual acuity, change in mean central retinal thickness, and need for photocoagulation therapy), and the drug was well-tolerated *(105)*.

In a subsequent retrospective analysis of 16 patients who entered the trial with retinal neovascularization, 8 of 13 who received pegaptanib showed complete regression of neovascularization or regression at 36 weeks *(106)*. None of the three patients with neovascularization in the sham group and none of four with neovascularization in the fellow eye showed complete regression. Among the eight patients whose neovascularization regressed with pegaptanib, three experienced progression at Week 52 following pegaptanib cessation at Week 30 *(106)*. Similar encouraging results, demonstrating regression in response to pegaptanib treatment, have since been reported in an open-label case series in patients with high-risk proliferative DR *(107)*.

Ranibizumab and Bevacizumab

Ranibizumab and bevacizumab, two nonselective agents that bind all VEGF isoforms, have been studied in small-scale trials as intravitreous treatments for DR and DME. Ranibizumab, a humanized antibody fragment engineered for high-affinity binding to VEGF *(108)*, has been examined in two pilot open-label studies, each involving 10 patients with DME *(109, 110)*. Both studies reported improvements in visual acuity and reductions in macular thickness; Nguyen et al. *(109)* reported no adverse events, while Chun et al. *(110)* encountered five cases of mild to moderate ocular inflammation.

Bevacizumab, a full-length monoclonal antibody related to ranibizumab that is approved for treatment of cancer *(108)*, was shown to be effective in small studies in inducing regression of iris *(111)* and retinal *(112)* neovascularization in patients with DR. In a case series involving patients with retinal and/or iris neovascularization, all 44 eyes with angiographically defined neovascularization that were treated with intravitreous bevacizumab (with doses ranging from 6.2 μg to 1.25 mg) showed a reduction in leakage within 1 week of injection; complete resolution of leakage was seen in 9 of the 11 cases of iris neovascularization and in 19 of 26 cases involving neovascularization of the disk *(113)*. In two patients receiving 1.25 mg, there was also some decrease in the leakage of retinal or iris neovascularization of the untreated fellow eye, indicating that systemic exposure may have occurred *(113)*.

These findings suggest that strategies targeting VEGF hold promise in treating DR and DME. Both pegaptanib and ranibizumab are clinically approved reagents for neovascular age-related macular degeneration after demonstrating acceptable tolerability profiles in pivotal randomized controlled trials. It remains to be established, however, whether their use in treating DR and DME, manifestations of a complex systemic disease, will also prove to be safe. With respect to bevacizumab, its safety as an intravitreous agent has yet to be examined in a controlled trial.

CONCLUSIONS

Since the initial proposal of Powell and Field *(1)* that DR is an inflammatory disease, both and preclinical clinical investigations have supported the importance of the influx of inflammatory cells, as well as the role of proinflammatory cytokines, in mediating both vascular damage and ischemia-induced neovascularization. These data support the concept that DR is a low-grade inflammatory disease. There is now strong evidence that VEGF, originally characterized as a promoter of angiogenesis, is itself a promoter of inflammatory processes, with the $VEGF_{165}$ isoform being especially potent in this respect. The perspective of DR as an inflammatory disease has already provided the basis for several therapeutic approaches, including VEGF-targeted agents, corticosteroids, and NSAIDs. There is every reason for optimism that additional studies of the roles played by VEGF and other inflammatory cytokines will lead to further advances, including the rational design of combinatorial approaches employing more than one therapeutic agent in the treatment of DR.

ACKNOWLEDGMENT

The development of this chapter was supported by (OSI) Eyetech and Pfizer Inc.

REFERENCES

1. Powell ED, Field RA. Diabetic retinopathy and rheumatoid arthritis. Lancet 1964;41:17–8.
2. Antonetti DA, Barber AJ, Bronson SK, et al. Diabetic retinopathy: seeing beyond glucose-induced microvascular disease. Diabetes 2006;55:2401–11.
3. Aiello LP, Avery RL, Arrigg PG, et al. Vascular endothelial growth factor in ocular fluid of patients with diabetic retinopathy and other retinal disorders. N Engl J Med 1994;331:1480–7.
4. Adamis AP, Miller JW, Bernal MT, et al. Increased vascular endothelial growth factor levels in the vitreous of eyes with proliferative diabetic retinopathy. Am J Ophthalmol 1994;118(4):445–50.
5. Demircan N, Safran BG, Soylu M, Ozcan AA, Sizmaz S. Determination of vitreous interleukin-1 (IL-1) and tumour necrosis factor (TNF) levels in proliferative diabetic retinopathy. Eye 2006;20:1366–9.
6. Funatsu H, Yamashita H, Shimizu E, Kojima R, Hori S. Relationship between vascular endothelial growth factor and interleukin-6 in diabetic retinopathy. Retina 2001;21:469–77.
7. Yuuki T, Kanda T, Kimura Y, et al. Inflammatory cytokines in vitreous fluid and serum of patients with diabetic vitreoretinopathy. J Diabetes Complications 2001;15:257–9.
8. Canataroglu H, Varinli I, Ozcan AA, Canataroglu A, Doran F, Varinli S. Interleukin (IL)-6, interleukin (IL)-8 levels and cellular composition of the vitreous humor in proliferative diabetic retinopathy, proliferative vitreoretinopathy, and traumatic proliferative vitreoretinopathy. Ocul Immunol Inflamm 2005;13:375–81.
9. Brooks HL Jr, Caballero S Jr, Newell CK, et al. Vitreous levels of vascular endothelial growth factor and stromal-derived factor 1 in patients with diabetic retinopathy and cystoid macular edema before and after intraocular injection of triamcinolone. Arch Ophthalmol 2004;122:1801–7.
10. Funatsu H, Yamashita H, Ikeda T, Nakanishi Y, Kitano S, Hori S. Angiotensin II and vascular endothelial growth factor in the vitreous fluid of patients with diabetic macular edema and other retinal disorders. Am J Ophthalmol 2002;133:537–43.

11. Patel JI, Hykin PG, Gregor ZJ, Boulton M, Cree IA. Angiopoietin concentrations in diabetic retinopathy. Br J Ophthalmol 2005;89:480–3.
12. Watanabe D, Suzuma K, Suzuma I, et al. Vitreous levels of angiopoietin 2 and vascular endothelial growth factor in patients with proliferative diabetic retinopathy. Am J Ophthalmol 2005;139:476–81.
13. Watanabe D, Suzuma K, Matsui S, et al. Erythropoietin as a retinal angiogenic factor in proliferative diabetic retinopathy. N Engl J Med 2005;353:782–92.
14. Hernandez C, Fonollosa A, Garcia-Ramirez M, et al. Erythropoietin is expressed in the human retina and it is highly elevated in the vitreous fluid of patients with diabetic macular edema. Diabetes Care 2006;29:2028–33.
15. Limb GA, Chignell AH, Green W, LeRoy F, Dumonde DC. Distribution of TNF alpha and its reactive vascular adhesion molecules in fibrovascular membranes of proliferative diabetic retinopathy. Br J Ophthalmol 1996;80:168–73.
16. Meleth AD, Agron E, Chan CC, et al. Serum inflammatory markers in diabetic retinopathy. Invest Ophthalmol Vis Sci 2005;46:4295–301.
17. Barber AJ, Lieth E, Khin SA, Antonetti DA, Buchanan AG, Gardner TW. Neural apoptosis in the retina during experimental and human diabetes. Early onset and effect of insulin. J Clin Invest 1998;102:783–91.
18. Mizutani M, Kern TS, Lorenzi M. Accelerated death of retinal microvascular cells in human and experimental diabetic retinopathy. J Clin Invest 1996;97:2883–90.
19. Esser P, Heimann K, Wiedemann P. Macrophages in proliferative vitreoretinopathy and proliferative diabetic retinopathy: differentiation of subpopulations. Br J Ophthalmol 1993;77:731–3.
20. Rungger-Brandle E, Dosso AA, Leuenberger PM. Glial reactivity, an early feature of diabetic retinopathy. Invest Ophthalmol Vis Sci 2000;41:1971–80.
21. Zeng XX, Ng YK, Ling EA. Neuronal and microglial response in the retina of streptozotocin-induced diabetic rats. Vis Neurosci 2000;17:463–71.
22. Krady JK, Basu A, Allen CM, et al. Minocycline reduces proinflammatory cytokine expression, microglial activation, and caspase-3 activation in a rodent model of diabetic retinopathy. Diabetes 2005;54:1559–65.
23. Miyamoto K, Khosrof S, Bursell SE, et al. Prevention of leukostasis and vascular leakage in streptozotocin-induced diabetic retinopathy via intercellular adhesion molecule-1 inhibition. Proc Natl Acad Sci USA 1999;96:10836–41.
24. Joussen AM, Poulaki V, Le ML, et al. A central role for inflammation in the pathogenesis of diabetic retinopathy. FASEB J 2004;18:1450–2.
25. Zhang J, Gerhardinger C, Lorenzi M. Early complement activation and decreased levels of glycosylphosphatidylinositol-anchored complement inhibitors in human and experimental diabetic retinopathy. Diabetes 2002;51:3499–504.
26. Joussen AM, Poulaki V, Mitsiades N, et al. Suppression of Fas-FasL-induced endothelial cell apoptosis prevents diabetic blood-retinal barrier breakdown in a model of streptozotocin-induced diabetes. FASEB J 2003;17:76–8.
27. Gerhardinger C, Costa MB, Coulombe MC, Toth I, Hoehn T, Grosu P. Expression of acute-phase response proteins in retinal Müller cells in diabetes. Invest Ophthalmol Vis Sci 2005;46:349–57.
28. Brownlee M. Biochemistry and molecular cell biology of diabetic complications. Nature 2001;414:813–20.
29. Sheetz MJ, King GL. Molecular understanding of hyperglycemia's adverse effects for diabetic complications. JAMA 2002;288:2579–88.
30. Caldwell RB, Bartoli M, Behzadian MA, et al. Vascular endothelial growth factor and diabetic retinopathy: pathophysiological mechanisms and treatment perspectives. Diabetes Metab Res Rev 2003;19:442–55.
31. Gardner TW, Antonetti DA, Barber AJ, LaNoue KF, Levison SW. Diabetic retinopathy: more than meets the eye. Surv Ophthalmol 2002;47:Suppl 2:S253–62.
32. Zheng L, Howell SJ, Hatala DA, Huang K, Kern TS. Salicylate-based anti-inflammatory drugs inhibit the early lesion of diabetic retinopathy. Diabetes 2007;56:337–45.
33. McLeod DS, Lefer DJ, Merges C, Lutty GA. Enhanced expression of intercellular adhesion molecule-1 and P-selectin in the diabetic human retina and choroid. Am J Pathol 1995;147:642–53.

34. Funatsu H, Yamashita H, Sakata K, et al. Vitreous levels of vascular endothelial growth factor and intercellular adhesion molecule 1 are related to diabetic macular edema. Ophthalmology 2005;112:806–16.
35. Lutty GA, Cao J, McLeod DS. Relationship of polymorphonuclear leukocytes to capillary dropout in the human diabetic choroid. Am J Pathol 1997;151:707–14.
36. Kim SY, Johnson MA, McLeod DS, Alexander T, Hansen BC, Lutty GA. Neutrophils are associated with capillary closure in spontaneously diabetic monkey retinas. Diabetes 2005;54:1534–42.
37. Schroder S, Palinski W, Schmid-Schonbein GW. Activated monocytes and granulocytes, capillary nonperfusion, and neovascularization in diabetic retinopathy. Am J Pathol 1991;139:81–100.
38. Miyamoto K, Hiroshiba N, Tsujikawa A, Ogura Y. In vivo demonstration of increased leukocyte entrapment in retinal microcirculation of diabetic rats. Invest Ophthalmol Vis Sci 1998;39:2190–4.
39. Barouch FC, Miyamoto K, Allport JR, et al. Integrin-mediated neutrophil adhesion and retinal leukostasis in diabetes. Invest Ophthalmol Vis Sci 2000;41:1153–8.
40. Song H, Wang L, Hui Y. Expression of CD18 on the neutrophils of patients with diabetic retinopathy. Graefes Arch Clin Exp Ophthalmol 2007;245:24–31.
41. Del Maschio A, Zanetti A, Corada M, et al. Polymorphonuclear leukocyte adhesion triggers the disorganization of endothelial cell-to-cell adherens junctions. J Cell Biol 1996;135:497–510.
42. Bolton SJ, Anthony DC, Perry VH. Loss of the tight junction proteins occludin and zonula occludens-1 from cerebral vascular endothelium during neutrophil-induced blood-brain barrier breakdown in vivo. Neuroscience 1998;86:1245–57.
43. Iijima K, Yoshikawa N, Connolly DT, Nakamura H. Human mesangial cells and peripheral blood mononuclear cells produce vascular permeability factor. Kidney Int 1993;44:959–66.
44. Freeman MR, Schneck FX, Gagnon ML, et al. Peripheral blood T lymphocytes and lymphocytes infiltrating human cancers express vascular endothelial growth factor: a potential role for T cells in angiogenesis. Cancer Res 1995;55:4140–5.
45. Gaudry M, Bregerie O, Andrieu V, El Benna J, Pocidalo MA, Hakim J. Intracellular pool of vascular endothelial growth factor in human neutrophils. Blood 1997;90:4153–61.
46. Horiuchi T, Weller PF. Expression of vascular endothelial growth factor by human eosinophils: upregulation by granulocyte macrophage colony-stimulating factor and interleukin-5. Am J Respir Cell Mol Biol 1997;17:70–7.
47. Joussen AM, Murata T, Tsujikawa A, Kirchhof B, Bursell SE, Adamis AP. Leukocyte-mediated endothelial cell injury and death in the diabetic retina. Am J Pathol 2001;158:147–52.
48. Boeri D, Maiello M, Lorenzi M. Increased prevalence of microthromboses in retinal capillaries of diabetic individuals. Diabetes 2001;50:1432–9.
49. Ishibashi T, Tanaka K, Taniguchi Y. Platelet aggregation and coagulation in the pathogenesis of diabetic retinopathy in rats. Diabetes 1981;30:601–6.
50. Yamashiro K, Tsujikawa A, Ishida S, et al. Platelets accumulate in the diabetic retinal vasculature following endothelial death and suppress blood-retinal barrier breakdown. Am J Pathol 2003;163:253–9.
51. Sharma NK, Gardiner TA, Archer DB. A morphologic and autoradiographic study of cell death and regeneration in the retinal microvasculature of normal and diabetic rats. Am J Ophthalmol 1985;100:51–60.
52. Segal MS, Shah R, Afzal A, et al. Nitric oxide cytoskeletal-induced alterations reverse the endothelial progenitor cell migratory defect associated with diabetes. Diabetes 2006;55:102–9.
53. Tepper OM, Galiano RD, Capla JM, et al. Human endothelial progenitor cells from type II diabetics exhibit impaired proliferation, adhesion, and incorporation into vascular structures. Circulation 2002;106:2781–6.
54. Caballero S, Sengupta N, Afzal A, et al. Ischemic vascular damage can be repaired by healthy, but not diabetic, endothelial progenitor cells. Diabetes 2007;56:960–7.
55. Ishida S, Usui T, Yamashiro K, et al. VEGF164-mediated inflammation is required for pathological, but not physiological, ischemia-induced retinal neovascularization. J Exp Med 2003;198:483–9.
56. Clauss M, Gerlach M, Gerlach H, et al. Vascular permeability factor: a tumor-derived polypeptide that induces endothelial cell and monocyte procoagulant activity, and promotes monocyte migration. J Exp Med 1990;172:1535–45.
57. Barleon B, Sozzani S, Zhou D, Weich HA, Mantovani A, Marme D. Migration of human monocytes in response to vascular endothelial growth factor (VEGF) is mediated via the VEGF receptor flt-1. Blood 1996;87:3336–43.

58. Usui T, Ishida S, Yamashiro K, et al. $VEGF_{164(165)}$ as the pathological isoform: differential leukocyte and endothelial responses through VEGFR1 and VEGFR2. Invest Ophthalmol Vis Sci 2004;45:368–74.
59. Harmey JH, Dimitriadis E, Kay E, Redmond HP, Bouchier-Hayes D. Regulation of macrophage production of vascular endothelial growth factor (VEGF) by hypoxia and transforming growth factor beta-1. Ann Surg Oncol 1998;5:271–8.
60. Grossniklaus HE, Ling JX, Wallace TM, et al. Macrophage and retinal pigment epithelium expression of angiogenic cytokines in choroidal neovascularization. Mol Vis 2002;8:119–26.
61. Espinosa-Heidmann DG, Suner IJ, Hernandez EP, Monroy D, Csaky KG, Cousins SW. Macrophage depletion diminishes lesion size and severity in experimental choroidal neovascularization. Invest Ophthalmol Vis Sci 2003;44:3586–92.
62. Sakurai E, Anand A, Ambati BK, van Rooijen N, Ambati J. Macrophage depletion inhibits experimental choroidal neovascularization. Invest Ophthalmol Vis Sci 2003;44:3578–85.
63. Tsutsumi C, Sonoda KH, Egashira K, et al. The critical role of ocular-infiltrating macrophages in the development of choroidal neovascularization. J Leukoc Biol 2003;74:25–32.
64. Ishida S, Yamashiro K, Usui T, et al. Leukocytes mediate retinal vascular remodeling during development and vaso-obliteration in disease. Nat Med 2003;9:781–8.
65. Koyama R, Nakanishi T, Ikeda T, Shimizu A. Catalogue of soluble proteins in human vitreous humor by one-dimensional sodium dodecyl sulfate-polyacrylamide gel electrophoresis and electrospray ionization mass spectrometry including seven angiogenesis-regulating factors. J Chromatogr B Anal Technol Biomed Life Sci 2003;792:5–21.
66. Gao BB, Clermont A, Rook S, et al. Extracellular carbonic anhydrase mediates hemorrhagic retinal and cerebral vascular permeability through prekallikrein activation. Nat Med 2007;13:181–8.
67. Joussen AM, Huang S, Poulaki V, et al. In vivo retinal gene expression in early diabetes. Invest Ophthalmol Vis Sci 2001;42:3047–57.
68. Starita C, Patel M, Katz B, Adamis AP. Vascular endothelial growth factor and the potential therapeutic use of pegaptanib (Macugen) in diabetic retinopathy. Dev Ophthalmol 2007;39:122–48.
69. Kuroki M, Voest EE, Amano S, et al. Reactive oxygen intermediates increase vascular endothelial growth factor expression in vitro and in vivo. J Clin Invest 1996;98:1667–75.
70. Lu M, Kuroki M, Amano S, et al. Advanced glycation end products increase retinal vascular endothelial growth factor expression. J Clin Invest 1998;101:1219–24.
71. Poulaki V, Joussen AM, Mitsiades N, Mitsiades CS, Iliaki EF, Adamis AP. Insulin-like growth factor-I plays a pathogenetic role in diabetic retinopathy. Am J Pathol 2004;165:457–69.
72. Hangai M, He S, Hoffmann S, Lim JI, Ryan SJ, Hinton DR. Sequential induction of angiogenic growth factors by TNF-alpha in choroidal endothelial cells. J Neuroimmunol 2006;171:45–56.
73. Ng EW, Adamis AP. Targeting angiogenesis, the underlying disorder in neovascular age-related macular degeneration. Can J Ophthalmol 2005;40:352–68.
74. Senger DR, Connolly DT, Van de Water L, Feder J, Dvorak HF. Purification and NH2-terminal amino acid sequence of guinea pig tumor-secreted vascular permeability factor. Cancer Res 1990;50:1774–8.
75. Aiello LP, Northrup JM, Keyt BA, Takagi H, Iwamoto MA. Hypoxic regulation of vascular endothelial growth factor in retinal cells. Arch Ophthalmol 1995;113:1538–44.
76. Famiglietti EV, Stopa EG, McGookin ED, Song P, LeBlanc V, Streeten BW. Immunocytochemical localization of vascular endothelial growth factor in neurons and glial cells of human retina. Brain Res 2003;969:195–204.
77. Blaauwgeers HG, Holtkamp GM, Rutten H, et al. Polarized vascular endothelial growth factor secretion by human retinal pigment epithelium and localization of vascular endothelial growth factor receptors on the inner choriocapillaris. Evidence for a trophic paracrine relation. Am J Pathol 1999;155:421–8.
78. Tolentino MJ, Miller JW, Gragoudas ES, et al. Intravitreous injections of vascular endothelial growth factor produce retinal ischemia and microangiopathy in an adult primate. Ophthalmology 1996; 103:1820–8.
79. Qaum T, Xu Q, Joussen AM, et al. VEGF-initiated blood-retinal barrier breakdown in early diabetes. Invest Ophthalmol Vis Sci 2001;42:2408–13.
80. Joussen AM, Poulaki V, Qin W, et al. Retinal vascular endothelial growth factor induces intercellular adhesion molecule-1 and endothelial nitric oxide synthase expression and initiates early diabetic retinal leukocyte adhesion in vivo. Am J Pathol 2002;160:501–9.

81. Miyamoto K, Khosrof S, Bursell SE, et al. Vascular endothelial growth factor (VEGF)-induced retinal vascular permeability is mediated by intercellular adhesion molecule-1 (ICAM-1). Am J Pathol 2000;156:1733–9.
82. Ishida S, Usui T, Yamashiro K, et al. $VEGF_{164}$ is proinflammatory in the diabetic retina. Invest Ophthalmol Vis Sci 2003;44:2155–62.
83. Taylor PC, Williams RO, Feldmann M. Tumour necrosis factor alpha as a therapeutic target for immune-mediated inflammatory diseases. Curr Opin Biotechnol 2004;15:557–63.
84. Navarro JF, Mora-Fernandez C. The role of TNF-alpha in diabetic nephropathy: pathogenic and therapeutic implications. Cytokine Growth Factor Rev 2006;17:441–50.
85. Cantor J, Haskins K. Effector function of diabetogenic CD4 Th1 T cell clones: a central role for TNF-alpha. J Immunol 2005;175:7738–45.
86. Kasama T, Miwa Y, Isozaki T, Odai T, Adachi M, Kunkel SL. Neutrophil-derived cytokines: potential therapeutic targets in inflammation. Curr Drug Targets Inflamm Allergy 2005;4:273–9.
87. Eizirik DL, Mandrup-Poulsen T. A choice of death–the signal-transduction of immune-mediated beta-cell apoptosis. Diabetologia 2001;44:2115–33.
88. Ruan H, Lodish HF. Insulin resistance in adipose tissue: direct and indirect effects of tumor necrosis factor-alpha. Cytokine Growth Factor Rev 2003;14:447–55.
89. Limb GA, Webster L, Soomro H, Janikoun S, Shilling J. Platelet expression of tumour necrosis factor-alpha (TNF-alpha), TNF receptors and intercellular adhesion molecule-1 (ICAM-1) in patients with proliferative diabetic retinopathy. Clin Exp Immunol 1999;118:213–8.
90. Ben-Mahmud BM, Mann GE, Datti A, Orlacchio A, Kohner EM, Chibber R. Tumor necrosis factor-alpha in diabetic plasma increases the activity of core 2 GlcNAc-T and adherence of human leukocytes to retinal endothelial cells: significance of core 2 GlcNAc-T in diabetic retinopathy. Diabetes 2004;53:2968–76.
91. Hawrami K, Hitman GA, Rema M, et al. An association in non-insulin-dependent diabetes mellitus subjects between susceptibility to retinopathy and tumor necrosis factor polymorphism. Hum Immunol 1996;46:49–54.
92. Joussen AM, Poulaki V, Mitsiades N, et al. Nonsteroidal anti-inflammatory drugs prevent early diabetic retinopathy via TNF-alpha suppression. FASEB J 2002;16:438–40.
93. Giraudo E, Primo L, Audero E, et al. Tumor necrosis factor-alpha regulates expression of vascular endothelial growth factor receptor-2 and of its co-receptor neuropilin-1 in human vascular endothelial cells. J Biol Chem 1998;273:22128–35.
94. Kern TS, Engerman RL. Pharmacological inhibition of diabetic retinopathy: aminoguanidine and aspirin. Diabetes 2001;50:1636–42.
95. Amrite AC, Ayalasomayajula SP, Cheruvu NP, Kompella UB. Single periocular injection of celecoxib-PLGA microparticles inhibits diabetes-induced elevations in retinal PGE_2, VEGF, and vascular leakage. Invest Ophthalmol Vis Sci 2006;47:1149–60.
96. Sun W, Gerhardinger C, Dagher Z, Hoehn T, Lorenzi M. Aspirin at low-intermediate concentrations protects retinal vessels in experimental diabetic retinopathy through non-platelet-mediated effects. Diabetes 2005;54:3418–26.
97. Kern TS, Miller CM, Du Y, et al. Topical administration of nepafenac inhibits diabetes-induced retinal microvascular disease and underlying abnormalities of retinal metabolism and physiology. Diabetes 2007;56:373–9.
98. ETDRS Study Group. Effects of aspirin treatment on diabetic retinopathy. ETDRS report number 8. Early Treatment of Diabetic Retinopathy Study Research Group. Ophthalmology 1991;98:5 Suppl:S757–65.
99. DAMAD Study Group. Effect of aspirin alone and aspirin plus dipyridamole in early diabetic retinopathy. A multicenter randomized controlled clinical trial. Diabetes 1989;38:491–8.
100. Jonas JB. Intravitreal triamcinolone acetonide: a change in a paradigm. Ophthalmic Res 2006; 38:218–45.
101. Penfold PL, Wen L, Madigan MC, King NJ, Provis JM. Modulation of permeability and adhesion molecule expression by human choroidal endothelial cells. Invest Ophthalmol Vis Sci 2002; 43:3125–30.
102. Matsuda S, Gomi F, Oshima Y, Tohyama M, Tano Y. Vascular endothelial growth factor reduced and connective tissue growth factor induced by triamcinolone in ARPE19 cells under oxidative stress. Invest Ophthalmol Vis Sci 2005;46:1062–8.

103. Sfikakis PP, Markomichelakis N, Theodossiadis GP, Grigoropoulos V, Katsilambros N, Theodossiadis PG. Regression of sight-threatening macular edema in type 2 diabetes following treatment with the anti-tumor necrosis factor monoclonal antibody infliximab. Diabetes Care 2005;28:445–7.
104. Markomichelakis NN, Theodossiadis PG, Sfikakis PP. Regression of neovascular age-related macular degeneration following infliximab therapy. Am J Ophthalmol 2005;139:537–40.
105. Cunningham ET Jr, Adamis AP, Altaweel M, et al. A phase II randomized double-masked trial of pegaptanib, an anti-vascular endothelial growth factor aptamer, for diabetic macular edema. Ophthalmology 2005;112:1747–57.
106. Adamis AP, Altaweel M, Bressler NM, et al. Changes in retinal neovascularization after pegaptanib (Macugen) therapy in diabetic individuals. Ophthalmology 2006;113:23–8.
107. Gonzalez V. Selective VEGF inhibition: effectiveness in modifying the progression of proliferative diabetic retinopathy. In: Annual Meeting of the American Academy of Ophthalmology; November 12, 2006; Las Vegas, Nevada; poster 309.
108. Ferrara N, Damico L, Shams N, Lowman H, Kim R. Development of ranibizumab, an anti-vascular endothelial growth factor antigen binding fragment, as therapy for neovascular age-related macular degeneration. Retina 2006;26(8):859–70.
109. Nguyen QD, Tatlipinar S, Shah SM, et al. Vascular endothelial growth factor is a critical stimulus for diabetic macular edema. Am J Ophthalmol 2006;142:961–9.
110. Chun DW, Heier JS, Topping TM, Duker JS, Bankert JM. A pilot study of multiple intravitreal injections of ranibizumab in patients with center-involving clinically significant diabetic macular edema. Ophthalmology 2006;113:1706–12.
111. Oshima Y, Sakaguchi H, Gomi F, Tano Y. Regression of iris neovascularization after intravitreal injection of bevacizumab in patients with proliferative diabetic retinopathy. Am J Ophthalmol 2006;142:155–8.
112. Mason JO III, Nixon PA, White MF. Intravitreal injection of bevacizumab (Avastin) as adjunctive treatment of proliferative diabetic retinopathy. Am J Ophthalmol 2006;142:685–8.
113. Avery RL, Pearlman J, Pieramici DJ, et al. Intravitreal bevacizumab (Avastin) in the treatment of proliferative diabetic retinopathy. Ophthalmology 2006;113:1695 e1–15.

14 Vascular Permeability in Diabetic Retinopathy

Vascular Permeability in Diabetic Retinopathy

David A. Antonetti, Heather D. VanGuilder, and Cheng Mao-Lin

CONTENTS

ABSTRACT

A hallmark of diabetic retinopathy is increased vascular permeability. The vasculature of the retina, which normally has tight control of the fluid and blood components that enter the retina, becomes leaky in diabetes leading to increased albumin flux into the retina, fluid accumulation, and macular edema, and over time may progress to hemorrhaging vessels. This chapter investigates our knowledge regarding the formation of the blood–brain and blood–retinal barrier. The molecular composition of the junctional complex that forms the basis of the blood–retinal barrier will be briefly reviewed and the changes that occur to the junctional complex in diabetes will be examined. Changes in permeability and the contribution of inflammatory cytokines in addition to vascular endothelial growth factor will be presented and potential therapies will be considered. It is the goal of this chapter that the reader will have a fundamental understanding of the development and structure of the blood–retinal barrier and know-ledge of our current understanding of the alterations to the junctional complex that contribute to vessel permeability in diabetic retinopathy.

From: *Contemporary Diabetes: Diabetic Retinopathy*
Edited by: E. Duh © Humana Press, Totowa, NJ

Key Words: Blood–retinal barrier (BRB); blood–brain barrier (BBB); claudin; occluding; permeability; tight junctions.

FORMATION OF THE BLOOD–RETINAL BARRIER

The central nervous system (CNS), including the brain and retina, require the development of a blood–neural barrier for proper neuronal function. In the retina this barrier includes the retinal pigment epithelium (RPE) and the vascular network that creates the capillary plexus in the ganglion cell layer and a deeper plexus extending from the inner plexiform layer through the inner nuclear layer to the outer plexiform layer *(1)*. The blood–brain and blood–retinal barrier (BRB) provide tight control of the nutrients, metabolic intermediates and fluid that enter the neural parenchyma and is often compromised in disease states. Formation of the blood–brain and BRBs requires a complex interaction of multiple cell types including the endothelial cells of the blood vessels, astrocytes, Müller cells, and pericytes.

Glia-Endothelial Interaction

Blood vessels in the CNS differentiate to form the BBB and BRB through signaling from the neural environment. One of the first demonstrations of the ability of neural tissue to induce formation of the BBB was achieved by Stewart and Wiley in 1981. The authors found that by transplanting the avascular neural tissue of Stage 13 quail brains into the coelomic cavity of 3-day chick embryos, the invading capillaries took on BBB characteristics *(2)*. Namely, the invading capillaries were able to exclude circulating trypan blue, tight junctions were increased as observed by electron microscopy, pinocytotic vesicles decreased, mitochondrial number increased to a density equal to that in the endothelium of neural capillaries, and two BBB markers, alkaline phosphatase and butyryl cholinesterase were elevated. However, somites grafted to the brain did not induce BBB of invading capillaries. These historic studies demonstrate that a component of neural tissue induces the formation of the BBB, supporting the theory that the capillary environment is critical for induction of capillary differentiation and development of the appropriate barrier properties. A similar experimental paradigm was utilized by Janzer et al. to reveal that astrocytes are capable of induction of the blood–brain/blood–retinal barriers *(3)*. Injection of astrocytes into the anterior chamber of the rat eye induced barrier properties as determined by reduced flux of the albumin-binding dye, Evans blue, in the vessels that invaded the astrocyte aggregates, as well as the iris proper. The astrocytes were also capable of inducing barrier properties in the vessels of chick chorioallantoic membranes. These studies support a role of astrocytes in the regulation of endothelial cell differentiation to the BRB and BRB. In the light of these experiments, it is interesting to note that while a number of epithelial cell lines develop strong ionic, solute, and fluid barriers such as the transformed retinal pigment epithelium cell line, ARPE19, there are no endothelial cell lines that reflect the very tight barrier of the BBB or BRB. However, a number of external signals such as astrocyte-conditioned media, angiopoietin 1, or glucocorticoids, can induce barrier properties in isolated retinal, and brain endothelial cells.

In vitro experiments provide evidence that glia directly contribute to endothelial differentiation of the BBB and BRB. These in vitro models were pioneered by Rubin et al., who demonstrated that astrocyte-conditioned media, along with cAMP analogues, stimulate barrier properties in endothelial cells *(4)*. Wolberg et al. further established that the combination of astrocytes and cAMP stimulate barrier properties and tight junction complexity in endothelial cells *(5)*. The role of cAMP signaling in the regulation of retinal endothelial barrier properties and alterations to this signaling pathway that may occur in diabetic retinopathy requires further study.

Astrocytes and Müller cells contact and ensheath the vascular plexus of the superficial region of the retina, but the deep capillary bed contacts only Müller cells. Tout et al. demonstrated that Müller cells are capable of inducing BRB properties similar to astrocyte induction. Transplantation of Müller cells into the anterior chamber of the rat eye cause Müller cell aggregates to form. These aggregates are vascularized and the invading blood vessels develop barrier properties preventing the flux of horseradish peroxidase or Evans Blue dye, similar to transplanted astrocytes but superior to those formed by meningeal cells *(6)*. Müller cell induction of BRB properties was further supported by co-culture experiments with retinal endothelial cells. Müller cell co-culture across 0.4 μm pore transwell filters increases barrier properties of endothelial cells demonstrated by decreased insulin flux and increased transendothelial electrical resis-tance *(7)*. Müller cell-conditioned media, however, did not provide the same effect *(7)*. Further, injection of Müller cells into the anterior chamber of the eye failed to restrict horseradish peroxidase permeability across adjacent vessels *(8)*. Thus, while astrocytes and Müller cells may both induce barrier properties, these studies may indicate important differences between these glial cells regarding barrier induction or maintenance.

Recent studies have identified a signal transduction adaptor molecule that promotes production of pro-barrier factors from astrocytes. Src-suppressed C kinase substrate or SSECKS in rodents, also termed gravin in humans, or AKAP12, coordinates signal transduction pathways by binding and organizing signaling molecules such as protein kinase C, protein kinase A, calmodulin, cyclins, and β-adrenergic receptors. In brain, SSECKS colocalizes with GFAP, indicating a glial expression pattern, and a recent report demonstrated that expression of SSECKS contributes to astrocytic induction of the BBB *(9)*. Overexpression of SSECKS reduces expression of vascular endothelial growth factor, apparently through reduced c-Jun and AP1 signaling and promoted angiopoietin-1 production. Angiopoietin-1 is a ligand for the Tie2 receptor, and is known to both stabilize blood vessels and protect vessels from VEGF-induced permeability *(10–12)*. The conditioned media from astrocytes overexpressing SSECKS blocks angiogenesis and promotes barrier properties of endothelial cells to a greater extent than astrocyte-conditioned media from mock-transfected cells. Further, antibodies to angio-poietin-1 blocked this barrier induction and conditioned media from astrocytes with siRNA to SSECKS-created endothelial cell barriers with greater permeability than control astrocyte-conditioned media. Additional studies of SSECKS/AKAP12 used expression studies and siRNA to demonstrate that SSECKS/AKAP12 downregulates HIF1α through the ubiquitin ligase von Hippel-Lindau and proteosomal degradation *(13)*. Together these studies demonstrate that glia play an important role in the induction of the BBB and BRB, but an understanding of the molecular mechanisms by which this differentiation proceeds is only beginning to be elucidated.

Time Course of Blood–Brain Barrier Development

Immunohistochemistry experiments of the developing brain and retina support a role for astrocyte expression of SSECKS in the formation of the BBB and BRB. Expression of the well-established tight junction proteins zonula occludens 1 (ZO-1), vascular endothelial growth factor and SSECKS were compared in developing mouse-brain cerebral cortex or the embryonic precursor, the neopallial cortex *(9)*. Expression of VEGF is present at embryonic Day 11.5 (E11.5) and increases through postnatal Day 3 (P3) but precipitously drops by P19 and is absent in adult. In contrast, ZO-1 is first detected at E15.5, while SSECKS could be detected at E16.5, and both proteins continue to increase expression through P19 and into adulthood. These results correlate well with the induction of the BBB during rat development, which dramatically increases barrier properties at E21 *(14)*. Using measures of electrical resistance across the brain vascular endothelium, a measure of ionic permeability, the brain vessels were found to increase resistance from 310 to 1,215 ohm × cm^2, which remained constant through adults. The results support a model in rodents in which SSECKS reduces VEGF expression in the brain as a phase of vessel growth ends and promotes formation of the tight junction complex that is stabilized by postnatal Day 21. However, it should be noted that other measures of permeability were found to demonstrate increased barrier properties after 21 days. Measures of potassium and urea flux revealed a dramatic drop in the influx rate constant from E21 to P2 that continued to slowly decrease to P50, suggesting further barrier changes after birth in rats *(15)*.

Quantitative immunohistochemical analysis of human retina in developing fetus demonstrates a similar pattern of BRB formation *(13)*. VEGF expression is observed at the 18th week of development in the retina but expression of the tight junction proteins occludin, ZO-2, and Claudin-1 as well as SSECKS/AKAP12, and angiopoietin 1 are not detectable at this time point. However, at the 24th week all these proteins were expressed and increased by the 27th week, while VEGF expression began to decrease at this time point and continued to decrease through the 39th week. These data support a role of SSECKS/AKAP12 in BRB formation through promotion of angiopoietin 1 expression, which subsequently promotes tight junction formation. However, angiopoietin 1 expression is not restricted to either the BBB or BRB, suggesting that additional signaling mechanisms contribute to barrier formation.

Pericyte Induction of the Blood–Retinal Barrier

In addition to glia, pericytes also induce barrier properties in retinal vascular endothelial cells. Pericytes are in close contact with the endothelial cells of the retinal capillaries and are encased by a common basal lamina *(16)*. In vitro studies using pericyte and endothelial cell lines demonstrated that pericytes secrete an angiopoietin 1 complex that induces expression of tight junction protein occludin *(17)*. Additionally, coculture of a rat brain endothelial cell line with a primary culture of rat brain pericytes decreases permeability to sodium fluorescein that is, in part, dependent on transforming growth factor β (TGF β), as demonstrated by using a blocking antibody. Finally, barrier induction is partially recapitulated by direct treatment with TGF β *(18)*.

Further evidence for a role of pericytes in the induction or maintenance of the BRB is found in platelet-derived growth factor B (PDGF) B or PDGF receptor β (PDGFR) β gene deletion studies. Endothelial cells of the BBB express PDGF B in order to recruit the pericytes, which express the PDGFR β. Gene deletion of either this ligand or receptor results in lethality at birth due to hemorrhaging and edema *(19, 20)*. The mice lack pericytes around the capillaries of the brain resulting in endothelial hyperplasia, increased capillary diameter, and abnormal ultrastructure. Further, VEGF A content increased, potentially contributing to the altered vessel structure and the observed hyperplasia. These studies suggest that pericyte recruitment by endothelial cells is necessary for normal vessel stabilization and barrier induction.

In summary, the BRB is formed by both retinal vasculature and the retinal pigmented epithelium. The vascular endothelium appears distinct from the epithelium, in that the endothelial cells require an external signal for induction of the BRB. Astrocytes, Müller cells, and pericytes all contribute to this complex signaling system, as shown schematically in Fig. 1. Further, communication and coordinated function between the vasculature, glia, and neurons suggests the existence of a functional neurovascular unit *(21)*.

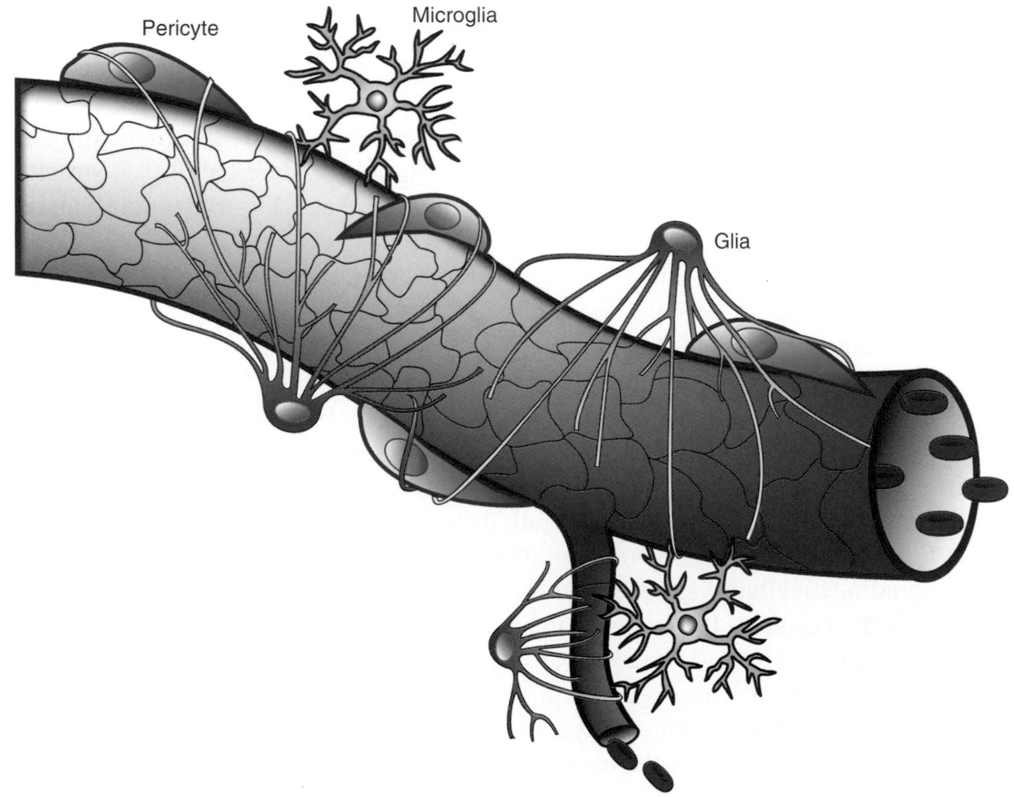

Fig. 1. Healthy retinal vasculature demonstrating cellular interactions Arterioles and capillaries provide oxygenated blood and nutrients to the inner neural retina. Astrocytes, Müller cells, and pericytes interact with the vasculature to induce barrier properties. Microglia also interact with the endothelium potentially to respond to changes in the blood components that cross into the retina. The molecular process of barrier induction in endothelial cells is poorly understood.

MOLECULAR COMPOSITION OF THE BLOOD–RETINAL BARRIER

Specialized Retinal Vessels Control Flux into Neural Tissue

The blood vessels of the CNS, including the retina, are different from blood vessels in other regions of the body. Vessels of the CNS lack fenestrations observed in highly permeable vessels such as the glomerular capillary wall *(22)* and choroid capillary plexus *(23)*. These fenestrations are a thinning of the capillary wall, bringing the apical and basal membranes in close apposition and promoting transcellular flux. This loss of endothelial cell fenestrations is one of the initial developmental steps of BBB formation *(24, 25)*. Additionally, the vessels of the CNS have reduced pinocytotic vesicles, also reducing transcellular transport *(26–28)*. These structural features allow specific control of transcellular permeability through specific mechanisms such as receptor-mediated endocytosis, and provide tight control of the fluids, nutrients, and metabolic precursors that enter the neural parenchyma.

Overview of Tight Junction Proteins

Paracellular flux is controlled by the presence and composition of the junctional complex, which includes both tight junctions and adherens junctions. In epithelial cells the adherens and tight junctions are easily discernable, but in the endothelium of the BBB and BRB these complexes cannot be differentiated at the ultrastructural level *(29, 30)*. Many studies of the tight junction have been carried out in epithelial cells and a number of reviews have detailed the molecular components of the tight junctions including *(31–34)*, and recently addressed by our group *(1)*. Here the overall structure of the tight junction is briefly reviewed and the changes that occur to the tight junction in diabetes are addressed.

Tight junctions are now known to be complex structures comprised of over 40 structural and regulatory proteins. Figure 2 provides a schematic of the vascular structure in the retina and a highly simplified view of the tight junction complex. (For a more detailed review of the tight junction proteins in the retina see the following review and text *(1, 35)*). Current concepts of the tight junctions suggest an organization of this complex array of proteins. Tight junctions are composed of both transmembrane proteins that create the connection to the adjoining cell, and organizing proteins that bind to multiple junctional proteins and link these proteins to the cytoskeleton.

The tight junction transmembrane proteins include junction adhesion molecules or JAM, occludin, tricellulin, and the claudin gene family. The most well-studied membrane-associated proteins that organize the junctional complex are the zonula occludens isoforms or ZO-1, -2, and -3 proteins. Recent studies using siRNA for the ZO isoforms reveals that this protein is necessary for proper assembly of the junctional complex *(36)*, confirming a role for these proteins as a scaffold. Other studies are beginning to elucidate the molecular function of the transmembrane proteins of the tight junction.

Claudins Confer Tight Junction Barrier Properties

Cell-culture experiments utilizing siRNA *(37)* or mutational analysis *(38)* and in vivo analysis of transgenic mice have demonstrated that claudins confer barrier properties to the tight junctions *(39–44)*. Claudins are a multigene family comprised of at least 24

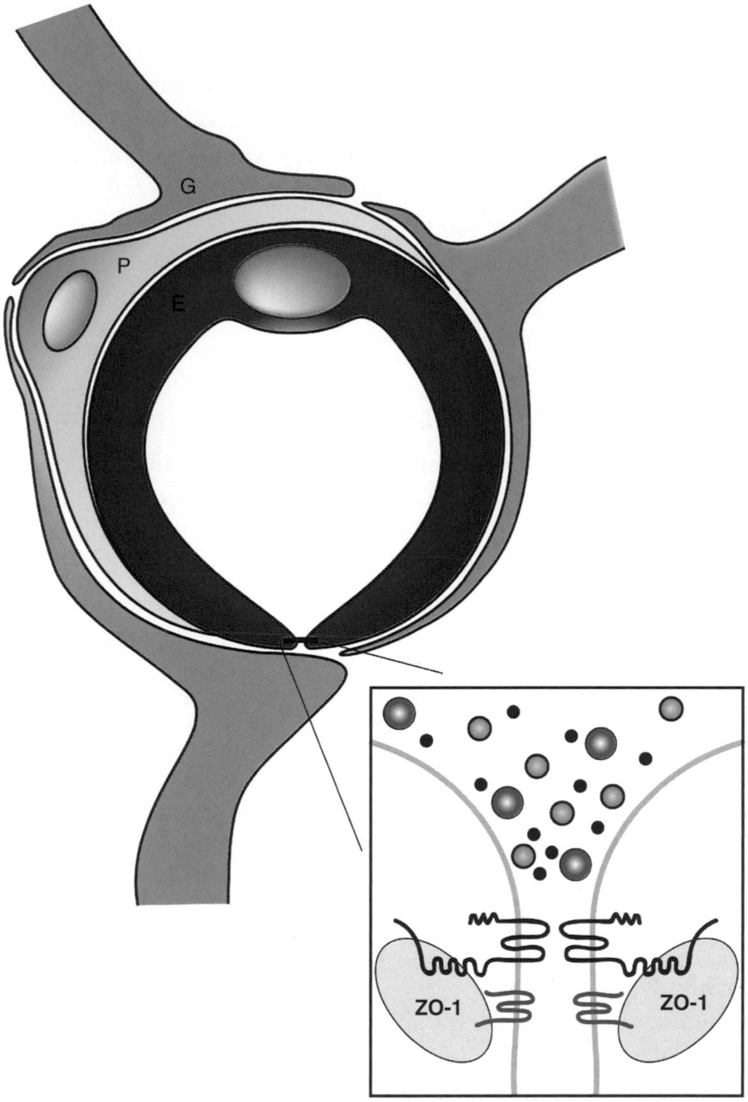

Fig. 2. Blood–retinal barrier is induced by glia and pericytes. Blood vessels are comprised of endothelial cells (E) and pericytes (P) that are contacted by glial processes (G). Together, the glia and pericytes induce the tight junction complex (*inset*). This highly simplified version of the tight junction emphasizes the transmembrane proteins occludin (longer cytoplasmic carboxy-tail) and claudins that create the barrier. The zonula occludens protein (ZO) connects these transmembrane proteins to the cytoskeleton. Tight junctions are now known to have over 40 proteins, and the contribution of these proteins to retinal endothelial barrier properties and the changes in these proteins that occur in diabetes are just beginning to be addressed. However, occludin phosphorylation state, cellular distribution, and content are all altered in diabetes.

isoforms *(45)*. The claudins are tetraspan transmembrane proteins with two extracellular loops and a short carboxy intracellular tail that interacts with the PDZ-1 domains of ZO-1, -2, and -3 *(46)*. The barrier property of a given tissue depends on the expression pattern of claudins. Claudins interact in both, a homologous and heterologous fashion, creating the barrier and simultaneously forming ion specific pores within the barrier *(47)*. Thus, charge-selective paracellular pores across the tight junction may be formed.

The expression pattern of claudins in the retina has only been partially characterized. The expression of Claudin 5 is largely restricted to the vasculature *(41)* and has been identified in retinal *(48)* and brain microvessels *(49)*. Gene deletion of Claudin 5 results in permeability to molecules less than 800 Da and neonatal lethality *(50)*. In chick retinal pigment epithelium, expression of Claudins 1, 2, and 5 was demonstrated by embryonic Day 14 at both the protein and mRNA level *(51)*. A comprehensive study of the expression pattern of claudins in the retina and changes in claudin expression in diabetic retinopathy is needed.

Occludin Regulates Barrier Properties

While claudins confer barrier properties to the tight junctions, occludin appears to regulate the cells response to the external signals that control barrier properties. Occludin content correlates well with barrier properties, and is higher in cells with a tighter barrier, such as the retinal endothelial cells of arterioles and capillaries, and lower in cells known to be more permeable, such as venous endothelial cells and endothelial cells of nonneuronal tissues *(48, 52, 53)*. Since occludin was the first transmembrane tight junction protein identified, and a number of expression studies suggested occludin contributed to barrier properties *(54, 55)* it was thought that this protein was a structural protein in tight junctions.

Studies of occludin knock-out mice changed the view of occludin. Occludin knock-out mice are viable and tight junctions appear normal, as assessed by electron microscopy. Studies of visceral endoderm cells originating from embryonic stem cells lacking occludin support the observations in knockout mice, that occludin is not required to maintain TJ structure *(56)*. However, the occluding-deficient mice do possess a diverse number of abnormalities, including postnatal growth retardation, male infertility, and inability of females to suckle their young, suggesting that this protein has an important regulatory function in several tissues that possess tight junctions. Additionally, salivary gland abnormalities, thinning of compact bone, brain calcium deposits, and hyperplasia of the gastric epithelium are other consequences of occludin gene deletion in mice *(57, 58)*. The role of occludin in regulation of epithelial cell division was further supported by the ability of exogenous occludin expression to revert the phenotype of raf transformed cells *(59)*. In studies conducted in our laboratory, antisense RNA to occludin induced the RPE cell line ARPE19 to increase cell division by approximately twofold (manuscript submitted). Therefore, occludin contributes to control of cell division in cells that express tight junctions. Understanding this process is just beginning and a role for occludin in controlling angiogenesis of the blood vessels of the CNS has not been investigated.

Recent studies using small inhibitory (siRNA) to reduce occludin expression reveal a regulatory role for this protein in the cell's response to changes in the environment as well as a direct contribution to barrier properties. A stable epithelial cell line with occludin gene expression almost completely reduced through siRNA, demonstrated increased permeability to small organic cations, such as ethanolamine and arginine *(60)*. But even more intriguing was the lack of normal response to cholesterol depletion. Cholesterol depletion dramatically reduced the electrical resistance of the cell monolayer and activates Rho, which is likely involved in cytoskeletal rearrangements conferring the cell's response. Both of these cholesterol responses are blocked in cells with occludin siRNA. These data suggest that occludin contributes to barrier properties and the ability of the cells to respond to environmental changes in the regulation of barrier properties.

Alterations in Occludin in Diabetic Retinopathy

Occludin in the retinal vasculature undergoes changes in phosphorylation, localization, and content with diabetes, which can be recapitulated in primary endothelial cell culture and VEGF treatment. Streptozotocin-induced diabetes reduces occludin content *(61)* and immunostaining at the endothelial cell borders *(48, 61, 62)*, while permeability to FITC-labeled albumin increases. This change in occludin content can be observed in primary retinal endothelial cells in response to VEGF treatment *(61)* and depends on urokinase plasminogen activator, suggesting extracellular proteolytic activity contributes to occludin degradation and permeability *(63)*. Similarly, diabetes reduces occludin content in the brain vasculature *(64)*.

Changes in occludin also occur in the RPE in response to permeabilizing factors. Treatment of RPE cells with hepatocyte growth factor (HGF) reduced tight junctions, decreased TER, and increased diffusion of fluorescently labeled marker from the apical to basolateral membrane. After 6 h of HGF treatment, occludin, Claudin-1, and α-catenin were redistributed from the membrane to the cytoplasm and ZO-1 immunostaining was reduced *(65)*. Interestingly, overexpression of HGF in RPE for 28 days resulted in chronic retinal detachment and retinal inflammation *(66)*.

Phosphorylation of occludin may provide a mechanism by which junctional properties are regulated. Treatment of endothelial cells with VEGF *(67, 68)*, histamine *(69)*, oxidized phospholipids *(70)*, monocyte chemoattractant protein-1 (MCP-1 or CCL2) *(71, 72)*, or shear stress *(73)* increased both serine/threonine phosphorylation of occludin and permeability. Furthermore, diabetes increases occludin phosphorylation in the rat retina similar to the VEGF-induced increase in BREC *(68)*. Conversely, in epithelial cells occludin phosphorylation may be associated with barrier tightening *(74)*. In these studies, dephosphorylation of occludin through protein phosphatase 2A and 1 are associated with promotion of barrier properties. These discrepancies may represent differences in the systems used or differences in the sites phosphorylated. Clearly, site identification and mutational analysis is necessary to pursue the functional meaning of occludin phosphorylation.

VE-CADHERIN AND DIABETIC RETINOPATHY

This chapter has focused on the tight junction complex, which is essential for the well-developed barrier properties of the BRB. However, adherens junction proteins also contribute to the barrier properties of the BRB. As mentioned earlier, the tight junction and adherens junction complex are not readily discernable at the ultrastructural level, as viewed by electron microscopy. However, vascular endothelial cadherin (VE-cadherin or cadherin 5) is a vascular constrained transmembrane protein of the adherens junction and is expressed in the retinal vasculature *(75)*. Injection of antibodies to VE-cadherin increases retinal permeability in vivo and causes primary retinal endothelial cells to separate in culture. Further, diabetes causes a reduction in VE-cadherin protein through matrix metalloprotease activity contributing to changes in permeability *(76)*. Also, in vascular endothelial cells without tight junctions, VEGF stimulation leads to VE-cadherin phosphorylation and endocytosis that controls endothelial permeability *(77)*. The tight junction complex and adherens junction may be viewed as resistors that act in series, each with distinct barrier properties. Diabetes alters both these complexes, contributing to increased permeability. The system is made more complex since there is a clear interaction of the two junctional complexes as demonstrated by the interaction of ZO-1 first with the adherens junction, from which point ZO-1 then organizes polymerization of the claudins of the tight junctions *(36)*.

PERMEABILITY IN DIABETIC RETINOPATHY

Diabetic retinopathy is characterized by increased vascular permeability as can be observed by fluorescein angiography. This change in permeability occurs during the early stages of the onset of diabetic retinopathy. Table 1 is a compilation of studies demonstrating that this change in vascular permeability can be recapitulated in rodent models of diabetes. There are limited studies that have failed to observe a difference in accumulation of marker in rodent models in diabetes but the majority of studies have observed an increase of 1.5- to 4.5-fold. This accumulation can be due to either increased flux into the retina, or decreased flux out of the retina. Further, passive flux is controlled by hydrostatic and oncotic pressure, as well as changes in vascular permeability (for a detailed discussion of fluid and solute movement across a vascular bed see *(78)*). Thus, changes in marker accumulation may be the result of a variety of vascular changes other than permeability alone. Indeed, increased solute accumulation in the retina elevates the tissue oncotic pressure, retaining fluid and likely contributing to macular edema. However, direct changes in endothelial cell culture permeability demonstrate a similar response to vascular endothelial growth factor addition *(79, 80)* suggesting the in vivo response is, at least in part, due to increased vessel permeability. A recent longitudinal study demonstrates the rate of diabetic retinopathy at 14 years is still over 70% *(81)*, and while the rate of proliferative retinopathy is on the decline, the rate of macular edema is on the rise *(82)*.

It should be emphasized that rodents lack a macula, and thus cannot completely model macular edema, which in humans is closely correlated with loss of vision *(83)*. However, the changes in vessel permeability observed in rodents and in the early stages of retinopathy in humans may be a first step toward macular edema. This altered barrier may set the stage for an ensuing event that leads to focal edema or hemorrhaging of retinal vessels. Much of the current research has focused on this change in vessel permeability. Future studies will need to address the issue as to the causes for progression from general leaky blood vessels, as observed by fluorescein angiography, to focal edema associated with vision loss. A recent study using mass spectrometry has identified carbonic anhydrase I from red blood cells in the vitreous of patients with hemorrhagic retinopathy, and further demonstrated that carbonic anhydrase stimulates the kallikrein pathway leading to bradykinin-induced endothelial permeability *(84)*. Thus, once established, hemorrhaging vessels further drive vascular permeability.

Table 1
Retinal Permeability in Streptozotocin-Induced Diabetes Rat Model

Time of diabetes	*Strain of rat*	*Permeability assay*	*Change in diabetes*	*References*
1 week	Sprague-Dawley	Evans Blue	1.7-fold	*(106)*
8 days	Long-Evans	Evans Blue	2.3-fold	*(107)*
8 days	Sprague-Dawley	Evans Blue	1.6-fold	*(108)*
8 days	Sprague-Dawley	Vitreous Protein	3.1-fold	*(109)*
8 days	Wistar	Vitreous Protein	2.8-fold	*(110)*
2 weeks	Brown-Norway	Evans Blue	2-fold	*(111)*
2 weeks	Brown-Norway	Evans Blue	3-fold	*(112)*
2 weeks	Long-Evans	Evans Blue	2.6-fold	*(88)*
2 weeks	Long-Evans	FITC-Dextran	4.1-fold	*(113)*
2 weeks	Sprague-Dawley	Alexa-Fluor 488-BSA	2-fold	*(114)*
2 weeks	Sprague-Dawley	Evans Blue	2.6-fold	*(115)*
2 weeks	Sprague-Dawley	FITC-BSA	3-fold	*(105)*
2 weeks	Wistar	Vitreous Fluorophotometry	1.6-fold	*(116)*
3 weeks	Long-Evans	FITC-Dextran	4.5-fold	*(117)*
1 and 4 weeks	Wistar	Evans Blue	1.4- and 1.4-fold	*(118)*
3 days to 4 weeks	Long-Evans	Isotope Dilution	2.9- to 10.7-fold	*(119)*
2 months	Sprague-Dawley	Vitreous Protein and FITC-Dextran	3.3- and 2.7-fold	*(120)*
3 months	Sprague-Dawley	Evans Blue and FITC-BSA	2.4- and 2.4-fold	*(121)*
3 months	Sprague-Dawley	FITC-BSA and Rhodamine-Dextran	1.6- and 1.1-fold	*(61)*
4 months	Brown-Norway	FITC-Dextran	2.5-fold	*(122)*
4 months	Sprague-Dawley	Isotope Dilution	2-fold	*(123)*
1 day to 16 weeks	Brown-Norway and S. Dawley	Evans Blue	1.9-fold (BN 16 weeks)	*(124)*
6 months	Sprague-Dawley	Isotope Dilution	2-fold	*(125)*
6 months	Sprague-Dawley	^{14}C-Sucrose	2.4-fold	*(126)*
6 months	Wistar	Fluroescein	3.7-fold	*(127)*
3 weeks, 6 and 13 months	Sprague-Dawley (Female)	Isotope Dilution	2.4-fold (13 months)	*(128)*
15 months	Sprague-Dawley	Fluroescein	2.7-fold	*(129)*

NEUROINFLAMMATION IS A CENTRAL PROCESS IN THE PATHOLOGY OF DIABETIC RETINOPATHY

The well-established elevation of vascular endothelial growth factor *(85)* may be part of a larger neuroinflammation in diabetic retinopathy. Neuroinflammation has been assigned various definitions; however, for the purpose of this chapter, neuroinflammation is defined as elevated expression of cytokines and chemokines, microglial activation, and leukostasis without necessarily including infiltration. Neuroinflammation has been identified as a component of a variety of neurodegenerative diseases. For example, elevated IL-1 has been found in ischemia, stroke, and in chronic CNS diseases such as Alzheimer's, Down's syndrome, multiple sclerosis, Parkinson's, HIV-associated dementia, amyotrophic lateral sclerosis, and epilepsy (reviewed in *(86)*). Further, IL-18 has been identified in ischemic stroke, multiple sclerosis and axonal injury (reviewed in *(87)*). Both of these interleukins are capable of generating a cascade of downstream responses similar to that observed in diabetic retinopathy. This inflammatory cascade includes elevated cytokines and chemokines such as MCP, a permeabilizing chemokine, and VEGF, induction of adhesion molecules such as PECAM and ICAM in endothelium and consequent leukostasis, adhesion of monocytes and polymorphonuclear cells leading to respiratory burst and generation of reactive oxygen species. Furthermore, the inflammatory response may include elevated FasL contributing to endothelial apoptosis *(88)*.

A number of studies support the hypothesis that diabetic retinopathy includes neuroinflammation. In a study of 543 Type I diabetic patients, elevated IL-6, TNF, and C-reactive peptide individually or combined was associated with retinopathy and cardiovascular disease, as was an association with elevated HbA_{1c}, LDL, triglycerides, and blood pressure *(89)*. Indeed, these inflammatory markers were specifically associated with nonproliferative diabetic retinopathy (NPDR). Another study of 93 patients revealed that levels of RANTES (chemokine CCL5) and SDF-1 (CXCL12) were elevated in serum associated with severe NPDR compared to nonsevere NPDR *(90)*. Immunocytochemistry of one retina revealed RANTES, MCP-1 (CCL2), and ICAM were elevated. IL-1β and TNFα were increased in the serum and vitreous of patients with proliferative diabetic retinopathy *(91)*. Antibodies associated with heat shock protein 65 are elevated in Type 1 diabetes with retinopathy recapitulating an increase in serum levels of this inflammatory marker in artherosclerotic disease *(92)*. Together, these studies provide compelling evidence that inflammatory markers, and in particular IL-1β, is elevated in the serum and vitreous of patients with proliferative and nonproliferative diabetic retinopathy.

Abundant data in animals further support a role for neuroinflammation in diabetic retinopathy. IL-1β protein was elevated in the retina of diabetic animals at 2 months *(93, 94)*. Gerhardinger et al. demonstrated that IL-1β mRNA was elevated in 6-month diabetic animals and by performing microchip array analysis of Muller cells isolated from control and diabetic retinas identified a series of acute phase and inflammatory markers that are responsive to IL-1 *(95)*. A series of elegant experiments demonstrated that leukostasis increases during streptozotocin-induced diabetes in mouse and rat models, and that deletion of the gene for the endothelial protein ICAM or its leukocyte binding partner CD18 ameliorated leukostasis after 11 months of diabetes and rectified vascular lesions in a galactosemic model *(96)*. Furthermore, in a 1-week model of diabetes, vascular permeability, leukostasis, CD18 and ICAM expression as well as NF-κB activation were all normalized by high-dose aspirin, or the COX-2 inhibitor, meloxicam, and by a soluble TNF receptor/Fc hybrid (entanercept), suggesting TNF and COX contribute to diabetic retinopathy *(97)*. Together, these animal models demonstrate a role for neuroinflammation in diabetic retinopathy and that interfering with this inflammatory response can alter the disease.

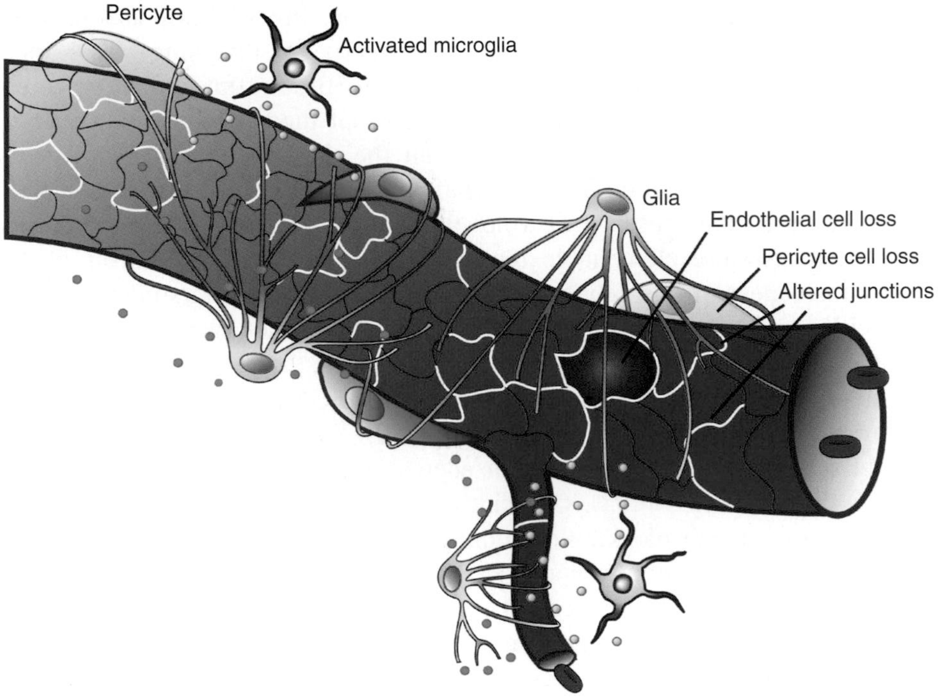

Fig. 3. Cellular and molecular changes in the retinal vasculature with diabetes. Diabetes leads to pericyte loss (*light-gray pericyte*), glial reactivity, and microglial activation (*retracted processes*). The loss of normal cell interactions and increased cytokine production (VEGF, TNFα, MCP and IL1β) increase endothelial cell death, and lead to alterations in tight junctions increasing permeability. Hemorrhaging blood vessels contribute carbonic anhydrase that further drives permeability through bradykinin activation.

The changes in retinal vascular permeability observed in diabetic retinopathy are caused, in part, by changes in cytokine/growth factor production. However, a role of oxidative stress leading to endothelial apoptosis has been proposed as a route of increased permeability as well. The relative contribution to vascular permeability of altered junctional complex compared to increased cell death has yet to be addressed. Further, the link between metabolic dysregulation and neuroinflammation requires more research. Figure 3 depicts a model of altered permeability including neuroinflammation and altered junctional permeability as well as cell death.

THERAPIES FOR VASCULAR PERMEABILITY IN DIABETIC RETINOPATHY

A number of potential therapies are currently under investigation for diabetic retinopathy that target vascular permeability. Glucocorticoids are well-established antiinflammatory compounds that may be effective in reversing or preventing the progression of macular edema, and are currently under investigation as a therapy for diabetic retinopathy *(98)*. Glucocorticoids are effective at reversing VEGF-induced permeability in animal models *(99)*. In addition to the antiinflammatory effect of glucocorticoids, our laboratory has demonstrated that these steroids also induce the synthesis and assembly of tight junctions and the dephosphorylation of occludin commensurate with a reduction in endothelial permeability *(100)*. Recent work in our laboratory revealed the presence of a novel enhancer element unlike the canonical glucocorticoid response element, in the occludin promoter that controls glucocorticoid responsiveness of this gene (manuscript submitted). Future studies may reveal more specific means to control expression of the tight junction proteins and barrier properties.

Protein kinase C β (PKCβ) acts downstream of VEGF *(101)* and inhibitors of this kinase can block VEGF-induced permeability *(102)*. Studies of PKCβ inhibitors have revealed effectiveness in treating macular edema in diabetic retinopathy and slowing progression of vision loss *(103)*. Cell-culture studies have demonstrated that PKCβ inhibitors are effective at blocking occludin phosphorylation in response to VEGF in endothelial cells, and can partially block VEGF-induced permeability *(68)*. Unfortunately, these inhibitors have not yet achieved FDA approval but may show greater effectiveness at increasing doses or in combination with other inhibitors. In addition to small molecule inhibitors the hormone pigment epithelium-derived growth factor has been shown to effectively reverse diabetes- and ischemia-induced permeability through the regulation of cytokine production *(104)*.

Finally, the use of neuroprotective agents has demonstrated effectiveness in reversing vascular permeability. The use of nonpsychotropic cannabidiol, which is neuroprotective, reversed the effects of diabetes on vascular permeability in streptozotocin-diabetic rats *(105)*. This effect highlights the intimate relationship of the BRB and the neural parenchyma.

SUMMARY AND CONCLUSIONS

Glia and pericytes interact with the endothelial cells of the blood vessels stimulating synthesis and the assembly of the junctional complex, reducing fenestrations and pinocytotic vessels and forming the BRB. Production of inflammatory cytokines and vascular endothelial growth factor alters the junctional complex and induces permeability in diabetic retinopathy. While a great deal is known regarding claudins in formation of the tight junctions, little is known about changes in the claudins in diabetic retinopathy. The tight junction protein occludin appears to contribute to the regulation of barrier properties, and may contribute to control of cell growth. This protein has been observed to increase in phosphorylation, relocate away from the cell border, and decrease in content with diabetic retinopathy. Also, the adherens junction protein VE-cadherin is reduced with diabetes associated with increased vessel permeability. Understanding the signaling pathways that alter the junctional complex provides therapeutic targets to prevent vessel permeability. Furthermore, understanding the mechanisms by which glucocorticoids and angiopoietin-1 induce barrier properties may lead to new therapies to restore barrier properties in diabetic retinopathy.

REFERENCES

1. Erickson KK, Sundstrom JM, Antonetti DA. Vascular permeability in ocular disease and the role of tight junctions. Angiogenesis 2007;10(2):103–17.
2. Stewart PA, Wiley MJ. Developing nervous tissue induces formation of blood-brain barrier characteristics in invading endothelial cells: a study using quail–chick transplantation chimeras. Dev Biol 1981;84(1):183–92.
3. Janzer RC, Raff MC. Astrocytes induce blood-brain barrier properties in endothelial cells. Nature 1987;325(6101):253–7.
4. Rubin LL, Hall DE, Porter S, et al. A cell culture model of the blood-brain barrier. J Cell Biol 1991;115(6):1725–35.
5. Wolburg H, Neuhaus J, Kniesel U, et al. Modulation of tight junction structure in blood-brain barrier endothelial cells. Effects of tissue culture, second messengers and cocultured astrocytes. J Cell Sci 1994;107 (Pt 5):1347–57.
6. Tout S, Chan-Ling T, Hollander H, Stone J. The role of Muller cells in the formation of the blood-retinal barrier. Neuroscience 1993;55(1):291–301.
7. Tretiach M, Madigan MC, Wen L, Gillies MC. Effect of Muller cell co-culture on in vitro permeability of bovine retinal vascular endothelium in normoxic and hypoxic conditions. Neurosci Lett 2005;378(3):160–5.
8. Small RK, Watkins BA, Munro PM, Liu D. Functional properties of retinal Muller cells following transplantation to the anterior eye chamber. Glia 1993;7(2):158–69.
9. Lee SW, Kim WJ, Choi YK, et al. SSeCKS regulates angiogenesis and tight junction formation in blood-brain barrier. Nat Med 2003;9(7):900–6.
10. Maisonpierre PC, Suri C, Jones PF, et al. Angiopoietin-2, a natural antagonist for Tie2 that disrupts in vivo angiogenesis [see comments]. Science 1997;277(5322):55–60.
11. Asahara T, Chen DH, Takahashi T, et al. Tie2 receptor ligands, angiopoietin-1 and angiopoietin-2, modulate VEGF-induced postnatal neovascularization. Circ Res 1998;83(3):233–40.
12. Thurston G, Rudge JS, Ioffe E, et al. Angiopoietin-1 protects the adult vasculature against plasma leakage. Nat Med 2000;6(4):460–3.
13. Choi YK, Kim JH, Kim WJ, et al. AKAP12 regulates human blood-retinal barrier formation by downregulation of hypoxia-inducible factor-1alpha. J Neurosci 2007;27(16):4472–81.
14. Butt AM, Jones HC, Abbott NJ. Electrical resistance across the blood-brain barrier in anaesthetized rats: a developmental study. J Physiol 1990;429:47–62.
15. Keep RF, Ennis SR, Beer ME, Betz AL. Developmental changes in blood-brain barrier potassium permeability in the rat: relation to brain growth. J Physiol 1995;488 (Pt 2):439–48.
16. Hughes S, Gardiner T, Baxter L, Chan-Ling T. Changes in pericytes and smooth muscle cells in the kitten model of retinopathy of prematurity: implications for plus disease. Invest Ophthalmol Vis Sci 2007;48(3):1368–79.
17. Hori S, Ohtsuki S, Hosoya K, Nakashima E, Terasaki T. A pericyte-derived angiopoietin-1 multimeric complex induces occludin gene expression in brain capillary endothelial cells through Tie-2 activation in vitro. J Neurochem 2004;89(2):503–13.
18. Dohgu S, Takata F, Yamauchi A, et al. Brain pericytes contribute to the induction and up-regulation of blood-brain barrier functions through transforming growth factor-beta production. Brain Res 2005;1038(2):208–15.
19. Hellstrom M, Gerhardt H, Kalen M, et al. Lack of pericytes leads to endothelial hyperplasia and abnormal vascular morphogenesis. J Cell Biol 2001;153(3):543–53.
20. Lindahl P, Johansson BR, Leveen P, Betsholtz C. Pericyte loss and microaneurysm formation in PDGF-B-deficient mice. Science 1997;277(5323):242–5.
21. Abbott NJ, Ronnback L, Hansson E. Astrocyte-endothelial interactions at the blood-brain barrier. Nat Rev Neurosci 2006;7(1):41–53.
22. Deen WM, Lazzara MJ, Myers BD. Structural determinants of glomerular permeability. Am J Physiol Renal Physiol 2001;281(4):F579–96.
23. Marmor MF. The Retinal Pigment Epithelium: Function and Disease. New York: New York Oxford University Press; 1998.

24. Bauer HC, Bauer H, Lametschwandtner A, Amberger A, Ruiz P, Steiner M. Neovascularization and the appearance of morphological characteristics of the blood-brain barrier in the embryonic mouse central nervous system. Brain Res Dev Brain Res 1993;75(2):269–78.
25. Fenstermacher J, Gross P, Sposito N, Acuff V, Pettersen S, Gruber K. Structural and functional variations in capillary systems within the brain. Ann N Y Acad Sci 1988;529:21–30.
26. Bertossi M, Virgintino D, Maiorano E, Occhiogrosso M, Roncali L. Ultrastructural and morphometric investigation of human brain capillaries in normal and peritumoral tissues. Ultrastruct Pathol 1997;21(1):41–9.
27. Coomber BL, Stewart PA. Three-dimensional reconstruction of vesicles in endothelium of blood-brain barrier versus highly permeable microvessels. Anat Rec 1986;215(3):256–61.
28. Sedlakova R, Shivers RR, Del Maestro RF. Ultrastructure of the blood-brain barrier in the rabbit. J Submicrosc Cytol Pathol 1999;31(1):149–61.
29. Shakib M, Cunha-Vaz JG. Studies on the permeability of the blood-retinal barrier. IV. Junctional complexes of the retinal vessels and their role in the permeability of the blood-retinal barrier. Exp Eye Res 1966;5(3):229–34.
30. Cunha-Vaz JG, Shakib M, Ashton N. Studies on the permeability of the blood-retinal barrier. I. On the existence, development, and site of a blood-retinal barrier. Br J Ophthalmol 1966;50(8):441–53.
31. Mitic LL, Anderson JM. Molecular architecture of tight junctions. Annu Rev Physiol 1998;60:121–42.
32. Mitic LL, van Itallie CM, Anderson JM. Molecular physiology and pathophysiology of tight junctions – I. Tight junction structure and function: lessons from mutant animals and proteins. Am J Physiol Gastrointest Liver Physiol 2000;279(2):G250-G4.
33. Fanning AS, Mitic LL, Anderson JM. Transmembrane proteins in the tight junction barrier. J Am Soc Nephrol 1999;10(6):1337–45.
34. Gonzalez-Mariscal L, Betanzos A, Nava P, Jaramillo BE. Tight junction proteins. Prog Biophys Mol Biol 2003;81(1):1–44.
35. Phillips BE, Antonetti DA. Retinal Vascular Disease. 1 ed. Berlin: Springer-Verlag; 2007.
36. Umeda K, Ikenouchi J, Katahira-Tayama S, et al. ZO-1 and ZO-2 independently determine where claudins are polymerized in tight-junction strand formation. Cell 2006;126(4):741–54.
37. Hou J, Gomes AS, Paul DL, Goodenough DA. Study of claudin function by RNA interference. J Biol Chem 2006;281:36117–23.
38. Colegio OR, Van Itallie CM, McCrea HJ, Rahner C, Anderson JM. Claudins create charge-selective channels in the paracellular pathway between epithelial cells. Am J Physiol Cell Physiol 2002;283(1):C142–7.
39. Furuse M, Fujita K, Hiiragi T, Fujimoto K, Tsukita S. Claudin-1 and -2: novel integral membrane proteins localizing at tight junctions with no sequence similarity to occludin. J Cell Biol 1998;141(7):1539–50.
40. Morita K, Furuse M, Fujimoto K, Tsukita S. Claudin multigene family encoding four-transmembrane domain protein components of tight junction strands. Proc Natl Acad Sci USA 1999;96:511–6.
41. Morita K, Sasaki H, Furuse M, Tsukita S. Endothelial claudin: Claudin-5/TMVCF constitutes tight junction strands in endothelial cells. J Cell Biol 1999;147(1):185–94.
42. Tsukita S, Furuse M. Occludin and claudins in tight-junction strands: leading or supporting players? Trends Cell Biol 1999;9(7):268–73.
43. Furuse M, Sasaki H, Fujimoto K, Tsukita S. A single gene product, claudin-1 or -2, reconstitutes tight junction strands and recruits occludin in fibroblasts. J Cell Biol 1998;143(2):391–401.
44. Furuse M, Hata M, Furuse K, et al. Claudin-based tight junctions are crucial for the mammalian epidermal barrier: a lesson from claudin-1-deficient mice. J Cell Biol 2002;156(6):1099–111.
45. Tsukita S, Furuse M, Itoh M. Multifunctional strands in tight junctions. Nat Rev Mol Cell Biol 2001;2(4):285–93.
46. Itoh M, Furuse M, Morita K, Kubota K, Saitou M, Tsukita S. Direct binding of three tight junction-associated MAGUKs, ZO-1, ZO-2 and ZO-3, with the COOH termini of claudins. J Cell Biol 1999;147(6):1351–63.
47. Tsukita S, Furuse M. Pores in the wall: claudins constitute tight junction strands containing aqueous pores. J Cell Biol 2000;149(1):13–6.

48. Barber AJ, Antonetti DA. Mapping the blood vessels with paracellular permeability in the retinas of diabetic rats. Invest Ophthalmol Vis Sci 2003;44(12):5410–6.
49. Liebner S, Fischmann A, Rascher G, et al. Claudin-1 and claudin-5 expression and tight junction morphology are altered in blood vessels of human glioblastoma multiforme. Acta Neuropathologica 2000;100(3):323–31.
50. Nitta T, Hata M, Gotoh S, et al. Size-selective loosening of the blood-brain barrier in claudin-5-deficient mice. J Cell Biol 2003;161(3):653–60.
51. Rahner C, Fukuhara M, Peng S, Kojima S, Rizzolo LJ. The apical and basal environments of the retinal pigment epithelium regulate the maturation of tight junctions during development. J Cell Sci 2004;117(15):3307–18.
52. Hirase T, Staddon JM, Saitou M, et al. Occludin as a possible determinant of tight junction permeability in endothelial cells. J Cell Sci 1997;110:1603–13.
53. Kevil CG, Okayama N, Trocha SD, et al. Expression of zonula occludens and adherens junctional proteins in human venous and arterial endothelial cells: role of occludin in endothelial solute barriers. Microcirculation 1998;5(2–3):197–210.
54. Balda MS, Whitney JA, Flores S, Gonzalez M, Cereijido M, Matter K. Functional dissociation of paracellular permeability and transepithelial electrical resistance and disruption of the apical-basolateral intramembrane diffusion barrier by expression of a mutant tight junction membrane protein. J Cell Biol 1996;134:1031–49.
55. McCarthy KM, Skare I, Stankewich MC, et al. Occludin is a functional component of the tight junction. J Cell Sci 1996;109:2287–98.
56. Saitou M, Fujimoto K, Doi Y, et al. Occludin-deficient embryonic stem cells can differentiate into polarized epithelial cells bearing tight junctions. J Cell Biol 1998;141(2):397–408.
57. Saitou M, Furuse M, Sasaki H, et al. Complex phenotype of mice lacking occludin, a component of tight junction strands. Mol Biol Cell 2000;11(12):4131–42.
58. Schulzke JD, Gitter AH, Mankertz J, et al. Epithelial transport and barrier function in occludin-deficient mice. Biochim Biophys Acta 2005;1669(1):34–42.
59. Wang Z, Mandell KJ, Parkos CA, Mrsny RJ, Nusrat A. The second loop of occludin is required for suppression of Raf1-induced tumor growth. Oncogene 2005;24(27):4412–20.
60. Yu AL, McCarthy KM, Francis SA, et al. Knock down of occludin expression leads to diverse phenotypic alterations in epithelial cells. Am J Physiol Cell Physiol 2005;288:C1231–41.
61. Antonetti D, Barber A, Khin S, et al. Vascular permeability in experimental diabetes is associated with reduced endothelial occludin content. Diabetes 1998;47:1953–9.
62. Barber AJ, Antonetti DA, Gardner TW. Altered expression of retinal occludin and glial fibrillary acidic protein in experimental diabetes. Invest Ophthalmol Vis Sci 2000;41(11):3561–8.
63. Behzadian MA, Windsor LJ, Ghaly N, Liou G, Tsai NT, Caldwell RB. VEGF-induced paracellular permeability in cultured endothelial cells involves urokinase and its receptor. Faseb J 2003;17(6):752–4.
64. Chehade JMHMJMAD. Diabetes-related changes in rat cerebral occludin and zonula occludens-1 (ZO-1) expression. Neurochem Res 2002;27(3):249–52.
65. Jin M, Barron E, He S, Ryan SJ, Hinton DR. Regulation of RPE intercellular junction integrity and function by hepatocyte growth factor. Investigative Ophthalmol Vis Sci 2002;43(8):2782–90.
66. Jin M, Chen Y, He S, Ryan SJ, Hinton DR. Hepatocyte growth factor and its role in the pathogenesis of retinal detachment. Invest Ophthalmol Vis Sci 2004;45(1):323–9.
67. Antonetti DA, Barber AJ, Hollinger LA, Wolpert EB, Gardner TW. Vascular endothelial growth factor induces rapid phosphorylation of tight junction proteins occludin and zonula occluden 1. A potential mechanism for vascular permeability in diabetic retinopathy and tumors. J Biol Chem 1999;274(33):23463–7.
68. Harhaj NS, Felinski EA, Wolpert EB, Sundstrom JM, Gardner TW, Antonetti DA. VEGF activation of protein kinase C stimulates occludin phosphorylation and contributes to endothelial permeability. Invest Ophthalmol Vis Sci 2006;47(11):5106–15.
69. Hirase T, Kawashima S, Wong EY, et al. Regulation of tight junction permeability and occludin phosphorylation by Rhoa-p160ROCK-dependent and -independent mechanisms. J Biol Chem 2001;276(13):10423–31.

70. DeMaio L, Rouhanizadeh M, Reddy S, Sevanian A, Hwang J, Hsiai TK. Oxidized phospholipids mediate occludin expression and phosphorylation in vascular endothelial cells. Am J Physiol Heart Circ Physiol 2006;290(2):H674–83.
71. Stamatovic SM, Dimitrijevic OB, Keep RF, Andjelkovic AV. Protein kinase C-alpha:Rhoa cross talk in CCL2-induced alterations in brain endothelial permeability. J Biol Chem 2006.
72. Stamatovic SM, Shakui P, Keep RF, et al. Monocyte chemoattractant protein-1 regulation of blood-brain barrier permeability. J Cereb Blood Flow Metab 2005;25(5):593–606.
73. DeMaio L, Chang YS, Gardner TW, Tarbell JM, Antonetti DA. Shear stress regulates occludin content and phosphorylation. Am J Physiol – Heart Circ Physiol 2001;281(1):H105–13.
74. Seth A, Sheth P, Elias BC, Rao R. Protein phosphatases 2A and 1 interact with occludin and negatively regulate the assembly of tight junctions in the CACO-2 cell monolayer. J Biol Chem 2007;282(15):11487–98.
75. Davidson MK, Russ PK, Glick GG, Hoffman LH, Chang MS, Haselton FR. Reduced expression of the adherens junction protein cadherin-5 in a diabetic retina. Am J Ophthalmol 2000;129(2):267–9.
76. Navaratna D, McGuire PG, Menicucci G, Das A. Proteolytic degradation of VE-cadherin alters the blood-retinal barrier in diabetes. Diabetes 2007;56(9):2380–7.
77. Gavard J, Gutkind JS. VEGF controls endothelial-cell permeability by promoting the beta-arrestin-dependent endocytosis of VE-cadherin. Nat Cell Biol 2006;8(11):1223–34.
78. Salathe EP, Venkataraman R. Interaction of fluid movement and particle diffusion across capillary walls. J Biomech Eng 1982;104(1):57–62.
79. Lakshminarayanan S, Antonetti DA, Gardner TW, Tarbell JM. Effect of VEGF on retinal microvascular endothelial hydraulic conductivity: the role of NO. Invest Ophthalmol Vis Sci 2000;41(13): 4256–61.
80. DeMaio L, Antonetti DA, Scaduto RC, Jr., Gardner TW, Tarbell JM. VEGF increases paracellular transport without altering the solvent-drag reflection coefficient. Microvasc Res 2004;68(3): 295–302.
81. LeCaire T, Palta M, Zhang H, Allen C, Klein R, D'Alessio D. Lower-than-expected prevalence and severity of retinopathy in an incident cohort followed during the first 4–14 years of type 1 diabetes: the Wisconsin Diabetes Registry Study. Am J Epidemiol 2006; 164(2):143–50.
82. Knudsen L, Lervang H, Lundbye-Christensen S, Gorst-Rasmussen A. The north jutland county diabetic retinopathy study population characteristics. Br J Ophthalmol 2006;90:1404–9.
83. Moss SE, Klein R, Klein BE. The 14-year incidence of visual loss in a diabetic population. Ophthalmology 1998;105(6):998–1003.
84. Gao BB, Clermont A, Rook S, et al. Extracellular carbonic anhydrase mediates hemorrhagic retinal and cerebral vascular permeability through prekallikrein activation. Nat Med 2007;13(2):181–8.
85. Aiello LP. Vascular endothelial growth factor and the eye: biochemical mechanisms of action and implications for novel therapies. Ophthalmic Research 1997;29(5):354–62.
86. Basu A, Krady JK, Levison SW. Interleukin-1: a master regulator of neuroinflammation. J Neurosci Res 2004;78(2):151–6.
87. Felderhoff-Mueser U, Schmidt OI, Oberholzer A, Buhrer C, Stahel PF. IL-18: a key player in neuroinflammation and neurodegeneration? Trends Neurosci 2005;28(9):487–93.
88. Joussen AM, Poulaki V, Mitsiades N, et al. Suppression of Fas-FasL-induced endothelial cell apoptosis prevents diabetic blood-retinal barrier breakdown in a model of streptozotocin-induced diabetes. Faseb J 2003;17(1):76–8.
89. Schram MT, Chaturvedi N, Schalkwijk CG, Fuller JH, Stehouwer CD. Markers of inflammation are cross-sectionally associated with microvascular complications and cardiovascular disease in type 1 diabetes–the EURODIAB Prospective Complications Study. Diabetologia 2005;48(2):370–8.
90. Meleth AD, Agron E, Chan CC, et al. Serum inflammatory markers in diabetic retinopathy. Invest Ophthalmol Vis Sci 2005;46(11):4295–301.
91. Demircan N, Safran BG, Soylu M, Ozcan AA, Sizmaz S. Determination of vitreous interleukin-1 (IL-1) and tumour necrosis factor (TNF) levels in proliferative diabetic retinopathy. Eye 2005.
92. Weitgasser R, Lechleitner M, Koch T, et al. Antibodies to heat-shock protein 65 and neopterin11 levels in patients with type 1 diabetes mellitus. Exp Clin Endocrinol Diabetes 2003;111(3):127–31.

93. Kowluru RA, Odenbach S. Role of interleukin-1beta in the development of retinopathy in rats: effect of antioxidants. Invest Ophthalmol Vis Sci 2004;45(11):4161–6.
94. Kowluru RA, Odenbach S. Role of interleukin-1beta in the pathogenesis of diabetic retinopathy. Br J Ophthalmol 2004;88(10):1343–7.
95. Gerhardinger C, Costa MB, Coulombe MC, Toth I, Hoehn T, Grosu P. Expression of acute-phase response proteins in retinal Muller cells in diabetes. Invest Ophthalmol Vis Sci 2005;46(1):349–57.
96. Joussen AM, Poulaki V, Le ML, et al. A central role for inflammation in the pathogenesis of diabetic retinopathy. Faseb J 2004;18(12):1450–2.
97. Joussen AM, Poulaki V, Mitsiades N, et al. Nonsteroidal anti-inflammatory drugs prevent early diabetic retinopathy via TNF-alpha suppression. Faseb J 2002;16(3):438–40.
98. Kuppermann BD, Blumenkranz MS, Haller JA, et al. Randomized controlled study of an intravitreous dexamethasone drug delivery system in patients with persistent macular edema. Arch Ophthalmol 2007;125(3):309–17.
99. Edelman JL, Lutz D, Castro MR. Corticosteroids inhibit VEGF-induced vascular leakage in a rabbit model of blood-retinal and blood-aqueous barrier breakdown. Exp Eye Res 2005;80(2):249–58.
100. Antonetti DA, Wolpert EB, DeMaio L, Harhaj NS, Scaduto RC. Hydrocortisone decreases retinal endothelial cell water and solute flux coincident with increased content and decreased phosphorylation of occludin. J Neurochem 2002;80:667–77.
101. Xia P, Aiello LP, Ishii H, et al. Characterization of vascular endothelial growth factor's effect on the activation of protein kinase C, its isoforms, and endothelial cell growth. J Clin Invest 1996;98(9):2018–26.
102. Aiello LP, Bursell SE, Clermont A, et al. Vascular endothelial growth factor-induced retinal permeability is mediated by protein kinase C in vivo and suppressed by an orally effective ß-isoform-selective inhibitor. Diabetes 1997;46:1473–80.
103. Aiello LP, Davis MD, Girach A, et al. Effect of ruboxistaurin on visual loss in patients with diabetic retinopathy. Ophthalmology 2006;113(12):2221–30.
104. Zhang SX, Wang JJ, Gao G, Shao C, Mott R, Ma JX. Pigment epithelium-derived factor (PEDF) is an endogenous antiinflammatory factor. Faseb J 2006;20(2):323–5.
105. El-Remessy AB, Al-Shabrawey M, Khalifa Y, Tsai NT, Caldwell RB, Liou GI. Neuroprotective and blood-retinal barrier-preserving effects of cannabidiol in experimental diabetes. Am J Pathol 2006;168(1):235–44.
106. Xu Q, Qaum T, Adamis AP. Sensitive blood-retinal barrier breakdown quantitation using Evans blue. Invest Ophthalmol Vis Sci 2001;42(3):789–94.
107. Poulaki V, Qin W, Joussen AM, et al. Acute intensive insulin therapy exacerbates diabetic blood-retinal barrier breakdown via hypoxia-inducible factor-1alpha and VEGF. J Clin Invest 2002;109(6):805–15.
108. Qaum T, Xu Q, Joussen AM, et al. VEGF-initiated blood-retinal barrier breakdown in early diabetes. Invest Ophthalmol Vis Sci 2001;42(10):2408–13.
109. Ayalasomayajula SP, Kompella UB. Celecoxib, a selective cyclooxygenase-2 inhibitor, inhibits retinal vascular endothelial growth factor expression and vascular leakage in a streptozotocin-induced diabetic rat model. Eur J Pharmacol 2003;458(3):283–9.
110. Carmo A, Cunha-Vaz JG, Carvalho AP, Lopes MC. Effect of cyclosporin-A on the blood–retinal barrier permeability in streptozotocin-induced diabetes. Mediators Inflamm 2000;9(5):243–8.
111. Zhang SX, Sima J, Shao C, et al. Plasminogen kringle 5 reduces vascular leakage in the retina in rat models of oxygen-induced retinopathy and diabetes. Diabetologia 2004;47(1):124–31.
112. Zhang SX, Sima J, Wang JJ, Shao C, Fant J, Ma JX. Systemic and periocular deliveries of plasminogen kringle 5 reduce vascular leakage in rat models of oxygen-induced retinopathy and diabetes. Curr Eye Res 2005;30(8):681–9.
113. Miyahara S, Kiryu J, Yamashiro K, et al. Simvastatin inhibits leukocyte accumulation and vascular permeability in the retinas of rats with streptozotocin-induced diabetes. Am J Pathol 2004;164(5):1697–706.
114. El-Remessy AB, Behzadian MA, Abou-Mohamed G, Franklin T, Caldwell RW, Caldwell RB. Experimental diabetes causes breakdown of the blood-retina barrier by a mechanism involving tyrosine nitration and increases in expression of vascular endothelial growth factor and urokinase plasminogen activator receptor. Am J Pathol 2003;162(6):1995–2004.

115. Xu X, Zhu Q, Xia X, Zhang S, Gu Q, Luo D. Blood-retinal barrier breakdown induced by activation of protein kinase C via vascular endothelial growth factor in streptozotocin-induced diabetic rats. Curr Eye Res 2004;28(4):251–6.
116. Takeda M, Mori F, Yoshida A, et al. Constitutive nitric oxide synthase is associated with retinal vascular permeability in early diabetic rats. Diabetologia 2001;44(8):1043–50.
117. Tamura H, Miyamoto K, Kiryu J, et al. Intravitreal injection of corticosteroid attenuates leukostasis and vascular leakage in experimental diabetic retina. Invest Ophthalmol Vis Sci 2005;46(4):1440–4.
118. Lawson SR, Gabra BH, Guerin B, et al. Enhanced dermal and retinal vascular permeability in streptozotocin-induced type 1 diabetes in Wistar rats: blockade with a selective bradykinin B1 receptor antagonist. Regul Pept 2005;124(1–3):221–4.
119. Miyamoto K, Khosrof S, Bursell SE, et al. Prevention of leukostasis and vascular leakage in streptozotocin-induced diabetic retinopathy via intercellular adhesion molecule-1 inhibition. Proc Natl Acad Sci USA 1999;96(19):10836–41.
120. Amrite AC, Ayalasomayajula SP, Cheruvu NP, Kompella UB. Single periocular injection of celecoxib-PLGA microparticles inhibits diabetes-induced elevations in retinal PGE2, VEGF, and vascular leakage. Invest Ophthalmol Vis Sci 2006;47(3):1149–60.
121. Chang YH, Chen PL, Tai MC, Chen CH, Lu DW, Chen JT. Hyperbaric oxygen therapy ameliorates the blood-retinal barrier breakdown in diabetic retinopathy. Clin Exp Ophthalmol 2006;34(6):584–9.
122. Muranaka K, Yanagi Y, Tamaki Y, et al. Effects of peroxisome proliferator-activated receptor gamma and its ligand on blood-retinal barrier in a streptozotocin-induced diabetic model. Invest Ophthalmol Vis Sci 2006;47(10):4547–52.
123. Osicka TM, Yu Y, Lee V, Panagiotopoulos S, Kemp BE, Jerums G. Aminoguanidine and ramipril prevent diabetes-induced increases in protein kinase C activity in glomeruli, retina and mesenteric artery. Clin Sci (Lond) 2001;100(3):249–57.
124. Zhang SX, Ma JX, Sima J, et al. Genetic difference in susceptibility to the blood-retina barrier breakdown in diabetes and oxygen-induced retinopathy. Am J Pathol 2005;166(1):313–21.
125. Gilbert RE, Kelly DJ, Cox AJ, et al. Angiotensin converting enzyme inhibition reduces retinal overexpression of vascular endothelial growth factor and hyperpermeability in experimental diabetes. Diabetologia 2000;43(11):1360–7.
126. Nakajima M, Cooney MJ, Tu AH, et al. Normalization of retinal vascular permeability in experimental diabetes with genistein. Invest Ophthalmol Vis Sci 2001;42(9):2110–4.
127. Hikichi T, Mori F, Nakamura M, et al. Inhibitory effects of bucillamine on increased blood-retinal barrier permeability in streptozotocin-induced diabetic rats. Curr Eye Res 2002;25(1):1–7.
128. Lightman S, Pinter G, Yuen L, Bradbury M. Permeability changes at blood-retinal barrier in diabetes and effect of aldose reductase inhibition. Am J Physiol 1990;259(3 Pt 2):R601–5.
129. Amano S, Yamagishi S, Kato N, et al. Sorbitol dehydrogenase overexpression potentiates glucose toxicity to cultured retinal pericytes. Biochem Biophys Res Commun 2002;299(2):183–8.

15 Retinal Neovascularization and the Role of VEGF

Elia J. Duh

CONTENTS

ABSTRACT

Diabetic retinopathy (DR) is a major cause of blindness in the United States and other industrialized countries. Retinal neovascularization is the hallmark of the proliferative stage of diabetic retinopathy and is a major cause of vision loss in diabetes. This chapter discusses our current knowledge regarding the mechanisms underlying retinal neovascularization in diabetic retinopathy, with a focus on the critical role played by vascular endothelial growth factor (VEGF). The current understanding of the stages of neovascularization is reviewed, beginning with the ischemic/hypoxic stimulus that is thought to

From: *Contemporary Diabetes: Diabetic Retinopathy*
Edited by: E. Duh © Humana Press, Totowa, NJ

play a critical role in the transition from nonproliferative to proliferative diabetic retinopathy. The evidence supporting the importance of VEGF in diabetic retinopathy is presented, including clinical, preclinical, and basic research studies. Furthermore, the regulation of VEGF expression in the retina as well as its actions at the cellular and molecular level is discussed in detail. In the light of VEGF's pathophysiologic importance in DR, the development of therapeutics targeting VEGF and its downstream actions is a promising approach for current and future treatment of proliferative diabetic retinopathy.

Key Words: Angiogenesis; endothelial cell; retinal neovascularization; VEGF.

INTRODUCTION

Despite improvements in medical management of diabetes and treatment of ocular complications, diabetic retinopathy (DR) remains the most common cause of severe visual loss in working-age adults in the United States and other industrialized countries. In the United States, DR results in blindness in over 10,000 individuals with diabetes per year *(1)*. Retinal neovascularization, the formation of new blood vessels from preexisting blood vessels, is a major underlying factor, and can cause severe vision loss from vitreous hemorrhage and tractional retinal detachment.

Significant research advances have been made regarding the mechanisms underlying the development of retinal neovascularization in DR. In particular, the identification of vascular endothelial growth factor (VEGF) as a major stimulus of retinal neovascularization has led to the development of therapies targeting this growth factor, and anti-VEGF treatments are being increasingly used in clinical management of patients with advanced diabetic retinopathy. This chapter is divided into two parts. The first part focuses on the current understanding of the mechanisms of angiogenesis, particularly with respect to diabetic retinopathy. The second part focuses on VEGF's critical role in retinal neovascularization, as well as its functional and biochemical properties, which provide insights with potentially important implications for anti-VEGF therapy in humans.

PROGRESSION OF NONPROLIFERATIVE TO PROLIFERATIVE DIABETIC RETINOPATHY

Diabetic retinopathy is clinically divided into two stages, nonproliferative diabetic retinopathy (NPDR) and proliferative diabetic retinopathy (PDR), which is characterized by retinal neovascularization (Figs. 1 and 2). As NPDR progresses, retinal capillary dropout occurs which results in progressive retinal ischemia and hypoxia. Ischemia and hypoxia are thought to play a critical role in the transition from nonproliferative to proliferative diabetic retinopathy. Indeed, the concept of ischemia and hypoxia as stimulators of retinal neovascularization arose over half a century ago *(2, 3)*, supported by clinical observations. For instance, neovascularization commonly occurs at the borders of perfused and nonperfused retina. In addition, retinal neovascularization is more common and severe in eyes with extensive capillary nonperfusion.

Ischemia and hypoxia result in the upregulation of various molecules that promote angiogenesis, including pro-angiogenic growth factors. Specifically, ischemic retinal cells secrete vasoproliferative growth factors which induce the formation of

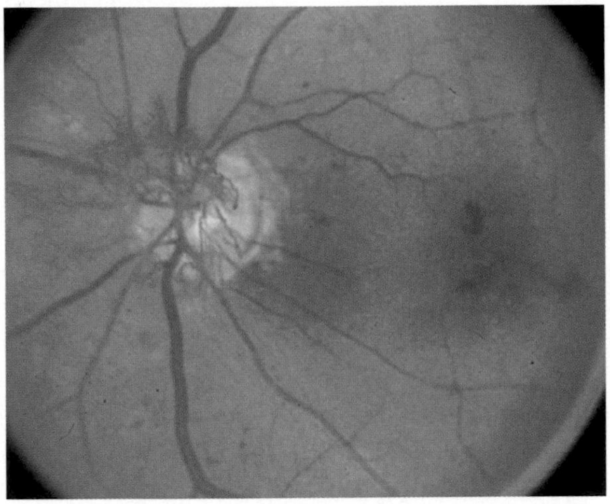

Fig. 1. Optic nerve head neovascularization in proliferative diabetic retinopathy.

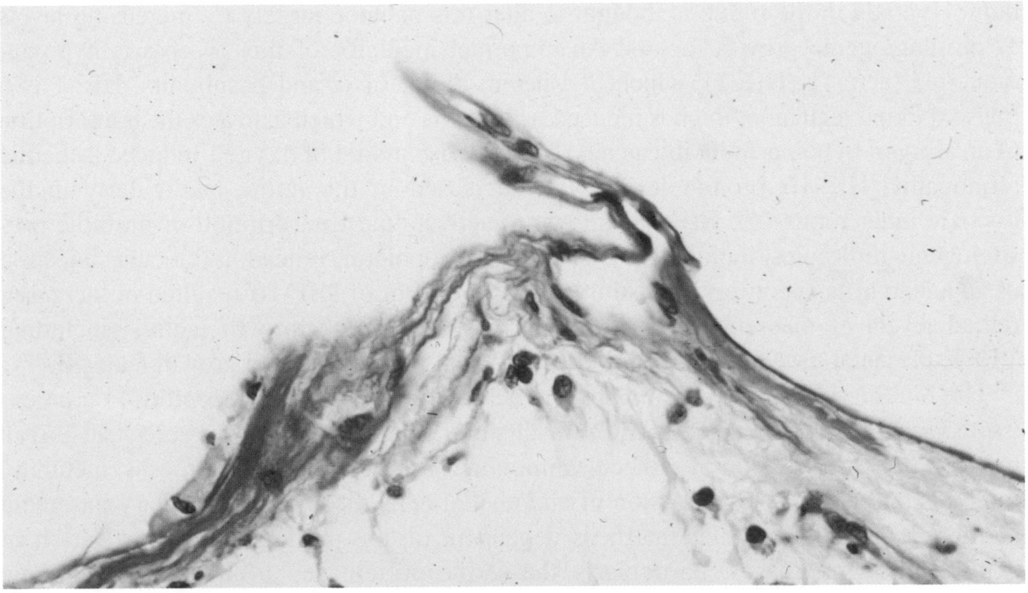

Fig. 2. Early retinal neovascularization in diabetes, with a new vessel extending from the retina into the vitreous. (Courtesy of W. Richard Green, MD.) H&E, original magnification ×160.

new blood vessels in the retina or iris. This neovascularization constitutes the hallmark of proliferative diabetic retinopathy. The new vessels grow along the retinal surface and along the vitreous scaffold of the posterior vitreous hyaloid. These new vessels are fragile and often bleed, resulting in preretinal as well as vitreous hemorrhage. In addition, glial tissue associated with the new vessels can contract, producing traction on the retina and eventually leading to retinal detachment. Vitreous hemorrhage and traction retinal detachment are the direct cause of most cases of severe vision loss in diabetic retinopathy.

STAGES OF ANGIOGENESIS

Angiogenesis, the formation of new blood vessels from existing vessels, occurs through a multi-step process, including: production of angiogenic growth factors by diseased tissue, binding of angiogenic growth factors to receptors on existing vascular endothelial cells (EC), activation of EC gene expression of pro-angiogenic molecules, EC invasion of surrounding tissue, EC migration and proliferation, formation of vascular tubes by EC, and stabilization of new blood vessels by mural cells. Each of these steps is potentially vulnerable to pharmacologic targeting, and anti-angiogenic therapies directed at various steps are under investigation *(4)*.

Under normal conditions, the vasculature is quiescent except during processes such as wound healing and the menstrual cycle, presumably due to a balance between inducers and inhibitors of angiogenesis *(5)*. A critical step in the initiation of angiogenesis arises from changes in the tissue milieu which leads to an imbalance between inducers and inhibitors, either from increased levels of inducers, decreased levels of inhibitors, or both. Hypoxia in the retina is thought to alter this balance largely by increasing levels of pro-angiogenic growth factors. An important mediator of this process is hypoxia-inducible factor 1 (HIF-1), which is a hetero-dimer of α and β subunits. HIF-1 is a transcriptional regulator which is induced by hypoxia and which activates the transcription of an array of hypoxia-inducible genes. In the mouse model of oxygen-induced ischemic retinopathy, HIF-1α protein levels were increased in the retina, particularly in the hypoxic inner retina *(6)*. HIF-1 is known to activate the transcription of multiple pro-angiogenic molecules, including VEGF and erythropoietin. Indeed, intraocular injection of an adenovirus encoding a constitutively-active form of HIF-1α resulted in increased retinal levels of messenger RNAs for various angiogenic growth factors, including VEGF, placental growth factor, angiopoietin-2, and platelet-derived growth factor-B *(7)*.

The binding of pro-angiogenic growth factors to their cognate receptor(s) on preexisting vascular endothelial cells (ECs) results in the activation of these cells, causing an increase in the expression of molecules important for the angiogenic process, including integrins and proteinases. Invasion of endothelial cells through the capillary basement membrane and extracellular matrix is dependent on the production and activation of extracellular proteinases, particularly the serine proteinase, urokinase plasminogen activator (uPA), as well as members of the matrix metalloproteinase (MMP) family. The expression of proteinase genes is induced by angiogenic growth factors including VEGF. In addition, the proteolytic process is induced by activation of pro-proteinases and downregulation of protease inhibitors. A detailed discussion of uPA and MMP's is provided in Chap. 16.

Dissolution of the capillary basement membrane and surrounding tissue is accompanied by endothelial cell migration. Growth factor-induced activation of endothelial cells leads to increased expression and activation of integrins, including $\alpha_v\beta_3$ and $\alpha_v\beta_5$ (see Chap. 16). These cell surface adhesion molecules play an important role in the attachment of endothelial cells to specific ligands in the extracellular matrix, including fibronectin, which serve as a scaffold for the migrating endothelial cells.

Activated endothelial cells proliferate and subsequently form vascular tubes. These immature vessels undergo further remodeling, with subsequent formation of a new basement membrane as well as recruitment of mural cells (pericytes or smooth muscle cells) to form a mature vessel. The recruitment of these mural cells is particularly important for the stabilization of the new blood vessels, and plays a critical role in the development of vessel resistance to regression *(8)*.

More recently, it has become appreciated that in addition to preexisting vascular endothelial cells, endothelial progenitor cells from the circulation may also play a role in retinal neovascularization. When hematopoietic stem cells (HSCs) containing a population of endothelial progenitor cells (EPCs) were administered by intravitreal injection into neonatal mouse eyes, there was stable incorporation of some of these cells into the developing retinal vasculature *(9)*. In addition, systemic administration of donor HSCs in an animal model of retinal venous occlusion resulted in incorporation of a subset of these cells into the retinal neovasculature *(10)*. Therefore, it is possible that EPCs may also play an important part in proliferative diabetic retinopathy, which may have therapeutic implications.

ANIMAL MODELS OF RETINAL NV: THE OXYGEN-INDUCED RETINOPATHY MODEL OF RETINAL NEOVASCULARIZATION

Existing animal models of diabetes have been limited by the absence of advanced lesions of diabetic retinopathy, including preretinal neovascularization. This is likely due in part to the shorter life span of these animals. Consequently, studies of retinal neovascularization have largely focused on animal models of retinopathy of prematurity. One of the most widely used animal models is the mouse model of oxygen-induced retinopathy (OIR) *(11)*.

Development of the retinal vasculature in mice occurs postnatally. In the mouse model of OIR, neonatal mice are exposed to high oxygen tensions (typically around 75%) from postnatal Day 7 (P7) until P12. This hyperoxic exposure results in retinal vessel regression and cessation of normal radial vessel growth. This vaso-obliteration leads to extensive retinal nonperfusion. The mice are then returned to room temperature at P12. The nonperfused retina becomes hypoxic, leading to the elaboration of angiogenic growth factors and retinal neovascularization, which is typically maximal by P17 *(12)*. Although this model clearly has important differences from proliferative diabetic retinopathy, it shares important similarities, most notably the induction of retinal neovascularization by retinal ischemia and hypoxia. The model has proven very useful in allowing the acquisition of insights into the pathogenesis of ischemic retinopathies, including PDR. Many studies have also been performed in related animal models of ROP, including the rat *(13)*.

VASCULAR ENDOTHELIAL GROWTH FACTOR

It has long been known that retinal neovascularization is strongly associated with retinal ischemia, based on clinical observations of ischemic retinopathies including diabetic retinopathy. Retinal capillary nonperfusion precedes neovascularization in these retinopathies *(14, 15)*. The degree of capillary nonperfusion correlates with the risk of neovascularization in branch retinal vein occlusion *(16)*. In 1948, Michaelson proposed that a diffusible angiogenic "factor X" released from areas of hypoxic retina, is responsible for neovascularization in diabetic retinopathy, as well as in other ischemic retinopathies *(2)*. In the 1990s, VEGF emerged as a strong candidate for "factor X," and subsequent research has strongly established VEGF as a major stimulator of retinal neovascularization in the ischemic retinopathies, including proliferative diabetic retinopathy.

Interest in VEGF's role in eye disease arose from earlier studies of VEGF's systemic role, including its contribution to tumor angiogenesis. VEGF is a homodimeric glycoprotein that is both a vasopermeability *(17)* and an angiogenesis factor *(18, 19)*. It was initially denoted as vasopermeability factor (VPF) based on its ability to increase microvascular permeability *(17)*. Indeed, in one assay of dermal microvascular permeability, VEGF was found to be 50,000 times as potent, on a molar basis, as histamine *(20)*. VEGF is mitogenic primarily for vascular endothelial cells *(19)*. The expression of VEGF has been found to be greatly increased in rapidly growing, highly vascularized tumors *(21)*, and inhibition of VEGF with a monoclonal antibody inhibited tumor growth in vivo *(22)*. Hypoxia induces VEGF expression in tumors and glial myogenic tumor cell lines *(23)*. VEGF binds two high affinity cell-surface tyrosine kinase receptors, in particular fms-like tyrosine kinase (Flt) and fetal live kinase 1 (Flk-1), deneted VEGFR-1 (Flt-1) and VEGFR-2 (KDR/FIk-7) both of which are expressed on vascular endothelial cells. VEGF and its receptors are critical for normal embryological development, and even heterozygous knockout of the VEGF gene results in embryonic lethality due to impairment of developmental angiogenesis *(24, 25)*. These characteristics of VEGF suggested that it might play a major role in mediating the microvascular complications observed in diabetic retinopathy, since they are also characterized by tissue ischemia, angiogenesis, and vascular permeability. Subsequent extensive studies in ocular cells, animal models, and patients have confirmed this, and they are detailed in the following paragraphs.

REGULATION OF VEGF EXPRESSION IN THE RETINA

Regulation of VEGF in Proliferative Diabetic Retinopathy

VEGF is produced by many cell types within the eye, including retinal pigment epithelial cells, pericytes, endothelial cells, glial cells, Muller cells, and ganglion cells *(26, 27)*. In the context of diabetic retinopathy, VEGF upregulation was first appreciated in the proliferative stage. In the mid-1990s, clinical studies demonstrated significantly increased intraocular concentrations of VEGF in specimens from patients with proliferative retinopathies, including diabetic retinopathy. In one investigation, 210 specimens of ocular fluid (vitreous and/or aqueous) were collected from 164 patients undergoing intraocular surgery, including 143 samples from patients with diabetes *(28)*. The patients with diabetes had different stages of retinopathy, including no retinopathy, nonproliferative retinopathy, quiescent proliferative retinopathy, and active proliferative retinopathy. VEGF concentrations were significantly elevated in both the vitreous and aqueous of patients with active proliferative diabetic retinopathy. In contrast, VEGF concentrations were low in a control group of patients with no neovascular disorder, and in diabetic patients with no retinopathy, nonproliferative retinopathy, or quiescent proliferative retinopathy. Six patients successfully underwent laser photocoagulation treatment for active proliferative retinopathy. In these six patients, intraocular VEGF concentrations were decreased by an average of 75% after treatment, as compared to before treatment *(28)*. Another study demonstrated similar findings measuring VEGF concentrations in vitreous specimens from 8 patients with PDR as compared to 12 control patients with no neovascular disorder *(29)*. These results have subsequently been corroborated by numerous studies.

Upregulation of VEGF levels has also been observed in animal models of retinal neovascularization. In the mouse model of oxygen-induced retinopathy, retinal VEGF RNA expression was increased by threefold within 12 h after commencement of relative retinal hypoxia, and the increase in VEGF expression persisted during the development of retinal neovascularization *(30)*. VEGF RNA was markedly increased in the inner nuclear layer, and confocal immunohistochemistry studies demonstrated that the VEGF-producing cells had a Muller-like morphology. Similar upregulation of VEGF was found in rat *(31)* and cat models of retinal neovascularization *(32, 33)*, as well as a primate model of iris neovascularization induced by laser occlusion of branch retinal veins *(34)*. These models all exhibit a temporal relationship between VEGF expression and ocular angiogenesis, with increased VEGF expression after the onset of retinal hypoxia, but before the development of neovascularization.

The role of hypoxia as an important stimulus for VEGF upregulation is supported by cell-culture studies. Hypoxia induces VEGF RNA expression in various ocular cell types *(27)*. Furthermore, VEGF induction is reversible upon return of the cells to normoxia. An important mediator of hypoxia-induced upregulation of VEGF expression is HIF-1, a hypoxia-induced transcription factor that is known to stimulate the transcription of multiple genes upregulated by hypoxia *(35)*. HIF-1 has been demonstrated to play an important role in the activation of VEGF transcription in cultured cells subjected to hypoxia *(36)*. Strong support for the involvement of HIF-1 in VEGF upregulation was provided by a study of mice in which the VEGF gene was replaced by a mutant VEGF gene containing a deletion of the HIF-1 binding site (hypoxia-response element) from the promoter region. Both wild-type and mutant mice were subjected to oxygen-induced retinopathy. In contrast to the wild-type mice, retinal VEGF RNA levels were not increased in the mutant mice. In addition, the mutant mice had significantly less retinal neovascularization *(37)*.

As noted earlier, laser photocoagulation has been demonstrated to reduce intraocular VEGF levels in patients with active proliferative retinopathy *(28)*. This has been corroborated in a study of aqueous specimens in patients with PDR undergoing panretinal photocoagulation *(38)*. In addition, immunohistochemical studies of postmortem eyes from individuals at different stages of diabetic retinopathy demonstrated that the intensity of VEGF immunostaining in diabetic retinas that had undergone laser photocoagulation (and exhibited no preretinal neovascularization) was similar to that in diabetic retinas without overt retinopathy *(39)*. A reduction in pro-angiogenic factors had long been suspected to underlie the therapeutic benefits of laser photocoagulation for PDR. The basis for this might be that the laser destroys cells responsible for production of pro-angiogenic factors including VEGF. However, a more attractive hypothesis is that laser-induced destruction of photoreceptor cells results in reduced oxygen consumption of the outer retina, allowing delivery of oxygen from the choriocapillaris to the inner layers of the retina. This idea is supported by studies of a mouse model of genetically induced photoreceptor degeneration. In this study, the mice did not develop retinal neovascularization when subjected to the experimental protocol of oxygen-induced retinopathy *(40)*. In addition, these mice did not exhibit the expected upregulation of retinal VEGF expression. A final idea concerning the basis for the therapeutic benefit of laser photocoagulation is the possible increase in levels of anti-angiogenic factors.

Regulation of VEGF in Nonproliferative Diabetic Retinopathy

Although upregulation of VEGF in diabetic retinopathy was first reported in the proliferative phase, it has become increasingly appreciated that VEGF levels are also elevated in nonproliferative diabetic retinopathy. Increased VEGF levels have been described in several studies of postmortem eyes of patients with NPDR compared with nondiabetic controls *(39–42)*. Furthermore, immunopositivity of VEGF was demonstrated in eyes with no anatomic evidence of retinal nonperfusion *(42)*. Increased VEGF levels have also been demonstrated in the vitreous of patients with nonproliferative diabetic retinopathy, particularly in the setting of macular edema *(43)*. Similarly, several investigators have demonstrated an increase in retinal VEGF levels in animal models of diabetic retinopathy *(44–46)*.

Several studies have provided a biochemical basis for VEGF upregulation in NPDR, linking this phenomenon to oxidative stress, and an increase in advanced glycation endproducts, two well-known consequences of diabetes in the retina. VEGF is upregulated by reactive oxygen intermediates in vitro *(47)*, and increased levels of reactive oxygen intermediates have been correlated with increased VEGF in diabetic rodents *(48)*. Furthermore, diabetes-induced increases in retinal VEGF protein are significantly reduced by antioxidant treatment *(49)*, strongly supporting the upregulation of VEGF by oxidative stress. Advanced glycation endproducts have also been demonstrated to upregulate VEGF expression in vitro. Interestingly, this AGE-induced upregulation was inhibited by antioxidant treatment *(50)*, further supporting the role of oxidative stress.

FUNCTIONAL ROLE OF VEGF IN RETINAL NV AND PROLIFERATIVE DIABETIC RETINOPATHY

In light of its important role in tumor angiogenesis, the evidence for dramatic upregulation of intraocular VEGF levels in PDR led to experiments to confirm its functional importance in retinal neovascularization. VEGF inhibition studies in animal models have established a causal relationship for VEGF in ocular neovascular processes. Several VEGF inhibitory molecules have been evaluated, including VEGF receptor chimeric proteins, neutralizing antibodies, and antisense phosphorothioate oligodeoxynucleotides.

VEGF receptor chimeric proteins were constructed containing the entire extracellular domain of VEGFR1 (the Flt receptor) or VEGFR2 (the Flk-1 receptor) joined with the heavy chain of IgG *(51)*. These chimeric proteins bind VEGF with the same affinity as the native receptors, and can therefore act as competitors for VEGF binding. Injection of these chimeric proteins into the mouse model of oxygen-induced retinopathy (discussed earlier) was performed just when the retinas became hypoxic. Retinal neovascularization was significantly reduced by either single or dual injections of either chimeric protein, with a mean suppression of approximately 50% *(52)* (Fig. 3).

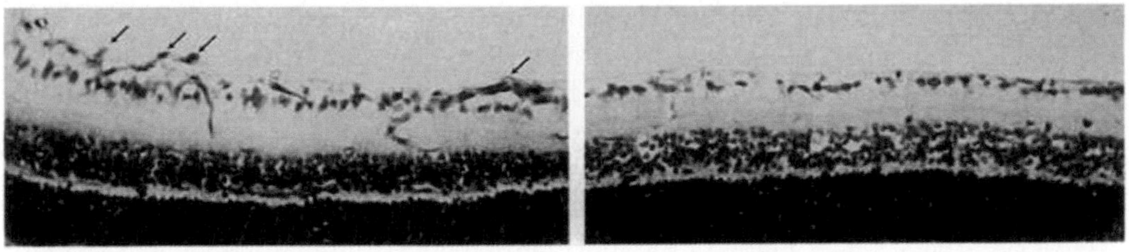

Fig. 3. Soluble VEGF receptor-IgG chimeric proteins reduce histologically evident ischemia-induced retinal neovascularization. Retinal ischemia was induced in C57BL/6J mice. The right eye of each mouse was injected with 250 ng of human CD4-IgG control chimeric protein on P12 and P14 (*left*). The left eye received intravitreal injections of 250 ng of human Flt-IgG chimera at the same times (*right*). Paraffin-embedded, periodic acid/Schiff reagent, and hematoxylin-stained 6 µm serial sections were obtained. Typical findings from corresponding retinal locations from both eyes of the same mouse are shown and are representative of all animals studied. Vascular cell nuclei internal to the inner limiting membrane represent areas of retinal neovascularization and are indicated with *arrows*. No vascular cell nuclei anterior to the internal limiting membrane are observed in normal, unmanipulated animals (from *(52)* with permission). × 50.

Antisense phosphorothioate oligodeoxynucleotides were also studied in the same model of oxygen-induced retinopathy. Two different VEGF antisense molecules were found to reduce retinal levels of VEGF protein by 40–66%, while decreasing new blood vessel growth by 25 and 31%, respectively, as compared to sense or noncomplementary mRNA controls *(53)*. Further investigation of VEGF inhibition was performed in a primate model of iris neovascularization, using VEGF neutralizing antibodies. In this study, intravitreal injections of VEGF neutralizing antibody administered every other day for 2 weeks resulted in inhibition of iris neovascularization as assessed by fluorescein iris angiograms *(54)*.

These initial studies strongly suggested that VEGF has a significant role in mediating retinal neovascularization in general and PDR in particular. Notably, the studies did not achieve complete inhibition of retinal neovascularization, suggesting either insufficient delivery of VEGF inhibitor or the role of other growth factors. In addition, it remains a significant question whether VEGF by itself is sufficient to stimulate retinal neovascularization. Intravitreal sustained release of VEGF-induced transient retinal NV in rabbits, but not primates *(55)*. Intraocular injections of VEGF in monkeys resulted in multiple vascular changes, including capillary nonperfusion, vessel dilation, and tortuosity, and disruption of the blood–retinal barrier. Preretinal neovascularization was observed in the peripheral retina that originated from superficial veins and venules, but neovascularization was not observed in the posterior pole *(56)*. Transgenic mice in which VEGF is produced by the photoreceptors exhibited very significant neovascularization that grew from the deep capillary bed of the retina and extended into the subretinal space, but not preretinal neovascularization (perhaps not surprising, since the VEGF was produced by the photoreceptors in this model) *(57)*. Conceivably, the ability of VEGF to stimulate preretinal neovascularization may depend on its levels and sustained presence. On the other hand, the presence of other pro-angiogenic factors or a reduction in anti-angiogenic molecules may be required. Nevertheless, the initial animal studies discussed earlier have demonstrated the significant role for VEGF and have been confirmed by multiple subsequent studies, including a study blocking VEGF receptor signaling *(58)*.

The emerging use of anti-VEGF therapies in patients has provided further suggestive evidence corroborating the important role of VEGF in proliferative diabetic retinopathy. For instance, a retrospective analysis was performed in a clinical trial evaluating the anti-VEGF aptamer, pegaptanib, for the treatment of diabetic macular edema (for further details, see Chap. 17). A subset of the study participants exhibited retinal neovascularization in the study eye at baseline. Eight of 13 patients receiving pegaptanib injection (including one which also received laser photocoagulation) had subsequent regression of neovascularization, compared with 0 of 3 in the sham treatment group. Notably, 4 of the 13 pegaptanib-treated patients also had neovascularization in the fellow (untreated) eye that did not regress. Although the study clearly had a small sample size, and indeed was not designed to directly address anti-VEGF and retinal neovascularization, it supports a direct effect of anti-VEGF treatment upon retinal neovascularization *(59)*. The strongest clinical evidence demonstrating a causative role for VEGF in ocular neovascularization comes from clinical trials demonstrating dramatic efficacy of anti-VEGF therapy for choroidal neovascularization in age-related macular degeneration *(60)*. Based on the body of experimental and clinical evidence, anti-VEGF treatments have emerged as a clinical option for the treatment of proliferative diabetic retinopathy, for instance in the context of neovascular glaucoma or vitreous hemorrhage.

BASIC VEGF BIOLOGY

The importance of VEGF as a stimulator of angiogenesis, both in ocular and systemic conditions, has driven intensive research efforts into its basic biology, including its mechanisms of action. In addition to improving our understanding of angiogenesis, these insights into VEGF biology have provided an array of targets for therapeutic manipulation. VEGF (also referred to as VEGF-A) is part of a gene family whose members include placental growth factor (PlGF) *(61)*, VEGF-B *(62)*, VEGF-C *(63, 64)*, and VEGF-D *(65)*. Each of these family members can interact with one or more of three VEGF receptors (Fig. 4).

VEGF has four primary isoforms, generated by alternative splicing of VEGF RNA, which contain 121, 165, 189, and 206 amino acids. These isoforms are referred to, respectively, as $VEGF_{121}$, $VEGF_{165}$, $VEGF_{189}$, and $VEGF_{206}$ *(66, 67)*. Of these, $VEGF_{165}$ is the predominant isoform. An important distinguishing property of the VEGF isoforms is their ability to bind heparin, conferred by heparin-binding peptides in exons 6 and 7 of the VEGF gene. $VEGF_{121}$ lacks both exons, does not bind heparin, and is freely diffusible. In contrast, $VEGF_{189}$ and $VEGF_{206}$ contain both exons and are almost completely bound by heparin-like moieties in the extracellular matrix. $VEGF_{165}$, which contains exon 7 but not 6, has intermediate properties.

RECEPTORS

There are two related high-affinity receptor tyrosine kinases for VEGF: VEGFR-1 (*fms*-like tyrosine kinase-1 or Flt-1) and VEGFR-2 (kinase insert domain-containing receptor or KDR). Both have seven extracellular immunoglobulin-like domains, a single

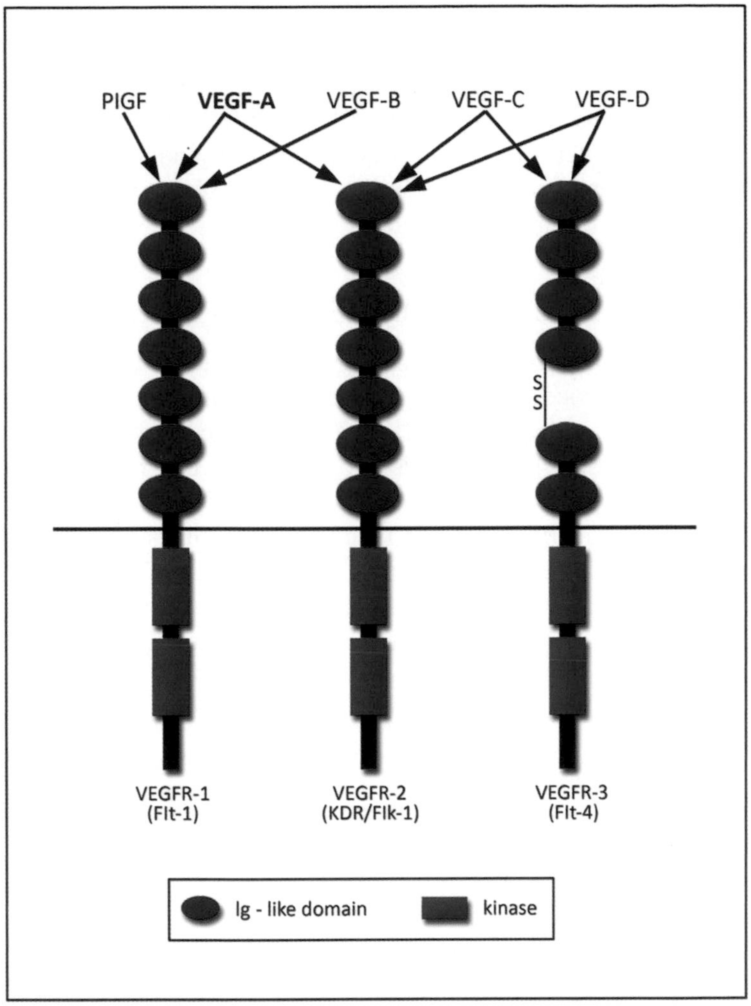

Fig. 4. VEGF receptors and their ligands. VEGF (also referred to as VEGF-A) binds two related receptor tyrosine kinases (RTKs), VEGFR-1 (also known as Flt-1) and VEGFR-2 (also known as KDR). Both VEGFR-1 and VEGFR-2 have an extracellular domain containing seven immunoglobulin-like loops (*ovals*), a single transmembrane region, and a cytoplasmic domain consisting of a single kinase domain (*rectangles*) interrupted by a non-catalytic region. VEGF-C and VEGF-D also bind to VEGFR2. Placental growth factor (PlGF) and VEGF-B bind only to VEGFR1. VEGFR3 (also known as Flt-4) is a member of the same family of receptor tyrosine kinases and binds VEGF-C and VEGF-D.

hydrophobic transmembrane domain, and a conserved intracellular tyrosine kinase domain which is interrupted by a kinase insert domain *(68, 69)*. Both VEGFR1 and VEGFR2 are autophosphorylating tyrosine kinases with binding affinities for VEGF in the low picomolar range. VEGFR-2 is known to be the major mediator of VEGF's mitogenic, angiogenic, and permeability-stimulating effects *(70)*. VEGFR-3 (*fms*-like-tyrosine kinase-4 or Flt-4) is also a member of the VEGFR family which is a receptor for VEGF-C and VEGF-D, but not VEGF *(64, 71)* (Fig. 4).

In addition to VEGFR1 and VEGFR2, neuropilin-1 (Npn-1) and neuropilin-2 (Npn-2) serve as coreceptors for VEGF. Neuropilin-1 *(72)* and neuropilin-2 *(73)* bind $VEGF_{165}$

with high affinity, but do not bind $VEGF_{121}$. The binding of $VEGF_{165}$ to these receptors is heparin-dependent. When coexpressed in cells with VEGFR2, neuropilin-1 enhances the binding of $VEGF_{165}$ to VEGFR2 as well as the stimulation of chemotaxis by $VEGF_{165}$. In addition, the inhibition of $VEGF_{165}$ binding to neuropilin-1 inhibits its binding to VEGFR2 as well as its mitogenic activity for endothelial cells *(72)*. These and other studies indicate that the neuropilins function in the enhancement of VEGF signaling and activation of endothelial cells.

VEGF'S MULTIPLE ACTIONS ON RETINAL ENDOTHELIAL CELLS

Consistent with its critical role in stimulating angiogenesis, VEGF stimulates multiple steps in the angiogenic process, including survival, migration, proliferation, tubulogenesis, and vascular permeability *(70, 74)*. These effects have been demonstrated in retinal microvascular endothelial cells in addition to numerous other endothelial cell types. Notably, retinal endothelial cells express cell surface VEGF receptors at a higher density than many other endothelial cell types *(75)*. VEGF has been demonstrated to stimulate retinal endothelial cell proliferation *(28)*, migration *(76)*, survival *(77, 78)*, and tubulogenesis *(79)*. In addition, VEGF stimulates retinal endothelial cell permeability *(80, 81)*. VEGF's vasopermeability properties in the retina are discussed in greater detail in Chap. 14.

MAIN SIGNALING PATHWAYS

The ability of VEGF to stimulate angiogenesis is dependent on its coordinate regulation of multiple endothelial cell activities. This is dependent on VEGF's ability to stimulate a network of intracellular signaling pathways. In endothelial cells, VEGFR-2 is the major mediator of VEGF signaling. Upon VEGF binding, VEGFR2 dimerizes, with one receptor, trans(auto)-phosphorylating tyrosine residues in the cytoplasmic domain of its partner *(74)*. The phosphorylated tyrosine residues can bind intracellular signaling molecules and initiate a cascade of signaling events leading to multiple cell responses promoting angiogenesis and vascular permeability.

Although VEGF activates multiple signaling pathways in endothelial cells, extensive research has focused on a few pathways that are thought to play particularly important roles (Fig. 5). VEGF stimulates endothelial cell proliferation primarily through stimulation of extracellular-signal-regulated protein kinases (ERK) 1 and 2, also known as p42/44 mitogen-activated protein (MAP) kinase. VEGF activation of VEGFR2 leads to tyrosine-phosphorylation of phospholipase C-γ (PLC-γ) *(82)*, which leads to the generation of inositol 1,4,5-trisphosphate and diacylgycerol (DAG). DAG activates protein kinase C, which in turn activates the Raf/MEK/ERK pathway, which plays a central role in endothelial cell mitogenesis *(82)*.

Activation of protein kinase C (PKC) is essential for VEGF's mitogenic effects on endothelial cells. The PKC family of serine-threonine kinases consists of multiple PKC isoforms, which differ in their regulatory and biochemical properties. Intravitreal administration of VEGF activates protein kinase C (PKC) in the retina, inducing membrane translocation of PKC isoforms α, βII, and δ *(83)*. PKC inhibitors block VEGF-induced activation of ERK1/2 *(84, 85)*, and endothelial cell proliferation *(86)*. Although

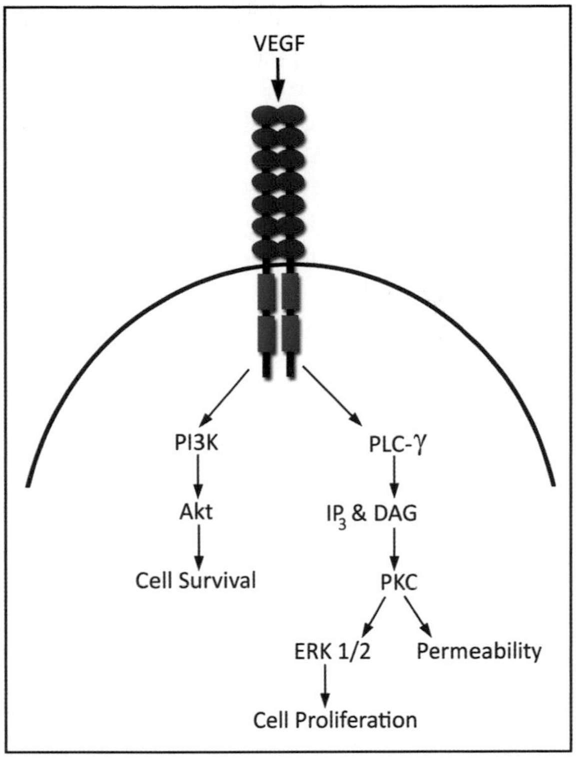

Fig. 5. VEGF signaling pathways. Most, and possibly all, of the biologically relevant VEGF signaling are mediated by VEGFR-2. Upon binding its ligand, VEGFR-2 undergoes receptor dimerization and autophosphorylation at multiple tyrosine residues in the intracellular domain. This leads to the activation of multiple signaling molecules, notably Akt, PKC, and ERK1/2. VEGF promotion of endothelial cell survival is largely dependent on PI 3-kinase (PI3K)-mediated activation of the anti-apoptotic kinase Akt. VEGF stimulates endothelial cell proliferation primarily through activation of ERK1/2. Binding of VEGF to VEGFR-2 leads to activation of PLC-γ, leading to generation of inositol 1,4,5-trisphosphate (IP_3) and diacylglycerol (DAG) and subsequent activation of PKC, which in turn mediates activation of ERK1/2. PKC (particularly PKC-β) also has an important role in VEGF's vasopermeability effects.

other PKC isoforms are likely to be important as well, particular attention has been placed on PKC-β. In bovine aortic endothelial cells, pharmacologic inhibition of PKC-β using the isoform selective inhibitor ruboxistaurin (LY333531) inhibited VEGF's mitogenic effect *(86)*. In addition to its role in VEGF's mitogenic effects, PKC-β appears to have an important role in VEGF's vasopermeability effects. Administration of ruboxistaurin strongly inhibited VEGF-induced retinal vascular permeability in vivo *(83)*. This effect was supported by an in vitro study, demonstrating that expression of a dominant negative PKCβII mutant significantly blocked VEGF-induced permeability of cultured retinal endothelial cells *(81)*.

The phosphatidylinositol 3′-kinase (PI3-kinase)/Akt signaling pathway is particularly important for VEGF's ability to promote endothelial cell survival. Activation of VEGFR2 leads to phosphorylation and activation of Akt/protein kinase B *(87)*, an anti-apoptotic kinase which mediates the promotion of cell survival by a variety of growth factors and cytokines. Akt then phosphorylates and inhibits Bad and caspase-9, proteins known to play a major role in promoting apoptosis. The importance of Akt in VEGF's survival effects are supported by experiments using dominant-negative mutant of Akt (DN-Akt). Overexpression of DN-Akt in endothelial cells completely blocked VEGF's survival effects; pharmacologic inhibition of PI3-kinase achieved the same effect *(87)*.

Although ERK1/2, PKC, and Akt have received particular attention with respect to VEGF signaling, it is likely that other signaling pathways contribute to VEGF's effects in stimulating angiogenesis. VEGF activates multiple other signaling molecules, including p38 mitogen-activated protein kinase, Src, and calcineurin *(74)*. The roles of these other pathways continue to be actively investigated.

OTHER ACTIONS OF VEGF

In addition to its initially demonstrated effects on vascular permeability and angiogenesis, there has been an increasing awareness that VEGF has additional effects as well. A consideration of these effects is important, both to fully realize the therapeutic potential of strategies targeting VEGF as well as the potential adverse effects.

Proinflammatory Effects of VEGF

VEGF has been found to have several proinflammatory properties, and this aspect of VEGF biology has received considerable attention with regard to diabetic retinopathy. As discussed earlier, VEGF is a very potent stimulator of vascular permeability *(20)*. VEGF acts directly on retinal endothelial cells to stimulate permeability *(80, 81)*, and intravitreous injections of VEGF promote blood–retinal barrier breakdown *(88)*. In an animal model, diabetes-induced blood retinal barrier breakdown was inhibited in a dose-dependent fashion by VEGF-TrapA_{40}, a fusion protein that contains binding domains from the VEGF receptors *(89)*. Intravitreal injections of VEGF increases retinal ICAM-1 levels *(90)*, and diabetes-induced increase in retinal ICAM-1 in an animal model was significantly reduced by treatment with VEGF-TrapA_{40}. VEGF plays a significant role in promoting leukocyte adhesion in the retinal vasculature *(91)*. In light of the possible role of proinflammatory pathways in the progression of diabetic retinopathy, these proinflammatory properties of VEGF could have important therapeutic implications (for a detailed discussion, see Chap. 13).

VEGF and Retinal Neuronal Development

The possible role of VEGF in the neural retinal development was raised by the identification of VEGF receptor expression in nonvascular cells of the retina. In developing mice, VEGFR1 mRNA was initially detected at postnatal Day 7 (P7) in the avascular retina, localized to the developing ganglion cell layer and inner nuclear layer. From P12 to P15, VEGFR1 mRNA was found in the inner nuclear layer and outer nuclear layer, consistent with a pattern of expression in Muller cells. VEGFR2 mRNA was first detected at P5, localized to the inner retinal layers. VEGFR2 mRNA was observed in the inner nuclear layer at P7 and in the inner and outer nuclear layers at P15. From P17 to P33, VEGFR1 and R2 became more localized in a vascular pattern, although VEGF receptor

RNA was still observed outside blood vessels. Isolated Muller cells were found to express both VEGFR1 and R2 *(92)*. Pharmacologic inhibition of VEGFR1 and R2 from P0 to P9 with a small molecule antagonist, SU5416, resulted in cell loss in the inner nuclear layer and ganglion cell layer, as compared with control mice *(92)*. This suggests that VEGF receptor activity may be important for normal retinal neural development.

VEGF and Neuroprotection

Research over the past few years indicates that VEGF has an additional role in neuroprotection *(93)*. VEGF stimulated axonal outgrowth and increased survival of both neurons and satellite cells in experiments with cultured superior cervical ganglia and dorsal root ganglia *(94)*. In explants of the ventral mesencephalon, VEGF treatment promoted the growth and survival of dopaminergic neurons and astrocytes *(95)*. Intriguing in vivo studies have implicated VEGF as a possible cause of motor neuron degeneration. A study of knock-in mice was performed, in which the VEGF gene promoter contained a deletion of the HIF-1 binding site (hypoxia-response element). These mice exhibited adult-onset motor neuron degeneration that was reminiscent of ALS. This neurodegeneration appeared to result from reduced neural vascular perfusion *(96)*. In addition, VEGF treatment of cultured motor neuron cells significantly reduced apoptosis induced by hypoxia, oxidative stress, and serum deprivation, indicating direct neuroprotective effects of VEGF. This survival effect was blocked by antibodies to neuropilin-1 and VEGFR2 *(96)*. Notably, variations in the VEGF gene that lower systemic VEGF expression increase the risk of ALS in humans *(97)*.

MODULATION OF VEGF ACTION BY OTHER GROWTH FACTORS

Although VEGF clearly plays a major role in stimulating retinal neovascularization, it is likely that other growth factors also play important roles, either independently or in concert with VEGF. For instance, a critical effect in VEGF modulation has been demonstrated for growth hormone (GH) and insulin-like growth factor-1 (IGF-1). IGF-1, which is known to mediate the growth promoting aspects of GH, has been demonstrated to modulate VEGF induction of endothelial cell signaling. In retinal endothelial cells, IGF-1 controlled the maximal VEGF stimulation of Akt *(78)*. In addition, antagonism of the IGF-1 receptor significantly inhibited VEGF stimulation of ERK1/2 in retinal endothelial cells *(98)*. These experiments suggest that IGF-1 plays a permissive role in VEGF action on angiogenesis. The importance of the GH/IGF-1 axis in retinal neovascularization is highlighted by studies using the oxygen-induced retinopathy model. In this model, retinal neovascularization was significantly decreased both in transgenic mice expressing a growth hormone antagonist gene and in normal mice treated with an inhibitor of growth hormone secretion *(99)*. Of note, GH inhibition did not reduce retinal expression of VEGF or VEGFR2. This inhibition of retinal neovascularization was reversed by systemic administration of IGF-1 *(99)*. Further experiments demonstrated that an IGF-1 receptor antagonist also suppressed retinal neovascularization in this model *(98)*.

A second growth factor that appears to modulate VEGF action on endothelial cells is placental growth factor, or PlGF. Placental growth factor is a member of the VEGF family of structurally related growth factors *(100)*. In contrast to VEGF-A (which binds both VEGFR-1 and VEGFR-2), PlGF specifically binds VEGFR-1. PlGF has been reported to enhance, or "amplify," VEGF-driven angiogenesis *(101)*, increasing VEGF induction of endothelial cell survival, migration, and proliferation. A molecular basis for this synergism was reported, in which PlGF activation of VEGFR1 results in intermolecular transphosphorylation of VEGFR2, thus amplifying VEGF-driven angiogenesis via VEGFR2 *(102)*. The potential importance of PlGF in PDR has been highlighted by experiments using mice deficient in PlGF, which have demonstrated that PlGF is required for pathologic retinal neovascularization in the oxygen-induced retinopathy model *(101)*. Furthermore, PlGF levels are significantly increased in the vitreous in PDR as compared to nonneovascular disease *(103, 104)*, and retinal PlGF protein is increased in the oxygen-induced retinopathy model *(105)*.

The ability of other growth factors to modulate VEGF action suggests that these growth factors might themselves be therapeutic targets for proliferative diabetic retinopathy. Indeed, somatostatin analogs that inhibit the GH/IGF-1 axis have been under investigation for the treatment of diabetic retinopathy.

CONCLUSION

The major role that VEGF plays in retinal neovascularization is now beyond question, in light of the preponderance of clinical, preclinical, and basic research studies. For this reason, the development and use of therapeutics targeting VEGF and its downstream actions is a promising approach for current and future treatment of proliferative diabetic retinopathy. At the same time, the multiple actions of VEGF warrant an awareness of the potential side effects of therapies targeting this molecule. In addition, it is highly likely that additional growth factors play important roles in retinal neovascularization in DR. Such growth factors might potentially have synergistic effects with VEGF or act at different steps in the neovascular process. Therefore, it will be important to continue investigations into the role of other growth factors, which themselves may serve as additional targets for therapy.

REFERENCES

1. Fong DS, Aiello LP, Ferris FL, III, Klein R. Diabetic retinopathy. Diabetes Care 2004;27(10): 2540–53.
2. Michaelson IC. The mode of development of the vascular system of the retina, with some observations on its significance for certain retinal disease. Trans Ophthalmol Soc UK 1948;68:137–80.
3. Ashton N, Ward B, Supell G. Effect of oxygen on developing retinal vessels with particular reference to the problem of retrolental fibroplasia. Br J Ophthalmol 1954;38:397–432.
4. Das A, McGuire PG. Retinal and choroidal angiogenesis: pathophysiology and strategies for inhibition. Prog Retin Eye Res 2003;22(6):721–48.
5. Hanahan D, Folkman J. Patterns and emerging mechanisms of the angiogenic switch during tumorigenesis. Cell 1996;86(3):353–64.
6. Ozaki H, Yu AY, Della N, et al. Hypoxia inducible factor-1alpha is increased in ischemic retina: temporal and spatial correlation with VEGF expression. Invest Ophthalmol Vis Sci 1999;40(1):182–9.
7. Kelly BD, Hackett SF, Hirota K, et al. Cell type-specific regulation of angiogenic growth factor gene expression and induction of angiogenesis in nonischemic tissue by a constitutively active form of hypoxia-inducible factor 1. Circ Res 2003;93(11):1074–81.

8. Chan-Ling T, Page MP, Gardiner T, Baxter L, Rosinova E, Hughes S. Desmin ensheathment ratio as an indicator of vessel stability: evidence in normal development and in retinopathy of prematurity. Am J Pathol 2004;165(4):1301–13.
9. Otani A, Kinder K, Ewalt K, Otero FJ, Schimmel P, Friedlander M. Bone marrow-derived stem cells target retinal astrocytes and can promote or inhibit retinal angiogenesis. Nat Med 2002;8(9):1004–10.
10. Grant MB, May WS, Caballero S, et al. Adult hematopoietic stem cells provide functional hemangioblast activity during retinal neovascularization. Nat Med 2002;8(6):607–12.
11. Smith LE, Wesolowski E, McLellan A, et al. Oxygen-induced retinopathy in the mouse. Invest Ophthalmol Vis Sci 1994;35(1):101–11.
12. Chen J, Smith LE. Retinopathy of prematurity. Angiogenesis 2007;10(2):133–40.
13. Madan A, Penn JS. Animal models of oxygen-induced retinopathy. Front Biosci 2003;8:d1030–43.
14. Gartner S, Henkind P. Neovascularization of the iris (rubeosis iridis). Surv Ophthalmol 1978;22(5):291–312.
15. Henkind P. Ocular neovascularization. The Krill memorial lecture. Am J Ophthalmol 1978;85(3):287–301.
16. Argon laser scatter photocoagulation for prevention of neovascularization and vitreous hemorrhage in branch vein occlusion. A randomized clinical trial. Branch Vein Occlusion Study Group. Arch Ophthalmol 1986;104(1):34–41.
17. Senger DR, Galli SJ, Dvorak AM, Perruzzi CA, Harvey VS, Dvorak HF. Tumor cells secrete a vascular permeability factor that promotes accumulation of ascites fluid. Science 1983;219(4587):983–5.
18. Keck PJ, Hauser SD, Krivi G, et al. Vascular permeability factor, an endothelial cell mitogen related to PDGF. Science 1989;246(4935):1309–12.
19. Leung DW, Cachianes G, Kuang WJ, Goeddel DV, Ferrara N. Vascular endothelial growth factor is a secreted angiogenic mitogen. Science 1989;246(4935):1306–9.
20. Senger DR, Connolly DT, Van de Water L, Feder J, Dvorak HF. Purification and NH2-terminal amino acid sequence of guinea pig tumor-secreted vascular permeability factor. Cancer Res 1990;50(6):1774–8.
21. Plate KH, Breier G, Weich HA, Risau W. Vascular endothelial growth factor is a potential tumour angiogenesis factor in human gliomas in vivo. Nature 1992;359(6398):845–8.
22. Kim KJ, Li B, Winer J, et al. Inhibition of vascular endothelial growth factor-induced angiogenesis suppresses tumour growth in vivo. Nature 1993;362(6423):841–4.
23. Shweiki D, Itin A, Soffer D, Keshet E. Vascular endothelial growth factor induced by hypoxia may mediate hypoxia-initiated angiogenesis. Nature 1992;359(6398):843–5.
24. Ferrara N, Carver-Moore K, Chen H, et al. Heterozygous embryonic lethality induced by targeted inactivation of the VEGF gene. Nature 1996;380(6573):439–42.
25. Carmeliet P, Ferreira V, Breier G, et al. Abnormal blood vessel development and lethality in embryos lacking a single VEGF allele. Nature 1996;380(6573):435–9.
26. Adamis AP, Shima DT, Yeo KT, et al. Synthesis and secretion of vascular permeability factor/vascular endothelial growth factor by human retinal pigment epithelial cells. Biochem Biophys Res Commun 1993;193(2):631–8.
27. Aiello LP, Northrup JM, Keyt BA, Takagi H, Iwamoto MA. Hypoxic regulation of vascular endothelial growth factor in retinal cells. Arch Ophthalmol 1995;113(12):1538–44.
28. Aiello LP, Avery RL, Arrigg PG, et al. Vascular endothelial growth factor in ocular fluid of patients with diabetic retinopathy and other retinal disorders. N Engl J Med 1994;331(22):1480–7.
29. Adamis AP, Miller JW, Bernal MT, et al. Increased vascular endothelial growth factor levels in the vitreous of eyes with proliferative diabetic retinopathy. Am J Ophthalmol 1994;118(4):445–50.
30. Pierce EA, Avery RL, Foley ED, Aiello LP, Smith LE. Vascular endothelial growth factor/vascular permeability factor expression in a mouse model of retinal neovascularization. Proc Natl Acad Sci U S A 1995;92(3):905–9.
31. Dorey CK, Aouididi S, Reynaud X, Dvorak HF, Brown LF. Correlation of vascular permeability factor/vascular endothelial growth factor with extraretinal neovascularization in the rat. Arch Ophthalmol 1996;114(10):1210–7.

32. Stone J, Chan-Ling T, Pe'er J, Itin A, Gnessin H, Keshet E. Roles of vascular endothelial growth factor and astrocyte degeneration in the genesis of retinopathy of prematurity. Invest Ophthalmol Vis Sci 1996;37(2):290–9.
33. Donahue ML, Phelps DL, Watkins RH, LoMonaco MB, Horowitz S. Retinal vascular endothelial growth factor (VEGF) mRNA expression is altered in relation to neovascularization in oxygen induced retinopathy. Curr Eye Res 1996;15(2):175–84.
34. Miller JW, Adamis AP, Shima DT, et al. Vascular endothelial growth factor/vascular permeability factor is temporally and spatially correlated with ocular angiogenesis in a primate model. Am J Pathol 1994;145(3):574–84.
35. Hirota K, Semenza GL. Regulation of angiogenesis by hypoxia-inducible factor 1. Crit Rev Oncol Hematol 2006;59(1):15–26.
36. Forsythe JA, Jiang BH, Iyer NV, et al. Activation of vascular endothelial growth factor gene transcription by hypoxia-inducible factor 1. Mol Cell Biol 1996;16(9):4604–13.
37. Vinores SA, Xiao WH, Aslam S, et al. Implication of the hypoxia response element of the Vegf promoter in mouse models of retinal and choroidal neovascularization, but not retinal vascular development. J Cell Physiol 2006;206(3):749–58.
38. Shinoda K, Ishida S, Kawashima S, et al. Clinical factors related to the aqueous levels of vascular endothelial growth factor and hepatocyte growth factor in proliferative diabetic retinopathy. Curr Eye Res 2000;21(2):655–61.
39. Boulton M, Foreman D, Williams G, McLeod D. VEGF localisation in diabetic retinopathy. Br J Ophthalmol 1998;82(5):561–8.
40. Lahdenranta J, Pasqualini R, Schlingemann RO, et al. An anti-angiogenic state in mice and humans with retinal photoreceptor cell degeneration. Proc Natl Acad Sci USA 2001;98(18):10368–73.
41. Lutty GA, McLeod DS, Merges C, Diggs A, Plouet J. Localization of vascular endothelial growth factor in human retina and choroid. Arch Ophthalmol 1996;114(8):971–7.
42. Amin RH, Frank RN, Kennedy A, Eliott D, Puklin JE, Abrams GW. Vascular endothelial growth factor is present in glial cells of the retina and optic nerve of human subjects with nonproliferative diabetic retinopathy. Invest Ophthalmol Vis Sci 1997;38(1):36–47.
43. Funatsu H, Yamashita H, Nakamura S, et al. Vitreous levels of pigment epithelium-derived factor and vascular endothelial growth factor are related to diabetic macular edema. Ophthalmology 2006;113(2):294–301.
44. Murata T, Nakagawa K, Khalil A, Ishibashi T, Inomata H, Sueishi K. The relation between expression of vascular endothelial growth factor and breakdown of the blood-retinal barrier in diabetic rat retinas. Lab Invest 1996;74(4):819–25.
45. Sone H, Kawakami Y, Okuda Y, et al. Ocular vascular endothelial growth factor levels in diabetic rats are elevated before observable retinal proliferative changes. Diabetologia 1997;40(6):726–30.
46. Gilbert RE, Vranes D, Berka JL, et al. Vascular endothelial growth factor and its receptors in control and diabetic rat eyes. Lab Invest 1998;78(8):1017–27.
47. Kuroki M, Voest EE, Amano S, et al. Reactive oxygen intermediates increase vascular endothelial growth factor expression in vitro and in vivo. J Clin Invest 1996;98(7):1667–75.
48. Ellis EA, Guberski DL, Somogyi-Mann M, Grant MB. Increased H2O2, vascular endothelial growth factor and receptors in the retina of the BBZ/Wor diabetic rat. Free Radic Biol Med 2000;28(1): 91–101.
49. Obrosova IG, Minchenko AG, Marinescu V, et al. Antioxidants attenuate early up regulation of retinal vascular endothelial growth factor in streptozotocin-diabetic rats. Diabetologia 2001; 44(9):1102–10.
50. Lu M, Kuroki M, Amano S, et al. Advanced glycation end products increase retinal vascular endothelial growth factor expression. J Clin Invest 1998;101(6):1219–24.
51. Park JE, Chen HH, Winer J, Houck KA, Ferrara N. Placenta growth factor. Potentiation of vascular endothelial growth factor bioactivity, in vitro and in vivo, and high affinity binding to Flt-1 but not to Flk-1/KDR. J Biol Chem 1994;269(41):25646–54.
52. Aiello LP, Pierce EA, Foley ED, et al. Suppression of retinal neovascularization in vivo by inhibition of vascular endothelial growth factor (VEGF) using soluble VEGF-receptor chimeric proteins. Proc Natl Acad Sci USA 1995;92(23):10457–61.

53. Robinson GS, Pierce EA, Rook SL, Foley E, Webb R, Smith LE. Oligodeoxynucleotides inhibit retinal neovascularization in a murine model of proliferative retinopathy. Proc Natl Acad Sci USA 1996;93(10):4851–6.
54. Adamis AP, Shima DT, Tolentino MJ, et al. Inhibition of vascular endothelial growth factor prevents retinal ischemia-associated iris neovascularization in a nonhuman primate. Arch Ophthalmol 1996;114(1):66–71.
55. Ozaki H, Hayashi H, Vinores SA, Moromizato Y, Campochiaro PA, Oshima K. Intravitreal sustained release of VEGF causes retinal neovascularization in rabbits and breakdown of the blood-retinal barrier in rabbits and primates. Exp Eye Res 1997;64(4):505–17.
56. Tolentino MJ, McLeod DS, Taomoto M, Otsuji T, Adamis AP, Lutty GA. Pathologic features of vascular endothelial growth factor-induced retinopathy in the nonhuman primate. Am J Ophthalmol 2002;133(3):373–85.
57. Okamoto N, Tobe T, Hackett SF, et al. Transgenic mice with increased expression of vascular endothelial growth factor in the retina: a new model of intraretinal and subretinal neovascularization. Am J Pathol 1997;151(1):281–91.
58. Ozaki H, Seo MS, Ozaki K, et al. Blockade of vascular endothelial cell growth factor receptor signaling is sufficient to completely prevent retinal neovascularization. Am J Pathol 2000;156(2): 697–707.
59. Adamis AP, Altaweel M, Bressler NM, et al. Changes in retinal neovascularization after pegaptanib (Macugen) therapy in diabetic individuals. Ophthalmology 2006;113(1):23–8.
60. Stone EM. A very effective treatment for neovascular macular degeneration. N Engl J Med 2006;355(14):1493–5.
61. Maglione D, Guerriero V, Viglietto G, Delli-Bovi P, Persico MG. Isolation of a human placenta cDNA coding for a protein related to the vascular permeability factor. Proc Natl Acad Sci USA 1991;88(20):9267–71.
62. Olofsson B, Pajusola K, Kaipainen A, et al. Vascular endothelial growth factor B, a novel growth factor for endothelial cells. Proc Natl Acad Sci USA 1996;93(6):2576–81.
63. Lee J, Gray A, Yuan J, Luoh SM, Avraham H, Wood WI. Vascular endothelial growth factor-related protein: a ligand and specific activator of the tyrosine kinase receptor Flt4. Proc Natl Acad Sci USA 1996;93(5):1988–92.
64. Joukov V, Pajusola K, Kaipainen A, et al. A novel vascular endothelial growth factor, VEGF-C, is a ligand for the Flt4 (VEGFR-3) and KDR (VEGFR-2) receptor tyrosine kinases. Embo J 1996;15(2):290–98.
65. Orlandini M, Marconcini L, Ferruzzi R, Oliviero S. Identification of a c-fos-induced gene that is related to the platelet-derived growth factor/vascular endothelial growth factor family. Proc Natl Acad Sci USA 1996;93(21):11675–80.
66. Tischer E, Mitchell R, Hartman T, et al. The human gene for vascular endothelial growth factor. Multiple protein forms are encoded through alternative exon splicing. J Biol Chem 1991; 266(18):11947–54.
67. Houck KA, Ferrara N, Winer J, Cachianes G, Li B, Leung DW. The vascular endothelial growth factor family: identification of a fourth molecular species and characterization of alternative splicing of RNA. Mol Endocrinol 1991;5(12):1806–14.
68. Terman BI, Carrion ME, Kovacs E, Rasmussen BA, Eddy RL, Shows TB. Identification of a new endothelial cell growth factor receptor tyrosine kinase. Oncogene 1991;6(9):1677–83.
69. Shibuya M, Yamaguchi S, Yamane A, et al. Nucleotide sequence and expression of a novel human receptor-type tyrosine kinase gene (flt) closely related to the fms family. Oncogene 1990;5(4):519–24.
70. Ferrara N, Gerber HP, LeCouter J. The biology of VEGF and its receptors. Nat Med 2003;9(6): 669–76.
71. Achen MG, Jeltsch M, Kukk E, et al. Vascular endothelial growth factor D (VEGF-D) is a ligand for the tyrosine kinases VEGF receptor 2 (Flk1) and VEGF receptor 3 (Flt4). Proc Natl Acad Sci USA 1998;95(2):548–53.
72. Soker S, Takashima S, Miao HQ, Neufeld G, Klagsbrun M. Neuropilin-1 is expressed by endothelial and tumor cells as an isoform-specific receptor for vascular endothelial growth factor. Cell 1998;92(6):735–45.

73. Gluzman-Poltorak Z, Cohen T, Herzog Y, Neufeld G. Neuropilin-2 is a receptor for the vascular endothelial growth factor (VEGF) forms VEGF-145 and VEGF-165. J Biol Chem 2000;275(38):29922.
74. Zachary I. VEGF signalling: integration and multi-tasking in endothelial cell biology. Biochem Soc Trans 2003;31(Pt 6):1171–7.
75. Thieme H, Aiello LP, Takagi H, Ferrara N, King GL. Comparative analysis of vascular endothelial growth factor receptors on retinal and aortic vascular endothelial cells. Diabetes 1995;44(1):98–103.
76. Duh EJ, Yang HS, Suzuma I, et al. Pigment epithelium-derived factor suppresses ischemia-induced retinal neovascularization and VEGF-induced migration and growth. Invest Ophthalmol Vis Sci 2002;43(3):821–9.
77. Wilson SH, Davis MI, Caballero S, Grant MB. Modulation of retinal endothelial cell behaviour by insulin-like growth factor I and somatostatin analogues: implications for diabetic retinopathy. Growth Horm IGF Res 2001;11 Suppl A:S53–9.
78. Hellstrom A, Perruzzi C, Ju M, et al. Low IGF-I suppresses VEGF-survival signaling in retinal endothelial cells: direct correlation with clinical retinopathy of prematurity. Proc Natl Acad Sci USA 2001;98(10):5804–8.
79. Im E, Venkatakrishnan A, Kazlauskas A. Cathepsin B regulates the intrinsic angiogenic threshold of endothelial cells. Mol Biol Cell 2005;16(8):3488–500.
80. Behzadian MA, Windsor LJ, Ghaly N, Liou G, Tsai NT, Caldwell RB. VEGF-induced paracellular permeability in cultured endothelial cells involves urokinase and its receptor. Faseb J 2003;17(6):752–4.
81. Harhaj NS, Felinski EA, Wolpert EB, Sundstrom JM, Gardner TW, Antonetti DA. VEGF activation of protein kinase C stimulates occludin phosphorylation and contributes to endothelial permeability. Invest Ophthalmol Vis Sci 2006;47(11):5106–15.
82. Matsumoto T, Claesson-Welsh L. VEGF receptor signal transduction. Sci STKE 2001; 2001(112):RE21.
83. Aiello LP, Bursell SE, Clermont A, et al. Vascular endothelial growth factor-induced retinal permeability is mediated by protein kinase C in vivo and suppressed by an orally effective beta-isoform-selective inhibitor. Diabetes 1997;46(9):1473–80.
84. Takahashi T, Ueno H, Shibuya M. VEGF activates protein kinase C-dependent, but Ras-independent Raf-MEK-MAP kinase pathway for DNA synthesis in primary endothelial cells. Oncogene 1999;18(13):2221–30.
85. Gliki G, Abu-Ghazaleh R, Jezequel S, Wheeler-Jones C, Zachary I. Vascular endothelial growth factor-induced prostacyclin production is mediated by a protein kinase C (PKC)-dependent activation of extracellular signal-regulated protein kinases 1 and 2 involving PKC-delta and by mobilization of intracellular Ca2+. Biochem J 2001;353(Pt 3):503–12.
86. Xia P, Aiello LP, Ishii H, et al. Characterization of vascular endothelial growth factor's effect on the activation of protein kinase C, its isoforms, and endothelial cell growth. J Clin Invest 1996;98(9):2018–26.
87. Gerber HP, McMurtrey A, Kowalski J, et al. Vascular endothelial growth factor regulates endothelial cell survival through the phosphatidylinositol 3′ ❑-kinase/Akt signal transduction pathway. Requirement for Flk-1/KDR activation. J Biol Chem 1998;273(46):30336–43.
88. Ishida S, Usui T, Yamashiro K, et al. VEGF164 is proinflammatory in the diabetic retina. Invest Ophthalmol Vis Sci 2003;44(5):2155–62.
89. Qaum T, Xu Q, Joussen AM, et al. VEGF-initiated Blood-Retinal Barrier Breakdown in Early Diabetes. Invest Ophthalmol Vis Sci 2001;42(10):2408–13.
90. Lu M, Perez VL, Ma N, et al. VEGF increases retinal vascular ICAM-1 expression in vivo. Invest Ophthalmol Vis Sci 1999;40(8):1808–12.
91. Joussen AM, Poulaki V, Qin W, et al. Retinal vascular endothelial growth factor induces intercellular adhesion molecule-1 and endothelial nitric oxide synthase expression and initiates early diabetic retinal leukocyte adhesion in vivo. Am J Pathol 2002;160(2):501–9.
92. Robinson GS, Ju M, Shih SC, et al. Nonvascular role for VEGF: VEGFR-1, 2 activity is critical for neural retinal development. Faseb J 2001;15(7):1215–7.

93. Storkebaum E, Lambrechts D, Carmeliet P. VEGF: once regarded as a specific angiogenic factor, now implicated in neuroprotection. Bioessays 2004;26(9):943–54.
94. Sondell M, Lundborg G, Kanje M. Vascular endothelial growth factor has neurotrophic activity and stimulates axonal outgrowth, enhancing cell survival and Schwann cell proliferation in the peripheral nervous system. J Neurosci 1999;19(14):5731–40.
95. Silverman WF, Krum JM, Mani N, Rosenstein JM. Vascular, glial and neuronal effects of vascular endothelial growth factor in mesencephalic explant cultures. Neuroscience 1999;90(4):1529–41.
96. Oosthuyse B, Moons L, Storkebaum E, et al. Deletion of the hypoxia-response element in the vascular endothelial growth factor promoter causes motor neuron degeneration. Nat Genet 2001;28(2):131–8.
97. Lambrechts D, Storkebaum E, Morimoto M, et al. VEGF is a modifier of amyotrophic lateral sclerosis in mice and humans and protects motoneurons against ischemic death. Nat Genet 2003;34(4):383–94.
98. Smith LE, Shen W, Perruzzi C, et al. Regulation of vascular endothelial growth factor-dependent retinal neovascularization by insulin-like growth factor-1 receptor. Nat Med 1999;5(12):1390–5.
99. Smith LE, Kopchick JJ, Chen W, et al. Essential role of growth hormone in ischemia-induced retinal neovascularization. Science 1997;276(5319):1706–9.
100. De Falco S, Gigante B, Persico MG. Structure and function of placental growth factor. Trends Cardiovasc Med 2002;12(6):241–6.
101. Carmeliet P, Moons L, Luttun A, et al. Synergism between vascular endothelial growth factor and placental growth factor contributes to angiogenesis and plasma extravasation in pathological conditions. Nat Med 2001;7(5):575–83.
102. Autiero M, Waltenberger J, Communi D, et al. Role of PlGF in the intra- and intermolecular cross talk between the VEGF receptors Flt1 and Flk1. Nat Med 2003;9(7):936–43.
103. Khaliq A, Foreman D, Ahmed A, et al. Increased expression of placenta growth factor in proliferative diabetic retinopathy. Lab Invest 1998;78(1):109–16.
104. Mitamura Y, Tashimo A, Nakamura Y, et al. Vitreous levels of placenta growth factor and vascular endothelial growth factor in patients with proliferative diabetic retinopathy. Diabetes Care 2002;25(12):2352.
105. Yao YG, Yang HS, Cao Z, Danielsson J, Duh EJ. Upregulation of placental growth factor by vascular endothelial growth factor via a post-transcriptional mechanism. FEBS Lett 2005;579(5):1227–34.

16 Beyond VEGF – Other Factors Important in Retinal Neovascularization: Potential Targets in Proliferative Diabetic Retinopathy

Arup Das, Deepti Navaratna, and Paul G. McGuire

CONTENTS

ABSTRACT

Retinal neovascularization (NV), or the formation of new blood vessels in the retina, is a leading cause of blindness in diabetics. Research advances have shed great insights into molecules that play an important role in retinal neovascularization, suggesting potential targets for therapeutic manipulation. Vascular endothelial growth factor (VEGF) is well-recognized as a major stimulus in retinal NV, and therapies directed against VEGF are currently being developed and used. However, a greater understanding of additional molecules regulating retinal NV has emerged. This chapter will review these molecules and discuss their potential importance to retinal neovascularization in diabetes. This discussion will include additional pro-angiogenic growth factors, extracellular proteinases, integrins, and

From: *Contemporary Diabetes: Diabetic Retinopathy*
Edited by: E. Duh © Humana Press, Totowa, NJ

endogenous inhibitors of neovascularization. The development of therapeutic strategies targeting these molecules may result in additional treatments for retinal neovascularization in diabetic retinopathy.

Key Words: Angiopoietin; angiostatin; basic fibroblast growth factor; endostatin,; erythropoietin; hepatocyte growth factor; insulin-like growth factor; integrin; matrix metalloproteinases; pigment epithelium-derived factor; retinal neovascularization; thrombospondin-1; tissue inhibitor of matrix metalloproteinases; transforming growth factor-β; tumor necrosis factor; urokinase plasminogen activator.

Retinal neovascularization or the formation of new blood vessels in the retina is a leading cause of blindness in diabetics. New blood vessels are fragile, and easily bleed into the vitreous, causing vitreous hemorrhage and eventually traction retinal detachment. It has been well accepted that hypoxia plays an important role in the initiation of the angiogenic process *(1, 2)*. Michaelson first hypothesized that a diffusible factor is released by the ischemic retina and can cause development of new blood vessels in the retina. Since then, several angiogenic growth factors have been identified: vascular endothelial growth factor (VEGF), basic fibroblast growth factor (bFGF), insulin-like growth factor (IGF), angiopoietin, erythropoietin, hepatocyte growth factor (HGF), and tumor necrosis factor (TNF) *(3, 4)*. These growth factors can cause cell proliferation, while increased integrins and proteinases are important in cell migration. Both cell proliferation and migration are essential steps in angiogenesis (Fig. 1). Although VEGF has been extensively studied in the pathogenesis of retinal angiogenesis one needs to be aware that there are other pathways and factors that are important in retinal angiogenesis. All the VEGF inhibitors (pegaptanib and ranibizumab) that have been so far approved by the FDA are used as anti-angiogenic agents in age-related macular degeneration. It is possible that inhibition of pathways other than VEGF, or combining anti-VEGF pathway with another agent may be more effective in controlling retinal neovascularization in diabetic retinopathy. The fact that most anti-VEGF therapies require several injections to make the new vessels regress and leak less makes a strong case for other molecules that need to be explored as potential targets in proliferative retinopathy *(5)*. The present chapter summarizes the molecules other than VEGF involved in retinal angiogenesis and pre-clinical studies emphasizing the importance of these molecules as potential targets in treatment of retinal neovascularization in diabetic retinopathy.

INSULIN-LIKE GROWTH FACTOR

The role of the pituitary and the importance of growth hormone in the development and progression of diabetic retinopathy have been recognized for a long time as regression of retinal neovascularization was seen after pituitary infarction *(6)*. Hypophysectomy was the first effective treatment for retinopathy but was discontinued because of the risk of severe hypoglycemia and later the development of more effective panretinal photocoagulation that it produced. This effect of pituitary ablation on diabetic retinopathy has been attributed to growth hormone (GH)/insulin-like growth factor-1 (IGF-1). Levels of serum IGF-1 in PDR patients were found to be almost twice the level in patients with no or minimal diabetic retinopathy *(7)*. Similarly, concentrations of IGF-1 in vitreous of

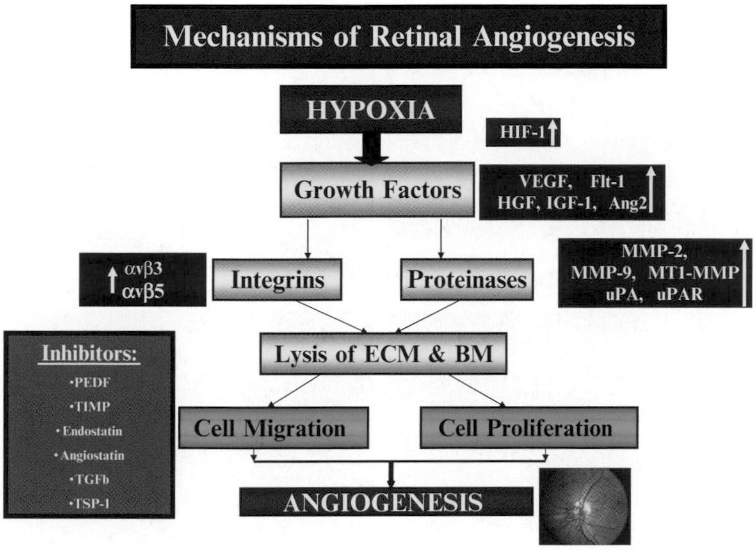

Fig. 1. Flow chart describing the mechanisms of retinal angiogenesis. The capillary non-perfusion results in hypoxia, which then upregulates the expression of growth factors either directly, or through HIF-1. Growth factors then increase the expression of integrins and proteinases, which result in endothelial cell migration. These factors also promote endothelial cell proliferation directly. Both cell migration and proliferation are essential steps in angiogenesis. There is a critical balance between angiogenesis promoters and endogenous inhibitors. Any destabilization in this balance may lead to angiogenesis (modified from *(5)* with permission).

patients with PDR undergoing vitrectomy were significantly higher than those in non-diabetics *(8)*. In a larger study, higher levels of serum IGF-1 were significantly associated with an increased frequency of PDR in the group using insulin *(9)*.

That the higher serum IGF-1 level may be a risk factor for the progression to proliferative retinopathy has been observed in several clinical studies. The Diabetes Control and Complications Trial (DCCT) has shown worsening of retinopathy in the tight glucose control group during the first 2 years of the trial *(10)*. This phenomenon of worsening of retinopathy has been attributed to the rise in serum IGF-1 concentration *(11)*. During continuous subcutaneous insulin infusion therapy, there has been a rise of serum IGF-1 over the first 4 months, which subsequently declined over the next 8 months.

The role of IGF-1 in retinal neovascularization has been extensively studied by Smith et al. Transgenic mice expressing a GH antagonist gene when exposed to oxygen-induced ischemia, show up to 44% inhibition of retinal neovascularization, and this could be reversed with exogenous IGF-1 administration (Fig. 2) *(12)*. These studies point towards a role of GH/IGF-1 in ischemia-induced retinal neovascularization. However, there was no reduction of VEGF mRNA or protein in response to inhibition of GH secretion or action in these treated animals. Interestingly, there was no increase in retinal NV in transgenic mice expressing increased GH levels.

Although VEGF has been shown to be an important factor in the development of retinal vessels, it is still not sufficient as knockout mice lacking IGF-1 have arrested retinal vascular development despite the presence of VEGF *(13)*. Studies have shown that

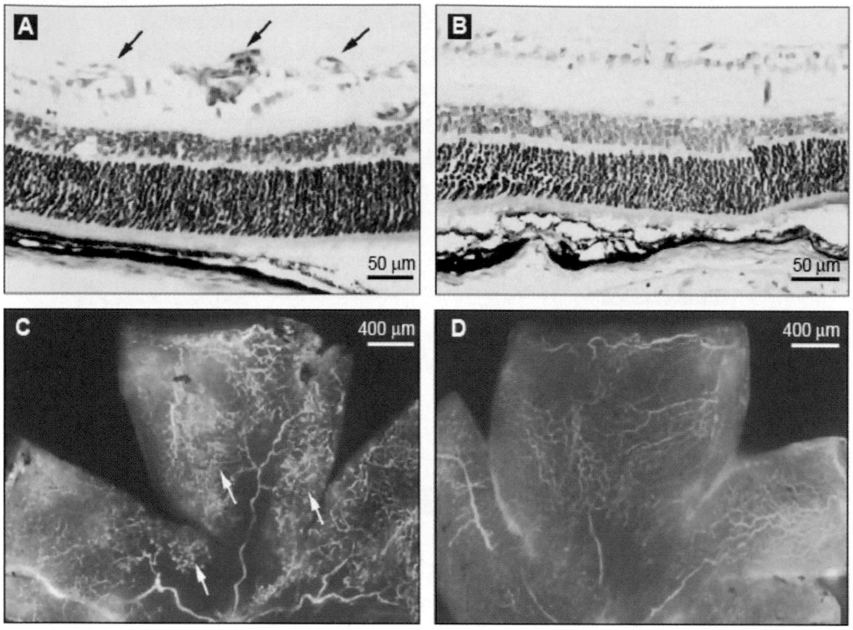

Fig. 2. Effect of GH inhibition on ischemia-induced retinal neovascularization (**A**). Cross section of an eye from a nontransgenic littermate mouse, showing retinal neovascularization internal to the inner limiting membrane (*arrows*) (**B**). Cross section of an eye from a GH antagonist G119K transgenic mouse. No vascular cell nuclei are apparent internal to the inner limiting membrane (**C**). Nontransgenic flat-mounted whole retina, showing extensive areas of retinal neovascularization *(14)* (bright fluorescence, indicated in part with *arrows*) that is significantly reduced in the retinas from the GH antagonist G119K transgenic mice (**D**) (reprinted from *(12)* with permission from AAAS).

premature infants who develop ROP have low levels of serum IGF-1 compared with infants without the disease *(14)*. Thus, IGF-1 is critical to normal retinal vascular development. Low levels of IGF-1 can predict ROP, and exogenously administered IGF-1 to restore normal levels might prevent ROP.

So, if all the evidence indicates that the IGF-1 plays a role in the pathogenesis of diabetic retinopathy, how does it work and contribute to angiogenesis? Intravitreal administration of IGF-1 has been shown to increase retinal Akt, JNK, HIF-1 alpha, NF-kappa B, AP-1 activity and VEGF levels *(15)*. IGF-1 may participate in the angiogenesis process by inducing retinal VEGF expression. Interestingly, IGF-1 has also been attributed to the increased leukostasis and blood–retinal barrier breakdown seen in diabetic animals. Normoglycemic, normoinsulinemic transgenic mice overexpressing IGF-1 in the retina develop loss of pericytes, and thickening of the basement membrane of retinal capillaries at 2 months *(16)*. At 6 months these animals develop intraretinal microvascular abnormalities and retinal neovascularization with subsequent rubeosis iridis and neovascular glaucoma. The neovascularization was found to be consistent with increased IGF-1 levels in aqueous humor and increased VEGF expression in retinal glial cells.

Because of the role played by IGF-1 in proliferative diabetic retinopathy, somatostatin analogues have been tested in PDR patients. Pilot studies using octreotide, by infusion pump or subcutaneous delivery, have shown decreased incidence of progression from severe nonproliferative diabetic retinopathy and early proliferative diabetic retinopathy into proliferative retinopathy *(17, 18)*. However, a short-term study using the growth hormone receptor antagonist pegvisomant alone in 25 patients with PDR for 3 months did not show any regression of new vessels *(19)*. The Sandostatin Study, a large-scale, multi-centered, randomized placebo-controlled clinical trial, has recently been completed looking at the effect of a long-acting somatostatin analogue, octreotide (Sandostatin LAR, Novartis) in patients with severe NPDR and early PDR. The octreotide was given by intramuscular injections (30 mg) every 4 weeks.

BASIC FIBROBLAST GROWTH FACTOR

Basic fibroblast growth factor (bFGF) (mol. wt. 18,000) which belongs to the family of heparin-binding growth factors has been implicated in retinal neovascularization. However, experiments with overexpression, or deficiency of bFGF have shown that bFGF may not be necessary for the development of retinal neovascularization *(20, 21)*.

The bFGF has been localized to the inner nuclear and ganglion cell layers of the adult retina *(22, 23)*. In the mouse model of oxygen-induced retinopathy, FGF-like peptides are elevated in the retinas during neovascularization *(24)*. One study has reported elevated levels of bFGF in the vitreous of patients with proliferative diabetic retinopathy *(25)*, while other studies have not found significant changes in bFGF levels in intraocular fluids of patients with diabetic retinopathy. This inconsistency about the bFGF levels in diabetic patients has been attributed to differences in the sensitivity of assays *(3)*. Immunocytochemical studies have reported the presence of bFGF in human retinal neovascular membranes. However, its role in the pathogenesis of retinal angiogenesis is under question, as only a minimal amount of bFGF is expressed in the basement membranes of new vessels in spite of their capacity to bind exogenous bFGF *(26, 27)*.

ANGIOPOIETIN

Angiopoietins are ligands for the Tie (Tyrosine kinase with Immunoglobulin and Epidermal growth factor homology) receptors, a class of endothelial specific tyrosine kinase receptors that have been shown to play an important role in vascular growth and development *(28)*. There are four members of the angiopoietin family. Ang-2 expression is upregulated during normal retinal development and retinal neovascularization in mice *(28–32)*. The expression of Ang-2 is greatest on day 17 (the time of the maximal angiogenic response) in the animal model of oxygen-induced retinopathy *(32)*. The in situ expression of Ang-2 was predominantly localized to cells within and near the inner nuclear layer, especially horizontal cells. Angiopoietin-2 promotes sensitivity to the angiogenic effects of VEGF in retinal vessels *(33)*. The stimulation of cultured retinal endothelial cells with Ang-1 and -2 resulted in the increased expression of MMP-9. Animals treated with the Tie-2 antagonist, muTek delta Fc showed a significant decrease (87%) in retinal NV, in addition to a concomitant decrease in MMP-9 expression in the retinas of treated animals *(32)*. Thus, the upregulation of proteinases like MMP-9 in retinal endothelial cells may be an important early response during development of retinal neovascularization.

What role does Ang-2 play in the pathogenesis of diabetic retinopathy? The vitreous levels of Ang-2 have been found to be significantly higher in patients with PDR than that in patients with nondiabetic ocular diseases *(34)*, and correlated significantly with that of VEGF in eyes with PDR. Both Ang-2 and VEGF levels in eyes with active PDR are higher than those with inactive PDR. Transgenic mice overexpressing human Ang-2 show a reduced coverage of capillaries with pericytes *(35)*. These animals, when exposed to the oxygen-induced retinopathy protocol, showed increased preretinal neovascularization. The newly formed intraretinal vessels were found to be pericyte deficient. Interestingly, Ang-2 is upregulated more than 30-fold in the retinas of diabetic rats, preceding the onset of pericyte loss *(36)*. Also, injection of Ang-2 into the eyes of normal rats induces a dose-dependent pericyte loss. Thus, upregulation of Ang-2 may play an important role in the loss of pericytes seen in early diabetic retinopathy.

As Ang-2 is critical for retinal angiogenesis, inhibition of the Ang-2/Tie-2 may be considered as another potential therapeutic approach for inhibiting retinal NV. A single intramuscular injection of adenovirus expressing the exTek gene (extracellular domain of the Tie-2 receptor) in the murine model of retinal NV can suppress retinal NV by 47% *(37)*. In the same model, systemic injection of the Tek delta Fc (the extracellular domain of the murine Tek receptor fused to the Fc portion of the murine IgG) that blocks binding of Ang-2 to the Tie-2 receptor can suppress retinal NV by 87% *(32)*.

ERYTHROPOIETIN

Erythropoietin is a glycoprotein that stimulates the formation of red blood cells, and shows angiogenic activity in vascular endothelial cells by stimulating cell proliferation and migration probably through erythropoietin receptors expressed in these cells. Vitreous erythropoietin level has been found to be significantly higher among patients with PDR compared to those without diabetes *(38)*. Interestingly, vitreous erythropoietin and VEGF levels were independently associated with PDR, and erythropoietin level was more strongly associated with the presence of PDR than was VEGF. Recent immunocytochemistry on human epiretinal membranes from patients with PDR shows strong expression of erythropoietin receptors in endothelial cells and stromal cells *(39)*.

Erythropoietin and VEGF levels were found to be upregulated in the animal model of retinal neovascularization, and inhibitors of erythropoietin suppress the neovascularization in vivo as well as endothelial cell proliferation in vitro *(38)*. The same group also observed that combined inhibition of VEGF and erythropoietin was more effective than inhibition of either alone in suppressing the endothelial cell proliferation. This definitely points out the role of more than one pathway in the pathogenesis of retinal angiogenesis and the rationale of using a combination therapy rather than using anti-VEGF therapy alone in the treatment of neovascularization *(40)*. As erythropoietin plays an important role as an endogenous retinal survival factor in protecting photoreceptors *(41)*, one needs to be cautious about the use of erythropoietin inhibitors in diabetic patients *(40)*.

HEPATOCYTE GROWTH FACTOR

Hepatocyte growth factor (HGF) has been reported to have angiogenic activity associated with tumor growth and wound healing *(42, 43)*. Levels of HGF in vitreous and aqueous fluids of PDR patients were found to be significantly elevated during the active stage *(44, 45)*. In a separate study, no correlation was found between serum and vitreous levels of HGF in diabetic patients, and the high HGF level in vitreous was attributed to intraocular synthesis of HGF in these patients *(46)*. These clinical observations raise the possibility of an important role for this growth factor in ocular angiogenesis. The function of HGF is dependent on the expression and activation of the Met receptor, a transmembrane tyrosine kinase encoded by the c-Met proto-oncogene *(47)*. In a mouse model of retinal angiogenesis, we have shown that HGF and c-Met are upregulated in the retinas, and the HGF was active as evidenced by the increased presence of the phophorylated form of c-Met in the tissues *(48)*. HGF stimulates the secretion of urokinase and expression of its receptor, uPAR in retinal endothelial cells. HGF also increases the migratory and invasive capacity of these cells which could be inhibited by the addition of the urokinase-derived peptide A6 *(48)*. Inhibition of c-Met results in a 70% decrease in retinal angiogenesis and a 40% decrease in urokinase activity in the retina (Fig. 3). Interestingly, HGF has been shown to increase retinal vascular permeability at physiologically relevant concentrations with a magnitude similar to that of VEGF without altering retinal hemodynamics *(49)*. Thus, HGF may play roles in both retinal angiogenesis and blood–retinal barrier alteration, and may be used as targets in diabetic retinopathy.

TUMOR NECROSIS FACTOR

Tumor necrosis factor, a 26 kDa transmembrane protein, has been shown to be expressed in retinas of human proliferative diabetic retinopathy *(50, 51)* and in animal models of retinal neovascularization *(51, 52)*. It is expressed mainly by Muller cells and inner nuclear layer and in the outer nuclear layer during the angiogenic phase as well *(52)*. TNFα is processed by a TNFα converting enzyme (TACE) to yield a 17 kDa soluble protein. TNFα functions through its binding to two receptors: p55, implicated in apoptosis and NFkB activation, and p75, involved with lymphocyte proliferation. TNFα increases the expression of several proteinases like MT1-MMP, MMP-3 and MMP-9 in cultured retinal microvascular endothelial cells. VEGF also plays a role in this process through its regulation of TNFα converting enzyme (TACE) and p55 mRNA in the vascular endothelial cells. The overlapping temporal expression of VEGF and TNFα suggests an interactive role of these two growth factors in the regulation of extracellular proteinases during the angiogenic process. Inhibition of TNFα significantly improves vascular recovery and reduces retinal neovascularization in the oxygen-induced retinopathy model *(53)*. Also, in animals with TNF receptor p55 deficiency there is significantly reduced vascularization in the same model *(54)*. TNFα has been shown to operate along with COX-2 in alteration of the blood–retinal barrier in early diabetic retinopathy, a newly recognized inflammatory disease *(55)*.

EXTRACELLULAR PROTEINASES

Endothelial cell migration and invasion through the capillary basement membrane and extracellular matrix (ECM) are crucial steps in the angiogenic process. This process is tightly coupled to the induction and activation of certain extracellular proteinases. Historically, two families of proteinases have been studied in this process – the serine

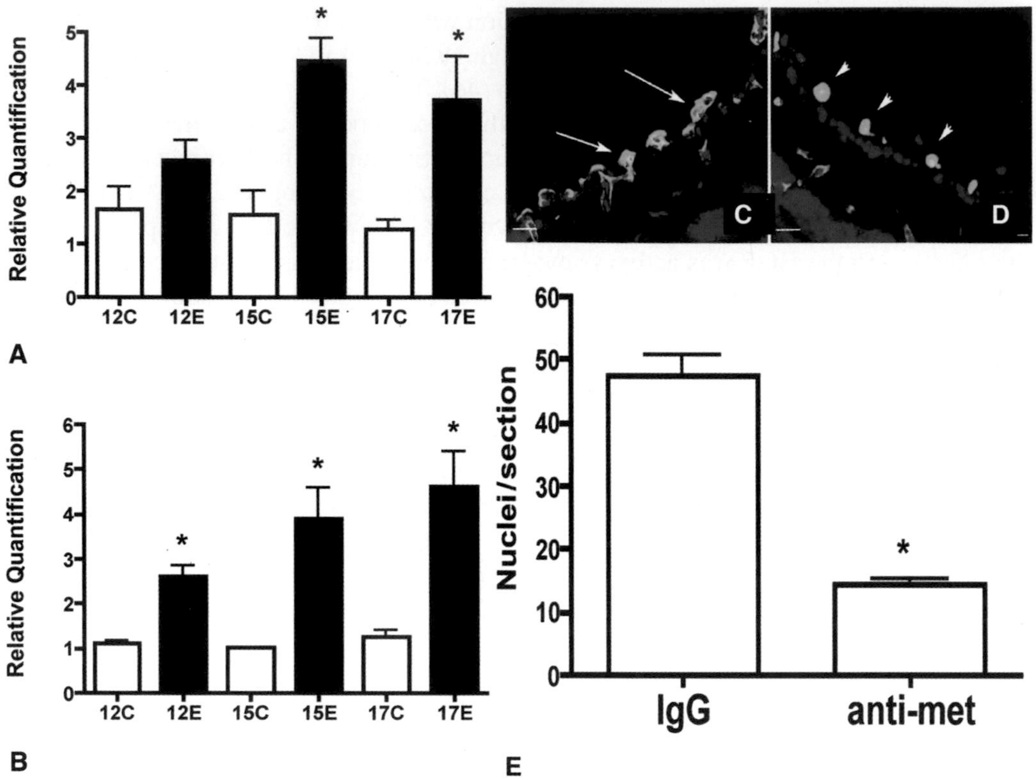

Fig. 3. Expression of HGF and c-Met mRNA in control and experimental OIR mice using the real-time comparative Ct method of quantitation. HGF mRNA levels in retinas from experimental animals was significantly elevated on days 15 ($P = 0.0093$) and 17 ($P = 0.0044$) compared with controls when new blood vessels were forming (**A**). The pattern of c-Met mRNA expression in experimental animals was similar (**B**). The level of c-Met mRNA increased significantly on day 12 ($P = 0.0043$) and persisted through day 15 ($P = 0.0126$) and day 17 ($P = 0.0121$). Samples are from day 12, 15, and 17 control (C) and experimental (E) animals; $n = 3$. *Significantly greater than control. Experimental mice were treated with a single intraocular injection of c-*met* neutralizing antibody on day 13 and were analyzed for new vessel formation. Representative images of retinas from normal IgG (**C**) and anti-c-*met*-treated (**D**) animals. Quantitation of new vessels reveals a 70% reduction in the degree of angiogenesis in the eyes treated with the c-*met* antibody (**e**). *Significantly less than IgG-treated animals ($P < 0.0001$). Bar, 10 μm. GF (reprinted from *(48)* with permission).

proteinase, urokinase plasminogen activator (uPA) and members of a family of zinc-dependent endopeptidases called matrix metalloproteinases (MMPs).

The Urokinase Plasminogen Activator System (uPA/uPAR System)

The urokinase plasminogen activator is present in endothelial cells in two molecular forms, a 54 kDa high molecular weight form and a 32 kDa low molecular weight form which lacks the amino terminal fragment of the protein *(56, 57)*. The amino terminal fragment contains the growth factor and kringle domains of the protein that mediate binding to uPAR and is postulated to play a role in cell proliferation *(58, 59)*. uPA is secreted as a zymogen (Pro-uPA) that is activated by autocatalytic cleavage upon binding to its receptor, uPAR. Active urokinase converts another zymogen, plasminogen to plasmin, a broad spectrum protease capable of degrading many components of the ECM. The invasive and migratory potential of endothelial cells is largely determined upon the pool of active urokinase available on the cell surface. The uPA/uPAR interaction represents a sensitive and flexible system to regulate proteolytic potential in endothelial cells. The amount of surface associated uPA might facilitate limited proteolysis of the matrix at the cell-attachment sites to facilitate directed cell migration or unleash large scale proteolytic events that culminate in widespread ECM remodeling (changes in growth factor sequestration, composition and adhesive properties).

The uPA system also plays an important role in the activation of several MMPs and in the release and activation of growth factors stored in the extracellular matrix *(60)*. Hypoxia, the classical stimulus for angiogenesis, has been found to increase the expression of uPAR *(61)*. The contribution of the uPA/uPAR system to angiogenesis has been studied in several animal models of tumor angiogenesis *(62, 63)*. Specific inhibitors of the urokinase system belonging to the serpin family of inhibitors have been characterized. Plasminogen activator inhibitors 1 and 2 (PAI-1 and PAI-2) regulate proteolytic activity by affecting uPAR availability on the cell surface, and inhibition of uPA activity directly *(59)*. PAI-1 null mice show decreased angiogenesis suggesting that PAI-1 is necessary for tumor cell invasion and neovascularization *(64, 65)* (Fig. 4).

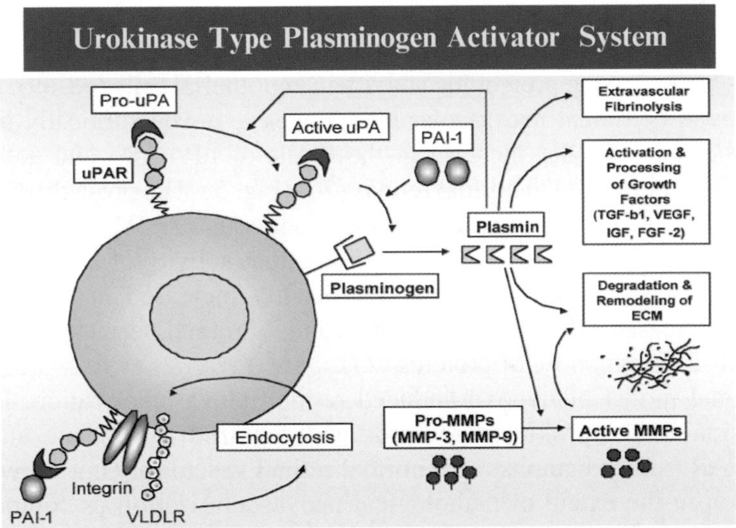

Fig. 4. Flow chart describing the role of the urokinase type plasminogen activator system in angiogenesis. The urokinase (uPA) binds to its receptor (uPAR) on the cell surface, and the active uPA coverts plasminogen to plasmin, which has a broad range of actions including ECM degradation and remodeling, extravascular fibrinolysis, activation and processing of growth factors, and activation of MMPs. The plasminogen activator inhibitor (PAI-1) inhibits the conversion of plasminogen to plasmin (modified from Fig. 1 in *(142)*).

Matrix Metalloproteinases

The matrix metalloproteinases are a family of zinc-dependent proteases, originally identified for their ECM degrading capabilities. At least 21 different types of MMPs have been identified to date. Based on their substrate specificity and cellular localization MMPs are grouped into the collagenases (MMP-1, MMP-8, and MMP-13), the gelatinases (MMP-2 and MMP-9), the stromelysins (MMP-3, MMP-10, MMP-11), and the non traditional MMPs (matrilysin/MMP-7, metalloelastase or MMP-12) and the membrane type MMPs,(MT-MMPs) *(66)*. There are at least five distinct types of MT-MMPs: MMP-12, -15, -16, -17 and -21 and MT1-MMP has been studied in relation to its ability to regulate focused matrix lysis and the activation of MMP-2 *(66)*. In addition to their capacity to degrade a large variety of ECM molecules, MMPs are known to process a number of bioactive molecules. MMPs regulate a variety of cell behaviors such as cell proliferation, migration, differentiation, apoptosis and host defense. In relation to retinal neovascularization, MMPs are implicated in the angiogenic process for their involvements in mainly endothelial cell migration and invasion and posttranslational modification of anti-angiogenic growth factor receptors.

Proteinases in Retinal Neovascularization

Significant upregulation of uPA (both the 54 and 32 kDa isoforms) along with increases in secretion and activation of MMP-2 and -9 were observed in the retinas of animals with neovascularization *(67)*. These results suggest that proteolytic activity and its regulatory mechanisms might play an important role in the angiogenic process. There has been increasing evidence that the plasminogen activators play an important role in the progression of this disease. Increased levels of VEGF and TPA have been accounted for in the vitreous fluid of patients with PDR *(68)*. Several growth factors such as HGF, TGF-B, VEGF and certain angiostatic drugs have been shown to induce angiogenesis by increasing proteolytic activity in endothelial cells *(48, 69)*. Examination of proteinases in epiretinal neovascular membranes removed surgically from humans with PDR showed a similar increase in the levels of uPA, pro and active forms of MMP-2 and -9 as compared to normal retinas *(70)* (Fig. 5). The pro-MMP2 and TIMP-2 have been reported in the normal and diabetic vitreous *(71, 72)*, and pro-MMP-9 in diabetic vitreous *(71)*. A recent study has shown that activity of both MMP-2 and its physiological activator MT1-MMP are significantly increased in retinas of diabetic animals, and increased MMP-2 activity compromises retinal pericyte survival possibly through MMP-2 action on ECM proteins *(73)*.

In an animal model of hypoxia-induced retinal neovascularization, it was found that expression of the urokinase receptor was required to mediate an angiogenic response. $uPAR^{-/-}$ mice demonstrated normal retinal vascularity but showed a significant reduction in the extent of pathological neovascularization as compared to wild type controls *(74)*. The expression of uPAR mRNA was upregulated in experimental animals during the active phase of angiogenesis and uPAR protein was localized to endothelial cells in the superficial layers of the retina. A peptide inhibitor of the urokinase system, A6, was able to reduce the extent of retinal neovascularization and uPAR expression in the experimental animals *(74)* (Fig. 6). In another study, the adenovirus-mediated delivery of a uPA/uPAR antagonist inhibited endothelial cell

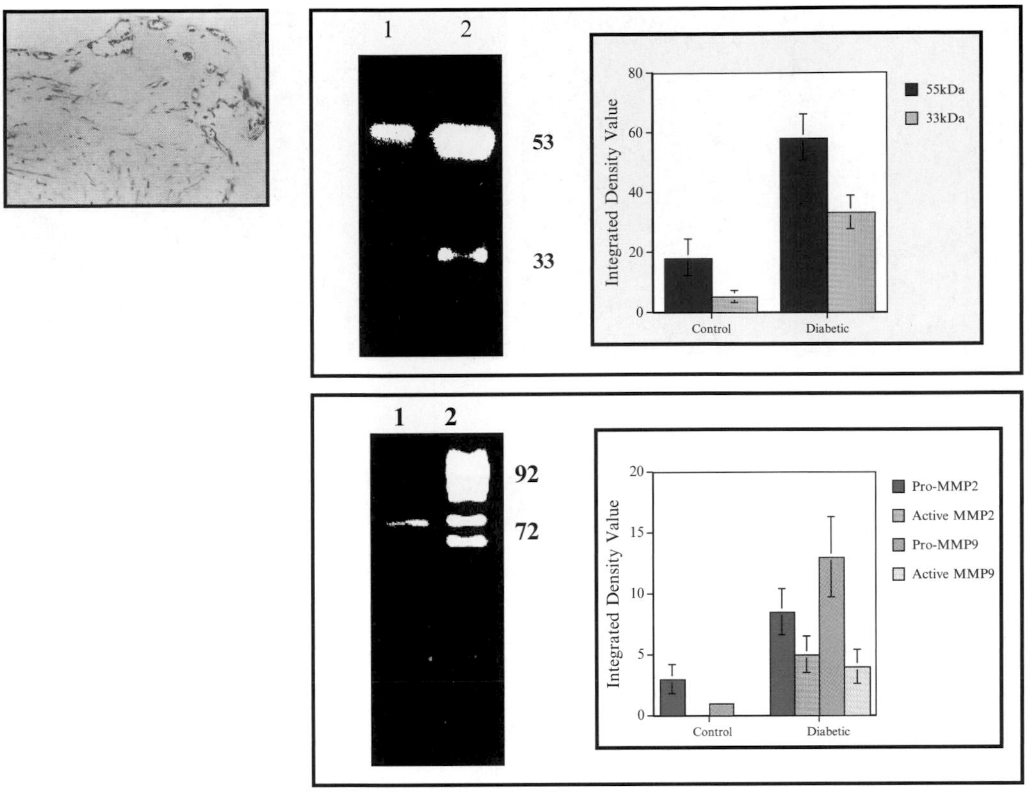

Fig. 5. Quantitation of urokinase (*top panel*) and MMPs (*bottom panel*) from normal donor eyes (control) and epiretinal neovascular membranes (diabetic) from patients with proliferative diabetic retinopathy. The levels of both high (53 kDa) and low (33 kDa) are significantly elevated in neovascular membranes compared with levels in normal retinas compared with normal retinas (control). Each panel also shows on the left side zymographic analysis extracts of retina and epiretinal membranes from PDR patients. The relative amounts of pro-MMP2 (72 kDa), active MMP2 (62 kDa), pro-MMP9 (84 kDa) and active MMP0 (84 kDa) were significantly higher in epiretinal membranes (diabetic) than in retinas of nondiabetic eyes (reprinted from *(70)* with permission).

migration and retinal neovascularization in a mouse model of ischemic retinopathy *(75)* These results suggest that inhibition of the urokinase receptor might be a promising target for anti-angiogenic therapy in the retina.

Induction of MMPs by several upstream pro-angiogenic factors such as angiopoietins, point to the central role played by MMPs in the angiogenic cascade *(32)*. Several recent studies indicate multiple roles for the matrix metalloproteinases in the molecular interplay of angiogenesis. In addition to their classic functions of ECM proteolysis, MMPs might control angiogenesis by their ability to control or modify the surface presentation of growth factor receptors and cell adhesion molecules. Notari et al. *(76)* showed that PEDF is a substrate for MMP-2 and -9 and that the downregulation of cell surface PEDF by proteolysis is a novel posttranslational mechanism by which the MMPs modulate endothelial survival and angiogenesis. Systemic injection of a broad-spectrum MMP inhibitor, BB-94 (1 mg/kg) in the murine model has been shown to

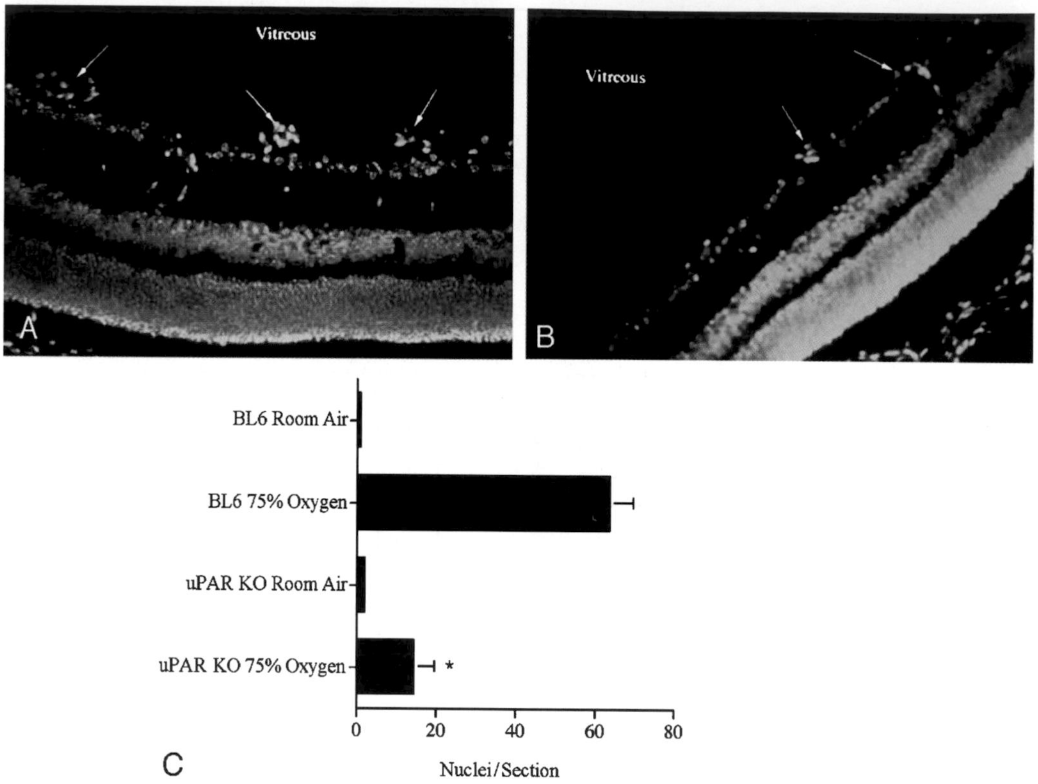

Fig. 6. Absence of the urokinase receptor uPAR reduced the extent of retinal neovascularization in the mouse. (**A**) Representative section of the retina from an experimental oxygen-treated P17 C57BL6 mouse demonstrating numerous neovascular tufts on the surface of the retina (*arrows*). (**B**) A similar section from an experimental oxygen-treated P17 uPAR$^{-/-}$ mouse with many fewer vascular tufts (*arrow*). (**C**) Quantitation of neovascularization in C57BL6 and uPAR$^{-/-}$ mice. The uPAR$^{-/-}$ mice demonstrated 73% less neovascularization compared with the normal C57BL6 mice. Values are the mean ± SEM for $n = 4$ mice in each group (eight eyes, 15–20 sections/eye). *Significantly less than in C57BL6 mice, $P < 0.01$ (reprinted from *(74)* with permission).

suppress retinal neovascularization by 72% *(67)* (Fig. 7). The retinas of BB-94 treated animals demonstrated a significant decrease in the levels of active forms of MMP-2 and MMP-9 compared to controls. In a mouse model of OIR, the extent of preretinal neovascularization was drastically reduced in MMP-2$^{-/-}$ (75%) and MMP-9$^{-/-}$ mice (44%) at postnatal day 19, compared to wild-type control mice. In the same study, the efficacy of three matrix metalloproteinase inhibitors with different selectivities was tested in a rat model of retinopathy of prematurity. Intravitreal injections of the MMP inhibitors resulted in a significant reduction in the angiogenic response in experimental animals in comparison with uninjected controls *(77)*. Elevated levels of ADAM-15/MMP-15, a membrane anchored glycoprotein and disintegrin, were reported in endothelial cells and Adam 15$^{-/-}$ mice demonstrated a major reduction in neovascularization in a model of retinopathy of prematurity *(78)*. The functional association of MMP-2 and $\alpha v\beta 3$ on the cell surface of angiogenic blood vessels points to the ability of MMPs to

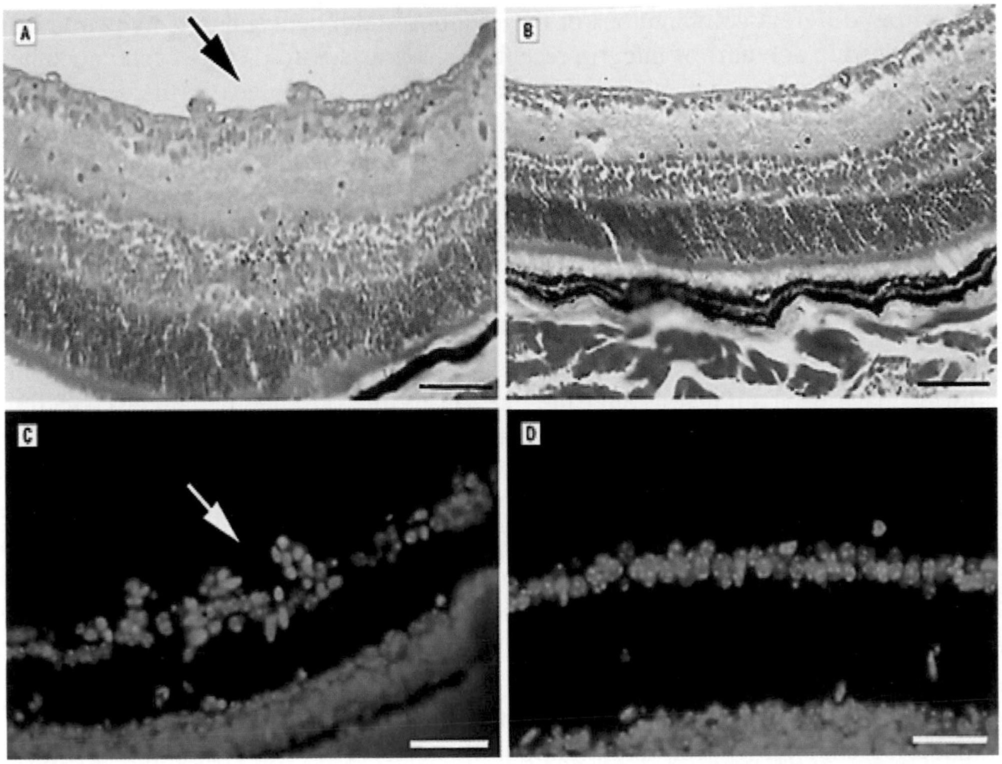

Fig. 7. Use of a matrix metalloproteinase inhibitor suppresses the development of retinal neovascularization. (**A**) Hematoxylin–eosin-stained cross section from the retina of a mouse exposed to 75% oxygen for 5 days followed by room air for an additional 5 days. Capillary tufts are present on the vitreal side of the inner limiting membrane, characteristic of the angiogenic response in this tissue (*arrow*). (**B**) Representative hematoxylin and eosin-stained section from the retina of an experimental mouse treated with BB-94m 1 mg/kg, on postnatal days 12, 14, and 16. (**C**) Similar section from an experimental animal stained with diamidinophenylindole showing individual endothelial cell nuclei that belongs to new vessels (*arrow*). (**D**) Similar section from the retina of a BB-94-treated mouse stained with diamidoniphenylindole showing a significant reduction in the number of neovascular nuclei. Only a single endothelial cell nucleus is present on the vitreal side of the inner limiting membrane. Scale bars: (**A**) and (**B**) – 166 μm; (**C**) and (**D**) – 113 μm (reprinted from *(67)* with permission).

regulate cell adhesion and integrin mediated behavior. A fragment of MMP-2, PEX has been shown to prevent this interaction, serving as a natural inhibitor of MMP-2 and has been reported to inhibit retinal neovascularization *(79)*. With the advent of more selective MMP inhibitors with reduced cytotoxicity, the inhibition of MMPs might prove to be a formidable therapeutic strategy for the future.

INTEGRINS

Integrins are a family of heterodimeric cell adhesion receptors that mediate cell-ECM and cell–cell signaling. Functional integrins consist of two non-covalently bound alpha and beta subunits dimers. About 20 different types of integrins have been identified arising from different combinations of the 18 alpha and 8 beta subunits known to date. The cytoplasmic domains of integrin receptors serve as scaffolds for several signaling/cytoskeletal molecules that mediate cellular responses to changes in the extracellular matrix. Integrins regulate cell adhesion, proliferation, migration and differentiation and hence are thought to be important in the pathogenesis of retinal neovascularization. Normal human retinas stain negatively for αvβ3 and αvβ5 while intense staining was seen in neovascular membranes from patients with diabetic retinopathy *(80–82)*. Neovascular ocular tissues from patients with PDR showed a selective upregulation of αvβ3 and αvβ5 integrins in the vascular beds of the retina and a systemically administered cyclic peptide antagonist was able to block the formation of new blood vessels with no effect on established blood vessels *(82)*. Anti-angiogenic and pro-angiogenic pathways have been studied to alter the integrin profile on endothelial cells. bFGF or TNF-α, induce αvβ3 signaling whereas VEGF, TGF-α or phorbol ester induce αvβ5 signaling in endothelial cells *(83)*. Thrombospondin-1, a multifunctional protein and anti-angiogenic factor has been reported to bind to α9β1, and this interaction promotes angiogenesis *(84)*. In addition to cytokine-directed therapies, integrins have emerged as promising targets for therapeutic intervention for most proliferative retinopathies. Several peptide and non-peptide antagonists have been tested in animal models of retinal angiogenesis and have been reported to inhibit retinal neovascularization *(81, 85, 86)*. However, Reynolds et al. *(87)* report that mice lacking β3 and β5 do not show suppressed tumor angiogenesis indicating that neither αvβ5 nor αvβ3 are required for pathological angiogenesis and highlight the need for further evaluation of integrin functions before anti-integrin therapy is favored.

ENDOGENOUS INHIBITORS OF NEOVASCULARIZATION

Angiogenic and anti-angiogenic factors interplay to maintain a guarded equilibrium in the normal physiology of the retinal vasculature. This balance is affected when the angiogenic factors outweigh endogenous inhibitors of angiogenesis in response to a pathological stimulus. Recently, several endogenous inhibitors have been identified; yet, a better understanding of the complex molecular events in the angiogenic process is warranted.

Pigment Epithelium Derived Growth Factor

Pigment epithelium derived growth factor (PEDF) was first purified from the conditioned media of human retinal pigmented epithelial cells and was characterized as a glycoprotein with a neuroprotective role in the retina *(88)*. Although PEDF shares homology with the serine proteinase inhibitor (Serpin) family, it lacks any native proteinase inhibiting activity itself *(89, 90)*. The Muller cells of the human retina secrete large amounts of PEDF and this secretion is purported to be oxygen-dependent. The neovasculature in the retina has been found to accumulate large amounts of it in the interstitium and surrounding fibrous tissue *(91)*. PEDF has been found in the subretinal fluid of patients with retinal detachment *(92)* and fibrovascular membranes in the eyes of patients with PDR *(91)*, and lower levels of PEDF were found in the vitreous fluid of patients with mild and severe diabetic retinopathy *(93)*. Vitreous PEDF protein was increased in perforated eyes or eyes with ocular injury and PEDF featured as a prominent player in the anti-angiogenic and neuroprotective mechanisms seen in such situations *(94, 95)*.

Historically, PEDF has been studied as the most potent antagonist to the mitogenic activities of VEGF in various models of angiogenesis and cell behavior studies. In a series of co-culture experiments, it was observed that the secretion of PEDF was higher in endothelial-Muller co-cultures than in Muller cells alone and VEGF exposure suppressed PEDF secretion *(96)*, pointing to a glial-endothelial crosstalk in modulation of PEDF levels *(97)*. In a mouse model of ischemia-induced retinal angiogenesis, the retinas with extensive neovascularization demonstrated a dramatic increase in VEGF mRNA and protein with a coupled decrease in PEDF levels, and the time course of this inverted VEGF/PEDF ratio correlated with the progression of this disease *(98)*. Human recombinant PEDF was able to block hypoxia-induced angiogenesis in a mouse model of retinal neovascularization, and PEDF inhibited VEGF-induced retinal endothelial cell proliferation and migration in cell culture *(99)*. Similar results were observed when an intravitreal injection of an adenoviral vector encoding PEDF resulted in decreased retinal neovascularization in mice, suggesting that PEDF gene therapy might be a useful approach in DR *(100)*.

Transforming Growth Factor-β

Transforming growth factor-β (TGF-β) is a soluble pleiotropic growth factor studied in the regulation of tumorigenesis and its contribution to the later stages of the angiogenic pathway. After initial endothelial cell proliferation, migration and invasion, the formation of the neovasculature involves the assembly of new vessel structures. This process includes investment of vessels with mural cells (pericytes or smooth muscle cells), generation of basement membrane and vascular regression. TGF-β plays an important role in the differentiation of vascularity by stabilizing the new blood vessels. In the context of the microvasculature, it is postulated that TGF-β functions at multiple steps including inhibition of endothelial cell proliferation and migration, as well as induction of pericyte/smooth muscle cell differentiation *(101)*.

Increased retinal expression of TGF-β along with other growth factors like VEGF was reported in diabetic human retinas *(102)*. Deficient activation and differential expression of TGF-β was observed in the vitreous fluid of patients with proliferative diabetic retinopathy *(103)*. Elevated expression of TGF-β was found in photocoagulated lesions of the rat retina and this correlated with vessel regression, indicating that the therapeutic effects of photocoagulation might be mediated through TGF-β *(104)*. Co-culture studies show that activation of TGF-β is seen after investment of endothelial tubes with pericytes, which stabilize blood vessels by inhibiting endothelial cell proliferation and migration and induce differentiation of pericytes *(105)*. Retinal glial cells were reported to upregulate TGF-β in response to hypoxia, and treatment of Muller cells with exogenous TGF-β was able to increase the expression of VEGF in a dose-dependent manner *(106)*. These results indicate that destabilization of existing blood vessels and stabilization of neo-vessels might involve close inter-cellular interactions between endothelial cells and mural cells, involving TGF-β.

Angiostatin and Endostatin

Angiostatin, a proteolytic fragment of plasminogen containing the first four kringle domains, is a potent inhibitor of angiogenesis *(107)*. Normal human vitreous was found to be devoid of angiostatin and the local release of angiostatin into the vitreous was seen in patients with PDR treated with laser photocoagulation *(108)*. Recombinant adeno-associated viral vector delivery of mouse angiostatin successfully suppressed experimental pre-retinal neovascularization in adult rats *(109)*. Intravitreal injection of angiostatin blocked retinal neovascularization in a murine model of oxygen-induced retinopathy *(110–111)* and in a separate study, lentivirus mediated expression of angiostatin efficiently inhibited retinal angiogenesis in the murine model *(112)*.

Endostatin is the C-terminal domain of type XVIII collagen, a component of most vascular basement membranes *(113)*. Endostatin has been shown to inhibit endothelial cell migration and induce apoptosis, thus leading to less vascularized tumors *(114)*. The concentrations of endostatin in aqueous humor and vitreous are significantly correlated with the degree and severity of diabetic retinopathy *(115)*. Abnormal maturation of retinal vasculature in endostatin/type XVII collagen deficient mice was seen with concomitant changes in retinal glial cells *(116)*. Retinal neovascularization was suppressed when endostatin was directly injected *(117)* or liposome mediated plasmids encoding endostatin gene were injected intravitreally into mice in a model of oxygen-induced retinopathy *(118)*. Subretinal injections of adenoviral vectors designed to deliver endostatin reduced vasopermeability and retinal neovascularization in mice suggesting that endostatin gene transfer might be effective in blocking both early and late retinal changes *(119)*.

Thrombospondin-1

Thrombospondin-1 (TSP-1) is a secreted glycoprotein found in the extra- and pericellular matrix and was originally identified in platelets. TSP-1 inhibits endothelial cell proliferation and migration, and is thus an anti-angiogenic molecule *(120)*. Many cell types secrete TSP-1 including endothelial cells and smooth muscle cells *(121, 122)*. TSP-1 interacts with extracellular matrix proteins and regulates the activation of several extracellular proteinases and latent TGF-β. In surgically removed epiretinal neovascular membranes from patients with PDR, TSP-1 localized to the endothelial cells of the retina, and plasmin-degraded products of TSP were found in the vitreous of these patients *(123)*. Microarray analysis of mouse eyes subjected to laser photocoagulation showed an upregulation of TSP-1 suggesting that long-term changes in gene expression are involved with laser therapy *(124)*. In a murine model of retinal neovascularization, the angiogenic peak coincided with an upregulation of TSP-1 mRNA. The same study reported that stimulation of bovine retinal microcapillary endothelial cells with VEGF induced TSP-1 expression and this might represent a negative feedback mechanism in ischemia-induced retinal changes *(125)*. Peptides derived from the TSP-1 molecule inhibited retinal angiogenesis in a rat model of retinopathy of prematurity *(126)*, and TSP-1 knockout mice exhibit decreased sensitivity to hyperoxia-induced vessel obliteration *(127)*. Ectopic expression of TSP-1 expression in the lens limited pre-retinal neovascularization in an oxygen-induced retinopathy model, and the TSP1 transgenic mice showed abnormal vascular patterning and density and increased levels of vessel obliteration *(128)*. These results point to the pivotal role played by TSP-1 in mechanisms regulating both vasculogenesis and angiogenesis.

Tissue Inhibitor of Matrix Metalloproteinases

Tissue inhibitors of matrix metalloproteinases (TIMPs) control local MMP activity in tissues by a direct 1:1 binding stoichiometry. Four TIMPs (TIMP-1, -2, -3, and -4) have been identified in vertebrates *(129)*, and their expression in relation to MMP is tightly regulated during tissue remodeling. ECM remodeling in response to a pathological stimulus, often involves unbalanced MMP activities and concomitant changes in TIMP levels. TIMP-1 primarily inhibits the activities of MMP-1, -3, and -9 and TIMP-2 inhibits MMP-2 *(130, 131)*. TIMP-3 is exclusively localized to the ECM and is relatively insoluble, pointing to its potential in preventing matrix lysis and desequestration of growth factors from the matrix. In the retinas of normal mice, TIMP-2 mRNA and protein levels have been found to increase steadily between postnatal days 13–17. This was in contrast to retinas of mice with hypoxia-induced retinal angiogenesis, in which TIMP-2 mRNA and protein remained low and significantly less than in retinas of 'room air' controls. A coincidental upregulation of MMP-2 and -9 and MT1-MMP mRNA was seen in experimental retinas as compared to 'age-matched room air' controls *(132)*. The normal human retina constitutively expresses MMP-1 and TIMP-2, while retinas with PDR stained positive for TIMP-1, -2, and -3 *(133)*. The role of TIMP-3 has been speculated in an age related macular degeneration. A point mutation of TIMP-3 gene has been implicated in patients with Sorsby's fundus dystrophy, an autosomal dominant macular disease with earlier onset of symptoms similar to those of ARMD and characterized by choroidal neovascularization *(134, 135)*.

CLINICAL IMPLICATIONS

Currently, the majority of the clinical trials in retinal diseases have targeted the VEGF molecule. So far two drugs, pegaptanib (Macugen), an aptamer against VEGF 165 and ranibizumab (Lucentis), a humanized monoclonal antibody fragment against all isoforms of VEGF have been approved by the FDA for use in exudative age-related macular degeneration. The Macugen DRS trial in PDR patients has shown regression of neovascularization in most of the patients by week 36 *(136)*. Short-term results with intravitreal bevacizumab (Avastin) suggest a rapid regression of retinal and iris neovascularization secondary to PDR *(137)*. A consistent biologic effect was noted, even with the lowest dose (6.2 μg) tested, and the observation of a possible therapeutic effect in the fellow eye raises concern of systemic side effects from treatment with intravitreal bevacizumab. The orally administered protein kinase C (PKC) beta isoform-selective inhibitor ruboxistaurin (RBX) in subjects with moderately severe to very severe nonproliferative diabetic retinopathy (NPDR) did not prevent progression to PDR *(138)*.

As the angiogenic cascade has been explored with more potential molecules involved, other therapeutic options using inhibitors other than VEGF inhibitors are being explored. At least in preclinical studies as pointed out in this chapter, many of these molecules have proved to be attractive targets for intervention in proliferative diabetic retinopathy. The rationale for searching other novel pathways is twofold. First, in macular degeneration patients, clinical experience shows that the drugs, ranibizumab or bevacizumab have to be administered every 4 weeks as complete regression is not possible with just a few injections. Repeated intravitreal injections have potential side effects of infection, vitreous hemorrhage and retinal detachment, and also there may be unknown potential side effects from continuous VEGF inhibition as VEGF has been shown to be a neuroprotective agent. Secondly, a combination therapy using more than one anti-angiogenic agent seems to be more attractive as one can attack different steps of the angiogenesis cascade rather than one. Such a combination therapy is common in glaucoma management where intraocular pressure-lowering agents are added one after another until the optimal therapeutic level is achieved. Also, the other scenario is possible where one can combine the current panretinal photocoagulation therapy with anti-VEGF or other anti-angiogenic agents.

What is the status of the antiangiogenic agents other than anti-VEGF agents that are promising in the treatment of proliferative diabetic retinopathy? The just completed Octreotide LAR Phase III study using the IGF-1 inhibitor, octreotide, has been shown to delay the progression of retinopathy, however the secondary endpoints of visual acuity and macular edema did not show any significant difference between placebo treated and octreotide treated patients *(139)*. The urokinase inhibitor, A6 (Angstrom Pharmaceuticals, San Diego, CA), which is currently in a Phase II clinical trial in ovarian carcinoma patients, has been shown to be a promising agent in both retinal and choroidal angiogenesis in pre-clinical studies. Our group has recently shown the therapeutic effects of A6 on increased retinal vascular permeability in diabetic animals *(140)*. Such a dual effect of A6 on both blood-retinal barrier and new vessels in diabetic retinopathy is an added advantage of this novel agent. Several MMP inhibitors, and integrin inhibitors are currently in clinical trial for different types of cancer *(141)*, and many of these agents have been shown to be effective in retinal angiogenesis as well.

New therapies involving pharmacological intervention of retinal angiogenesis are currently being developed. These therapies, or a combination of them, would probably be more effective than the current destructive laser modalities. As we develop new drugs for anti-angiogenic effects, one needs to consider the fact that factors other than VEGF are also critical in the angiogenesis cascade, and one should target against these "other" molecules as well.

ACKNOWLEDGMENTS

Supported by National Institutes of Health RO1 12604-08 and Juvenile Diabetes Research Foundation International.

REFERENCES

1. Michaelson M. The mode of the development of the vascular system of the retina with some observations on Trans Ophthalmol Soc UK 1948; 68:137–180.
2. Ashton N. Retinal vascularization in health and disease. Am J Ophthalmol 1957; 44:7–17.
3. D'Amore PA. Mechanisms of retinal and choroidal angiogenesis. Invest Ophthalmol Vis Sci 1994; 35:3974–3979.
4. Casey R, Li WW. Factors controlling ocular angiogenesis. Am J Ophthalmol 1997; 124:521–529.

5. Das A, McGuire PG. Retinal and choroidal angiogenesis: pathophysiology and strategies for inhibition. Progr Retinal Eye Res 2003; 22:721–748.
6. Poulsen JE. The Houssay phenomenon in man: recovery from retinopathy in a case of diabetes with Simmond's disease. Diabetes 1953; 2:7–12.
7. Merimee TJ, Zapf J, Froesch ER. Insulin-like growth factors: studies in diabetics with and without retinopathy. N Eng J Med 1983; 309:527–530.
8. Grant MB, Russell B, Fitzgerald C et al. Insulin-like growth factors in vitreous: studies in control and diabetic subjects with neovascularization. Diabetes 1986; 35:416–420.
9. Dills DG, Moss SE, Klein R et al. Association of IGF-1 levels with increased retinopathy in late-onset diabetes. Diabetes 1991; 40:1725–1730.
10. The Diabetes Control and Complications Trial Research Group. The effect of intensive treatment of diabetes on the development and progression of long-term complications in insulin-dependent diabetes mellitus. N Engl J Med 1993;329:977–86.
11. Hyer SL, Sharp PS, Sleightholm M et al. Progression of diabetic retinopathy and changes in serum insulin-like growth factor 1(IGF 1) during continuous subcutaneous insulin infusion. Horm Metabol Res 1989; 21:18–22.
12. Smith LEH, Kopchick JJ, Chen W et al. Essential role of growth hormone in ischemia-induced retinal neovascularization. Science 1997; 276:1706–1709.
13. Hellstrom A, Perruzzi C, Ju M et al. Low IGF-1 suppresses VEGF-survival signaling in retinal endothelial cells: direct correlation with clinical retinopathy of prematurity. Proc natl Acad Sci USA 2001; 98:5804–5808.
14. Smith LEH. Pathogensis of retinopathy of prematurity. Semin Neonatol 2003; 8:469–473.
15. Poulaki V, Joussen AM, Mitsiades N et al. Insulin-like growth factor-1 plays a pathogenic role in diabetic retinopathy. Am J Pathol 2004; 165:457–469.
16. Ruberte J, Ayuso E, Navarro M et al. Increased ocular levels of IGF-1 in transgenic mice lead to diabetes-like eye disease. J Clin Invest 2004; 113:1149–1157.
17. McCombe M, Lightman S, Eckland DJ et al. Effect of a long-acting somatostatin analogue (BIM23014) on proliferative diabetic retinopathy: a pilot study. Eye 1991; 5:569–575.
18. Grant MB, Mames RN, Fitzgerald C et al. The efficacy of octrotide in the therapy of severe nonproliferative diabetic retinopathy – a randomized controlled study. Diabetes Care 2000; 23:504–509.
19. Growth Hormone Antagonist for Proliferative Diabetic Retinopathy Study Group. The effect of a growth hormone receptor antagonist drug on proliferative diabetic retinopathy. Ophthalmology 2001; 108:2266–2272.
20. Ozaki H, Okamoto N, Ortega S et al. Basic fibroblast growth factor is neither necessary nor essential for the development of retinal neovascularization. Am J Pathol 1998; 153:757–765.
21. Yamada H, Yamada E, Kwak N et al. Cell injury unmasks a latent proangiogenic phenotype in mic with incrased expression of FGF-2 in the retina. J Cell Physiol 2000; 185:135–142.
22. Gao H, Hollyfield JG. Basic fibroblast growth factor (bFGF) immunolocalization in the rodent outer retina demonstarted with anti-rodent bFGF antibodies. Brain Res 1992; 585:355–360.
23. Kostyk SK, D'Amore PA, Herman IM et al. Optic nerve injury alters basic fibroblast growth factor localization in the retina and optic nerve. J Neurosci 1994; 14:1441–1449.
24. Nyberg F, Hahnenberger P, Jakobson AM et al. Enhancement of FGF-like ploypeptides in the retina of newborn mice exposed to hyperoxia. FEBS Lett 1990; 267:75–77.
25. Sivalingam A, Kenny J, Brown GC et al. Basic fibroblast growth factor levels in the vitreous of pateints with proliferative diabetic retinopathy. Arch Ophthalmol 1990; 108: 869–872
26. Hanneken A, DeJuan E, Lutty GA et al. Altered distribution of basic fibroblast growth factor in diabetic retinopathy. Arch Ophthalmol 1991; 109:1005–1011.
27. Frank RN, Amin RH, Eliott D et al. Basic fibroblast growth factor and vascular endothelial growth factor are present in epiretinal and choroidal neovascular membranes. Am J Ophthalmol 1996; 122:393–403.
28. Sato TN, Qin Y, Kozak CA et al. Tie-1 and Tie-2 define another class of putative receptor tyrosine kinase genes expressed in early embryonic vascular system. Proc Natl Acad Sci USA 1993; 90:9355–9358.
29. Oh H, Takagi H, Suzuma K et al. Hypoxia and vascular endothelial growth factor selectively upregulate angiopoietin-2 in bovine microvascular endothelial cells. J Biol Chem 1999; 274:15732–15739.

30. Oh H, Takagi H, Takagi C et al. The potential angiogenic role of macrophages in the formation of choroidal neovascular memebranes. Invest Ophthalmol Vis Sci 1999; 40:1891–1898.
31. Hackett SF, Ozaki H, Strauss RE et al. Angiopoietin-2 expression in the retina: upregulation during physiologic and pathological neovascularization. J Cell Physiol 2000; 184:275–284.
32. Das A, Fanslow W, Cerretti D et al. Angiopoietin/Tek interactions regulate MMP-9 expression and retinal neovascularization. Lab Invest 2003; 83:1637–1645.
33. Oshima Y, Deering T, Oshima S et al. Angiopoietin-2 enhances retinal vessel sensitivity to vascular endothelial growth factor. J Cell Physiol 2004; 199:412–417.
34. Watanabe D, Suzuma K, Suzuma I et al. Vitreous levels of angiopoietin-2 and vascular endothelial growth factor in patients with proliferative diabetic retinopathy. Am J Ophthalmol 2005; 139:476–481,
35. Feng Y, vom Hagen Pfister F et al. Impaired pericyte recruitment and abnormal retinal angiogenesis as a result of angiopoietin2 overexpression. Thromb Haemost 2007; 97:99–108.
36. Hammes HP, Lin J, Wagner P et al. Angiopoietin-2 causes pericyte dropout in the normal retina: evidence for involvement in diabetic retinopathy. Diabetes 2004; 53:1104–10.
37. Hangal M, Moon YS, Kitaya N et al. Systemically expressed soluble Tie2 inhibits intraocular neovascularization. Hum Gene Ther 2001; 12:1311.
38. Watanabe D, Suzuma K, Matsui S et al. Erythropoietin as a retinal angiogenic factor in proliferative diabetic retinopathy. N Eng J Med 2005; 353:782–792.
39. Kase S, Saito W, Ohgami K et al. Expression of erythropoietin receptor in human epiretinal membrane of proliferative diabetic retinopathy. Br J Ophthalmol 2007; May 23 Epub.
40. Aiello LPA. Angiogenic pathways in diabetic retinopathy. N Eng J Med 2005; 353:839–841.
41. Becerra SP, Amaral J. Erythropoietin – an endogenous retinal survival factor. N Eng J Med 2002; 347:1968–1970.
42. Bevan D, Fan TP, Edwards D et al. Diverse and potent activities of HGF/SF in skin wound repair. J Pathol 2004; 203:831–838.
43. Maulik G, Shirkhande A, Kijima T et al. Role of the hepatocyte growth factor receptor, c-Met, in oncogenesis and potential for therapeutic inhibition. Cytokine Growth Factor Rev 2002; 13:41–59.
44. Katsura Y, Okano T, Noritake M et al. Hepatocyte growth factor in vitreous fluid of patients with proliferative diabetic retinopathy and other retinal disorders. Diabetes Care 1998; 21:1759–1763.
45. Shinoda K, Ishida S, Kawashima S et al. Comparison of the levels of hepatocyte growth factor and vascular endothelial growth factor in aqueous fluid and serum with grades of retinopathy in patients with diabetes mellitus. Br J Ophthalmol 1999; 83:834–837.
46. Canton A, Burgos R, Hernandez C et al. Hepatocyte growth factor in vitreous and serum from patients with proliferative diabetic retinopathy. 2000; 84:732–735.
47. Birchmeier C, Birchmeier W, Gherardi E et al. Met, metastasis, motility and more. Nat Rev Mol Cell Biol 2003; 4:915–925.
48. Colombo ES, Menicucci G, McGuire PG, Das A. Hepatocyte growth factor/scatter factor promotes retinal angiogenesis through increased urokinase expression. 2007; 48:1793–1800.
49. Clermont AC, Cahill M, Salti H et al. Hepatocyte growth factor induces retinal vascular permeability via MAP-kinase and PI-3 kinase without altering retinal hemodynamics. Invest Ophthalmol Vis Sci 2006; 47:2701–2708.
50. Limb GA, Chignell AH, Green W et al. Distribution of TNF and its reactive vascular adhesion molecules in fibrovascular membranes of PDR. Br J Ophthalmol 1996; 80:168–173.
51. Armstrong D, Yeda T, Yeda T et al. Lipid hydroperoxide stimulates retinal neovascularization in rabbit retina through expression of tumor necrosis factor alpha, vascular endothelial growth factor, and platelet-derived growth factors. Angiogenesis 1998; 1:93–104.
52. Majka S, McGuire PG, Das A. Regulation of matrix metalloproteinase expression by tumor necrosis factor in a murine model of retinal neovascularization. Invest Ophthalmol Vis Sci 2002; 43:260–266.
53. Gardiner TA, Gibson DS, de Gooyer TE et al. Inhibition of tumor necrosis factor-alpha improves physiological angiogenesis and reduces pathological neovascularization in ischemic retinopathy. Am J Pathol 2005; 166:637–644.
54. Kociok N, Radetzky S, Krohne TU et al. Pathological but not physiological retinal neovascuularization is altered in TNF-Rp55-receptor-deficient mice. Invest Ophthalmol Vis Sci 2006; 47:5057–5065.

55. Joussen AM, Poulaki V, Mitsiades N et al. Non-steroidal anti-inflammatory drugs prevent early diabetic retinopathy via TNF-alpha suppression. FASEB 2002; 16:438–440.
56. Manchanda N, Schwartz BS. Single chain urokinase: augmentation of enzymatic activity upon binding to monocytes. J Biol Chem 1991; 266:14580–14584.
57. Quax P, van Muijen G, Weening-Verhoeff E et al. Metastatic behavior of human melanoma cell lines in nude mice correlates with urokinase type plasminogen activator, its type inhibitor, urokinase-mediated matrix degradation. J Cell Biol 1991; 115:191–199.
58. Rabbani SA, Desjardins J, Bell AW et al. An amino terminal fragment of urokinase isolated from a prostate cancer cell line is mitogenic for osteoblast-like cells. Biochem Biophys Res Commun 1990; 173:1058–1064.
59. Blasi R. Urokinase and urokinase receptor: a paracrine/autocrine system regulating cell migration and invasiveness. Bioassays 1993; 15:105–111.
60. Rabbani SA, Mazar AP. The role of plasminogen activator system in angiogenesis and metastasis. Surg Oncol Clin N Am 2001; 10:393–415.
61. Kroon ME, Koolwijk P, van DerVecht B et al. Urokinase receptor expression on human microvascular endothelial cells is increased by hypoxia: implications for capillarylike tube formation in a fibrin matrix. Blood 2000; 96:2775–2783.
62. Evans CP, Elfman F, Parangi S et al. Inhibition of prostate cancer neovascularization and growth by urokinase plasminogen activator receptor blockade. Cancer Res 1997; 57:3594–3599.
63. Li H, Lu H, Griscelli F et al. Adenovirus-mediated delivery of a uPA/uPAR antagonist suppresses angiogenesis-dependent tumor growth and dissemination in mice. Gen Ther 1998; 5:1105–1113.
64. Bajou K, Noel A, Gerrard RD et al. Absence of host plasminogen activator inhibitor 1 prevents cancer invasion and vascularization. Nat Med 1998; 4:923–928.
65. Bajou K, Masson V, Gerrad RD et al. The plasminogen activator inhibitor PAI-1 controls in vivo tumor vascularization by interaction with proteases, not vitronectin: implications for antiangiogenic strategies. J Cell Biol 2001; 152:777–784.
66. Pepper MS. Role of the matrix metalloproteinase and plasminogen activator-plasmin systems in angiogenesis. Arterioscler Thromb Vasc Biol 2001; 21:1104–1117.
67. Das A, McLamore A, Song W, McGuire PG. Retinal neovascularization is suppressed with a MMP inhibitor. Arch Ophthalmol 1999; 117:498–503.
68. Hattenbach LO, Allers A, Gumbel HO et al. Vitreous concentrations of TPA and plasminogen activator are associated with VEGF in proliferative diabetic vitreo retinopathy. Retina 1999; 19:383–389.
69. Yoshikawa H, Ishibashi T, Hata Y et al. The suppressive effect of tecogalan sodium on in vitro angiogenesis via the periendothelial proteolytic activities. Ophthalmic Res 2000; 32:261–269.
70. Das A, McGuire PG, Eriqat C et al. Human diabetic neovascular membranes contain high levels of urokinase and metalloproteinase enzymes. Invest Ophthalmol Vis Sci 1999; 40:809–813.
71. Brown D, Hamidi H, Bahri S et al. Characterization of an endogenous metalloproteinase in human vitreous. Curr Eye Res 1994; 13:639–647.
72. De La Paz MA, Itoh H, Toth CA et al. Matrix metalloproetinases and their inhibitors in human vitreous. Invest Ophthalmol Vis Sci 1998; 39:1256–1260.
73. Yang R, Liu H, Williams I et al. Matrix metalloproteinase-2 expression and apoptogenic activity in retinal pericytes: implications in diabetic retinopathy. Ann NY Acad Sci 2007; 1103:196–201.
74. McGuire PG, Jones TR, Talarico et al. The urokinase/urokinase receptor system in retinal neovascularization: inhibition by A6 suggests a new therapeutic target. Invest Ophthalmol Vis Sci 2003; 44:2736–2742.
75. Le Gat L, Gogat K, Bouquet C et al. In vivo adenovirus-mediated delivery of a uPA/uPAR antagonist reduces retinal neovascularization in a mouse model of retinopathy. Gene Ther 2003; 10:2098–2103.
76. Notari L, Miller A, Martinez A et al. Pigment epithelium-derived factor is a substrate for matrix metalloproteinase type 2 and type 9: implications for downregulation in hypoxia. Invest Ophthalmol Vis Sci 2005; 46:2736–2747.
77. Barnett JM, McCollum GW, Fowler JA et al. Pharmacologic and genetic manipulation of MMP-2 and MMP-9 affects retinal neovascularization in rodent models of OIR. Invest Ophthalmol Vis Sci 2007; 48:907–915.
78. Horiuchi K, Weskamp G, Lum L et al. Potential role of ADAM15 in pathological neovascularization in mice. Mol Cell Biol 2003; 23:5614–5624.

79. Brooks PC, Silletti S, von Schalscha TL et al. Disruption of angiogenesis by PEX, a noncatalytic metalloproteinase fragment with integrin binding activity. Cell 1998; 92:391–400.
80. Robbins SG, Bren RB, Wilson DJ et al. Immunolocalizations of integrins in proliferative retinal membranes. Invest Ophthalmol Vis Sci 1994; 35:3475–3485.
81. Luna J, Tobe T, Mousa SA et al. Antagonists of integrin avb3 inhibit retinal neovascularization in amurine model. Lan Invest 1996; 75:563–573.
82. Friedlander M, Theesfeld CL, Sugita M et al. Involvement of integrins avb3 and avb5 in ocular neovascular diseases. Proc Natl Acad Sci USA 1996; 93:9764–9769.
83. Friedlander M, Brooks PC, Shaffer RW et al. Definition of two angiognic pathways by distinct av integrins. Science 1995; 270:1500–1502.
84. Staniszewska I, Zaveri S, Del Valle L et al. Interaction of alpha9beta1 integrin with thrombospondin-1 promotes angiogenesis. Cic Res 2007; 100:1308–1316.
85. Wilkinson-Berka JL, Jones D, Taylor G et al. SB-267268, a nonpeptidic antagoinist of alpha v beta 3 and alpha v beta 5 integrins, reduces angiogenesis and VEGF expression in a mouse model of retinopathy of prematurity. Invest Ophthalmol Vis Sci 2006; 47:1600–1605.
86. Hammes HP, Brownlee M, Jonczyk A et al. Subcutanteous injection of a cyclic peptide antagonist of vitronectin receptor-type integrins inhibits retinal neovascularization. Nat Med 1996; 2:529–533.
87. Reynolds LE, Wyder L, Lively JC et al. Enhanced pathological angiogenesis in mice lacking beta3 integrin or beta3 and beta5 integrins. Nat Med 2002; 8:27–34.
88. Tombran-Tink J, Chader G, Johnson LV. PEDF: a pigment epithelium derived factor with potent neuronal differentiatitive activity. Exp Eye Res 1991; 53:411–414.
89. Steele F, Chader G, Johnson LV et al. Pigment epithelium derived factor: neurotrophic activity and identification as a member of the serine protease inhibitor gene family. Proc Natl Acad Sci USA 1993; 90:1526–1530.
90. Becerra SP, Sagasti A, Spinella P et al. Pigment epithelium derived factor behaves like a noninhibitory serpin. Neurotropic activity does not require the serpin reactive loop. J Biol Chem 1995; 270:24992–24999.
91. Matsouka M, Ogata N, Minamino K et al. Expression of pigment epithelium derived factor and vascular endothelial growth factor in fibrovascular membranes from patients with proliferative diabetic retinopathy. Jpn J Ophthalmol 2006; 50:116–120.
92. Abdiu O, Olivestedt G, Berglin L et al. Detection of PEDF in subretinal fluid of retinal detachment: possible role in the prevention of subretinal neovascularization. Preliminary results. Ophthalmic Res 2006; 38:189–192.
93. Ogata N, Nishikawa M, Nishimura T et al. Unbalanced vitreous levels of pigment epithelium-derived factor and vascular endothelial growth factor in diabetic retinopathy. Am J Ophthalmol 2002; 134:348–353.
94. Penn JS, McCollum GW, Barnett JM et al. Angiostatic effect of penetrating ocular injury: role of pigment epithelium-derived factor. Invest Ophthalmol Vis Sci 2006; 47:405–414.
95. Stitt AW, Graham D, Gardiner TA. Ocular wounding prevents pre-retinal neovascularization and upregulates PEDF expression in the inner retina. Mol Vis 2004; 10:432–438.
96. Eichler W, Yafai Y, Keller T et al. PEDF derived from glial Muller cells: a possible regulator of retinal angiogenesis. Exp Cell Res 2004; 299:68–78.
97. Yafai Y, Lange J, Wiedemann P et al. Pigment epithelium derived factor acts as an opponent of growth-stimulatory factors in retinal glial-endothelial cell interactions. Glia 2007; 55:642–651.
98. Gao G, Li Y, Fant J et al. Difference in ischemic regulation of vascular endothelial growth factor and pigment epithelium derived factor in Brown Norway and Sprague Dawley rats contributing to different susceptibilities to retinal neovascularization. Diabetes 2002; 51:1218–1225.
99. Duh EJ, Yang HS, Suzuma I et al. Pigment epithelium derived factor suppresses ischemia-induced retinal neovascularization and VEGF-induced migration and growth. Invest ophthalmol Vis Sci 2002; 43:821–829.
100. Mori K, Duh E, Gehlbach P et al. Pigment epithelium derived factor inhibits retinal and choroidal neovascularization. J Cell Physiol 2001; 188:252–263.
101. Darland DC, D'Amore PA. Blood vessel maturation: vascular development comes of age. J Clin Invest 1999; 103:157–158.

102. Spirin KS, Saghizadeh M, Lewin SL et al. Basement membrane and growth factor gene expression in normal and diabetic human retinas. Curr Eye Res 1999; 18:490–499.
103. Sprager J, Meyer-Schwwickerath R, Klein M et al. Deficient activation and different expression of transforming growth factor beta isoforms in active proliferative diabetic retinopathy and neovascular eye diseases. Exp Clin Endocrinol Diabetes 1999; 107:21–28.
104. Yamamoto C, Ogata N, Yi X et al. Immunolocalization of transforming growth factor beta during wound repair in rat retina after laser photocoagulation. Graefes Arch Clin Exp Ophthalmol 1998; 236:41–46.
105. Antonelli-Orlidge A, Sauders KB, Smith SR et al. An activated form of transforming growth factor b is produced by co-cultures of endothelial cells and pericytes. Proc Natl Acad Sci USA. 1989; 86:4544–4548.
106. Behzadian MA, Wang XL, Al-Shabrawey M, Caldwell RB. Effects of hypoxia on glial cell expression of angiogenesis-regulating factors VEGF and TGF-beta. Glia 1998; 24:216–225.
107. O'Reilly MS, Holmgree L, Shing Y et al. Angiostatin: a novel angiogenesis inhibitor that mediates the suppression of metastases by a Lewistrong lung carcinoma. Cell 1994; 79:315–328.
108. Spranger J, Hammes HP, Preissner KT et al. Release of the angiogenesis inhibitor angiostatin in patients with proliferative diabetic retinopathy: association with retinal photocoagulation. Diabetologia 2000; 43:1404–1407.
109. Lai CC, Wu WC, Chen SL et al. Recombinant adeno-associated virus vector expressing angiostatin inhibits preretinal neovascularization in adult rats. Ophthalmic Res 2005; 37:50–56.
110. Drixler TA, Borel Rinkes IH, Ritchie et al. Angiostatin inhibits pathological but not physiological retinal angiogenesis. Invest Ophthalmol Vis Sci 2001; 42:3325–3330.
111. Meneses PI, Hajjar KA, Berns KI et al. Recombinant angiostatin prevents retinal neovascularization in a murine proliferative retinopathy model. Gene Ther 2001; 8:646–648.
112. Igrashi T, Miyake K, Kato K et al. Lentivirus-mediated expression of angiostatin efficeintly inhibits neovascularization in a murine proliferative retinopathy model. Gene Ther 2003; 10:219–226.
113. Kalluri R. Basement membranes: structure, assembly and role in tumor angiogenesis. Nat Rev Cancer 2003; 3:422–433.
114. O'Reilly MS, Boehm T, Shing Y et al. Endostatin: an endogenous inhibitor of angiogenesis and tumor grwoth. Cell 1997; 88:277–285.
115. Noma H, Funatsu H, Yamashita H et al. Regulation of angiogenesis in diabetic retinopathy: possible balance between vascular endothelial growth factor and endostatin. Arch Ophthalmol. 2002; 120:1075–1080.
116. Hurskainen M, Eklund L, Hagg PO et al. Abnormal maturation of the retinal vasculature in type XVIII collagen/endostatin deficient mice and changes in retinal glial cells due to lack of collagen types XV and XVIII. FASEB J 2005; 19:1564–1566.
117. Zhang M, Yang Y, Yan M et al. Downregulation of vascular endothelial growth factor and integrin beta3 by endostatin in a mouse model of retinal neovascularization. Exp Eye Res 2006; 82:74–80.
118. Wang W, Xie LX, Dong XG et al. Trandfer of endostatin gene for inhibition of retinal angiogenesis in mice. Zhonghua Yan Ke Za Zhi 2006; 42:111–115.
119. Takahashi K, Saishin Y, Saishin Y et al. Intraocular expression of endostatin reduces VEGF-induced retinal vascular permeability, neovascularization, and retinal detachment. FASEB J 2003; 17:896–898.
120. Lawler J. Thrombospondin-1 as an endogenous inhibitor of angiogenesis and tumor growth. J Cell Mol Med 2002; 6:1–12.
121. McPherson J, Sage H, Bornstein P. Isolation and characterization of a glycoprotein secreted by aortic endothelial cells in culture: apparent identity with platelet thrombospondin. J Biol Chem 1981; 256:11330–11336.
122. Majack RA, Cook SC, Bornstein P. Platelet-derived growth factor and heparin-like glycosoaminoglycans regulate thrombospondin synthesis and deposition in the matrix by smooth muscle cells. J Cell Biol 1985; 101:1059–1070.
123. Esser P, Weller M, Heimann K et al. Thrombospondin and its importance in proliferative retinal diseases. Fortschr Ophthalmol 1991; 88:337–340.
124. Binz N, Graham CE, Simpson K et al. Long-term effect of therapeutic laser photocoagulation on gene expression of the eye. FASEB J 2006; 20:383–385.

125. Suzuma K, Takagi H, Otani A et al. Expression of thrombospondin-1 in ischemia-induced retinal neovascularization. Am J Pathol 1999; 154:343–354.
126. Shafiee A, Penn JS, Krutzsch HC et al. Inhibition of retinal angiogenesis by peptides derived from thrombospondin-1. Invest Ophthalmol Vis Sci 2000; 41:2378–2388.
127. Wang S, Wu Z, Sorenson CM et al. Thrombospondin-1-deficient mice exhibit increased vascular density during retinal vascular development and are less sensitive to hyperoxia-mediated vessel obliteration. Dev Dyn 2003; 228:630–642.
128. Wu Z, Wang S, Sorenson CM et al. Attenuation of retinal vascular development and neovascularization in transgenic mice overexpressing thrmbospondin-1 in the lens. Dev Dyn 2006; 235:1908–1920.
129. Brew K, Dinakarpandian D, Nagase H. Tissue inhibitors of metalloproteinases: evolution, structure and function. Biochim Biophys Acta. 2000; 1477:267–283.
130. Moses M, Langer R. 1991. A metalloproteinase inhibitor as an inhibitor of neovascularization. J Cell Biochem 47, 230–235.
131. Baramova E, Foidart JM. 1995. Matrix metalloproteinase family. Cell Biol Int 19, 239–242.
132. Majka S, McGuire PG, Colombo S, Das A. The balance between proteinases and inhibitors in a murine model of proliferative retinopathy. Invest Ophthalmol Vis Sci 2001; 42:210–215.
133. Salzmann J, Limb GA, Khaw PT et al. Matrix metalloproteinases and their natural inhibitors in fibrovascular membranes of proliferative diabetic retinopathy. Br J Ophthalmol 2000; 84:1091–1096.
134. Weber BHF, Vogt G, Pruett RC et al. Mutations in the tissue inhibitor of metalloproteinases-3 (TIMP-3) in patients with Sorsby's fundus dystrophy. Nat Genet 1994; 8:352–356.
135. Farris RN, Apte SS, Luhert PJ et al. Accumulations of tissue inhibitor metalloproteinases-3 in human eyes with Sorsby's fundus dystrophy or retinitis pigmentosa. Br J Ophthalmol 1998; 82:1329–1334.
136. Adamis A, Altaweel M, Bressler NM et al. Changes in retinal neovascularization after pegaptanib (Macugen) therapy in diabetic individuals. Ophthalmol 2006; 113:23–28.
137. Avery RL, Pearlman J, Pieramici J et al. Intravitreal bevacizumab (Avastin) in the treatment of proliferative diabetic retinopathy. Ophthalmology 2006; 113:1695–1670.
138. The PKC-DRS Study Group. The effect of ruboxistaurin on visual loss in patients with moderately severe to very severe nonproliferative diabetic retinopathy: initial results of the Protein Kinase C beta Inhibitor Diabetic Retinopathy Study (PKC-DRS) multicenter randomized clinical trial. Diabetes. 2005; 54:2188–97.
139. Grant MB. ADA Presentation, June 2007.
140. Navaratna D, Meniciccu G, McGuire P, Das A. Urokinase and its receptor – A Novel Therapeutic Target in Diabetic Retinopathy. #0099-OR. ADA Meeting, June, 2007, Chicago.
141. Folkman J. Angiogenesis: an organizing principle for drug discovery? Nat Rev Drug Discov 2007;6:273–86.

III Emerging Treatments and Concepts in Diabetic Retinopathy

III

17 Anti-VEGF Therapy as an Emerging Treatment for Diabetic Retinopathy

Diana V. Do, Julia A. Haller, Anthony P. Adamis, Carla Striata, Quan Dong Nguyen, Syed Mahmood Shah, and Antonia M. Joussen

CONTENTS

ABSTRACT

Anti-VEGF therapies are currently under investigation for diabetic maculopathy. Both clinical and preclinical findings have implicated vascular endothelial growth factor (VEGF) in the pathophysiology of diabetic macular edema (DME). VEGF is involved both in vascular integrity and leakage as well as neovascularization. VEGF levels are elevated in the vitreous of patients with diabetic macular edema, and in animal models elevated VEGF levels in the eye coincide with breakdown of the blood-retinal barrier. Two VEGF antagonists are FDA approved for the clinical treatment of neovascular age-related macular degeneration: pegaptanib and ranibizumab. Phase II data for pegaptanib are available demonstrating a superior visual acuity for treated patients compared to the sham group as well as a reduced retinal thickness and a reduced need for laser therapy. Phase I data for ranibizumab in diabetic macular edema demonstrated a reduction in excess retinal thickness and improvement in visual acuity. Phase II studies are underway to compare ranibizumab and laser photocoagulation.

Key Words: Bevacizumab; Diabetic macular edema; Pegaptanib; Proliferative diabetic retinopathy; Ranibizumab; VEGF.

From: *Contemporary Diabetes: Diabetic Retinopathy*
Edited by: E. Duh © Humana Press, Totowa, NJ

INTRODUCTION

Diabetic retinopathy is the most prevalent cause of vision loss among adults of working age, and diabetic macular edema (DME) is the most common cause of moderate vision loss in individuals with diabetes mellitus *(1)*, especially in patients with type 2 diabetes *(2)*. Diabetic retinopathy accounts for an estimated 15–17% of the 2.7 million cases of blindness in the European Union *(3)*. In the United States, an estimated 4.1 million individuals aged 40 years and older are affected by diabetic retinopathy, with nearly 900,000 having vision-threatening disease *(4)*.

There are two major causes that lead to deterioration of vision in diabetic retinopathy: (1) direct damage to the retinal vasculature and (2) development of retinal neovascularization. Severe visual loss in patients with diabetes occurs primarily as a consequence of retinal neovascularization and complications resulting from intraocular angiogenesis such as vitreous hemorrhage or tractional retinal detachment; moderate visual loss results primarily from DME related to altered permeability of the retinal vasculature.

Currently, laser photocoagulation is the standard of care in treating retinal complication s of diabetes, and while it has contributed significantly to reducing the incidence of severe vision loss, it is basically a destructive intervention that does not address the underlying pathophysiology. The mechanism by which scatter laser photocoagulation reduces proliferative retinopathy is not known. It has been proposed that light energy absorbed by melanin in the retinal pigment epithelium destroys highly metabolically active outer retinal cells, reducing retinal oxygen consumption and facilitating improved oxygen diffusion from the choriocapillaris through the laser scars *(5)*. By destroying a portion of viable retina, laser therapy also lessens the metabolic load and therefore the absolute need for oxygen.

However, laser treatment is accompanied by frank destruction of neural tissue and can lead to night blindness, visual field constriction, and dyschromatopsia. A progression in the severity of retinopathy after treatment is not uncommon *(2)*. There is thus a need for newer therapies with fewer side effects, especially approaches that counter retinopathic change through targeting the underlying pathophysiology of DR, rather than relying on *ex post facto* ablation.

Metabolic control, intraocular steroids, and novel pharmacological therapy such as vascular endothelial growth (VEGF) factor blockers may help to decrease DME and may reverse vision loss associated with this disease. This chapter reviews the pathogenesis of DME, the rationale for the role of anti-VEGF agents, and preliminary clinical studies on the use of ranibizumab (Lucentis™, Genentech Inc., South San Francisco, CA) and pegaptanib (Macugen, OSI/Eyetech, New York, NY) for DME.

Pathogenesis

DME occurs from leakage of plasma into the central retina, resulting in thickening of the retina because of excess interstitial fluid. The excess interstitial fluid within the macula results in stretching and distortion of photoreceptors which eventually leads to decreased vision. Histopathological studies have demonstrated that microaneurysms are likely to be responsible for focal leakage that may be seen in eyes with DME. Microaneurysms are thought to form because of hyperglycemia-induced pericyte death, which weakens the walls of retinal vessels resulting in the formation of small aneurysms which lose their barrier qualities and leak *(6)*. In addition to focal leakage caused by microaneurysms, eyes with DME may also demonstrate diffuse leakage from retinal capillaries that do not show visible structural changes such as microaneurysms. This pattern of diffuse leakage may be due to microscopic damage to retinal vessels that is not visible in images obtained during fluorescein angiography. It is possible that diffuse leakage results from the presence of excessive amounts of permeability factors.

Vascular Endothelial Growth Factor (VEGF)

Retinal hypoxia has been implicated in the pathogenesis of DME *(7)*. Hypoxia causes increased expression of VEGF, a potent inducer of vascular permeability that has been shown to cause leakage from retinal vessels *(8, 9)*. VEGF was isolated independently by two groups, first as a vascular permeability factor *(10)* and second as a potent endothelial cell mitogen *(11)*.

The VEGF family, which includes VEGF-A, VEGF-B, VEGF-C, VEGF-D, VEGF-E and placental growth factor, plays an important role in angiogenesis and vascular permeability *(10–12)*, among other things. Studies have demonstrated that VEGF-A is a primary activator of angiogenesis and vascular permeability, whereas other VEGF family members play a lesser role in angiogenesis. Nine VEGF-A isoforms are produced through alternate splicing of the mRNA of the human VEGF-A gene: $VEGF_{121}$, $VEGF_{145}$, $VEGF_{148}$, $VEGF_{162}$, $VEGF_{165}$, $VEGF_{165b}$, $VEGF_{183}$, $VEGF_{189}$, and $VEGF_{206}$. *(13)*. Among the nine isoforms, $VEGF_{165}$ is the most abundantly expressed VEGF-A isoform, and it plays a critical role in angiogenesis. However, other isoforms, such as $VEGF_{121}$, $VEGF_{183}$, and $VEGF_{189}$, are also commonly expressed in various tissues *(14)*. Although investigations during the 1980s suggested numerous proangiogenic and antiangiogenic factors, only VEGF convincingly showed all the characteristics of a necessary and sufficient inducer of angiogenesis *(15)*.

VEGF in Physiological and Pathological Angiogenesis

Over the past 15 years, an extensive body of research has established that VEGF is a key regulator of both physiological and pathological angiogenesis, playing a variety of roles in promoting blood vessel growth and vascular permeability (Table 1). Alternative splicing of the human gene yields at least 6 biologically active isoforms; each composed of 121, 145, 165, 183, 189, and 206 amino acids *(15)*.

Table 1
Actions of VEGF in Promoting Angiogenesis

Endothelial cell mitogen
- Endothelial cell survival factor
- Chemoattractant for bone marrow-derived endothelial cells
- Chemoattractant for monocyte lineage cells
- Inducer of synthesis of endothelial nitric oxide synthase, and consequent elevation of nitric oxide, itself a promoter of angiogenesis
- Inducer of synthesis of enzymes promoting blood vessel extravasation
  - Matrix metalloproteinases
  - Plasminogen activator

Table 2
Additional Physiological Processes Involving VEGF

- Bone growth
- Wound healing
- Female reproductive cycling
- Vasorelaxation
- Glomerulogenesis
- Protection of hepatic cells
- Skeletal muscle regeneration
- Neural survival factor
- Trophic support of choriocapillaris

In addition to its role as a potent endothelial cell mitogen, VEGF serves as an endothelial cell survival factor *(16)* and as a chemoattractant for bone marrow-derived endothelial cells *(17–19)*. VEGF also induces the synthesis of several enzymes whose actions affect angiogenesis, including the matrix metalloproteinases and plasminogen activator *(20–22)*. VEGF induces nitric oxide synthase, leading to upregulation of nitric oxide, a stimulator of angiogenesis *(23, 24)*. In addition, VEGF acts as a chemoattrac-tant for monocyte lineage cells *(25)*. which are believed to contribute to pathological ocular neovascularization *(26, 27)* and to promote local adhesion of leukocytes and subsequent injury to the vascular endothelium *(28, 29)*.

It is important to note, however, that the family of VEGF isoforms is much more than a promoter of angiogenesis as it acts in a wide variety of cellular processes *(30–44)* Table 2). In this regard, intravenous administration of VEGF inhibitors have been associated with an increased incidence of hypertension, proteinuria, bleeding and thromboembolic events. *(45–48)*

VEGF IN OCULAR NEOVASCULARIZATION

An extensive series of clinical and preclinical investigations has confirmed that VEGF plays a central role in promoting ocular neovascularization *(49–56)*. Clinical studies have demonstrated elevated ocular levels of VEGF in patients with anterior segment neovascularization *(49)*, retinal vein occlusion *(49)*, neovascular glaucoma *(57)*, retinopathy of prematurity *(58)*, and DME *(59–62)*. In other studies, increased expression of VEGF was detected within the maculae of patients with age-related macular degeneration *(63)* and in choroidal neovascular membranes *(64–66)*

A variety of models have been employed to demonstrate that blockage of VEGF and its receptors can inhibit the development of ocular neovascularization. In one of the first preclinical studies, Miller et al. *(67)* reported that experimentally induced retinal vein occlusion in monkeys resulted in iris neovascularization and an associated increase in ocular VEGF levels. Injection of anti-VEGF antibodies was shown to prevent the neovascularization of the monkey iris that normally followed laser occlusion of the vein *(51)*, and antibodies or their Fab fragments were also effective in preventing choroidal neovascularization in a photocoagulation-induced model in monkeys *(54)* and in a rat corneal wound model *(68)*. Other approaches to inactivate VEGF to prevent ocular neovascularization included administration of soluble VEGFR chimeric proteins by injection *(53)*, expression from an adenovirus vector *(69)*, injection of pegaptanib (Ishida et al. 2003), and injection of an anti-VEGF antisense oligonucleotide *(82)*.

VEGF AND DIABETIC RETINOPATHY

Animal studies have demonstrated that VEGF-A plays a vital role in the pathogenesis of ocular diseases in which neovascularization and increased vascular permeability occur, such as proliferative diabetic retinopathy, macular edema, and neovascular AMD *(50, 62)*. Overexpression of VEGF-A has been reported to cause ocular neovascularization and macular edema in monkeys *(71)*. In addition, elevated levels of VEGF-A have been identified in the vitreous of patients with diabetic retinopathy *(49, 62)* and higher VEGF-A levels are found in the vitreous and aqueous humor of patients with DME *(50)*. Evidence from animal and clinical studies has clearly demonstrated a pathological role for overexpression of VEGF; therefore anti-VEGF therapies are likely to have an important role in the treatment of DME and proliferative diabetic retinopathy.

The pathophysiology of diabetic retinopathy is complex, with the products of several biochemical pathways being potential mediators in the relationship between hyperglycemia and retinal vascular damage. These include polyols, advanced glycation end products and reactive oxygen intermediates *(65, 66)* Anatomical correlates of the progression of DR include death of capillary pericytes, basement membrane thickening, and entrapment of leukocytes, leading to capillary blockages and local hypoxia *(66, 72)* Upregulation of VEGF is likely to occur either directly, through stimulation by metabolites such as advanced glycation end-products *(73)* and reactive oxygen intermediates *(74)*, or indirectly, through the local hypoxia induced by capillary dropout. VEGF is synthesized by a wide range of retinal cell types *(52, 75, 76)* and this synthesis is significantly increased in hypoxic conditions *(42, 52, 77)* Clinical findings have confirmed that VEGF levels are elevated in both DR *(49, 50, 59, 62, 78, 79)* and DME *(59–61, 80)*. $VEGF_{165}$, the most abundant isoform of VEGF is principally responsible for diabetes-associated ocular pathology *(81, 82)*

It is now well established that increases in ocular concentrations of VEGF are closely linked both to the aberrant growth of new vessels and to increased vascular permeability resulting in tissue edema. This edema further exacerbates the vision loss associated with diabetic retinopathy (Table 3) and other ocular conditions such as neovascular age-related macular degeneration (AMD). The increase in permeability reflects several VEGF-mediated processes, including induction of fenestrations in the endothelium (Roberts and Palade 1997) *(83)*, dissolution of tight junctions *(84)*, and the promotion of adherence to the retinal vasculature by leukocytes which then act to damage the endothelium *(29, 81)*

Clinical Application of Anti-VEGF Drugs

Currently, there are three VEGF inhibitors commonly used in the treatment of proliferative retinopathies and AMD: pegaptanib (Macugen, OSI/Eyetech), bevacizumab (Avastin, Genentech), and ranibizumab (Lucentis, Genentech). While both pegaptanib and ranibizumab are approved for neovascular AMD in the U.S. and many European countries, neither of the agents is as yet approved for the treatment of diabetes- related

Table 3
Key Findings Linking VEGF to Pathophysiology of Diabetic Retinopathy

- VEGF levels are elevated in eyes of patients with diabetic retinopathy (DR) and DME
- Experimental elevation of VEGF in normal primate eyes induces many changes typical of DR, including formation of microaneurysms and exudation following blood retinal barrier breakdown
- Studies with rodent models of diabetes have revealed that DR is associated with increases in retinal VEGF levels which underlie a local inflammation and consequently result in vascular damage and leakage
- One VEGF isoform (VEGF165 in humans, VEGF164 in rodents) is especially important in mediating this inflammation
- Elevation of retinal levels of VEGF164 occur in parallel with blood retinal barrier breakdown in diabetic rodents
- Intravitreous injection of VEGF164 induces blood retinal barrier breakdown in normal animals more potently than VEGF120

Table 4
Pegaptanib

- Nuclease-resistant RNA aptamer, specific for the VEGF165 isoform
- Inhibits VEGF165-mediated cellular actions, including increases in vascular permeability and endothelial cell proliferation
- Intravitreous pegaptanib is approved as a treatment for neovascular AMD
- Intravitreous pegaptanib can reverse blood retinal barrier breakdown in diabetic rodents
- Intravitreous pegaptanib inhibits pathological, but not physiological vascularization

eye disease. Both pegaptanib and ranibizumab are currently under investigation in prospective clinical trials for the treatment of diabetic retinopathy.

Pegaptanib

Pegaptanib is a nuclease resistant, pegylated 28-nucleotide RNA aptamer which binds to the $VEGF_{164/165}$ isoform at high affinity (200 pM), while showing little activity toward the $VEGF_{120/121}$ isoform *(85)* (Table 4). Pegaptanib includes a 40 kD polyethylene glycol moiety at the 5′ terminal *(86)* a change which prolongs intravitreal half-life *(87)*

Pegaptanib inhibits $VEGF_{164/165}$ from binding to its cellular receptors, preventing the initiation of downstream signaling events. In experiments with cultured endothelial cells, pegaptanib inhibited the induction of mitogenesis by $VEGF_{165}$, but not by $VEGF_{121}$, consistent with pegaptanib's specificity for $VEGF_{165}$ *(88)*. In addition, in the Miles assay for vascular permeability, the VEGF-induced increase in vascular leakage was inhibited by 83% when VEGF was pre-incubated with 0.1 μM pegaptanib *(86)*. In subsequent studies, using a rodent model of retinopathy of prematurity, intravitreous injection of pegaptanib was shown to inhibit pathological neovascularization, but not the physiological vascularization of the retina *(82)* suggesting that pegaptanib treatment might be relatively harmless to the normal retinal vasculature. Further evidence of pegaptanib's sparing of physiological tissues came from studies of retinal ischemia, in which $VEGF_{120}$ was shown to be sufficient to exert a neuroprotective effect *(89)*. Most importantly for DR, in experiments with diabetic rodents, intravitreous injection of pegaptanib was shown to cause restoration of the blood retinal barrier *(82)*.

The V.I.S.I.O.N. study *(90),* which comprised two pivotal phase 3 trials, has already demonstrated that intravitreous administration of pegaptanib is effective in treating neovascular AMD, and is associated with a low risk of serious adverse events such as endophthalmitis, traumatic lens injury or retinal detachment; where these occurred they were related to the injection procedure, rather than the drug on study by itself. An important safety finding is that there was no evidence that pegaptanib was associated with major systemic adverse events, such as hypertension, thromboembolism or serious hemorrhage, that have been reported with systemically administered VEGF blockade. The results of the V.I.S.I.O.N. study led to pegaptanib's approval for neovascular AMD by regulatory authorities in several countries including the United States, Canada, and Europe.

Taken together with the data implicating $VEGF_{165}$ in the pathophysiology of diabetic retinopathy and DME, and the positive safety record of pegaptanib in clinical trials *(91)*, a Phase 2 clinical trial to examine pegaptanib's utility as a treatment for DME was conducted.

Bevacizumab

Bevacizumab (Avastin®, Genentech, Inc. South San Francisco) is a full-length humanized murine monoclonal antibody against the VEGF molecule. The amino acid sequence of this antibody is 93% of human origin and 7% murine *(92)*. Bevacizumab is approved by the Food and Drug Administration (FDA) for the treatment of metastatic colorectal cancer in combination with 5-fluorouracil and is in Phase III trials for advanced breast cancer and advanced renal cancer *(48, 93)*. VEGF selectively stimulates endothelial cells by binding to two receptors, VEGFR-1 and VEGF-R2, which respond in typical fashion to ligand binding by activation of signal transduction cascades *(15)*. Bevacizumab can theoretically inhibit the activity of both receptors *(94)*. Recently off-label use of intravitreal bevacizumab has been described in patients with neovascular AMD and proliferative diabetic retinopathy *(95–98)*. Intravitreal bevacizumab caused regression of neovascularization secondary to proliferative diabetic retinopathy, and resulted in decreased excess retinal thickness from neovascular AMD and short-term improvements in visual acuity *(96–98)*. Additional prospective studies with intravitreal bevacizumab for DME and neovascular AMD are currently underway.

Ranibizumab

Ranibizumab (Lucentis™; Genentech, Inc., South San Francisco, Calif) is a recently FDA-approved humanized antigen-binding fragment (Fab) designed to bind and inhibit all VEGF-A isoforms and the biologically active degradation product, $VEGF_{110}$. The vitreous half-life of ranibizumab after intravitreal administration in monkeys is 3 days with very low systemic exposure following intravitreal administration in both humans and monkeys *(99, 100)*.

Phase I/II/III clinical trials in patients with choroidal neovascularization (CNV) secondary to AMD have shown intravitreal injection of ranibizumab to be safe and well tolerated. In addition, two pivotal phase III clinical trials (**M**inimally Classic/Occult Trial of the **A**nti-VEGF Antibody **R**anibizumab **In** the Treatment of **N**eovascular **AMD** [MARINA] Trial and the **An**ti-VEGF Antibody for the Treatment of Predominantly Classic **Chor**oidal Neovascularization in AMD [ANCHOR]) demonstrated the efficacy of ranibizumab in patients with neovascular AMD; these studies were the first to show visual acuity improvement, not just a stabilization of visual acuity, in individuals with neovascular AMD.

The MARINA Trial was a randomized, double-masked, sham-controlled clinical trial of patients with minimally classic or occult with no classic CNV secondary to AMD who were treated with monthly intravitreal ranibizumab (0.3 or 0.5 mg) or sham injections for 24 months. In the MARINA trial, approximately 90–92% of ranibizumab-treated patients lost fewer than 15 letters of VA compared with 53% of sham-injected patients after 24 months *(101)*. In addition, at 24 months of follow-up, approximately 33% of ranibizumab-treated patients experienced visual improvement of 15 or more letters compared with 4% of the sham-injected patients.

The ANCHOR Trial was a randomized, double-masked, sham-controlled clinical trial of patients with predominantly classic CNV secondary to AMD treated with intravitreal ranibizumab (0.3 or 0.5 mg) and sham photodynamic therapy (PDT) or sham injection and PDT (monthly administration for ranibizumab and every 3 months for PDT) for 24 months. After 12 months of follow-up, 94 and 96% of ranibizumab-treated patients (0.3 and 0.5 mg, respectively) lost fewer than 15 letters of VA compared with 64% of PDT-treated patients *(102)*. In addition, 36% and 40% of ranibizumab-treated patients experienced visual improvement of 15 or more letters (0.3 and 0.5 mg, respectively) compared with 6% of PDT-treated patients.

Use of Anti-VEGF Therapies in Diabetic Retinopathy

Phase 2 Trial – Intravitreous Pegaptanib as a Treatment for DME

Pegaptanib was evaluated in a randomized, sham-controlled, double-masked, dose-ranging, multi-center phase 2 trial which enrolled 172 patients 18 years and older with type I or type II diabetes, visual acuity (VA) between 20/50 and 20/320, and DME affecting the center of the macula (Table 5). *(103)* Only patients for whom focal/grid laser could be deferred for at least 16 weeks in the study eye, even though focal/grid laser was indicated, were enrolled. Principal exclusion criteria included photocoagulation or other retinal treatments within the previous 6 months, abnormalities interfering with VA measurements and fundus photography, severe cardiac disease, clinically significant peripheral vascular disease, uncontrolled hypertension, and glycosylated hemoglobin levels ≥13%.

Patients were randomized to 4 treatment arms (0.3, 1, 3 mg pegaptanib or sham injection), with stratification by study site, size of the thickened retina area (≤2.5 disc areas vs. >2.5 disc areas), and baseline VA (ETDRS letter score ≥58 vs. < 58). Injections were given at baseline and every 6 weeks thereafter for a minimum of 3 from baseline to week 12. Additional injections to a total maximum of 6 injections were allowed at

Table 5
Pegaptanib Phase 2 Trial for Diabetic Macular Edema

- Phase 2 trial, randomizing 172 patients with DME to pegaptanib (0.3, 1 and 3 mg) or sham injection
- Pegaptanib treatment shown superior to sham for all prespecified endpoints, including measurements of VA, retinal thickness and need for further additional photocoagulation therapy for DME
- Mean changes in VA at week 36 in the 0.3 mg pegaptanib treatment group was + 4.7 letters compared to –0.4 letters for sham
- Eight of 13 pegaptanib-treated patients with revascularization in the "study" eye experienced its regression during the trial; regression of revascularization was not seen in any of 3 sham treated patients or in the 4 "fellow" eyes (Altaweel et al. 2006)
- Pegaptanib was well tolerated, with only one case of endophthalmitis occurring among 652 injections (0.15%)
- No evidence that pegaptanib treatment was associated with systemic adverse events

investigator's discretion from week 18 to 30. Focal/grid laser photocoagulation was allowed also at investigator's discretion after week 12. Main efficacy assessments were made at week 36, or 6 weeks after the last injection. Refraction, VA assessment, an ophthalmologic examination, optical coherence tomography (OCT), and color fundus photography were conducted at baseline and at each visit, while fluorescein angiography was carried out at baseline and 6 weeks after the last injection. Overall, 169 patients received at least one injection, and over 90% of patients in each treatment group completed the study. Pre-specified efficacy criteria included VA, retinal thickness as measured by OCT, and the need for photocoagulation therapy. In addition, patients found to show diabetic neovascularization at baseline were evaluated for the impact of pegaptanib treatment upon its advance or regression *(103)*.

Principal Endpoints – VA, Retinal Thickness, Retinal Volume, and Need for Photocoagulation

Pegaptanib treatment was superior to sham injection, according to all pre-specified endpoints. Mean change in VA in the 0.3 mg pegaptanib-treated group was + 4.7 letters, compared to –0.4 letters for sham ($P = 0.04$). Pegaptanib treatment also resulted in more patients gaining ≥ 0, ≥ 5, ≥ 10, and ≥ 15 letters of VA (Fig. 1). Mean change in center point (foveal) retinal thickness was $-68\,\mu m$ in the 0.3 mg pegaptanib arm, compared to $+ 3.7\,\mu m$ in the sham group ($P = 0.02$) and pegaptanib treatment resulted in significantly more patients experiencing decreases in thickness of ≥ 75 and $\geq 100\,\mu m$). As well, macular volume decreased $0.58\,mm^3$ in the 0.3 mg pegaptanib arm, but increased $0.12\,mm^3$ with sham ($P = 0.009$) (Data on file, (OSI) Eyetech Inc. and Pfizer Inc. 2005). OCT center point thickness at baseline and change in thickness from baseline to week 36 had a modest correlation with VA at baseline or change in VA from baseline to week 36 (R squared = 0.18). Lastly, in the 0.3 mg pegaptanib arm, only 25% of patients required further treatment with photocoagulation, compared to 48% in the sham group ($P = 0.042$) *(103)*.

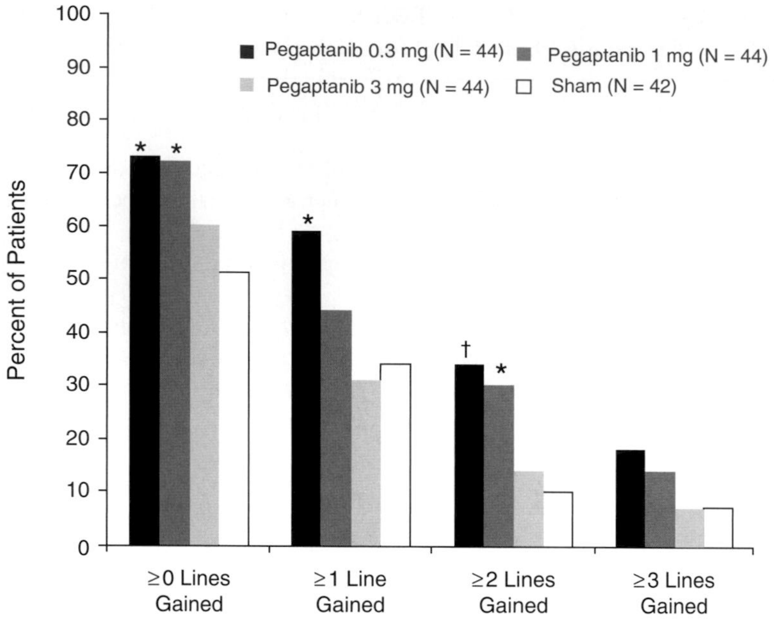

Fig. 1. Stabilization or improvement of visual acuity after pegaptanib. Percentage of subjects with maintenance of or improvement in visual acuity based on ETDRS lines gained. Subjects treated with 0.3 mg pegaptanib were more likely to have improvements in visual acuity compared to higher doses of pegaptanib (1 or 3 mg) or sham treatments (from Macugen Diabetic Retinopathy Study Group *(103)*).

Retinal Neovascularization – Retrospective Analysis

Fundus photographs were graded in a masked fashion for the presence of neovascularization. A retrospective analysis was done to evaluate the effects of pegaptanib on retinal neovascularization. Nineteen patients in all were found to have retinal revascularization in the study eye, 16 of whom were available for full analysis. Thirteen patients had received pegaptanib while the other 3 received sham injections. Four of the 13 pegaptanib-treated patients also had neovascularization in the fellow eye. At 36 weeks, 8 of the 13 patients in the pegaptanib groups (61%) showed regression of neovascularization, as assessed by fundus photography, while no regression was seen in the 3 sham-treated patients, or in the 4 fellow eyes. Three of the 8 patients with regressed neovascularization experienced a recurrence between weeks 36 and 52, after pegaptanib therapy was discontinued (Fig. 2) *(104)*.

Safety

Pegaptanib was well tolerated at all administered doses. Adverse events were transient, and associated with the injection procedure, rather than the drug of study. One case of endophthalmitis occurred among 652 injections (0.15% per injection); it was successfully treated and resolved, without severe loss of vision *(103)*. There was no evidence that pegaptanib treatment was associated with systemic thromboembolic events or cardiac, gastrointestinal or hemorrhagic complications There is an ongoing randomized, double-masked, multicenter, phase 2/3 study assessing the safety and

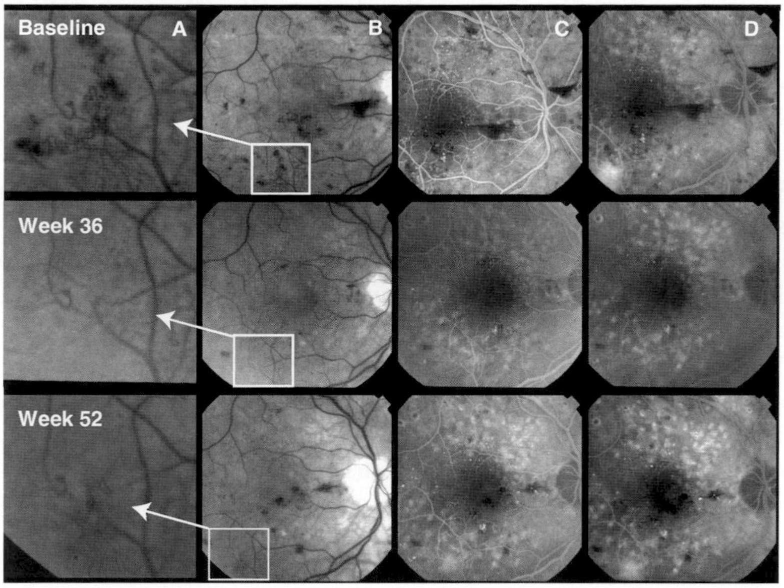

Fig. 2. Changes in retinal neovascularization after pegaptanib. First row, Baseline visit shows magnification of retinal neovascularization elsewhere (NVE) (**A**), the location of the neovascularization along the inferotemporal arcade (red-free photograph) (**B**), areas of capillary nonperfusion in the early-phase frame (fluorescein angiogram) (**C**), and leakage from the NVE in the late-phase frame (fluorescein angiogram) (**D**). Second row, At week 36, after 6 periodic pegaptanib injections and 6 weeks since the most recent injection, there is seen regression of NVE on red-free photographs (**A**, **B**), less apparent microaneurysms in the early phase (**C**), and regression of leakage from NVE in the late phase (**D**). Third row, 52 weeks after study entry and 22 weeks since the last pegaptanib injection, there is seen reappearance of NVE on red-free photographs (**A**, **B**) and reappearance of leakage from NVE in early- and late-phase frames (**C**) (from Macugen Diabetic Retinopathy Study Group *(104)*).

efficacy of pegaptanib compared with non-treatment control (sham injection) for the treatment of DME with foveal involvement.

Clinical Experience with Bevacizumab in Diabetic Retinopathy

Several published studies have demonstrated a biological effect of intravitreal bevacizumab in proliferative diabetic retinopathy and diabetic macular edema. The majority of these studies are limited by their retrospective nature and short follow-up period.

Avery and colleagues retrospectively evaluated the use of intravitreal bevacizumab in patients with retinal neovascularization due to proliferative diabetic retinopathy *(96)*. In 44 eyes treated with intravitreal bevacizumab (6.2 μg–1.25 mg), retinal neovascularization demonstrated on fluorescein angiography had complete (or at least partial) reduction in leakage within 1 week after the injection. Complete resolution of angiographic leakage from neovascularization of the disc was noted in 19 of 26(73%) eyes, and leakage of iris neovascularization completely resolved in 9 of 11 (82%) eyes. The leakage was noted to diminish as early as 24 h after injection. Recurrence of fluorescein leakage varied and was seen as early as 2 weeks in one case, whereas in other cases, no recurrent leakage was noted at the last available follow-up of 11 weeks. No ocular or systemic adverse events were noted.

Retrospective case series of bevacizumab as an adjunct for intraoperative use in diabetic tractional retinal detachment repair *(105)* or in eyes with proliferative retinopathy and non-clearing vitreous hemorrhage *(97)* have been reported. Similarly, intracameral injection of bevacizumab for iris rubeosis *(106, 107)* has been noted to have a beneficial short-term effect. Although there was a regression of the rubeotic vessels present as early as 1 week after injection, no persistent effect on intraocular pressure in cases of neovascular glaucoma is yet proven.

In a prospective, consecutive, non-comparative case series, 51 consecutive patients (26 females and 25 males; mean age, 64 years) with diffuse diabetic macular oedema were treated with intravitreal bevacizumab *(108)*. Inclusion criteria were determined independently of the size of oedema, retinal thickness, VA, age, metabolic control, type of diabetes, or previous treatments beyond a 6-month period. All patients had undergone previous treatments, such as focal laser therapy (35%), full-scatter panretinal laser therapy (37%), vitrectomy (12%), and intravitreal triamcinolone (33%). Sixteen patients (70%) received at least two intravitreal injections of bevacizumab during the study period. Mean central retinal thickness by OCT was 501 μm (range, 252–1,031 μm) at baseline and decreased to 425+/– 180 μm at 2 weeks (P = 0.002) after bevacizumab, 416+/– 180 μm at 6 weeks (P = 0.001), and 377+/– 117 μm at 12 weeks (P = 0.001). VA, as measured by ETDRS letters, did not improve significantly through the follow-up period.

A phase II randomized multicenter clinical trial of intravitreal bevacizumab for diabetic macular oedema was performed by the Diabetic Retinopathy Clinical Research Network (DRCR.net) *(110)*. This study involved 121 eyes from 121 individuals with diabetic macular oedema involving the center of the macula based on clinical examination, best-corrected Snellen VA equivalent ranging from 20/32 to 20/320, OCT central subfield thickness (CST) greater than or equal to 275 μm, and no history of treatment for DME in the prior 3 months. Of the 121 subjects, 109 met criteria for inclusion in the analyses. Subjects were randomized to 1 of 5 treatment groups, with 19–24 subjects per group: (A) focal laser photocoagulation at baseline, (B) intravitreal injection of 1.25 mg of bevacizumab at baseline and 6 weeks, (C) intravitreal injection of 2.5 mg of bevacizumab at baseline and 6 weeks, (D) intravitreal injection of 1.25 mg of bevacizumab at baseline and sham injection at 6 weeks, or (E) intravitreal injection of 1.25 mg of bevacizumab at baseline and 6 weeks with focal photocoagulation at 3 weeks. Follow-up visits were performed at 3, 6, 9, 12, 18, 24, 41, and 70 weeks, and a report was published for analysis of central subfield thickness (CST) and VA during the first 12 weeks *(110)*.

Both the 1.25- and 2.5 mg bevacizumab-treated eyes had a greater reduction in central retinal thickness at 3 weeks, compared to the control group receiving photocoagulation. However, the photocoagulation group showed improvement in these parameters with longer follow-up, so that there were no meaningful differences in CST observed for bevacizumab compared to photocoagulation after the 3-week time point. About half of the eyes demonstrated what was deemed to be a response to bevacizumab (greater than an 11% decrease in retinal thickness compared to baseline). With regard to VA, there was an approximately 1 line greater improvement with both bevacizumab doses on average compared to photocoagulation throughout the 12 weeks.

In the 12 week time-frame, there was not a large difference in effect between the 2 doses of bevacizumab. Interestingly, the reduction in retinal thickness associated with bevacizumab at 3 weeks appeared to plateau or decrease in most eyes between the

3- and 6-week visits, suggesting that 6 weeks might be too long for an optimal initial injection interval. A similar phenomenon was observed after the second injection of bevacizumab. Combining photocoagulation with bevacizumab did not result in any apparent short-term benefit.

This study also monitored for any possible adverse effects, although the safety evaluation was limited by the small sample size and short follow-up duration. In the subjects treated with bevacizumab, there were several cases of systemic cardiovascular or renal adverse effects (including two cases of myocardial infarction), all of which occurred in subjects with related pre-existing medical conditions. However, the sample sizes were too small to attribute cause of any systemic events to the drug. In addition, there was 1 case of injection-related endophthalmitis in 185 injections, but no important ocular complications attributable to the bevacizumab.

This study therefore indicates a short-term response in reduction of retinal thickness from bevacizumab injection. Definitive determinations of a clinically meaningful benefit of intravitreal bevacizumab for DME will require a large phase III randomized clinical trial. This will also be required to provide definitive conclusions regarding safety. No significant safety concerns have arisen to date, but most of the published data on bevacizumab and diabetic eye disease is limited to retrospective case series and anecdotal case reports.

Ranibizumab in Diabetic Macular Edema

Nguyen and colleagues conducted an open-label study (**R**anibizumab for **E**dema of the m**A**cula in **D**iabetes: A Phase 1 Study – the **READ-1 Study**) to investigate the effect of intravitreal injections of ranibizumab in patients with DME *(109)*. Intraocular injections of 0.5 mg of ranibizumab were administered at entry to the study and at 1, 2, 4, and 6 months after entry. The injection regimen was selected to assess the effect of 3 monthly injections and then determine the impact of increasing the time interval between injections to 2 months for the last 2 injections. The primary outcome measure was foveal thickness measured by OCT at 7 months compared to baseline. Secondary outcome measures were macular volume measured by OCT and VA measured by the protocol of the Early Treatment Diabetic Retinopathy Study (ETDRS) at 7 months compared to baseline, and ocular and systemic safety.

Among the 10 subjects (5 men and 5 women) initially enrolled, pertinent baseline characteristics included: 8 eyes that had received at least two sessions of focal/grid laser photocoagulation not less than 5 months prior to study entry (range 5–120 months), 3 eyes that had received intraocular steroids not less than 10 months prior to entry (range 10–20 months), and a mean foveal thickness of 503 ± 115 μm (range 326–729 μm) at baseline, indicating the presence of severe, chronic DME that was poorly responsive to standard therapies.

Effect on Foveal Thickness and Macular Volume

Compared to baseline, mean foveal thickness was reduced by 246 μm at the primary endpoint of the study (7 months after the first ranibizumab injection), representing an elimination of 85% of the excess foveal thickness that had been present at baseline. In addition, mean macular volume was reduced from 9.22 mm^3 at baseline to 7.47 mm^3 at 7 months, a

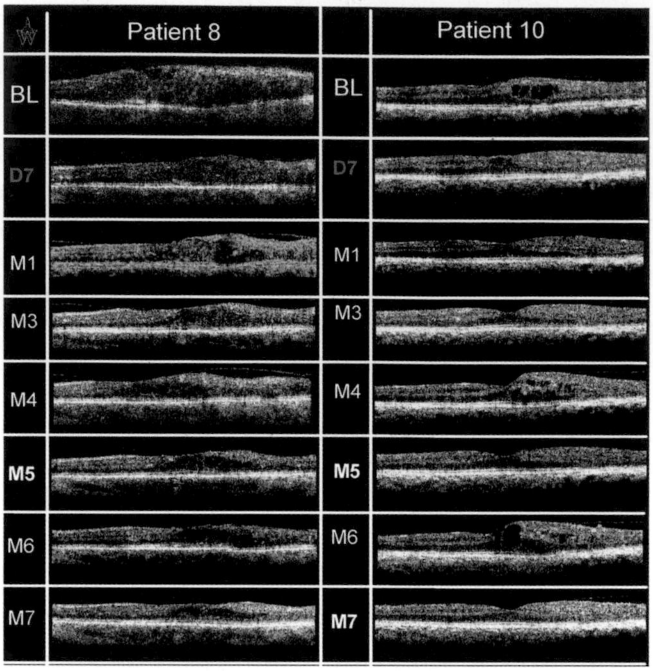

Fig. 3. Horizontal cross sectional optical coherence tomography (OCT) scans at all time points for patients #8 and #10 to illustrate two patterns of response over time. Ranibizumab injections were administered at baseline, month 1 (M1), month 2, month 4 (M4), and month 6 (M6). Seven days after the first intraocular injection of 0.5 mg of Ranibizumab (D7), patient 8 showed an immediate improvement in the appearance of the OCT scan with less intraretinal cystoid spaces and a reduction in excess retinal thickening. Patient 8 continued to have a reduction in excess retinal thickness throughout the course of the study. By month 7 (M7), which was the primary endpoint of the study, patient 8 had eliminated most of the excess retinal thickness. Like patient 8, patient 10 also showed substantial improvement at D7 compared to baseline with resolution of several large cysts. At M4 and M6, 2 months after the third and fourth injections, respectively, the scan showed significant deterioration in patient 10. However, 1 month after injection at M4 and M6, there was marked improvement at M5 and M7, respectively.

reduction of 1.75 mm^3 which was statistically significant ($P = 0.009$). This reduction constituted 77% of the excess macular volume that was present at baseline. OCT scans from two subjects whose DME showed responses to ranibizumab are shown in Fig. 3.

Effect on Visual Acuity

Throughout each study time point, mean and median visual acuities were better than those at baseline. At the primary endpoint (7 months after the initial ranibizumab injection), mean and median visual acuity improved by 12.3 and 11 letters in the initial 10 subjects, which represents an improvement of a little more than 2 lines. Figure 4 provides updated visual acuity data on the final 18 subjects who participated in the READ study and shows the mean and median visual acuity improved by 10 letters (2 lines) at 7 months.

In this study cohort, there was a strong correlation (R^2 value of 0.78) between visual acuity and foveal thickness as measured by OCT. However, the rate of change of these two outcome measures was different, and rapid changes in foveal thickness were

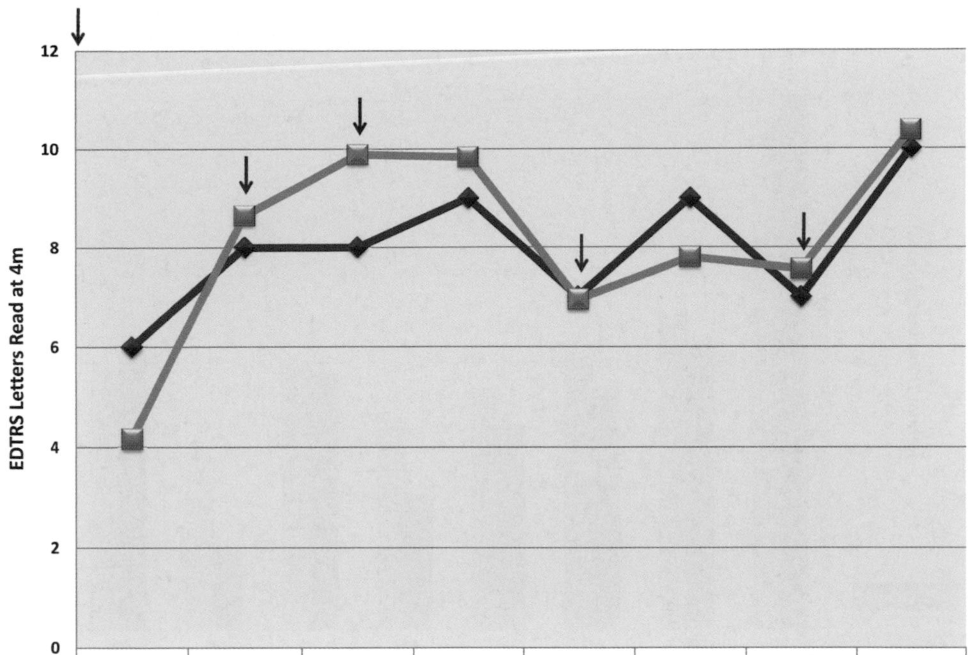

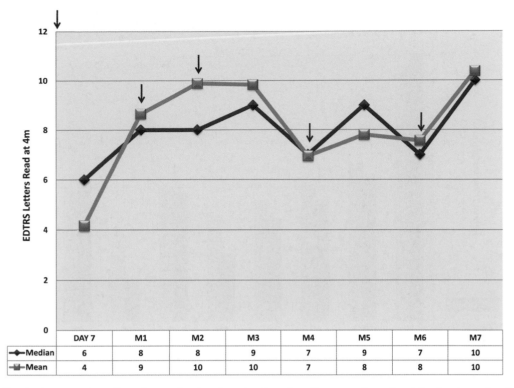

	DAY 7	M1	M2	M3	M4	M5	M6	M7
Median	6	8	8	9	7	9	7	10
Mean	4	9	10	10	7	8	8	10

Fig. 4. Mean and median change in visual acuity from baseline at each study visit after intravitreal ranibizumab for diabetic macular edema. Mean change (*squares*) and median change (*diamonds*) in visual acuity were measured in the number of letters that were read on the Early Treatment Diabetic Retinopathy Study (ETDRS) visual acuity chart. The *arrows* show times of intraocular injection of 0.5 mg of Ranibizumab. At the primary endpoint (7 months) there was an improvement of 10 letters in mean visual acuity and 10 letters in median visual acuity among the 18 participants.

associated with more gradual improvements in visual acuity. Figure 5 shows the reduction in excess retinal thickness through 7 months of follow-up in the final 18 participants. Further studies are underway to investigate the correlation between visual acuity and retinal thickness as measured by OCT.

Intraocular injections of ranibizumab were tolerated well with no ocular inflammation or adverse events. There were no systemic adverse events; no thromboembolic events, cerebral vascular accidents, nor myocardial infarctions. Capillary nonperfusion was measured by image analysis on baseline and month 6 fluorescein angiograms with the investigator masked with respect to time point. The mean area of nonperfusion was 0.19812 disc areas at baseline and 0.19525 at 6 months. Therefore, no significant change in capillary nonperfusion was seen throughout the study.

The READ-2 Study, a multi-center phase 2 randomized clinical trial investigating the bioactivity and safety of ranibizumab for DME is underway in the United States. The three treatment arms in the study include: (1) ranibizumab, (2) ranibizumab with focal laser photocoagulation, and (3) focal laser photocoagulation with deferred ranibizumab. Preliminary results are expected in 2008.

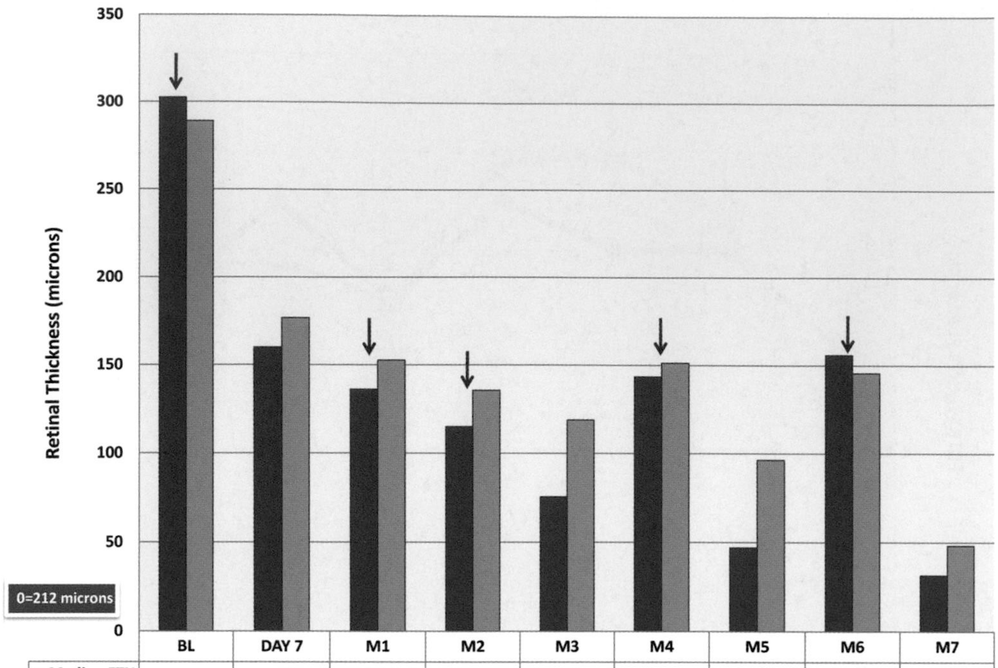

	BL	DAY 7	M1	M2	M3	M4	M5	M6	M7
Median FTH	303	160	136	115	76	144	47	156	32
Mean FTH	289	177	153	136	119	151	96	146	48

Fig. 5. The mean excess foveal thickness at each study visit after ranibizumab for diabetic macular edema. Each bar represents the mean or median value for excess foveal thickness for all 18 patients at the designated study visit. The arrows show when intraocular injections of 0.5 mg of ranibizumab were administered. Compared to baseline, foveal thickness was reduced by 241 μm at the primary endpoint of the study, constituting elimination of over 80% of the excess foveal thickness that had been present at baseline.

Another clinical trial investigating ranibizumab for diabetic retinopathy is also under way, A double-masked, multicenter, phase II study assessing the safety and efficacy of ranibizumab (0.3 and 0.5 mg intravitreal injections) compared with non-treatment control (sham injection) for the treatment of DME is recruiting patients in the United States as well as in Europe, New Zealand and Asia.

The primary objective is to explore whether ranibizumab treatment is superior to non-treatment in reducing macular edema from baseline to Month 6 in patients diagnosed with DME. Results are expected in 2009.

Finally, the Diabetic Retinopathy Clinical Research Network (DRCR.net) is conducting a randomized, multicenter clinical trial investigating intravitreal ranibizumab or triamcinolone acetonide in combination with laser photocoagulation for diabetic macular edema. This study will involve subjects with DME involving the center of the macula (with OCT central subfield thickness greater than 250 μ) responsible for visual acuity of 20/32 or worse. The objective is to determine which is a better treatment approach for DME: laser alone, laser combined with intravitreal triamcinolone, laser combined with intravitreal ranibizumab, or intravitreal ranibizumab alone. Patient recruitment for this study began in March 2007. The primary efficacy outcome will be visual acuity at 12 months adjusted for the baseline acuity, with secondary outcomes being the change in retinal thickening of central subfield and retinal volume (measured by OCT) as well as number of injections in the first year. Safety outcomes will include injection-related events, ocular drug-related events, and systemic drug-related events.

SUMMARY

Treatment of DME is complex and involves both systemic and ocular therapies. Although focal laser photocoagulation is considered the gold standard for the treatment of macular edema, novel therapies directed at decreasing vascular permeability at the molecular level with anti-VEGF agents have shown beneficial effects in early clinical trials. Results from phase 2 clinical studies should provide further information on the efficacy and safety of VEGF inhibitors in diabetic retinopathy. Inhibitors of VEGF are likely to play a therapeutic role for the treatment of both DME and proliferative diabetic retinopathy.

REFERENCES

1. Klein R. Retinopathy in a population-based study. Trans Am Ophthalmol Soc 1992;90:561–594
2. Caldwell RB, Bartoli M, Behzadian MA, El-Remessy AE, Al-Shabrawey M, Platt DH, Caldwell RW. Vascular endothelial growth factor and diabetic retinopathy: pathophysiological mechanisms and treatment perspectives. Diabetes Metab Res Rev 2003;19:442–455
3. Resnikoff S, Pascolini D, Etya'ale D, Kocur I, Pararajasegaram R, Pokharel GP, Mariotti SP. Global data on visual impairment in the year 2002. Bull World Health Organ 2004;82:844–851
4. Kempen JH, O'Colmain BJ, Leske MC, Haffner SM, Klein R, Moss SE, Taylor HR, Hamman RF. The prevalence of diabetic retinopathy among adulats in the United States. Arch Ophthalmol 2004;122:552–563
5. Stefanson E. The therapeuthic effects on retinal laser treatment and vitrectomy. A theory based on oxygen and vascular physiology. Acta Ophthalmol Scnad 2001;79:435–440
6. Moore J, Bagby S, Ireland G, et al. Three dimensional analysis of microaneurysms in the human diabetic retina. Anat J 1999;194:89–100
7. Nguyen QD, Shah SM, Van Anden E, et al. Supplemental inspired oxygen improves diabetic macular edema; a pilot study. Invest Ophthalmol Vis Sci 2003;45:617–624
8. Ozaki H, Hayashi H, Vinores SA, et al. Intravitreal sustained release of VEGF causes retinal neovascularization in rabbits and breakdown of the blood-retinal barrier in rabbits and primates. Exp Eye Res 1997;64:505–517
9. Derevjanik NL, Vinores SA, Xiao W-H, et al. Quantitative assessment of the integrity of the blood-retinal barrier in mice. Invest Ophthalmol Vis Sci 2002;43:2462–2467
10. Senger DR, Galli SJ, Dvorak AM, et al. Tumor cells secrete a vascular permeability factor that promotes accumulation of ascites fluid. Science 1983;219:983–985
11. Leung DW, Cachianes G, Kuang WJ, Goeddel DV, Ferrara N. Vascular endothelial growth factor is a secreted angiogenic mitogen. Science 1989;246:1306–1309
12. Olofsson B, Korpelainen E, Pepper MS, et al. Vascular endothelial growth factor B (VEGF-B) binds to VEGF receptor-1 and regulates plasminogen activator activity in endothelial cells. Proc Natl Acad Sci USA 1998;95:11709–11714
13. Takahashi H, Shibuya M. The vascular endothelial growth factor (VEGF)/VEGF receptor system and its role under physiological and pathological conditions. Clin Sci (Lond) 2005;109(3):227–241
14. Houck KA, Ferrara N, Winer J, et al. The vascular endothelial growth factor family: identification of a fourth molecular species and characterization of alternative splicing of RNA. Mol Endocrinol 1991;5:1806–1814
15. Ferrara N. Vascular endothelial growth factor: basic science and clinical progress. Endocr Rev 2004;25:581–611

16. Alon T, Hemo I, Itin A, Pe'er J, Stone J, Keshet E. Vascular endothelial growth factor acts as a survival factor for newly formed retinal vessels and has implications for retinopathy of prematurity. Nat Med 1995;1:1024–1028
17. Skillings JR, Johnson DH, Miller K, Kabbinavar F, Bergsland E, Holmgren E, Holden SN, Hurwitz H, Scappaticci F. Arterial thromboembolic events (ATEs) in a pooled analysis of 5 randomized, controlled trials (RCTs) of bevacizumab (BV) with chemotherapy [abstract]. J Clin Oncol 2005;23:3019
18. Asahara T, Takahashi T, Masuda H, Kalka C, Chen D, Iwaguro H, Inai Y, Silver M, Isner JM. VEGF contributes to postnatal neovascularization by mobilizing bone marrow-derived endothelial progenitor cells. EMBO J 1999;18:3964–3972
19. Lyden D, Hattori K, Dias S, Costa C, Blaikie P, Butros L, Chadburn A, Heissig B, Marks W, Witte L, Wu X, Hicklin D, Zhu Z, Hackett NR, Crystal RG, Moore MA, Hajjar KA, Manova K, Benezra R, Rafii S. Impaired recruitment of bone-marrow-derived endothelial and hematopoietic precursor cells blocks tumor angiogenesis and growth. Nat Med 2001;7:1194–1201
20. Pepper MS, Ferrara N, Orci L, Montesano R. Vascular endothelial growth factor (VEGF) induces plasminogen activators and plasminogen activator inhibitor-1 in microvascular endothelial cells. Biochem Biophys Res Commun 1991;181:902–906
21. Lamoreaux WJ, Fitzgerald ME, Reiner A, Hasty KA, Charles ST. Vascular endothelial growth factor increases release of gelatinase A and decreases release of tissue inhibitor of metalloproteinases by microvascular endothelial cells in vitro. Microvasc Res 1998;55:29–42
22. Hiratsuka S, Nakamura K, Iwai S, Murakami M, Itoh T, Kijima H, Shipley JM, Senior RM, Shibuya M. MMP9 induction by vascular endothelial growth factor receptor-1 is involved in lung-specific metastasis. Cancer Cell 2002;2:289–300
23. Uhlmann S, Friedrichs U, Eichler W, Hoffmann S, Wiedemann P. Direct measurement of VEGF-induced nitric oxide production by choroidal endothelial cells. Microvasc Res 2001;62:179–189
24. Papapetropoulos A, Garcia-Cardena G, Madri JA, Sessa WC. Nitric oxide production contributes to the angiogenic properties of vascular endothelial growth factor in human endothelial cells. J Clin Invest 1997;100:3131–3139
25. Clauss M, Gerlach M, Gerlach H, Brett J, Wang F, Familletti PC, Pan YC, Olander JV, Connolly DT, Stern D. Vascular permeability factor: a tumor-derived polypeptide that induces endothelial cell and monocyte procoagulant activity, and promotes monocyte migration. J Exp Med 1990;172:1535–1545
26. Ishida S, Usui T, Yamashiro K, Kaji Y, Ahmed E, Carrasquillo KG, Amano S, Hida T, Oguchi Y, Adamis AP. VEGF164 is proinflammatory in the diabetic retina. Invest Ophthalmol Vis Sci 2003a;44:2155–2162
27. Usui T, Ishida S, Yamashiro K, Kaji Y, Poulaki V, Moore J, Moore T, Amano S, Horikawa Y, Dartt D, Golding M, Shima DT, Adamis AP. VEGF 164(165) as the Pathological Isoform: differential leukocyte and endothelial responses through VEGFR1 and VEGFR2. Invest Ophthalmol Vis Sci 2004;45:368–374
28. Miyamoto K, Khosrof S, Bursell SE, Moromizato Y, Aiello LP, Ogura Y, Adamis AP. Vascular endothelial growth factor (VEGF)-induced retinal vascular permeability is mediated by intercellular adhesion molecule-1 (ICAM-1). Am J Pathol 2000;156:1733–1739
29. Joussen A, Murata T, Tsujikawa A, Kirchhof B, Bursell S-E, Adamis AP. Leukocyte-mediated endothelial cell injury and death in the diabetic retina. Am J Pathol 2001;158:147–152
30. Ryan AM, Eppler DB, Hagler KE, Bruner RH, Thomford PJ, Hall RL, Shopp GM, O'Neill CA. Preclinical safety evaluation of rhuMAbVEGF, an antiangiogenic humanized monoclonal antibody. Toxicol Pathol 1999;27:78–86
31. Gerber HP, Vu TH, Ryan AM, Kowalski J, Werb Z, Ferrara N. VEGF couples hypertrophic cartilage remodeling, ossification and angiogenesis during endochondral bone formation. Nat Med 1999;5:623–628
32. Nissen NN, Polverini PJ, Koch AE, Volin MV, Gamelli RL, DiPietro LA. Vascular endothelial growth factor mediates angiogenic activity during the proliferative phase of wound healing. Am J Pathol 1998;152:1445–1452
33. Deodato B, Arsic N, Zentilin L, Galeano M, Santoro D, Torre V, Altavilla D, Valdembri D, Bussolino F, Squadrito F, Giacca M. Recombinant AAV vector encoding human VEGF165 enhances wound healing. Gene Ther 2002;9:777–785
34. Fraser HM, Wilson H, Rudge JS, Wiegand SJ. Single injections of vascular endothelial growth factor trap block ovulation in the macaque and produce a prolonged, dose-related suppression of ovarian function. J Clin Endocrinol Metab 2005;90:1114–1122

35. Liu MH, Jin H, Floten HS, Ren Z, Yim AP, He GW. Vascular endothelial growth factor-mediated, endothelium-dependent relaxation in human internal mammary artery. Ann Thorac Surg 2002;73:819–824
36. Kitamoto Y, Tokunaga H, Tomita K. Vascular endothelial growth factor is an essential molecule for mouse kidney development: glomerulogenesis and nephrogenesis. J Clin Invest 1997;99:2351–2357
37. LeCouter J, Moritz DR, Li B, Phillips GL, Liang XH, Gerber HP, Hillan KJ, Ferrara N. Angiogenesis-independent endothelial protection of liver: role of VEGFR-1. Science 2003;299:890–893
38. Arsic N, Zacchigna S, Zentilin L, Ramirez-Correa G, Pattarini L, Salvi A, Sinagra G, Giacca M. Vascular endothelial growth factor stimulates skeletal muscle regeneration in vivo. Mol Ther 2004;10:844–854
39. Oosthuyse B, Moons L, Storkebaum E Beck H, Nuyens D, Brusselmans K, Van Dorpe J, Hellings P, Gorselink M, Heymans S, Theilmeier G, Dewerchin M, Laudenbach V, Vermylen P, Raat H, Acker T, Vleminckx V, Van Den Bosch L, Cashman N, Fujisawa H, Drost MR, Sciot R, Bruyninckx F, Hicklin DJ, Ince C, Gressens P, Lupu F, Plate KH, Robberecht W, Herbert JM, Collen D, Carmeliet P. Deletion of the hypoxia-response element in the vascular endothelial growth factor promoter causes motor neuron degeneration. Nat Genet 2001;28:131–138
40. Storkebaum E, Lambrechts D, Carmeliet P. VEGF: once regarded as a specific angiogenic factor, now implicated in neuroprotection. Bioessays 2004;26:943–954
41. Nishijima K, Ng YS, Zhong L, Bradley J, Schubert W, Jo N, Akita J, Samuelsson SJ, Robinson GS, Adamis AP, Shima DT Vascular endothelial growth factor-A is a survival factor for retinal neurons and a critical neuroprotectant during the adaptive response to ischemic injury. Am J Pathol 2007;171(1):53–67
42. Blaauwgeers HG, Holtkamp GM, Rutten H, Witmer AN, Koolwijk P, Partanen TA, Alitalo K, Kroon ME, Kijlstra A, van Hinsbergh VW, Schlingemann RO. Polarized vascular endothelial growth factor secretion by human retinal pigment epithelium and localization of vascular endothelial growth factor receptors on the inner choriocapillaris. Evidence for a trophic paracrine relation. Am J Pathol 1999;155:421–428
43. Marneros AG, Fan J, Yokoyama Y, Gerber HP, Ferrara N, Crouch RK, Olsen BR. Vascular endothelial growth factor expression in the retinal pigment epithelium is essential for choriocapillaris development and visual function. Am J Pathol 2005;167:1451–1459
44. Peters S, Heiduschka P, Julien S, Ziemssen F, Fietz H, Bartz-Schmidt KU. Tübingen Bevacizumab Study Group, Schraermeyer U Ultrastructural findings in the primate eye after intravitreal injection of bevacizumab. Am J Ophthalmol 2007;143(6):995–1002
45. Kabbinavar F, Hurwitz HI, Fehrenbacher L, Meropol NJ, Novotny WF, Lieberman G, Griffing S, Bergsland E. Phase II, randomized trial comparing bevacizumab plus fluorouracil (FU)/leucovorin (LV) with FU/LV alone in patients with metastatic colorectal cancer. J Clin Oncol 2003;21:60–65
46. Kabbinavar FF, Schulz J, McCleod M, Patel T, Hamm JT, Hecht JR, Mass R, Perrou B, Nelson B, Novotny WF. Addition of bevacizumab to bolus fluorouracil and leucovorin in first-line metastatic colorectal cancer: results of a randomized phase II trial. J Clin Oncol 2005;23:3697–3705
47. Hurwitz H, Fehrenbacher L, Novotny W, Cartwright T, Hainsworth J, Heim W, Berlin J, Baron A, Griffing S, Holmgren E, Ferrara N, Fyfe G, Rogers B, Ross R, Kabbinavar F. Bevacizumab plus irinotecan, fluorouracil, and leucovorin for metastatic colorectal cancer. N Engl J Med 2004;350:2335–2342
48. Miller KD, Chap LI, Holmes FA, Cobleigh MA, Marcom PK, Fehrenbacher L, Dickler M, Overmoyer BA, Reimann JD, Sing AP, Langmuir V, Rugo HS. Randomized phase III trial of capecitabine compared with bevacizumab plus capecitabine in patients with previously treated metastatic breast cancer. J Clin Oncol 2005;23:792–799
49. Aiello LP, Avery RL, Arrigg PG, Keyt BA, Jampel HD, Shah ST, Pasquale LR, Thieme H, Iwamoto MA, Park JE, Nguyen HV, Aiello LM, Ferrara N, King GL. Vascular endothelial growth factor in ocular fluid of patients with diabetic retinopathy and other retinal disorders. N Engl J Med 1994;331:1480–1487
50. Adamis AP, Miller JW, Bernal MT, D'Amico DJ, Folkman J, Yeo TK, Yeo KT. Increased vascular endothelial growth factor levels in the vitreous of eyes with proliferative diabetic retinopathy. Am J Ophthalmol 1994;118:445–450
51. Adamis AP, Shima DT, Tolentino MJ, Gragoudas ES, Ferrara N, Folkman J, D'Amore PA, Miller JW. Inhibition of vascular endothelial growth factor prevents retinal ischemia-associated iris neovascularization in a nonhuman primate. Arch Ophthalmol 1996;114:66–71

52. Aiello LP, Northrup JM, Keyt BA, Takagi H, Iwamoto MA. Hypoxic regulation of vascular endothelial growth factor in retinal cells. Arch Ophthalmol 1995a;113:1538–1544
53. Aiello LP, Pierce EA, Foley ED, Takagi H, Chen H, Riddle L, Ferrara N, King GL, Smith LEH. Suppression of retinal neovascularization in vivo by inhibition of vascular endothelial growth factor (VEGF) using soluble VEGF-receptor chimeric proteins. Proc Natl Acad Sci USA 1995b;92: 10457–10461
54. Krzystolik MG, Afshari MA, Adamis AP, Gaudreault J, Gragoudas ES, Li W, Connolly E, O'Neill CA, Miller JW. Prevention of experimental choroidal neovascularization with intravitreal anti-vascular endothelial growth factor antibody fragment. Arch Ophthalmol 2002;120:338–346
55. Tolentino MJ, Miller JW, Gragoudas ES, Chatzistefanou K, Ferrara N, Adamis AP. Vascular endothelial growth factor is sufficient to produce iris neovascularization and neovascular glaucoma in a nonhuman primate. Arch Ophthalmol 1996a;114:964–970
56. Tolentino MJ, Miller JW, Gragoudas ES, Jakobiec FA, Flynn E, Chatzistefanou K, Ferrara N, Adamis AP. Intravitreous injections of vascular endothelial growth factor produce retinal ischemia and microangiopathy in an adult primate. Ophthalmology 1996b ;103:820–1828
57. Tripathi RC, Li J, Tripathi BJ, Chalam KV, Adamis AP. Increased level of vascular endothelial growth factor in aqueous humor of patients with neovascular glaucoma. Ophthalmology 1998;105:232–237
58. Lashkari K, Hirose T, Yazdany J, McMeel JW, Kazlauskas A, Rahimi N. Vascular endothelial growth factor and hepatocyte growth factor levels are differentially elevated in patients with advanced retinopathy of prematurity. Am J Pathol 2000;156:1337–1344
59. Funatsu H, Yamashita H, Ikeda T, Nakanishi Y, Kitano S, Hori S. Angiotensin II and vascular endothelial growth factor in the vitreous fluid of patients with diabetic macular edema and other retinal disorders. Am J Ophthalmol 2002;133:537–543
60. Funatsu H, Yamashita H, Ikeda T, Mimura T, Eguchi S, Hori S. Vitreous levels of interleukin-6 and vascular endothelial growth factor are related to diabetic macular edema. Ophthalmology 2003;110:1690–1696
61. Funatsu H, Yamashita H, Sakata K, Noma H, Mimura T, Suzuki M, Eguchi S, Hori S. Vitreous levels of vascular endothelial growth factor and intercellular adhesion molecule 1 are related to diabetic macular edema. Ophthalmology 2005;112:806–816
62. Funatsu H, Yamashita H, Noma H, et al. Increased levels of vascular endothelial growth factor and interleukin-6 in the aqueous humor of diabetics with macular edema. Am J Ophthalmol 2002;133:70–77
63. Kliffen M, Sharma HS, Mooy CM, Kerkvliet S, de Jong PT. Increased expression of angiogenic growth factors in age-related maculopathy. Br J Ophthalmol 1997;81:154–162
64. Lopez PF, Sippy BD, Lambert HM, Thach AB, Hinton DR. Transdifferentiated retinal pigment epithelial cells are immunoreactive for vascular endothelial growth factor in surgically excised age-related macular degeneration-related choroidal neovascular membranes. Invest Ophthalmol Vis Sci 1996;122:393–403
65. Frank RN, Amin RH, Eliott D, Puklin E, Abrams GW. Basic fibroblast growth factor and vacular endothelial growth facto rare present in epiretinal and choroidal neovascular membranes. Invest Ophthalmol Vis Sci 1996;122:393–403
66. Grossniklaus HE, Ling JX, Wallace TM, Dithmar S, Lawson DH, Cohen C, Elner VM, Elner SG, Sternberg P Jr. Macrophage and retinal pigment epithelium expression of angiogenic cytokines in choroidal neovaskularization. Mol Vis 2002;8:119–126
67. Miller JW, Adamis AP, Shima DT, D'Amore PA, Moulton RS, O'Reilly MS, Folkman J, Dvorak HF, Brown LF, Berse B, Yeo T-K, Yeo K-T. Vascular endothelial growth factor/vascular permeability factor is temporally and spatially correlated with ocular angiogenesis in a primate model. Am J Pathol 1994;145:574–584
68. Amano S, Rohan R, Kuroki M, Tolentino M, Adamis AP. Requirement for vascular endothelial growth factor in wound- and inflammation-related corneal neovascularization. Invest Ophthalmol Vis Sci 1998;39:18–22
69. Honda M, Sakamoto T, Ishibashi T, et al. Experimental subretinal neovascularization is inhibited by adenovirus-mediated soluble VEGF/flt-1 receptor gene transfection: a role of VEGF and possible treatment for SRN in age-related macular degeneration. Gene Ther 2000;11:978–985
70. Bhisitkul RB, Robinson GS, Moulton RS et al. An antisense oligonucleotide against vascular endothelial growth factor in a nonhuman primate model of iris neovascularization. Arch Ophthalmol 2005;123:214–219

71. Lebherz C, Maguire AM, Auricchio A, et al. Nonhuman primate models for diabetic ocular neovascularization using AAV2-mediated overexpression of vascular endothelial growth factor. Diabetes 2005;54:1141–1149
72. Miyamoto K, Hiroshiba N, Tsujikawa A, Ogura Y. In vivo demonstration of increased leukocyte entrapment in retinal microcirculation of diabetic rats. Invest Ophthalmol Vis Sci 1998;39:2190–2194
73. Kuroki M, Voest EE, Amano S, Beerepoot LV, Takashima S, Tolentino M, Kim RY, Rohan RM, Colby KA, Yeo KT, Adamis AP. Reactive oxygen intermediates increase vascular endothelial growth factor expression in vitro and in vivo. J Clin Invest 1996;98:1667–1675
74. Lu M, Kuroki M, Amano S, Tolentino M, Keough K, Kim I, Bucala R, Adamis AP. Advanced glycation end products increase retinal vascular endothelial growth factor expression. J Clin Invest 1998;101:1219–1224
75. Adamis AP, Shima DT, Yeo KT, Yeo TK, Brown LF, Berse B, D'Amore PA, Folkman J. Synthesis and secretion of vascular permeability factor/vascular endothelial growth factor by human retinal pigment epithelial cells. Biochem Biophys Res Commun 1993;193:631–638
76. Famiglietti EV, Stopa EG, McGookin ED, Song P, LeBlanc V, Streeten BW. Immunocytochemical localization of vascular endothelial growth factor in neurons and glial cells of human retina. Brain Res 2003;969:195–204
77. Shima DT, Adamis AP, Ferrara N, Yeo KT, Yeo TK, Allende R, Folkman J, D'Amore PA. Hypoxic induction of endothelial cell growth factors in retinal cells: identification and characterization of vascular endothelial growth factor (VEGF) as the mitogen. Mol Med. 1995;1(2):182–93
78. Boulton M, Foreman D, Williams G, McLeod D. VEGF localisation in diabetic retinopathy. Br J Ophthalmol 1998;82:561–568
79. Malecaze F, Clamens S, Simorre-Pinatel V, Mathis A, Chollet P, Favard C, Bayard F, Plouet J. Detection of vascular endothelial growth factor messenger RNA and vascular endothelial growth factor-like activity in proliferative diabetic retinopathy. Arch Ophthalmol 1994;112:1476–1482
80. Brooks HL Jr, Caballero S Jr, Newell CK, Steinmetz RL, Watson D, Segal MS, Harrison JK, Scott EW, Grant MB. Vitreous levels of vascular endothelial growth factor and stromal-derived factor 1 in patients with diabetic retinopathy and cystoid macular edema before and after intraocular injection of triamcinolone. Arch Ophthalmol 2004;122:1801–1807
81. Joussen AM, Adamis AP. Inflammation as a stimulus for vascular leakage and proliferation. In: Joussen AM, Gardner TW, Kirshhof B, Ryan SJ (eds) Retinal vascular disease. Springer, Berlin, 2007
82. Ishida S, Usui T, Yamashiro K, Kaji Y, Amano S, Ogura Y, Hida T, Oguchi Y, Ambati J, Miller JW, Gragoudas ES, Ng YS, D'Amore PA, Shima DT, Adamis AP. VEGF164-mediated inflammation is required for pathological, but not physiological, ischemia-induced retinal neovascularization. J Exp Med 2003b;198:483–489
83. Roberts WG, Palade GE. Neovasculature induced by vascular endothelial growth factor is fenestrated. Cancer Res 1997;57:765–772
84. Antonetti D, Barber AJ, Hollinger LA, Wolpert EB, Gardner TW. Vascular endothelial growth factor induces rapid phosphorylation of tight junction proteins occludin and zonula occluden 1. J Biol Chem 1999;274:23463–23467
85. Ng EWM, Shima DT, Calias P, Cunningham ET Jr, Guyer DR, Adamis AP. Pegaptanib, a targeted anti-VEGF aptamer for ocular vascular disease. Nat Rev/Drug Discov 2006;5:123–32
86. Ruckman J, Green LS, Beeson J, Waugh S, Gillette WL, Henninger DD, Claesson-Welsh L, Janjic N. 2′ h-Fluoropyrimidine RNA-based aptamers to the 165-amino acid form of vascular endothelial growth factor (VEGF165). Inhibition of receptor binding and VEGF-induced vascular permeability through interactions requiring the exon 7-encoded domain J Biol Chem 1998;273:20556–20567
87. Drolet DW, Nelson J, Tucker CE, Zack PM, Nixon K, Bolin R, Judkins MB, Farmer JA, Wolf JL, Gill SC, Bendele RA. Pharmacokinetics and safety of an anti-vascular endothelial growth factor aptamer (NX1838) following injection into the vitreous humor of rhesus monkeys. Pharm Res 2000;17:1503–1510
88. Bell C, Lynam E, Landfair DJ, Janjic N, Wiles ME. Oligonucleotide NX1838 inhibits VEGF165-mediated cellular responses in vitro. In Vitro Cell Dev Biol Anim 1999;35:533–542
89. Shima DT, Nishijima K, Jo N, Adamis AP. VEGF-mediated neuroprotection in ischemic retina. Invest Ophthalmol Vis Sci 2004;45:E-Abstract 3270
90. Gragoudas ES, Adamis AP, Cunningham ET Jr, Feinsod M, Guyer DR. VEGF Inhibition Study in Ocular Neovascularization Clinical Trial Group Pegaptanib for neovascular age-related macular degeneration. N Engl J Med (2004);351:2805–2816

91. The Eyetech Study Group Anti-vascular endothelial growth factor therapy for subfoveal choroidal neovascularization secondary to age-related macular degeneration: phase II study results. Ophthalmology 2003;110:979–986
92. Presta LG, Chen H, O'Connor SJ et al. Humanization of an anti-VEGF monoclonal antibody for the therapy of solid tumors and other disorders. Cancer Res 1997;57:4593–4599
93. Yang JC, Haworth RM, Sherry RM et al. A randomized trial of bevacicumab, an anti-VEGF antibody, for metastatic renal cancer. N Engl J Med 2003;349:427–434
94. Ellis LM, Curley SA, Grothey A. Surgical resection after downsizing of colorectal liver metastasis in the era of Bevacicumab. J Clin Oncol 2005;23:4853–4855
95. Aisenbrey S, Ziemssen F, Volker M, Gelisken F, Szurman P, Jaissle G, Grisanti S, Bartz-Schmidt KU. Intravitreal bevacizumab (Avastin) for occult choroidal neovascularization in age-related macular degeneration. Graefes Arch Clin Exp Ophthalmol 2007;245:941–948
96. Avery RL, Pearlman J, Pieramici DJ, Rabena MD, Castellarin AA, Nasir MA, Giust MJ, Wendel R, Patel A. Intravitreal bevacizumab (Avastin) in the treatment of proliferative diabetic retinopathy. Ophthalmology 2006;113(10):1695.e1–15
97. Spaide RF, Fisher YL. Intravitreal bevacizumab (Avastin) treatment of proliferative diabetic retinopathy complicated by vitreous hemorrhage. Retina 2006;26(3):275–278
98. Spaide RF, Laud K, Fine HF, Klancnik JM Jr, Meyerle CB, Yannuzzi LA, Sorenson J, Slakter J, Fisher YL, Cooney MJ. Intravitreal bevacizumab treatment of choroidal neovascularization secondary to age-related macular degeneration. Retina 2006;26(4):383–390
99. Gaudreault J, Fei D, Rusit J, et al. Preclinical pharmacokinetics of ranibizumab (rhuFabV2) after a single intravitreal administration. Invest Ophthalmol Vis Sci 2005;46:726–733
100. Rosenfeld PJ, Schwartz SD, Blumenkranz MS, et al. Maximum tolerated dose of a humanized anti-vascular endothelial growth factor antibody fragment for treating neovascular age-related macular degeneration. Ophthalmology 2005;112:1048–1053
101. Rosenfeld PJ, Brown DM, Heier JS, et al. Ranibizumab for neovascular age-related macular degeneration: 2-year results of the MARINA Study. N Engl J Med 2006;355:1419–1431
102. Brown DM, Kaiser PK, Michels M et al. Ranibizumab versus verteporfin for neovascular age-related macular degeneration. N Engl J Med 2006;355:1432–1444
103. Cunningham ET Jr, Adamis AP, Altaweel M, Aiello LP, Bressler NM, D'Amico DJ, Goldbaum M, Guyer DR, Katz B, Patel M, Schwartz SD. Macugen Diabetic Retinopathy Study Group. A phase II randomized double-masked trial of pegaptanib, an anti-vascular endothelial growth factor aptamer, for diabetic macular edema. Ophthalmology 2005;112(10):1747–1757
104. Adamis AP, Altaweel M, Bressler NM, Cunningham ET Jr, Davis MD, Goldbaum M, Gonzales C, Guyer DR, Barrett K, Patel M. Macugen Diabetic Retinopathy Study Group. Changes in retinal neovascularization following pegaptanib (Macugen) therapy in diabetic individuals. Ophthalmology 2006;113(1):23–28
105. Chen E, Park CH. Use of intravitreal bevacizumab as a preoperative adjunct for tractional retinal detachment repair in severe proliferative diabetic retinopathy. Retina 2006;26(6):699–700. No abstract available
106. Grisanti S, Biester S, Peters S, Tatar O, Ziemssen F, Bartz-Schmidt KU. Tuebingen Bevacizumab Study Group. Intracameral bevacizumab for iris rubeosis. Am J Ophthalmol 2006;142(1):158–160
107. Silva Paula J, Jorge R, Alves Costa R, Rodrigues Mde L, Scott IU. Short-term results of intravitreal bevacizumab (Avastin) on anterior segment neovascularization in neovascular glaucoma. Acta Ophthalmol Scand. 2006;84(4):556–557
108. Haritoglou C, Kook D, Neubauer A, Wolf A, Priglinger S, Strauss R, Gandorfer A, Ulbig M, Kampik A. Intravitreal bevacizumab (Avastin) therapy for persistent diffuse diabetic macular edema. Retina 2006;26(9):999–1005
109. Nguyen QD, Tatlipinar S, Shah SM, Haller JA,Quinlan E, Sung JU, Zimmer-Galler I, Do DV, Campochiaro PA. Vascular endothelial growth factor is a critical stimulus for diabetic macular edema. Am J Ophthalmol 2006;142(6):961–969
110. Diabetic Retinopathy Clinical Research Network, Scott IU, Edwards AR, Beck RW, Bressler NM, Chan CK, Elman MJ, Friedman SM, Greven CM, Maturi RK, Pieramici DJ, Shami M, Singerman LJ, Stockdale CR. A phase II randomized clinical trial of bevacizumab for diabetic macular edema. Ophthalmology 2007;114(10):1860–1867

18 Clinical Trials in Protein Kinase C-β Inhibition in Diabetic Retinopathy

Jennifer K. Sun, Rola Hamam, and Lloyd P. Aiello

CONTENTS

ABSTRACT

Protein kinase C (PKC) activation plays a key role in the development of microvascular complications in diabetes, including diabetic retinopathy. Vision loss in patients with diabetes stems from the development of ocular complications that include diabetic macular edema (DME), and proliferative diabetic retinopathy (PDR). Even with timely intervention, a large number of patients lose vision from diabetic eye disease each year, necessitating an ongoing effort toward exploring new and more effective approaches for the prevention and treatment of diabetic retinopathy (DR). Clinical trials of PKC inhibition for diabetic retinopathy have focused largely on the oral PKC-β inhibitor, ruboxistaurin (RBX). Preclinical studies of RBX in animal models demonstrated amelioration of diabetes-induced abnormalities in retinal circulation, vascular permeability, and leukocyte adhesion. Subsequent clinical studies, consisting of multiple multicenter, double-masked, randomized, placebo-controlled trials have consistently demonstrated

From: *Contemporary Diabetes: Diabetic Retinopathy*
Edited by: E. Duh © Humana Press, Totowa, NJ

that RBX reduces long-term visual loss, increases visual gain, slows progression of diabetic macular edema, and reduces the need for initial macular laser photocoagulation in patients with advanced nonproliferative DR (NPDR). However, RBX does not halt the progression of diabetic retinopathy. RBX has been well-tolerated with a favorable safety profile. Additional studies with this drug are currently ongoing to provide additional supporting data on its beneficial effects in diabetic macular edema and vision loss.

Key Words: Diabetes; Diabetic retinopathy; Macular edema; Protein kinase c; LY333531; Ruboxistaurin; Clinical trials.

INTRODUCTION

Despite the proven efficacy of treatments such as laser photocoagulation in reducing visual loss and improving anatomic outcomes, diabetic retinopathy remains the leading cause of blindness in the working-age population *(1)*. Vision loss primarily stems from the development of diabetic ocular complications including diabetic macular edema (DME) and proliferative diabetic retinopathy (PDR). Given appropriate treatment, a significant proportion of visual loss associated with diabetes can be prevented. However, even with timely intervention, a large number of patients lose vision from diabetic eye disease each year, necessitating ongoing efforts to explore new and more effective approaches for prevention and treatment of diabetic retinopathy (DR). Preclinical studies have demonstrated that protein kinase C (PKC) activation likely plays a key role in the development of diabetic microvascular complications. Human clinical trials have subsequently shown some degree of benefit of the oral PKC-beta inhibitor, ruboxistaurin in preventing vision loss, reducing progression of DME, and decreasing the need for macular focal/grid laser photocoagulation in patients with diabetes.

PROTEIN KINASE C-β

Multiple studies have demonstrated the association between poor glycemic control and development of severe diabetic ocular complications. The Diabetes Control and Complications Trial (DCCT) *(2, 3)* and the United Kingdom Prospective Diabetes Study (UKPDS) *(4)* in particular highlighted the importance of strict glycemic control in preventing the development of DR in both Type 1 and Type 2 diabetic patients over time.

The hyperglycemia associated with diabetes causes an increase in advanced glycation end-products (AGE), as well as reactive oxygen species *(5)*. Increases in these molecules in turn lead to formation of diacylglycerol (DAG), a physiologic activator of protein kinase c (PKC) *(6)*. In addition, hyperglycemia leads to *de novo* synthesis of DAG *(7, 8, 9)*. Increases in DAG result in activation of the PKC serine/threonine kinase family of enzymes, which alter the activity of key signaling proteins throughout the body by phosphorylation.

There are at least 12 isoforms of PKC that play roles in the signaling pathways of multiple growth factors, hormones, neurotransmitters, and cytokines *(10, 11)*. Various isoforms are localized and activated differentially in various tissues within the body. Studies have shown that among the different isoforms, PKC-beta is the predominant one activated in diabetic vascular tissues *(12–15)*. Chapter 8 includes a thorough discussion of the molecular mechanisms involved in PKC's actions on retinal blood flow, extracellular matrix, basement membrane, vascular permeability, and angiogenesis. Some of these mechanisms involve both upstream and downstream effects on vascular endothelial growth factor (VEGF) *(16, 17)*, a molecule with a primary role in diabetes-induced retinal neovascularization and vascular permeability.

PKC INHIBITION WITH RUBOXISTAURIN

Early nonselective inhibitors of PKC, such as H-7, GF109203X, chelerythrine, and staurosporine *(18)*, were demonstrated to have wide-ranging toxicity that prevented their use in clinical trials. An orally administered kinase inhibitor PKC412 with nonselective PKC inhibition activity was evaluated in subjects with DME *(19)*. A randomized, multicenter, double-masked, parallel-group study evaluated 141 subjects with DME receiving placebo or one of three doses of PKC412 for up to three months. Fundus photographs ($p = 0.032$) and OCT ($p = 0.039$) demonstrated reduction in retinal thickness after PKC412 treatment, as compared with placebo. There was also a small improvement in visual acuity at three months in the high-dose group. Further clinical development of this compound was not pursued due to gastrointestinal side effects (diarrhea, nausea, vomiting), altered glycemic control, and liver toxicity.

However, the identification of beta isoform of PKC as a key molecular target in diabetes-induced microvascular alterations led to a subsequent detailed investigation of LY333531, also called ruboxistaurin (RBX). RBX is a highly selective inhibitor of the beta isoform of PKC, with at least a fiftyfold higher affinity for PKC-beta than for other PKC isoforms (α, γ, δ, ε, η, and ζ) *(20)*. The drug is readily orally bioavailable, and was shown in animal studies to ameliorate abnormalities in retinal circulation in diabetic rats *(21, 22)*. In other preclinical rat studies, RBX reduced intraocular neovascularization in an ischemic model of retinopathy, reduced VEGF-associated retinal vascular permeability, and decreased leukocyte adhesion within the retinal vasculature *(23, 24)*.

EARLY CLINICAL TRIALS WITH RBX

Phase 1 studies tested both single and multiple dosing regimens of RBX in multiple patient populations, including healthy volunteers, the elderly, and those with diabetes *(25, 26)*. Initial pharmacokinetic data were obtained, and the drug was demonstrated to have a favorable safety profile in doses up to 32 mg per day or more for 30 days.

A double-masked, placebo-controlled, parallel, randomized, Phase 2 study examined the effect of treatment with RBX on retinal blood flow and retinal circulation time in diabetic subjects *(27)*. Retinal hemodynamic parameters were assessed using fluorescein dye dilution technique and scanning laser ophthalmoscopy. This study enrolled 29 patients with Type 1 or Type 2 diabetes, duration of diabetes < 10 years, and no to minimal DR. Subjects were treated with either RBX or placebo for 28 days. Treatment with 16 mg RBX twice daily ameliorated diabetes-induced prolongation of retinal mean circulation time. Placebo treated subjects had an exacerbation of the mean retinal circulation time abnormality during this period with a change of $+0.16 \pm 0.80$ s. In contrast, RBX-treated patients experienced normalization of mean retinal circulation time by -0.68 ± 0.73 s ($p = 0.046$) (Fig. 1). A similar, although not statistically significant,

Derby Hospitals NHS Foundation Trust
Library and Knowledge Service

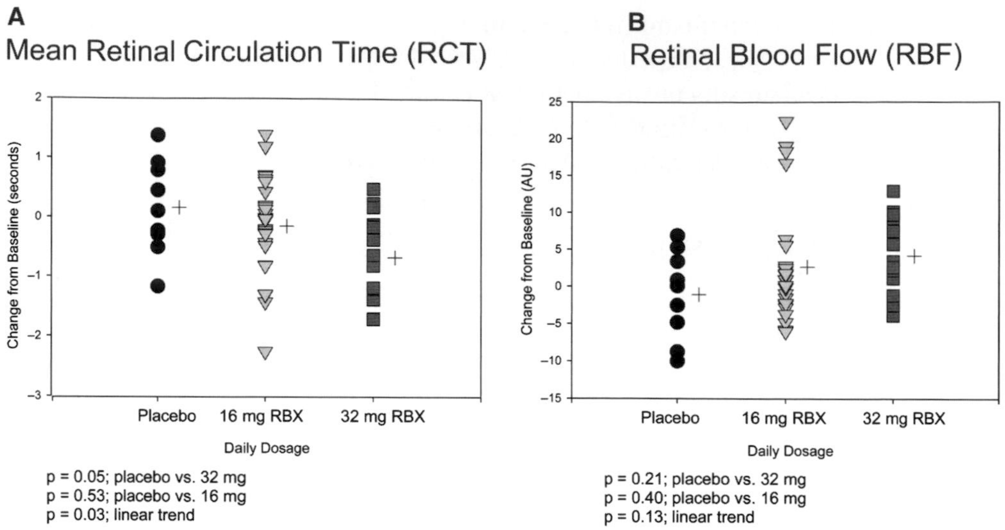

Fig. 1. Pharmacodynamic effect of RBX on mean RCT (*left*) and retinal blood flow (*right*). Changes from baseline of measurements of mean retinal circulation time (**A**) and retinal blood flow (**B**) for each eye are indicated for each RBX dose. The mean value for each group is noted (+). *AU* arbitrary units. (From Fig. 1 in *(27)*. Reproduced with permission of *Investigative Ophthalmology and Visual Science*).

beneficial effect of RBX treatment was observed regarding retinal blood flow. This study provided the first direct evidence that the oral drug, RBX was bioavailable to retinal blood vessels in the human and could also favorably impact diabetes-induced retinal vascular hemodynamic abnormalities.

RBX EFFECTS ON VISUAL OUTCOMES AND DIABETIC MACULAR EDEMA

Till date, results from three multicenter, double-masked, randomized, placebo-controlled trials have been published regarding the effects of RBX on visual outcomes and macular edema in patients with diabetes. The first two of these studies, the Protein Kinase C β Inhibitor Diabetic Retinopathy Study (PKC-DRS) and the Protein Kinase C β Inhibitor Diabetic Macular Edema Study (PKC-DMES) were initiated in 1998, and completed in 2002 *(28)*. Overall, individual studies as well as meta-analysis performed of combined data from these three trials support a modest beneficial effect of RBX on diabetes-associated vision loss, reduced need for macular laser photocoagulation, and increased rates of visual gain. It appears that these benefits are likely mediated primarily through RBX's effects on DME, although there is some evidence for a direct effect as well. In contrast, none of the trials show any reduction in the rate of retinopathy severity progression.

The PKC-DRS trial evaluated the safety and efficacy of three different doses (8 mg per day, 16 mg per day, and 32 mg per day) of RBX in 252 subjects with moderately severe to very severe NPDR *(29)*. The primary end-point for the study was progression of DR over three years, but additional efficacy measures included moderate visual loss (MVL), defined as a doubling of the visual angle (equivalent to the loss of three or more

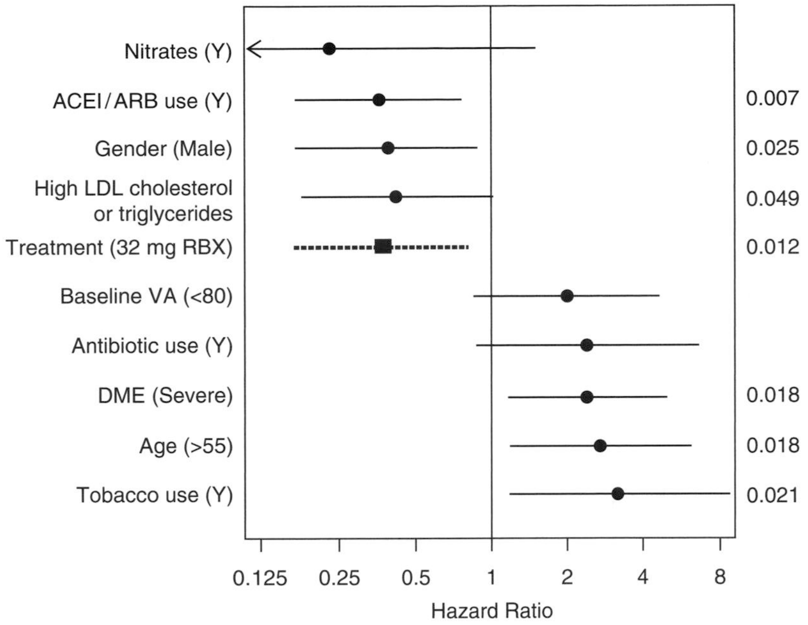

Fig. 2. Cox proportional hazard model for MVL. Severe DME is defined as retinal thickening (or adjacent hard exudates) located at or within 100 μm of the center of the macula. Horizontal bars indicate 95% CIs, and *P* values are indicated to the right. (From Fig. 6 in *(29)*. Reproduced with permission from *The American Diabetes Association*).

lines on the ETDRS chart), and sustained MVL (SMVL), defined as MVL compared to baseline that was present at two consecutive visits at least six months apart. A beneficial effect of RBX was found with regard to the secondary study outcomes of MVL and SMVL. When compared with placebo, treatment with 32 mg per day of RBX resulted in a significantly lower rate of occurrence of MVL ($p = 0.038$) and a nonstatistically significant trend toward a reduced rate of SMVL. Subgroup analysis revealed that SMVL was reduced in RBX-treated (32 mg per day) vs. control subjects who had DME at baseline ($p = 0.017$) or more severe retinopathy (ETDRS level 53, $p = 0.024$). Multivariable Cox proportional hazard analysis confirmed that RBX (32 mg per day) treatment was independently associated with a reduction in risk of MVL as compared with placebo (hazard ratio 0.37 [95% CI 0.17–0.80], $p = 0.012$) (Fig. 2).

The PKC-DMES Trial evaluated the hypothesis that RBX treatment would delay the progression of DME and/or the use of macular focal/grid laser photocoagulation in patients with DME greater than 1/6 of a disc area at baseline located within 2 disc diameters, but farther than 300 μm from the center of the macula *(30)*. Additional eligibility criteria included the presence of mild to moderately severe NPDR, visual acuity of 20/32 or better, and no history of prior laser photocoagulation treatment. The composite primary endpoint was defined as either: (1) progression to sight-threatening DME (development of macular thickening or adjacent hard exudates within 100 μm of the fovea, or development of retinal thickening within 300 μm of the fovea if the distance of baseline DME from the fovea was 1,300 μm or farther) or (2) application of focal/grid laser photocoagulation for treatment of DME in the study eye.

Six hundred and eighty-six patients were randomized to placebo or RBX treatment (4, 16, or 32 mg per day) over 30 months. Both univariate analyses and multivariable Cox proportional hazards analysis revealed that there was no significant difference between treatment and placebo groups in terms of time to occurrence of the composite primary endpoint, or in the total percentage of patients who attained this endpoint. However, secondary analysis demonstrated that the risk of progression to sight-threatening DME was significantly reduced in the 32 mg per day RBX-treated group as compared with placebo when adjusted for covariates including body mass index, baseline visual acuity, mean arterial blood pressure, presence of clinically significant macular edema (CSME), type of DM, and hemoglobin A1c worse than 10% (hazard ratio 0.66 [95% CI 0.47–0.93], p = 0.02).

Based upon the PKC-DRS results showing a beneficial effect of RBX on visual acuity but no effect on retinopathy progression, the primary objective of a subsequent third study, the Protein Kinase C Diabetic Retinopathy Study 2 (PKC-DRS2), was amended prior to any data analysis or investigator/subject unmasking. Although the PKC-DRS2 was originally designed to examine the effect of RBX treatment on progression of DR to PDR, the primary study endpoint was changed after consultation with the US Food and Drug Administration to assess differences in SMVL between diabetic patients on 32 mg per day of RBX vs. those on placebo *(31)*. This study enrolled 685 subjects who had at least 1 study eye with moderately severe to severe NPDR, no history of previous scatter photocoagulation, and best corrected visual acuity measuring at least 45 letters on the ETDRS chart (Snellen equivalent of 20/125 or better). Prior treatment for DME in the study eye was allowed by the eligibility criteria, as was the presence of any current level of DME. The PKC-DRS2 demonstrated a 40% risk reduction in SMVL in the RBX group compared with the placebo group. SMVL occurred in 5.5% of RBX-treated subjects and 9.1% of placebo-treated subjects (p = 0.034). Eye-level analysis revealed a similar risk reduction (45%, p = 0.011) when comparing the RBX and placebo groups. Furthermore, treatment with RBX vs. placebo was associated with improvement in several secondary outcomes, including a higher proportion of subjects whose visual acuity improved by three or more lines on the ETDRS chart from baseline to endpoint (4.9% vs. 2.4%, p = 0.027), a lower proportion of patients whose visual acuity was reduced by three or more lines from baseline to endpoint (6.7% vs. 9.9%, p = 0.044) (Fig. 3), a reduction in the number of patients where DME progressed from center-threatening (CSME > 100 μm from the fovea) to center-involved (50% vs. 68%, P = 0.003), and a reduction in the use of focal/grid laser photocoagulation in patients without prior history of laser at baseline (28.0% vs. 37.9%, p = 0.008) *(31)*.

Subsequent meta-analysis of data from all three trials demonstrated a consistently modest beneficial effect of RBX on SMVL *(32)*. Data combined from the PKC-DRS and PKC-DRS2 trials evaluating a total of 813 patients and 1,392 eyes showed that SMVL occurred significantly more often in placebo-treated subjects, compared with RBX-treated patients (10.2% vs. 6.1%, respectively, p = 0.011). Compared with placebo-treated patients, RBX-treated patients were more likely to gain ≥ 15 letters (2.4% vs. 4.7%) and less likely to lose ≥ 15 letters (11.4% vs. 7.4%, respectively) in visual acuity on the ETDRS chart (p = 0.012). DME was the primary cause of SMVL in 60–100% of study eyes. Among eyes without prior history of focal/grid photocoagulation at baseline,

A

Category	Placebo N=573	32 mg RBX N=571	Chi-Square P-Value*	Overall P-Value**
≥+15 Letters (Improvement)	14 (2.4%)	28 (4.9%)	0.027	0.005
+14 to -14 Letters (No Change)	502 (87.6%)	505 (88.4%)	0.665	
≥-15 Letters (Worsening)	57 (9.9%)	38 (6.7%)	0.044	

B

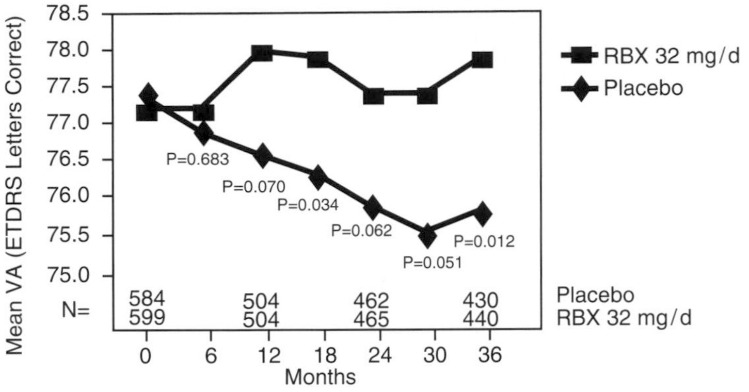

Fig. 3. Ruboxistaurin (RBX) treatment effects on visual acuity (VA). (**A**) Categorical analysis of changes in VA from baseline to end point in study eyes. *Placebo versus RBX. **Wilcoxon–Mann–Whitney. (**B**) Demonstration of the difference in mean change from baseline VA between RBX- and placebo-treated groups. *P* values are for differences between treatment groups in mean change from baseline. *d* day; *ETDRS* Early Treatment Diabetic Retinopathy Study. (From Fig. 2 in *(31)*. Reproduced with permission from Elsevier).

fewer RBX-treated eyes (26.7%) required subsequent macular laser than did placebo-treated eyes (35.6%; p = 0.008). Meta-analysis of the three RBX trials in DR that included the PKC-DMES, PKC-DRS and PKC-DRS2 also found a beneficial effect of RBX on SMVL.

RBX AND PROGRESSION OF DIABETIC RETINOPATHY

Both the PKC-DRS and PKC-DRS2 demonstrated no significant effect of RBX on progression of DR. The primary endpoint of the PKC-DRS was a composite of progression of DR by three or more steps in the ETDRS retinopathy person severity scale for patients with two study eyes, progression of DR by two or more steps in the ETDRS retinopathy person severity scale for patients with only one study eye, or treatment with scatter laser photocoagulation for DR in a study eye *(29)*. In this study, there was no significant difference between treatment groups in terms of time to DR progression as defined by the composite primary endpoint or in terms of cumulative percentage of patients who reached the primary endpoint (Fig. 4). There was also no significant difference between treatment groups when the components of the composite endpoint were analyzed individually, that is, separate analyses were performed for the progression of DR and application of laser photocoagulation. The PKC-DRS2 similarly showed

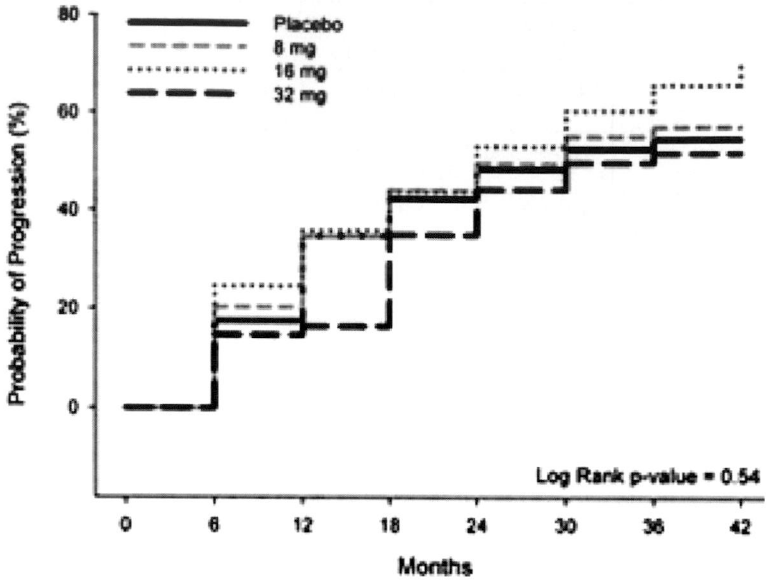

Fig. 4. Effect of RBX on time to progression of DR or to application of PRP. (From Fig. 2 in *(29)*. Reproduced with permission from *The American Diabetes Association*).

that RBX treatment had no demonstrable effect on DR progression to PDR or the application of scatter photocoagulation *(31)*.

ONGOING TRIALS WITH RBX

There are currently three ongoing clinical trials assessing RBX as a treatment for diabetic ocular complications *(33)*. One of these studies, entitled "The Effect of Ruboxistaurin on Clinically Significant Macular Edema", is actively enrolling patients. This trial tests the hypothesis that treatment with RBX will reduce the baseline-to-endpoint change in retinal thickness as measured by OCT in patients with noncenter-involving CSME over the course of 18 months *(34)*. Two other studies have finished patient recruitment and are in follow-up phase. Patients in the "Reduction in the Occurrence of Center-Threatening Diabetic Macular Edema Study" receive either placebo or 32 mg per day RBX for three years. The primary endpoint for this study is the development of center-threatening DME (i.e., DME that extends to within 100 µm of the macular center) *(35)*. The third ongoing trial is an extension of the previous PKC-DRS2 study, in which patients who completed participation and who might benefit from further treatment with RBX are receiving open-label RBX (32 mg per day) for up to two additional years *(36)*. The primary study objective is to evaluate the effect of RBX on the occurrence of SMVL. Secondary objectives are to evaluate the long-term effect of RBX treatment on SMVL using Visit 1 of the PKC-DRS2 as baseline, and to examine effect of withdrawing RBX on vision loss during the time period that elapsed between the end of the PKC-DRS2 and the beginning of this study (approximately 18 months).

RBX AND OTHER, NONOCULAR COMPLICATIONS OF DIABETES

The role of RBX in preventing and/or treating diabetic microvascular complications other than DR has also been investigated. Several studies have evaluated the effect of PKC-β inhibition on nephropathy and neuropathy, but definitive conclusions regarding the role of PKC-β in these conditions are still pending.

Preclinical nephropathy studies in animal models of Type 1 and Type 2 diabetes have demonstrated efficacy of RBX in decreasing urinary albumin, normalizing the glomerular filtration rate (GFR), and preventing tubulointerstitial pathology, glomerulosclerosis, transforming growth factor-β overexpression, mesangial expansion, and osteopontin expression *(22, 37, 38, 39)*. Human clinical trials have also shown trends consistent with amelioration of diabetic nephropathy by PKC-β inhibition. A randomized, double-masked, placebo-controlled clinical trial enrolled 123 subjects with Type 2 diabetes and baseline albuminuria *(40)*. After one year of treatment of 32 mg per day RBX, urinary albumin/creatinine ratio (ACR) was reduced in the RBX-treated group compared with the placebo group (fall in ACR of 24 vs. 9%, respectively). The estimated GFR did not decline as significantly in the RBX group compared with the placebo group (-2.5 ± 1.9 mL min^{-1} per 1.73 m^2 vs. -4.8 ± 1.8 mL min^{-1} per 1.73 m^2). However, this pilot trial was not powered sufficiently to demonstrate a significant difference between the two treatment arms.

Another Phase 2 trial examined the effect of RBX on symptomatic diabetic peripheral neuropathy *(41)*. This was a double-masked, placebo-controlled trial that randomized 250 patients to 32 mg per day RBX, 64 mg per day RBX, or placebo for one year. No relationship was seen between RBX treatment and the primary endpoint of vibration detection threshold. However, in the 83 patients who had clinically significant neuropathic symptoms at baseline, a statistically significant reduction was found in the Neuropathy Total Symptom Score-6 (NTSS-6) in the 64 mg per day group as compared to the placebo group ($p = 0.025$). RBX treatment appeared to be of benefit for the subgroup of patients with less severe symptomatic diabetic peripheral neuropathy by relieving sensory symptoms and improving nerve fiber function ($p = 0.006$). In a recent study of 20 placebo and 20 RBX (32 mg d^{-1}) treated patients with diabetic peripheral neuropathy, there was RBX benefit in NTSS-6 ($p = 0.03$) *(42)*. To date, larger phase three trials have not been performed to replicate these findings.

SAFETY PROFILE OF RBX

Recently, safety data were reported from the combined outcome of 11 placebo-controlled, double-masked clinical trials with RBX *(43)*. Overall, RBX appears well-tolerated with a favorable safety profile. Data evaluated 1,396 subjects treated with 32 mg per day RBX as compared to data from 1,408 subjects given placebo. The cumulative proportions of patients who experienced one or more serious adverse events were 20.8% in RBX and 23.2% in the placebo group. No mortality event within the overall cohort was directly attributed to RBX. There were 21 deaths in the RBX-treated group and 30 in the placebo group. Common adverse drug reactions were dyspepsia (2.7% placebo, 4.3% RBX) and increased blood creatine phosphokinase (0.3% placebo, 1.0% RBX), although these levels did not exceed the normal range. The drug-discontinuation rate due to adverse events was equivalent between the treatment groups (4% placebo, 3% RBX).

CLINICAL STATUS OF RBX

RBX continues to be investigated in Phase 3 clinical trials. It is not currently commercially available for clinical use. In August, 2006, the US FDA issued an approvable letter regarding RBX, but required submission of further Phase 3 clinical data before proceeding with approval *(44)*. An application by Eli Lilly and Company to the European Agency for the Evaluation of Medicinal Products (EMEA) for marketing authorization for RBX was withdrawn in March, 2007 *(45)*. This withdrawal did not affect the status of ongoing clinical trials for the use of RBX in diabetic complications.

CONCLUSIONS

Clinical trials of PKC inhibition for DR have focused primarily on the oral PKC-β inhibitor, ruboxistaurin. Multiple multicenter, double-masked, randomized, placebo-controlled trials have demonstrated a tendency toward a modest benefit in preventing long-term visual loss, increasing rates of visual gain, reducing progression of DME, and less need for initial macular laser photocoagulation in patients with advanced NPDR. However, RBX clearly does not appear to halt the progression of DR. RBX is well-tolerated with a favorable safety profile. Additional phase clinical 3 trials will be required for regulatory approval of the drug in the United States. Phase 3 clinical studies of RBX are currently ongoing to help clarify its role in the treatment of DME and the prevention of vision loss in patients with diabetes.

REFERENCES

1. Centers for Disease Control and Prevention. National diabetes fact sheet: general information and national estimates on diabetes in the United States, 2003. Rev ed. Atlanta, GA: U.S. Department of Health and Human Services, Centers for Disease Control and Prevention, 2004.
2. DCCT Research Group. The effect of intensive treatment of diabetes on the development and progression of long-term complications in insulin-dependent diabetes mellitus. The diabetes Control and complications Trial Research Group. N Engl J Med 1993;329:977–986.
3. Diabetes Control and Complications Trial Research Group. Progression of retinopathy with intensive versus conventional treatment in the Diabetes Control and Complications Trial. Ophthalmology 1995;102:647–661.
4. UKPDS Group. Intensive blood-glucose control with sulphonyl ureas or insulin compared with conventional treatment and risk of complications in patients with type 2 diabetes (UKPDS 33). UK Prospective Diabetes Study (UKPDS0 Group). Lancet 1998;352:837–853.
5. Friedman EA. Advanced glycosylated end products and hyperglycemia in the pathogenesis of diabetic complications. Diabetes Care 1999;22 Suppl 2:B65–B71.
6. Giugliano D, Ceriello A, Paolisso G. Oxidative stress and diabetic vascular complications. Diabetes Care 1996;19:257–267.
7. Nishizuka Y. Intracellular signaling by hydrolysis of phospholipids and activation of protein kinase C. Science 1992;258:607–614.
8. Nishizuka Y. Protein kinase C and lipid sinaling for sustained cellular responses. FASEB 1995;9:484–496.
9. Liscovitch M, Cantley LC. Lipid second messengers. Cell 1994;77:329–334.
10. Nishizuka Y. Intracellular signaling by hydrolysis of phospholipids and activation of protein kinase C. Science 1992;258:607–614.
11. Way KJ, Chou E, King GL. Identification of PKC-isoform-specific biological actionsusing pharmacological approaches. Trends Pharmacol Sci 2000;21:181–187.

12. Inoguchi T, Battan R, Handler E, et al. Preferential elevation of protein kinase C isoform beta II and diacylglycerol levels in the aorta and heart of diabetic rats: differential reversibility to glycemic control by islet cell transplantation. Proc Natl Acad Sci USA 1992;89:11059–11063.
13. Kunisaki M, Bursell SE, Umeda F, et al. Normalization of diacylglycerol-protein kinase C activation by vitamin E in aorta of diabetic rats and cultured rat smooth muscle cells exposed to elevated glucose levels. Diabetes 1994;43:1372–1377.
14. Shiba T, Inoguchi T, Sportsman JR, et al. Correlation of diacylglcerol level and protein kinase C activity in rat retina to retinal circulation. Am J Phsiol 1993;265:E783–E793.
15. Inoguchi T, Xia P, Kunisaki M, et al. Insulin's effect on protein kinase C and diacylglycerol inducted by diabetes and glucose in vascular tissues. Am J Physiol 1994;267:E369–E379.
16. Aiello LP, Bursell SE, Clermont A, et al. Vascular endothelial growth factor-induced retinal permeability is mediated by protein kinase C in vivo and suppressed by an orally effective beta-isoform-selective inhibitor. Diabetes 1997;46:1473–1480.
17. Xia P, Aiello LP, Ishii H, et al. Characterization of vascular endothelial growth factor's effect on the activation of protein kinase C, its isoforms, and endothelial cell growth. J Clin Invest 1996;98:2018–2026.
18. Way KJ, Katai N, King GL. Protein kinase C and the development of diabetic vascular complications. Diabet Med 2001;18:949–959.
19. Campochiaro PA; C99-PKC412-003 Study Group. Reduction of diabetic macular edema by oral administration of the kinase inhibitor PKC412. Invest Ophthalmol Vis Sci. 2004;45:922–931.
20. Ishii H, Jirousek MR, Koya D, et al. Amelioration of vascular dysfunctions in diabetic rats by an oral PKC β inhibitor. Science 1996;272:728–731.
21. Bursell SE, Takagi C, Clermont AC, et al. Specific retinal diacylglycerol and protein kinase C beta isoform modulation mimics abnormal retinal hemodynamics in diabetic rats. Invest Ophthalmol Vis Sci 1997;38:2711–2720.
22. Ishii H, Jirousek MR, Koya D, et al. Amelioration of vascular dysfunctions in diabetic rats by an oral PKC β inhibitor. Science 1996;272:728–731.
23. Danis RP, Bingaman DP, Jirousek M, et al. Inhibition of intraocular neovascularization cuased by retinal ischemia in pigs by PKC-beta inhibition with LY 333531. Invest Ophthalmol Vis Sci 1998;39:17–179.
24. Nonaka A, Kiryu J, Tsujikawa A, et al. PKC-eta inhibitor (LY 333531) attenuates leukocyte entrapment in retinal microcirculation of diabetic rats. Invest Ophthalmol Vis Sci 2000;41:2707–2706.
25. Demolle D, deSuray JM, Onkelinx C. Pharmacokinetics and safety of multiple oral doses of LY333531, a PKC beta inhibitor, in healthy subjects. Clin Parmacol Ther 1999;65:189.
26. Demolle D, de Suray JM, Vandenhend F, et al. LY333531 single escalating oral dose study in healthy volunteers. Diabetologia 1998;41 (Suppl 1):A354.
27. Aiello LP, Clermont A, Arora V, et al. Inhibition of PKC β by oral administration of ruboxistaurin is well tolerated and ameliorates diabetes-induced retinal hemodynamic abnormalities in patients. Invest Ophthalmol Vis Sci 2006;47:86–92.
28. Clarke M, Dodson PM. PKC inhibition and diabetic microvascular complications. Best Pract Res Clin Endocrinol Metab 2007;21:573–86.
29. The PKC-DRS Study Group. The effect of ruboxistaurin on visual loss in patients with moderately severe to very severe nonproliferative diabetic retinopathy: initial results of the Protein Kinase C beta Inhibitor Diabetic Retinopathy Study (PKC-DRS) multicenter randomized clinical trial. Diabetes 2005;54:2188–2197.
30. PKC-DMES Study Group. Effect of ruboxistaurin in patients with diabetic macular edema: thirty-month results of the randomized PKC-DMES clinical trial. Arch Ophthalmol 2007;125:318–324.
31. PKC-DRS2 Group, Aiello LP, Davis MD, et al. Effect of ruboxistaurin on visual loss in patients with diabetic retinopathy. Ophthalmology 2006;113:2221–2230.
32. Aiello LP, Vignati L, Sheetz MJ. Oral PKC β inhibition using ruboxistaurin: efficacy, safety, and causes of vision loss among 813 patients (1,392 eyes) with diabetic retinopathy in the PKC-DRS and the PKC-DRS2 and meta-analyses of 3 ruboxistaurin trials (1,736 eyes). Unpublished data.
33. Trials involving ruboxistaurin. At ClinicalTrials.gov: A service of the U.S. National Institutes of Health. http://www.clinicaltrials.gov/ct2/results?term=ruboxistaurin&show_flds=Y (Accessed on January 14, 2008).

34. The Effect of Ruboxistaurin on Clinically Significant Macular Edema. At ClinicalTrials.gov: A service of the U.S. National Institutes of Health. http://www.clinicaltrials.gov/ct2/show/NCT00090519?term=ruboxis taurin&rank = 5 (Accessed on January 14, 2008).
35. Reduction in the Occurrence of Center-Threatening Diabetic Macular Edema. At ClinicalTrials.gov: A service of the U.S. National Institutes of Health. http://www.clinicaltrials.gov/ct2/show/ NCT00090519?term = ruboxistaurin&rank = 5 (Accessed on January 14, 2008).
36. Treatment for Completers of the Study B7A-MC-MBCM. At ClinicalTrials.gov: A service of the U.S. National Institutes of Health. http://www.clinicaltrials.gov/ct2/show/NCT00266695?term = ruboxist-aurin&rank = 2 (Accessed on January 14, 2008).
37. Koya D, Jirousek MR, Lin YW, et al. Characterization of protein kinase C β isoform activation on the expression of transforming growth factor- β extracellular matrix components and prostanoids in the glomeruli of diabetic rats. J Clin Invest 1997;100:115–126.
38. Kelly DJ, Xhang Y, Hepper C, et al. Protein kinase C β in hibition attenuates the progression of experimental diabetic nephropathy in the presence of continued hypertension. Diabetes 2003;52:512–518.
39. Koya D, Haneda M, Nadagawa H, et al. Amelioration of accelerated diabetic mesangial expansion by treatment with a PKC β in hibitor in diabetic db/db mice, a rodent model for type 2 diabetes. FASEB J 2000;14:439–447.
40. Tuttle KR Bakris GL, Toto RD, et al. The effect of ruboxistaurin on nephropathy in type 2 diabetes. Diabetes Care 2005;28:2686–2690.
41. Vinik AI, Bril V, Kemplar P, et al. Treatment of symptomatic diabetic peripheral neuropathy with the protein kinase C beta-inhibitor ruboxistaurin mesylate during a 1 year, randomized, placebo-controlled, double-blind clinical trial. Cinical Therapeutics 2005;27:1164–1180.
42. Casellini CM, Barlow PM, Rice AL, et al. A 6-month, randomized, double-masked, placebo-controlled study evaluating the effects of the protein kinase c-β inhibitor ruboxistaurin on skin microvascular blood flow and other measures of diabetic peripheral neuropathy. Diabetes Care 2007;30:896–902.
43. McGill JB, King GL, Berg PH, et al. Clinical safety of the selective PKC-beta inhibitor, ruboxistaurin. Expert Opin Drug Saf. 2006;5(6):835–45.
44. Approvable Letter Issued By FDA For Arxxant(R) (ruboxistaurin Mesylate) For Diabetic Retinopathy. At Medical News Today. http://www.medicalnewstoday.com/articles/50029.php (Accessed on January 16, 2008).
45. Withdrawal of ARXXANT™ (ruboxistaurin), 32 mg, film-coated tablets. http://www.emea.europa.eu/ humandocs/PDFs/EPAR/arxxant/arxxant_withdrawal_letter.pdf (Accessed January 16, 2008)

19 The Role of Intravitreal Steroids in the Management of Diabetic Retinopathy

Mark C Gillies

CONTENTS

ABSTRACT

The use of steroids for the treatment of diabetic macular edema has been a major recent breakthrough in the management of retinal diseases. First studied in animal models in the 1980s, intravitreal triamcinolone acetonide (IVTA) was first used in human eyes at the Save Sight Institute in Sydney for exudative macular degeneration. When early observations suggested that its effect on macular disease was more marked against exudation than neovascularization, it was used for diabetic macular edema with remarkable effects, which could be appreciated particularly using optical coherence tomography. A placebo-controlled randomized clinical trial reported a beneficial effect of IVTA treatment on best-corrected visual acuity and central macular thickness after 3 months that persisted out to 2 years. Glaucoma medication was required in 15/34 (44%) of IVTA-treated eyes, and removal of steroid-induced posterior subcapsular cataract was required in 55%, mostly in the second year of the study. There was one case of infectious endophthalmitis which responded well to prompt treatment. IVTA can be considered, for example, in eyes with macular edema secondary to focal parafoveal or severe diffuse leak, prior to cataract surgery, or in eyes with macular

From: *Contemporary Diabetes: Diabetic Retinopathy*
Edited by: E. Duh © Humana Press, Totowa, NJ

edema and high-risk proliferative diabetic retinopathy for which immediate pan-retinal photocoagulation is required. Further research is warranted to determine the safest and most efficacious dose of IVTA, and into how ocular steroid therapy can be combined with both retinal laser treatment and the new anti-vascular endothelial growth factor treatments for the safest and most efficacious outcomes for patients.

Key Words: Adverse events; Diabetic macular edema; Intravitreal therapy; Triamcinolone acetonide.

Diabetic macular edema (DME) is the main cause of vision impairment in people with diabetes *(1)*. In the Wisconsin Epidemiologic Study of Diabetic Retinopathy, macular edema developed in 20% of people with type I diabetes over a 10-year period *(2)*. Laser treatment has been proven effective in reducing the risk of visual loss from DME and is widely employed, but it is also inherently destructive. Progressive loss of vision occurred in up to 26% of patients with DME despite laser treatment in the Early Treatment of Diabetic Retinopathy Study *(3)*. Thus an intervention that could reduce DME in patients who were failing laser treatment would prevent many cases of blindness in people with diabetes.

There has been increased recognition lately that features of chronic inflammation, such as adhesion of leukocytes to the retinal vasculature and migration into the retina, may play a role in the pathogenesis of diabetic retinopathy *(4)*. Glucocorticoids have also been widely used for the treatment of edema in the brain and the lung. Since the blood–brain barrier is similar to the blood–retinal barrier, the long-standing use of corticosteroids in the treatment of brain edema, which is possibly mediated through suppression of vascular endothelial growth factor secretion *(5)*, suggests they should be evaluated for the treatment of macular edema. In asthma, which is also characterized by increased vascular leak, steroids have been found to reduce vascular leak *(6)* and to suppress the release of endothelial cell activators. However, long-term systemic administration of steroids in people with diabetes would cause problems with glycemic control and elevate the risk of other adverse events to unacceptable levels. Intraocular administration of steroids has the potential to give extended doses of a drug at high local concentrations with minimal risks of systemic complications. Local delivery of high-dose long-acting steroids by periocular and orbital injections has been standard treatment for various inflammatory conditions of the eye for many years *(7,8)*.

Intravitreal therapy with triamcinolone acetonide was first proposed as a treatment for ocular angiogenesis in a series of animal studies mainly performed by Machemer's group at Duke University in the 1980s *(9)*. Triamcinolone acetonide was chosen because its unique crystalline nature resulted in slow release of the drug over several months, and its vehicle appeared safe when injected into animal eyes *(10,11)*.

The first report of its use in humans was by Penfold et al. from the Save Sight Institute in Sydney, in which intravitreal triamcinolone acetonide (IVTA) was used to treat a group of patients with exudative age-related macular degeneration (AMD) *(12)*. IVTA was a popular treatment for subfoveal neovascularization for a while, particularly since there were no other treatments at that time that might stabilize or improve vision in such eyes, but its use waned with the advent of photodynamic therapy with verteporfin, the safety and efficacy of which had been proven by a phase III randomized clinical trial; at the same time, a randomized clinical trial of intravitreal triamcinolone detected no benefit for AMD with classic choroidal neovascularization *(13)*. These studies did, however, establish that IVTA had a manageable, albeit significant, adverse event profile, thus providing a foundation for clinical trials of IVTA for other macular diseases.

Subsequent animal studies suggested that IVTA might be efficacious for macular edema. Detecting the leak of a gadolinium-based marker into the vitreous, Wilson et al. found that intravitreal, but not sub-Tenon's, triamcinolone significantly attenuated blood–retinal barrier breakdown caused by argon-laser panretinal photocoagulation in the rabbit eye *(14)*. Edelman et al. found that a single intravitreal 2 mg dose of IVTA completely blocked VEGF-induced retinal and iris leakage for 45 days after VEGF165 was injected intravitreally in Dutch Belt rabbits, while indomethacin had no effect *(15)*.

CLINICAL EFFICACY

The first report of the clinical use of IVTA for DME came from Jonas et al. in 2001 *(16)*. This was quickly confirmed by a number of short case series which were extremely useful at the time. Martidis et al. presented a series of 16 eyes with DME treated with 4 mg IVTA with 1 month follow-up for 14 eyes and 6 months for 8. Snellen visual acuity improved in association with reduction of central macular thickness *(17)*. Similarly, Jonas et al. reported improvement in Snellen visual acuity and fluorescein leakage in 26 eyes of 20 patients treated with 25 mg of triamcinolone in 0.2 ml with a mean follow-up of 6 months *(16)*.

The subsequent explosion of short-term, uncontrolled studies of IVTA for practically every conceivable acquired macular condition has, however, added little more information, particularly for DME. Once efficacy has been suggested in phase I/II studies, interventions need to be tested in randomized clinical trials. As experience with AMD demonstrated, the apparent initial efficacy of interventions for macular disease frequently does not stand up to the scrutiny of a formal, double-masked clinical trial in which primary end points are prospectively identified and measured by trained observers.

The Triamcinolone for Diabetic Macular Edema study (TDMO), also conducted at the Save Sight Institute, was the first randomized clinical trial that was adequately powered to test the hypothesis that an intravitreal injection of triamcinolone acetonide would be beneficial for DME that had failed laser treatment. It was also the first study published to follow patients for long enough (2 years) to provide a realistic estimation of the risks of treatment.

The TDMO study was a prospective, double-masked, placebo-controlled randomized clinical trial that enrolled 69 eyes of 43 patients, with 34 eyes receiving active treatment and 35 placebo. The procedure was designed to be performed in the office under sterile conditions with topical and subconjunctival anesthesia. Triamcinolone acetonide (0.1 ml of 40 mg ml^{-1}) was injected through the pars plana using a 27G needle. Patients with persistent DME involving the central fovea persisting for 3 months or more after adequate laser treatment and best-corrected visual acuity in the affected eye(s) of 6/9 or worse were included. Eyes randomized to placebo received a subconjunctival injection of saline. The main outcome measures were improvement of best-corrected Log MAR visual acuity by five or more letters and incidence of moderate or severe adverse events. Retreatment was considered at each visit as long as treatments

Table 1
Effect of Triamcinolone on Change in Eye Outcomes 3 Months from Baseline[a]

Characteristic	*Triamcinolone* *(N = 33)*	*Placebo* *(N = 32)*	*P–value**
Visual acuity – no. (%)			0.001
Gain of 10 or more letters	8 *(24)*	3 *(9)*	
Gain of 5–9 letters	10 *(30)*	2 *(6)*	
No change (gain or loss < 5 letters)	14 *(42)*	20 *(34)*	
Loss of 5–9 letters	0	4 *(13)*	
Loss of 10 or more letters	1 *(3)*	3 *(9)*	
Contact lens grading macula edema: no. (%)			< 0.0001
	1 *(3)*	0	
Reduction by 3 grades	11 *(33)*	0	
Reduction by 2 grades	13 *(39)*	5 *(16)*	
Reduction by 1 grade	8 *(24)*	21 *(66)*	
No change	0	6 *(19)*	
Increase of 1 grade			
Gain in visual acuity – letters	5.0 ± 1.2	−0.1 ± 1.5	0.008
Reduction in central retinal thickness – μm	152 ± 27 (*N* = 21)	36 ± 17 (*N* = 20)	< 0.0001

(Reprinted from *(18)* with permission)
[a]Plus-minus values are means ± SE
* *P*-value using generalized estimating equations (GEE) to allow for correlations between paired eyes

were at least 6 months apart. Eyes with a reduction of visual acuity of at least five letters from previous peak value and persistent central macular thickness greater than 250 μm received retreatment with study medication. If visual acuity had not improved significantly when measured 4 weeks later and macular thickening persisted, then fluorescein angiography was performed and further laser treatment was applied if the investigator thought it would be beneficial.

The data were analyzed at 3 months to ensure that a single treatment was in fact efficacious in the short term *(18)*. Vision improved by five or more letters in 18/33 (55%) eyes treated with IVTA that completed this visit compared with 5/32 (16%) eyes treated with placebo ($P = 0.002$) (Table 1). Central macular thickness decreased by a mean of 152 μm in the treated eyes compared with 36 μm in placebo-treated eyes. One IVTA-treated eye developed infectious endophthalmitis, which was promptly treated with persistent improvement of visual acuity compared with baseline throughout the study.

After 2 years, the beneficial effect of IVTA continued to hold up *(19)*. Vision had improved by five or more letters in 19/34 (56%) IVTA-treated eyes compared with 9/35 (26%) eyes treated with placebo ($P = 0.006$). Only 6/34 (18%) treated eyes lost five or more letters compared with 13/35 (37%) untreated eyes. The mean improvement in visual acuity was 5.7 (95% CI: 1.4–9.9) letters more in the IVTA-treated eyes than in those treated with placebo (Table 2). The mean number of injections received in the IVTA-treated group was 2.6 with a maximum of 5 possible (Table 3). Although some of the placebo-treated eyes had done well, emphasizing the importance of randomized

Table 2
Effect of Triamcinolone on Change in Eye Outcomes 24 Months from Baseline

Characteristic	*Triamcinolone (N = 34)*	*Placebo (N = 35)*	*P-Value*
Visual acuity – *n* (%)			0.013*
Gain of 15 or more letters	4 (12%)	1 (3%)	
Gain of 10–14 letters	3 (9%)	3 (9%)	
Gain of 5–9 letters	12 (35%)	5 (14%)	
No change (gain or loss < 5 letters)	9 (26%)	13 (37%)	
Loss of 5–9 letters	3 (9%)	4 (11%)	
Loss of 10–14 letters	2 (6%)	5 (14%)	
Loss of 15 or more letters	1 (3%)	4 (11%)	
Gain in visual acuity – letters	3.1	−2.9	0.01**
Reduction in central retinal thickness – μm[a]	125	71	0.009**

(Reprinted from *(19)* with permission)
[a]*N* = 21 for each group
**P*-value from exact Mantel–Haenszel trend test
***P*-value using generalized estimating equations (GEE) to allow for correlations between paired eyes

Table 3
Distribution of Number of Treatments Given by Treatment Group for Patients Completing 2-year Follow-up

Number of treatments	*Triamcinolone (N = 31)*	*Placebo (N = 29)*
1	6 (19%)	11 (38%)
2	9 (29%)	13 (45%)
3	10 (32%)	4 (14%)
4	4 (13%)	1 (3%)
5	2 (6%)	0
Mean	2.6	1.8
Median	3	2

Mantel–Haenszel trend test $\chi_1^2 = 7.57$, $P = 0.006$ (reprinted from *(19)* with permission)

clinical trials for treatments for DME, IVTA treatment had roughly doubled the chance of improving vision and halved the risk of visual loss. The mean improvement in visual acuity was not especially large. However, many eyes in the study had 20/30 vision on entry. If only eyes with 20/40 visual acuity had been accepted, then improvements would likely have been greater. The study continues, with 5-year visits to be completed by March 2008.

It has been reported that repeated intravitreal injections may not be as effective as the initial treatment *(20)*. However, we have yet to find any evidence of this. In the TDMO study, the mean number of injections was 2.4 over 2 years with a total potential of 5. We found that there was no difference in the reduction in central macular thickness and improvement in visual acuity in eyes receiving 4–5 injections compared with the first injection *(21)*. It is possible that the effect of steroids may wane over 3–5 years; this will be evident from the 5-year TDMO study data to be released in 2008.

SAFETY

IVTA treatment confers a high risk of cataract and elevated intraocular pressure (IOP), which increases as more injections are given. After one injection in eyes with exudative AMD, we found significant development or progression of posterior subcapsular cataract in 8/33 (25%) phakic IVTA-treated eyes compared with 0/22 placebo-treated eyes *(22)*. Elevated IOP ≥ 5 mmHg was found in 32/75 (43%) IVTA-treated eyes compared with 3/76 (4%) placebo-treated eyes, with glaucoma medication required in 21 (28%) treated vs. 1 (1%) untreated. No eyes required trabeculectomy. In the TDMO study, in which a mean of 2.6 IVTA injections were received by the treatment group, cataract surgery was required (exclusively for progressive posterior subcapsular opacification) in 15/28 (54%) treated vs. 0/21 (0%) untreated eyes that were phakic at baseline. An increase of intraocular pressure of ≥ 5 mmHg was observed in 23/34 (68%) treated compared with 3/30 (10%) untreated eyes, with glaucoma medication required in 15/34 (44%) treated vs. 1/30 (3%) untreated eyes. Two (6%) treated eyes required trabeculectomy. Cataracts did not become significant in most cases until over a year after treatment had started, indicating the critical importance of long-term studies of steroid treatment if an accurate indication of safety is to be obtained. Thus it appears that multiple injections are associated with an increased risk of developing at least visually significant cataract, and probably elevation of the intraocular pressure as well. It is worth noting, however, that interventions are already routinely employed by ophthalmologists that cause cataract, the removal of which is known to exacerbate the condition being treated. Pars plana vitrectomy, which is required, for example, for the removal of epiretinal membranes, results in the eventual formation of significant cataract in up to 67% of eyes *(23)*.

We have studied the results of removal of the 15 triamcinolone-induced cataracts that developed in eyes of participants in the TDMO study (unpublished data). In all eyes, IVTA was given at the time of surgery. Mean visual acuity had improved after 6 months but mean central macular thickness remained the same. Two (15%) eyes undergoing cataract surgery suffered aggravation of macular edema and loss of >15 letters. Thus visual outcomes after removal of IVTA-induced cataract seem generally good; however, a small proportion of patients may do badly. We suspect that administering IVTA 4–6 weeks prior to surgery in order to control the DME first might reduce the risk of poor outcomes. However, this warrants further research.

Other adverse events associated with IVTA are uncommon but still need to be considered. At the Sydney Eye Hospital, where we have administered approximately 1,500 treatments with IVTA over the last 15 years, we have encountered "pseudo-endophthalmitis" *(13,18)* in around 1:100 injections, and true infectious endophthalmitis in around 1:500. We have had one case of retinal detachment and no cases of vitreous hemorrhage or damage to the lens. The nature of the cause of IVTA-related "pseudo-endophthalmitis" remains obscure. Acute loss of vision is noticed by the patient in some cases immediately following the injection – in these, we suspect that there may be partial blocking of the drug in the barrel of the needle, resulting in a spraying of a suspension of crystals throughout the vitreous. In other cases it may be indistinguishable from infectious endophthalmitis, except that pain and inflammation may be absent. Paracentesis for microscopy and culture as well as the injection of intravitreal antibiotics may be required in these cases. Vitreous opacification in some cases can occasionally take months to clear even if it is not infectious.

PHARMACOLOGY

The formulation of triamcinolone acetonide that we have used and is widely employed elsewhere was originally developed for use in skin and the musculoskeletal system rather than the eye. It is possible that the vehicle, the preservatives, or even the drug itself will have a toxic effect on the retina in the long term. We have not had any evidence of long-term ocular toxicity (apart from the conventional steroid-related events as described) in patients treated with IVTA over the last 15 years at the Sydney Eye Hospital, although systematic follow-up has not been for greater than 3 years. Whilst the present formulation appears to be relatively safe in human eyes, the development and validation of a formulation specifically for use in the eye would be a significant advance.

PHARMACOKINETICS

Formal studies on the duration of action of intravitreal triamcinolone in the human eye are not available. The most commonly used dose of 4 mg appears to have been chosen because it is the amount of the highest concentration of the drug that is commercially available that can safely be injected into the eye (i.e., 0.1 ml of a 40 mg ml^{-1} solution). Since the crystalline nature of triamcinolone acetonide allows its extended release, it is likely that vitreous levels are about the same with different amounts injected, but larger doses might last longer. Audren et al. conducted a phase 2 trial comparing 4 mg vs. 2 mg IVTA for diffuse DME with 16 patients per group *(24)*. No significant difference was found with respect to central macular thickness, visual acuity, or intraocular pressure up to 24 weeks. Median time to recurrence of the DME was shorter for the 2 mg group at 16 weeks, compared with 20 weeks for the 4 mg group ($P = 0.11$). A significant difference may have been found with larger numbers. This group also conducted pharmacokinetic modeling of a 4 mg intravitreal injection of triamcinolone using central macular thickness as the pharmacodynamic parameter. The mean estimated half-life of triamcinolone ± SD was 15.4 ± 1.9 days, and the mean maximum duration of its effect was 140 ± 17 days *(24)*. We have found that a dose of 1 mg seems to have equivalent short-term efficacy compared with 4 mg, although it wears off much earlier (6–8 weeks compared with 4–6 months, unpublished data). Lam et al. studied the response to 4, 6, and 8 mg IVTA *(25)*. They felt that higher doses may have prolonged the duration of visual improvement and reduction in DME. Spandau et al. reached the same conclusions when they studied doses of 2, 5, and 13 mg, but numbers were small and the duration of follow-up was as short as 3 months in some eyes *(26)*. Further studies are warranted to investigate the safest and most efficacious dose of IVTA for DME.

ROUTE OF ADMINISTRATION

There are some data that suggest that triamcinolone given periocularly can also be efficacious. Tunc et al. randomized 60 eyes with DME to receive macular photocoagulation alone or combined with a posterior sub-Tenon's capsule injection of triamcinolone *(27)*. The vision of both groups had improved 18 weeks later, but significantly more so in the eyes that received triamcinolone. Shimura et al. presented convincing evidence that posterior sub-Tenon's capsule triamcinolone stabilized both vision and macular thickness in 20 patients requiring panretinal photocoagulation for proliferative diabetic retinopathy in both eyes who received triamcinolone therapy in just one eye *(28)*. Bakri and Kaiser found in a retrospective uncontrolled analysis of 63 eyes of 50 patients with refractory DME that vision remained stable or improved over a 12-month period after posterior sub-Tenon's capsule triamcinolone injections *(29)*. By contrast, Bonini-Filho et al. studied 28 eyes randomized to receive either sub-Tenon's capsule or intravitreal triamcinolone for DME and followed for 24 weeks. Both mean visual acuity and central macular improved in the intravitreal group, while neither improved in the sub-Tenon's group. The mean elevation of IOP was the same for both groups. It appears that triamcinolone is somewhat more efficacious and longer lasting when injected intravitreally compared with sub-Tenon's capsule. However, we do consider the latter route in eyes that have had their vitreous removed.

One potential advantage of periocular therapy is safety. Certainly the risk of infectious endophthalmitis is greatly reduced, although steroid-related adverse events may not be much lower. Helm and Holland reported development of significant cataract in 4/11 (36%) phakic eyes 10 months to 4 years after treatment with posterior sub Tenon's capsule triamcinolone for uveitis, as well as significant elevation of the intraocular pressure in 6/20 (30%) eyes studied *(30)*.

THE EFFECT OF VASCULAR ENDOTHELIAL GROWTH FACTOR INHIBITORS ON INTRAVITREAL STEROID THERAPY

Proof of principle that VEGF inhibitors may be efficacious in the management of DME was provided by a phase II, 36 week clinical trial in which patients receiving six weekly injections of pegaptanib sodium (0.3 mg) had better VA outcomes, were more likely to show reduction in central retinal thickness, and were deemed less likely to need additional therapy with photocoagulation at follow-up *(31)*. Given the central role of VEGF in the pathogenesis of DME *(32)*, similar results attesting to the short-term efficacy of VEGF inhibitors are anticipated in the near future from studies of ranibizumab and bevacizumab.

There are presently insufficient data to judge whether VEGF inhibitors will be superior to steroids for DME. Certainly they do not cause the high risk of steroid-related adverse events such as cataract and elevated IOP, but there is suspicion that they may be neurotoxic locally and also that they may confer an increased risk of systemic thromboembolic events *(13,19,33)*. These risks have not been studied closely in the population with chronic DME, which is already known to have an increased mortality. The frequent injections (every 4–6 weeks) for a presumably extended period that may be required with the currently available anti-VEGF compounds confer an increased risk of injection-related complications such as infectious endophthalmitis. It is possible that a low-dose combination of steroids with a VEGF inhibitor might be the safest and most efficacious treatment for DME, but this hypothesis is yet to be tested.

COMBINATION WITH LASER TREATMENT

With a number of different therapeutic options becoming available to clinicians, it is likely in the future that a combination of treatments will be used for macular disease. The first place to start with steroids will be laser treatment. As with any medical treatment, DME tends to recur after triamcinolone wears off. Applying laser treatment a few weeks after IVTA allows less laser energy to be used if the edema has settled. It also means that the retinal capillaries are closer to the retinal pigmented epithelium, which is where laser has its poorly understood effect. These are, however, only theoretical considerations; whether there really is a benefit to combining laser with IVTA will need to be tested in clinical trials.

Results of studies combining laser treatment with IVTA so far are conflicting. Kang et al. randomized 86 eyes with DME to receive IVTA alone or with laser applied 3 weeks after the injection. Both groups had improved vision and macular thickness after 3 weeks, but the laser-treated group did better after 3 and 6 months *(34)*. This study randomized patients depending on whether the hospital identifying number was odd or even, so the investigator would have known which group the patient would enter before enrolling the patient. This may also have affected "masked" observers. The data are, however, consistent with those of Tunc et al. described above, who felt that sub-Tenon's triamcinolone had been helpful for patients undergoing macular photocoagulation for DME *(27)*. On the other hand, Avitabile et al. did not find any benefit in adding laser to IVTA in around 63 eyes randomized to receive laser, IVTA, or both and followed for 6–12 months, suggesting that IVTA could be used as primary treatment in patients with cystoid macular edema *(35)*. This study included 15 eyes with retinal vein occlusion. While it allowed re-treatment with IVTA, it did not test the hypothesis that laser treatment might reduce the need for further treatment with IVTA. The Australian Retinal Collaboration is conducting a study in which 85 eyes have been randomized to receive IVTA vs. placebo followed by laser. This study will complete 1 year follow-up in early 2008.

CLINICAL GUIDELINES

How do these data translate into routine clinical practice? With its significant adverse event profile, IVTA is used only occasionally and exclusively for advanced cases of DME (Table 4). It would very uncommonly be used in eyes with normal vision. As a general rule, IVTA treatment is always a more attractive option in pseudophakic eyes because these eyes cannot develop cataract, which is the most significant associated adverse event.

Macular edema that has failed laser treatment. This is the commonest indication. In these eyes there is usually a history of multiple laser treatments over several years to the extent that the only untreated areas are in the parafoveal zone that is too close to the fovea to treat with photocoagulation.

Table 4
Conditions for which Intravitreal Triamcinolone Therapy may be Considered

Clinical situations in which intravitreal triamcinolone might be considered for the treatment of diabetic macular edema
– Failed laser treatment
– Focal parafoveal leak
– Widespread heavy diffuse leak
– Coexistent high-risk proliferative retinopathy
– Uncontrolled edema prior to cataract surgery
– Juxtafoveal hard exudate with heavy leak

Macular Edema Caused by Focal Parafoveal Leak

Sometimes macular edema is caused by leak that is simply too close to the fovea to treat safely. If there is just one microaneurysm leaking in this location, a light burn on its anterior margin may suffice, but photocoagulation may not be safe if there are several leaking points. Even if one can successfully treat leakage close to the fovea with photocoagulation in the short term, there is a risk that the atrophy associated with the laser burn will expand into the fovea over years. This is an unpredictable response that varies from patient to patient.

Widespread Heavy Diffuse Leak

Severe diffuse macular edema (Fig. 1) often does not respond well to grid photocoagulation. Where visual acuity is markedly decreased to the extent that it is interfering with the patient's ability to drive, read, or work, treatment with IVTA may be more likely to improve vision.

Macular Edema and High-Risk Proliferative Retinopathy

Patients presenting with macular edema and preretinal haemorrhage cannot have panretinal photocoagulation deferred until the edema is controlled by macular laser treatment, even though the pan retinal treatment is likely to exacerbate the edema. Treatment with IVTA in these eyes when the panretinal treatment is commenced will settle the edema and improve vision in most cases while the proliferative disease is treated. Focal treatment of the macula should be considered if appropriate after the edema has settled based on a pre-IVTA angiogram.

Macular Edema Prior to Cataract Surgery

Sometimes patients with diabetes will present with macular edema and cataract that is so dense that laser treatment to control the edema preoperatively is not possible. Cataract surgery in such cases often results in severe exacerbation of the maculopathy. Removal of the cataract in these eyes can usually be performed safely under cover of triamcinolone. We believe that it is better to control the edema with IVTA around 1 month prior to surgery rather than to give the two treatments simultaneously.

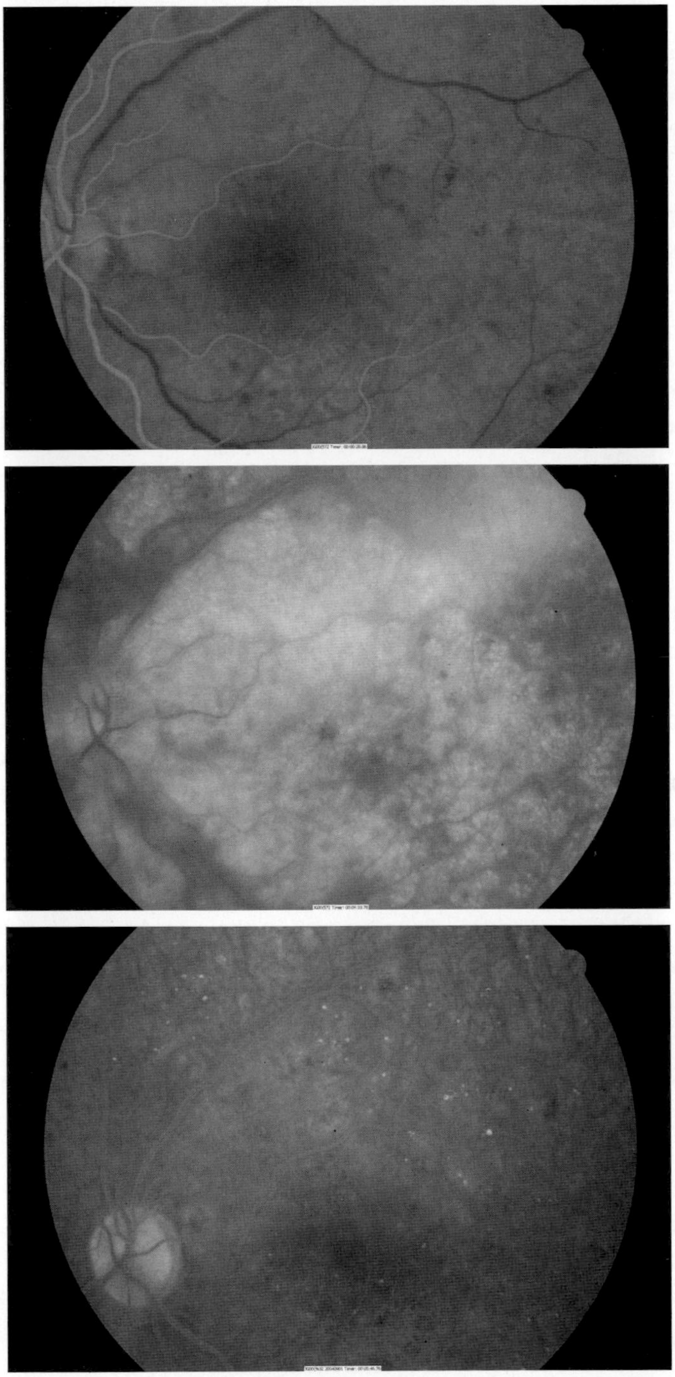

Fig. 1. Early-phase fluorescein angiogram of a 48-year-old man with an 11-year history of type 2 diabetes whose glycosylated hemoglobin had fallen from 14.8 to 7.8% over the preceding 6 months after being started on insulin treatment. Grid pattern photocoagulation is evident in the inferior macula. Visual acuity was 20/120. Late-phase angiogram (4 min 20 s) of the same eye showing heavy diffuse leak. Late-phase angiogram (5 min 45 s) 3 months after an intravitreal injection of triamcinolone acetonide. Visual acuity improved to 20/25. This eye received 6 more injections of triamcinolone over 45 months. On each occasion, visual acuity had fallen to 20/50 or less, and after each injection it improved to 20/40 or better. The cataract was removed after the fourth injection. Treatment of elevated intraocular pressure was not required. The patient's glycosylated hemoglobin has remained under 8%, blood pressure is consistently less than 140/90 mmHg, and renal function is normal. The other eye has a similar history. This man was able to return to work one week after treatment with intravitreal triamcinolone.

JUXTAFOVEAL HARD EXUDATE WITH HEAVY LEAK

Laser treatment of heavy leakage may temporarily increase the amount of macular hard exudate; if this precipitates in the fovea, it can lead to subfoveal fibrosis and permanent damage *(36)*. We used morphometric techniques developed for the grading of drusen to examine the effect of IVTA on hard exudate in the 42 eyes that had it at baseline in the TDMO study *(37)*. In 21 triamcinolone-treated eyes the average amount of lipid had decreased significantly 3 months after the injection (although in two IVTA-treated eyes there was an increase in lipid deposition), whereas in the placebo-treated group it had increased slightly. We now consider IVTA when we believe that there is a high risk that laser treatment will lead to precipitation of lipid at the fovea.

CONTROL OF SYSTEMIC RISK FACTORS

IVTA lasts for an extended period, usually 6 months, but macular edema will return in most cases necessitating re-treatment. Systemic disease is poorly controlled in most patients receiving treatment. It is essential that risk factors are reviewed in detail with the patient, and that a letter is sent to the patient's general practitioner warning of the risk of loss of vision. Consultation with an endocrinologist should be considered if it has not already taken place. Targets should be set to lower the glycosylated hemoglobin to less than 8%, and less than 7% if possible, and the blood pressure to less than 140/90 mmHg even if three medications are required. Excessively high glycosylated hemoglobin levels (>10%) should be lowered gradually to avoid exacerbation of the retinopathy by "early worsening". In many cases, the simple act of putting needles in their eyes is enough to finally make patients take their diabetes seriously.

THE FUTURE OF INTRAVITREAL STEROID THERAPY

New formulations of steroid for injection into the eye to control macular disease include a preservative-free form of triamcinolone acetonide and a slow-release formulation of dexamethasone (Posurdex). Preservative-free triamcinolone is being tested in a phase III randomized clinical trial for DME conducted by the Diabetic Retinopathy Clinical Research network. It will also provide new information on whether a lower dose (1 mg) might be equally efficacious. An ongoing phase III study of Posurdex for DME will establish whether this preparation is efficacious and also whether it has a lower risk of steroid-related adverse events than triamcinolone.

REFERENCES

1. Kohner EM. Diabetic retinopathy. Clin Endocrinol Metab 1977;6:345–75.
2. Klein R, Klein BE, Moss SE, Cruickshanks KJ. The Wisconsin Epidemiologic Study of Diabetic Retinopathy. XV. The long-term incidence of macular edema. Ophthalmology 1995;102:7–16.
3. Early photocoagulation for diabetic retinopathy. ETDRS report number 9. Early Treatment Diabetic Retinopathy Study Research Group. Ophthalmology 1991;98:766–85.
4. Adamis AP. Is diabetic retinopathy an inflammatory disease? Br J Ophthalmol 2002;86:363–5.

5. Heiss JD, Papavassiliou E, Merrill MJ, et al. Mechanism of dexamethasone suppression of brain tumor-associated vascular permeability in rats. Involvement of the glucocorticoid receptor and vascular permeability factor. J Clin Invest 1996;98:1400–8.
6. Van de Graaf EA, Out TA, Roos CM, Jansen HM. Respiratory membrane permeability and bronchial hyperreactivity in patients with stable asthma. Effects of therapy with inhaled steroids. Am Rev Respir Dis 1991;143:362–8.
7. Coles RS, Krohn DL, Breslin H, Braunstein R. Depo-Medrol in treatment of inflammatory diseases. Am J Ophthalmol 1962;54:407–11.
8. Sturman RM, Laval J, Sturman MF. Subconjunctival triamcinolone acetonide. Am J Ophthalmol 1966;61:155–66.
9. Chandler DB, Hida T, Sheta S, Proia AD, Machemer R. Improvement in efficacy of corticosteroid therapy in an animal model of proliferative vitreoretinopathy by pretreatment. Graefe's Arch Clin Exp Ophthalmol 1987;225:259–65.
10. Hida T, Chandler D, Arena JE, Machemer R. Experimental and clinical observations of the intraocular toxicity of commercial corticosteroid preparations. Am J Ophthalmol 1986;101:190–5.
11. McCuen BW, II, Bessler M, Tano Y, Chandler D, Machemer R. The lack of toxicity of intravitreally administered triamcinolone acetonide. Am J Ophthalmol 1981;91:785–8.
12. Penfold PL, Gyory JF, Hunyor AB, Billson FA. Exudative macular degeneration and intravitreal triamcinolone. A pilot study. Aust N Z J Ophthalmol 1995;23:293–8.
13. Gillies MC, Simpson JM, Luo W, et al. A randomized clinical trial of a single dose of intravitreal triamcinolone acetonide for neovascular age-related macular degeneration: one-year results. Arch Ophthalmol 2003;121:667–73.
14. Wilson CA, Berkowitz BA, Sato Y, Ando N, Handa JT, de Juan E, Jr. Treatment with intravitreal steroid reduces blood-retinal barrier breakdown due to retinal photocoagulation. Arch Ophthalmol 1992;110:1155–9.
15. Edelman JL, Lutz D, Castro MR. Corticosteroids inhibit VEGF-induced vascular leakage in a rabbit model of blood-retinal and blood-aqueous barrier breakdown. Exp Eye Res 2005;80:249–58.
16. Jonas JB, Kreissig I, Sofker A, Degenring RF. Intravitreal injection of triamcinolone for diffuse diabetic macular edema. Arch Ophthalmol 2003;121:57–61.
17. Martidis A, Duker JS, Greenberg PB, et al. Intravitreal triamcinolone for refractory diabetic macular edema. Ophthalmology 2002;109:920–7.
18. Sutter FK, Simpson JM, Gillies MC. Intravitreal triamcinolone for diabetic macular edema that persists after laser treatment: three-month efficacy and safety results of a prospective, randomized, double-masked, placebo-controlled clinical trial. Ophthalmology 2004;111:2044–9.
19. Gillies MC, Sutter FK, Simpson JM, Larsson J, Ali H, Zhu M. Intravitreal triamcinolone for refractory diabetic macular edema: two-year results of a double-masked, placebo-controlled, randomized clinical trial. Ophthalmology 2006;113:1533–8.
20. Chan CK, Mohamed S, Shanmugam MP, Tsang CW, Lai TY, Lam DS. Decreasing efficacy of repeated intravitreal triamcinolone injections in diabetic macular oedema. Br J Ophthalmol 2006;90:1137–41.
21. Gillies MC, Islam A, Zhu M, Larsson J, Wong TY. Efficacy and safety of multiple intravitreal triamcinolone injections for refractory diabetic macular oedema. Br J Ophthalmol 2007;91:1323–26.
22. Gillies MC, Simpson JM, Billson FA, et al. Safety of an intravitreal injection of triamcinolone: results from a randomized clinical trial. Arch Ophthalmol 2004;122:336–40.
23. Hsuan JD, Brown NA, Bron AJ, Patel CK, Rosen PH. Posterior subcapsular and nuclear cataract after vitrectomy. J Cataract Refract Surg 2001;27:437–44.
24. Audren F, Lecleire-Collet A, Erginay A, et al. Intravitreal triamcinolone acetonide for diffuse diabetic macular edema: phase 2 trial comparing 4 mg vs 2 mg. Am J Ophthalmol 2006;142:794–99.
25. Lam DS, Chan CK, Mohamed S, et al. A prospective randomised trial of different doses of intravitreal triamcinolone for diabetic macular oedema. Br J Ophthalmol 2007;91:199–203.
26. Spandau UH, Derse M, Schmitz-Valckenberg P, Papoulis C, Jonas JB. Dosage dependency of intravitreal triamcinolone acetonide as treatment for diabetic macular oedema. Br J Ophthalmol 2005; 89:999–1003.
27. Tunc M, Onder HI, Kaya M. Posterior sub-Tenon's capsule triamcinolone injection combined with focal laser photocoagulation for diabetic macular edema. Ophthalmology 2005;112:1086–91.

28. Shimura M, Yasuda K, Shiono T. Posterior sub-Tenon's capsule injection of triamcinolone acetonide prevents panretinal photocoagulation-induced visual dysfunction in patients with severe diabetic retinopathy and good vision. Ophthalmology 2006;113:381–7.
29. Bakri SJ, Kaiser PK. Posterior subtenon triamcinolone acetonide for refractory diabetic macular edema. Am J Ophthalmol 2005;139:290–4.
30. Helm CJ, Holland GN. The effects of posterior subtenon injection of triamcinolone acetonide in patients with intermediate uveitis. Am J Ophthalmol 1995;120:55–64.
31. Cunningham ET, Jr., Adamis AP, Altaweel M, et al. A phase II randomized double-masked trial of pegaptanib, an anti-vascular endothelial growth factor aptamer, for diabetic macular edema. Ophthalmology 2005;112:1747–57.
32. Qaum T, Xu Q, Joussen AM, et al. VEGF-initiated blood-retinal barrier breakdown in early diabetes. Invest Ophthalmol Vis Sc 2001;42:2408–13.
33. van Wijngaarden P, Coster DJ, Williams KA. Inhibitors of ocular neovascularization: promises and potential problems. JAMA 2005;293:1509–13.
34. Kang SW, Sa HS, Cho HY, Kim JI. Macular grid photocoagulation after intravitreal triamcinolone acetonide for diffuse diabetic macular edema. Arch Ophthalmol 2006;124:653–8.
35. Avitabile T, Longo A, Reibaldi A. Intravitreal triamcinolone compared with macular laser grid photocoagulation for the treatment of cystoid macular edema. Am J Ophthalmol 2005;140(4):695–702.
36. Lovestam-Adrian M, Agardh E. Photocoagulation of diabetic macular oedema–complications and visual outcome. Acta Ophthalmol Scand 2000;78(6):667–71.
37. Larsson J, Kifley A, Zhu M, et al. Rapid reduction of hard exudates in eyes with diabetic retinopathy after intravitreal triamcinolone – Data from a randomized, placebo controlled clinical trial. In: Acta Ophthalmologica, in press

20 Antagonism of the Growth Hormone Axis as a Therapeutic Strategy for Diabetic Retinopathy

Alexander V. Ljubimov, Michael E. Boulton, Sergio Caballero, and Maria B. Grant

CONTENTS

Abstract

Drugs targeting somatostatin (SST) receptors have been long recognized as having promise for treating proliferative diabetic retinopathy (PDR) by a systemic mechanism of action involving inhibition of the insulin-like growth factor-1 (IGF-1)–growth hormone (GH) axis. However, the clinical outcome has not been uniformly favorable, and it appears that these drugs may be most beneficial in patients with severely ischemic eyes. Many patients that received benefit, however, required high dosage regimens with doses well above those used for lowering systemic GH in acromegaly patients. Thus, local rather than systemic effects of SST analogs may be more important clinically. This is suggested from the data showing the presence of SST receptors (SSTR) in ocular targets such as vascular endothelium and retinal pigment epithelium and demonstrating direct anti-angiogenic effects of SST analogs, particularly octreotide, in various endothelial cell types (including human retinal endothelial cells). For the SST analog octreotide, high doses may be required owing to inadequate penetration by this peptide drug through the blood–retinal barrier (BRB) after systemic administration, supporting the need to develop small-molecule SSTR agonists with better BRB penetration. High doses of octreotide may be needed because of the drug's low affinity towards the other key anti-angiogenic SSTR subtype, SSTR-3. Thus, SSTR agonists have the potential to treat neovascular ocular diseases when given by a systemic as well as

From: *Contemporary Diabetes: Diabetic Retinopathy*
Edited by: E. Duh © Humana Press, Totowa, NJ

an ocular route; however, a need remains to develop more potent and selective agents and to explore local ocular delivery of these agents and their combinations.

Key Words: Diabetes; Diabetic retinopathy; Growth hormone; Insulin-like growth factor 1; Octreotide Somatostatin.

OVERVIEW

In this chapter, we will review the rationale for use of somatostatin (SST) analogs and provide a historical perspective on the role of growth hormone (GH) in diabetic retinopathy (DR). We will define the molecular pharmacology underlying the anti-angiogenic effects of SSTR agonists and examine local versus systemic efficacy in ocular disease models as a basis for application of somatostatinergic therapy of neovascular ocular disease. To this end, the expression of SSTR subtypes in various target tissues such as endothelium and retinal pigment epithelial (RPE) cells will be discussed. Current SST receptor (SSTR) peptide and small-molecule agonists will be considered, as will their receptor selectivity and functional anti-angiogenic activity. The potential advantage of using receptor agonists targeted to SSTRs of type 2 vs. type 3 will be debated. In vitro and in vivo animal studies comparing established vs. newest SST analogs will be discussed. Finally, an overview of all clinical trials will be presented. Particular attention will be given to the recent studies performed with long-acting release octreotide (Sandostatin LAR), and attempts will be made to explain why this agent so successfully treated some patients yet the study failed to achieve key end points required for FDA approval as a treatment for DR.

INTRODUCTION AND HISTORICAL PERSPECTIVE

Growth Hormone and Diabetic Retinopathy

One of the best-studied endocrine axes, the SST–growth hormone-releasing hormone (GHRH)–GH axis (typically referred to as the GH axis), provides the target for the use of SST analogs as therapeutic agents. The GH axis starts in the central nervous system, which secretes a series of neurotransmitters, catecholamines, and serotonergic and cholinergic substances that cause the hypothalamus to synthesize GHRH and SST. The anterior pituitary secretes GH, which results in the synthesis of insulin-like growth factor -1 (IGF-1) mainly by the liver and fat but also by many other tissues *(1)*. Serum GH mediates its proliferative effects by stimulating both systemic and local IGF-1 production.

Considerable evidence supports a role for GH in the progression of DR *(2, 3)*. Controlling excess GH can slow the progression of this disease *(4)*. The initial observation by Poulsen in a patient whose severe proliferative diabetic retinopathy (PDR) regressed following pituitary infarction *(5)* led to the initiation of hypophysectomy, pituitary yttrium implantation, or α-particle pituitary radiation for treatment of PDR. Clinical trials indicated that the greater the degree of GH decrease, the greater the degree of eye disease regression and preservation of vision. Merimee provided additional support for the role of GH in neovascularization by observing that GH-deficient dwarfs with diabetes were free of microvascular complications after being followed for more than 25 years *(6)*.

The IGF-1 System and Retinopathy

IGF-1 mediates the growth promoting effects of GH. The IGF system is complex and includes not only IGF-1, IGF-2, and their receptors (IGF-1R and IGF-2R), but also IGF binding proteins (IGFBPs) *(7–9)*. IGF-1 can enhance cellular uptake of glucose in select tissues by acting like insulin. By increasing intracellular glucose, IGF-1 can act as a growth factor as well as a progression factor, being a key signal for cells going into the mitotic cycle (Fig. 1). The effects of IGF-1 are mediated by IGF-1R and modulated by complex interactions with IGFBPs, which themselves are also regulated at multiple levels. Circulating IGF-1 is generated by the liver, fat, kidney, and other tissues under the control of GH and local factors *(10)*. Six well-characterized IGFBPs function as transporter proteins and storage pools for IGF-1 in a tissue- and developmental stage-specific manner. Phosphorylation, proteolysis, polymerization, and cell or matrix association regulate the functions of IGFBPs *(11)*. IGFBPs have been shown to either stimulate or inhibit IGF-1 action, with IGFBP-1, -3, and -5 stimulating IGF-1 action in some systems *(11)*.

IGFBP-3 is the best-studied and most abundant IGFBP. It carries 75% or more of serum IGF-1 and IGF-2 in heterotrimeric complexes that also contain the acid-labile subunit (ALS) *(11)*. ALS, IGFBP-3, and IGF-1 form the ternary complex that serves as the IGF storage pool in the plasma. Free or binary complexes (without ALS) are believed to exit the circulation rapidly, whereas ternary complexes appear to be confined to the vascular compartment. Besides these key endocrine effects, IGFBP-3 has autocrine and paracrine actions affecting cell mobility, adhesion, apoptosis, survival, and the cell cycle *(12)*. Like the other IGFBPs, IGFBP-3 also has IGF-1-independent effects. IGFBP-3 is increased in hypoxic conditions; it can enhance angiogenesis in some systems and inhibit it in others *(13, 14)*, thereby demonstrating potentially contradictory effects on the vasculature. Recently we demonstrated that IGFBP-3 promotes endothelial precursor cell migration, differentiation, and capillary formation in vitro *(13)*. Targeted overexpression of IGFBP-3 by hematopoietic precursors protected the vasculature from damage and promoted proper vascular repair after hyperoxic insult in the oxygen-induced retinopathy mouse model. IGFBP-3 expression may represent a physiological adaptation to ischemia, and potentially this protein may serve as a therapeutic for treatment of ischemic conditions. Lofqvist *et al.* recently showed a dose-dependent increase in vessel survival and retinal vessel re-growth with increasing levels of IGFBP-3 *(14)*. In premature infants, lower IGF-1 and IGFBP-3 correlated with more severe retinopathy of prematurity (ROP). These authors conclude, as we also have, that IGFBP-3 helps to prevent oxygen-induced vessel loss and promote vascular regrowth after vascular destruction in vivo, and that an increase in vessel survival prevents hypoxia-induced neovascularization and ROP. They also find that the IGFBP-3 effect is independent of IGF-1 *(14)*. Whereas the effect of IGFBP-3 on the retinal vasculature of the diabetic individual is not known, IGF-1 has been strongly implicated in both health and disease of the retinal vasculature.

IGF-1 stimulates numerous events associated with both physiological and pathological neovascularization including endothelial cell proliferation, migration, and tube formation *(15–18)*. IGF-1 is required for normal retinal vascular development since this process is arrested in its absence despite the presence of vascular endothelial growth factor (VEGF) *(19)*. Development of ROP is associated with low levels of IGF-1, as the lack

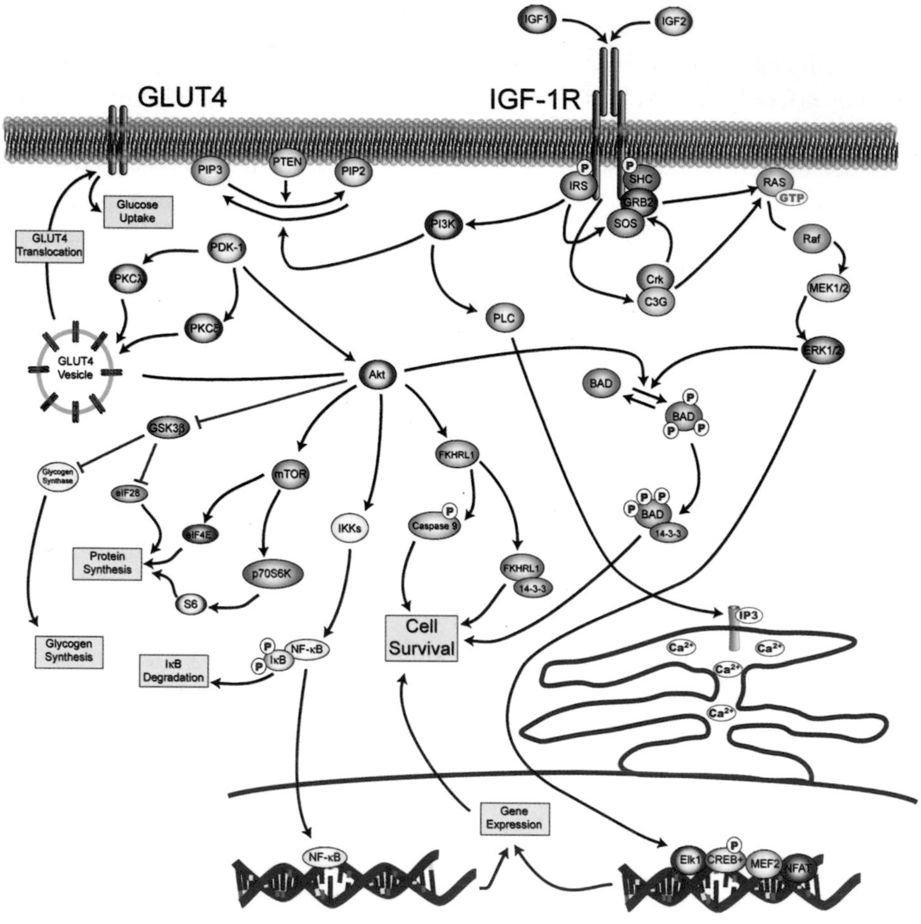

Fig. 1. IGF receptor signaling. The IGF-1R plays an important signaling role in many tissues and cell types. IGF-1R, like the closely related insulin receptor, is a heterotetrameric receptor tyrosine kinase consisting of two extracellular α subunits and two transmembrane β subunits. The kinase catalytic domains are in the cytoplasmic regions of the β subunits. IGF-1R is activated by binding of the growth factor ligand IGF-1 (or the lower-affinity ligand IGF-2) to the extracellular domain of the receptor. Ligand binding promotes a conformational change in the β subunits, which stimulates the intrinsic tyrosine kinase activity of the receptor. A key step in the activation process is the autophosphorylation of three tyrosines in the activation loop, a flexible segment within the catalytic domain of the kinase. The activated IGF-1R kinase phosphorylates cellular substrates such as IRS-1 and IRS-2, initiating a number of signaling pathways, including the phosphatidylinositol 3-kinase (PI-3K)/Akt and Erk/MAPK pathways. Glucose transport is an essential physiological process that is characteristic of all eukaryotic cells. The transport of glucose into cells occurs via specific proteins (GLUTs). A number of GLUT isoforms have been identified, and their cellular distribution appears related to the metabolic demands of the tissue including the retina. GLUT-4, which under basal conditions resides primarily in intracellular compartments, is recruited to the plasma membrane/t-tubules in response to physiological stimuli, such as insulin, IGF-1, exercise, and hypoxia. IGF-1 can mediate many of the metabolic effects of insulin.

of IGF-1 in early neonatal period leads to the development of avascular retina, which subsequently results in ROP *(20)*; In diabetes, the action of IGF-1 in local repair of damaged vascular tissues is highly relevant *(21)*. Unregulated IGF-1 expression can lead to pathological neovascularization *(17, 22)* and IGF-1R antagonists are able to suppress retinal neovascularization in vivo by inhibiting VEGF signaling *(23)*.

Numerous clinical reports support a role for IGF-1 in DR. Kohner and Daneman were the first to note that DR developed with improved diabetes control in young patients with initially poor control *(24)*. In a case report, Chantelau observed a rise in serum IGF-1 preceding the acute progression of DR in a pre-pubertal patient with chronic insulin deficiency *(25)*. Furthermore, adult diabetic patients on intense insulin therapy showed an improvement in hemoglobin A1C from >11 to <8% within 5 months with a concomitant increase in serum IGF-1 levels of 70–220% and worsening of their retinopathy from mild to severe non-proliferative *(25)*. Chantelau hypothesized that adequate insulinization of the liver resulted in increased levels of IGF-1, which promotes retinal neovascularization *(25, 26)*. This was also observed during the early years of the Early Treatment Diabetic Retinopathy Study (ETDRS) in the patients receiving intensive insulin therapy *(27)*. Diabetic patients demonstrated increased IGF-1 levels, with the highest levels found in patients with PDR. In patients who had undergone vitrectomy after laser treatment, intravitreal VEGF levels were reduced but not the IGF-1 levels *(28)*. Interestingly, however, diabetic animal studies suggest that increased IGF-1 and VEGF may represent an attempt by Müller cells to preserve retinal neural cells, which start getting lost early in diabetes *(29)*.

The Role of SST in Diabetic Retinopathy

SST is a natural peptide hormone that affects the release of a number of other hormones, such as GH, glucagon, insulin, and gastrin. In addition to inhibiting pituitary GH secretion and suppressing GHRH secretion, SST also inhibits secretion of the thyroid stimulating hormone (TSH). SST influences processes besides hormone secretion including neurotransmission, cell proliferation, smooth muscle contraction, nutrient absorption, and inflammation. SST is synthesized from a pro-hormone and is secreted by the paraventricular and arcuate nuclei in the hypothalamus into the portal vascular system at the median eminence. SST is also synthesized by pancreatic delta cells in the islets of Langerhans, by gastrointestinal cells, and by the retina. SST is secreted in two forms. One is a peptide of 14 amino acids and the other is a peptide of 28 amino acids. SST acts via five specific receptors (SSTR1–5). After binding SST, the SSTRs generate a transmembrane signal. This results in a reduction of the calcium concentration and activation of tyrosine phosphatases.

SST is a postreceptor antagonist of growth factors acting by inhibition of signal transduction *(30)*. SST and SSTRs have been shown to be produced in the retina. SST also appears to have an effect on fluid transport from the RPE cells to the choroid, a process that is important in the development of diabetic macular edema. Thus one would predict that SST analogs can stabilize the BRB in patients with diabetic macular edema, which has been confirmed *(30)*.

Rationale for the Clinical use of Octreotide

Previously, therapies for neovascular ocular disease relied exclusively on laser treatment, e.g., panretinal photocoagulation (PRP) for PDR. Whereas PRP remains the standard of care for PDR, angiogenic inhibitors are emerging as important therapies.

The classical endocrine action of SST to inhibit pituitary GH release is mediated by both SSTR2 and SSTR5; however, the SSTRs present in the eye are SSTR1, 2, and 3. Octreotide, the most widely used SST analog, is a stable peptide analog drug, has high activity towards SSTR2, good activity towards SSTR5, moderate activity towards SSTR3, and is essentially inactive towards SSTR1 and SSTR4. Octreotide is currently the leading SST drug, which has been approved for treating acromegaly, a disease characterized by the hypersecretion of GH, and the symptomatic treatment of diverse hypersecretory (functional) neuroendocrine tumors. Octreotide inhibits the pituitary release of GH from the tumor and lowers IGF-1 plasma levels. As overproduction of GH and IGF-1 plays an important role in the pathogenesis of DR, octreotide has been under investigation for the treatment of DR.

Octreotide acts via paracrine and autocrine effects on retinal endothelial cells (Fig. 2) *(31)*. It binds to the SSTR and inhibits endothelial cell proliferation stimulated by growth factors like VEGF and IGF-1. One source of VEGF is the RPE cells. These cells play a crucial role in the regulation of outer retinal homeostasis *(32)*. Among its many functions are maintenance of the outer BRB and polarized secretion of growth factors. The RPE cells express both SST and functional SSTRs. There is general agreement from immunohistochemical staining of eye sections and cell culture analyses that the RPE cells express SSTR1 and SSTR2 *(33–36)*, with one report suggesting that the human D407 RPE cell line also expresses SSTR5 *(36)*. The specific SSTR2 subtype active in the RPE is open to some debate because both SSTR2A *(35)* and SSTR2B *(36)* have been identified. The secretion of SST together with the expression of active SSTRs suggests that SST plays an autocrine role in the regulation of RPE function in addition to RPE-derived SST acting as a paracrine effector for neighboring cells. An autocrine role is supported by the observations that (a) the SST analog octreotide inhibits RPE cell proliferation and migration at levels between 10 nM and 10 μM *(37, 38)*; (b) the SST and SSTR2 selective agonist MK678 increases NO production in cultured RPE cells whereas this is blocked by the SSTR2 antagonist CYN-154806 *(36)*; (c) both SST and octreotide inhibit IGF-IR phosphorylation and decrease VEGF production in cultured human RPE cells *(34)*; and (d) octreotide improves RPE BRB function and increases fluid flow across the RPE, which may suggest a role for octreotide in the treatment of diabetic macular edema *(39)*. The paracrine role for SST is currently unclear, but it is likely to regulate retinal and choroidal endothelial cells by the mechanisms discussed in the previous sections. In addition, a recent study indicates that SST may modulate activated macrophages *(40)*. Neutralization of SST in RPE-conditioned medium suppressed NO production by activated macrophages suggesting that SST may play a role in damping down ocular conditions with an inflammatory component such as AMD as well as reducing the availability of angiogenic factors.

In preclinical studies, octreotide also directly inhibited endothelial cell proliferation indicating that it has additional mechanisms of antiangiogenic action, probably by direct SSTR-mediated inhibition *(31)*.

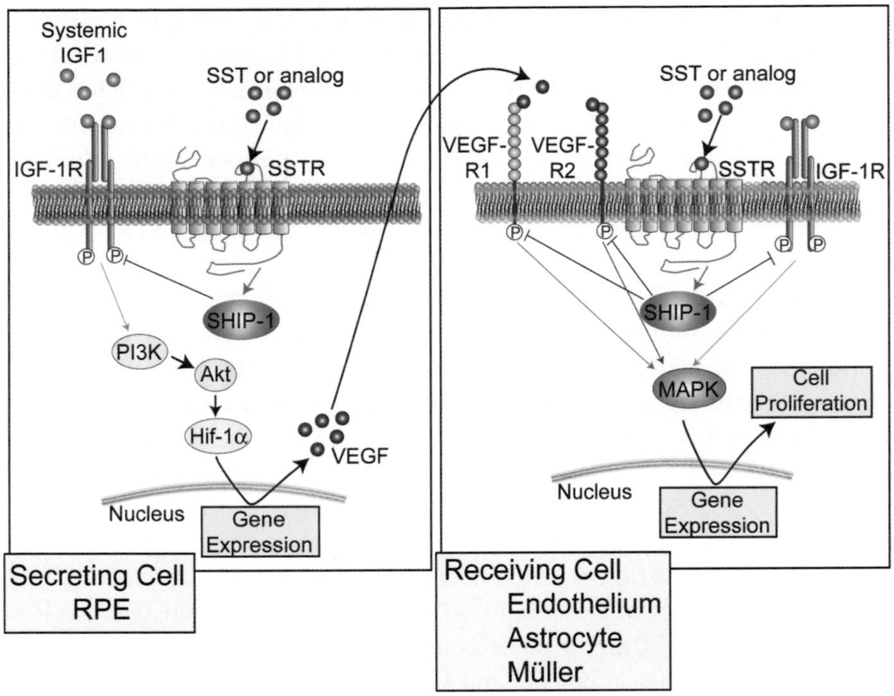

Fig. 2. SST analogs such as octreotide act via paracrine and autocrine effects on retinal endothelial cells and RPE cells. SST or an SST analog binds to the SSTR on endothelial cells and inhibits endothelial cell proliferation stimulated by growth factors like VEGF and IGF-1. RPE cells play a crucial role in the regulation of outer retinal homeostasis. Systemic IGF-1 can stimulate IGF-1 receptors present on RPE cells to express VEGF. VEGF then can stimulate retinal endothelial cells via VEGFR1 or VEGFR2. SST or its analogs can block the activation of IGF-1 receptor in RPE cells resulting in a decrease in VEGF expression, which leads to less VEGF-induced endothelial proliferation. This is one of the mechanisms of SST analog inhibition of angiogenesis.

CLINICAL EVIDENCE FOR SST AS A THERAPEUTIC FOR PDR

In vitro and in vivo studies have confirmed that SST analogs are potent inhibitors of GH and IGF-1. Octreotide was found to reduce elevated levels of GH and IGF-1. Octreotide showed a positive effect on DR in several small, controlled trials and case reports.

In a study of 18 patients with persistent PDR with vitreous hemorrhage after laser treatment, a significantly reduced incidence of vitreous hemorrhages and number of vitrectomies was observed in the group treated with octreotide *(41)*. The dose used was 300 μg per day in three divided doses. In the treated group of nine patients, 78% showed an improvement in contrast to the control group. In the octreotide group visual acuity was stable, whereas it significantly decreased in the control group. Neovascularization decreased in 85% of the patients in the treated group and was stable in 15%, and in the control group neovascularization increased in 42% and was unchanged in 58%.

We studied the effect of octreotide in type 1 and 2 diabetics with pre-proliferative and early proliferative DR. In the treated group, significantly fewer patients developed high risk characteristics. In only 1 of the 22 eyes was laser treatment required in contrast to 9 of 24 eyes in the control group. An important limitation in our study was the use of the maximally tolerated dose of the drug. Moreover, patients were simultaneously treated with thyroid hormone. This was justified based on octreotide's ability to suppress TSH with prolonged use and on the enhancement of SSTR expression by thyroid hormone *(42)*.

Recently, two Phase III, multi-center, double-masked, placebo-controlled study trials that included both type 1 and 2 diabetic patients who were ETDRS stages 47–61 were completed. The patients were treated with the long-acting octreotide (Sandostatin LAR, Novartis), which was injected intramuscularly once a month. The studies were initiated in 1999 and completed in 2006; when combined, these studies represent the largest investigation to date in moderate to severe NPDR to low-risk PDR patients. At completion, study 802 evaluated 585 patients at 61 European sites and study 804 evaluated 313 patients at 36 sites in North America and Brazil. The patients received randomized therapy for on average 4 years, with some patients being treated up to 6 years. For these studies, patients were randomized to receive either Sandostatin LAR at 20 or 30 mg in study 802 and 30 mg or placebo in study 804. Ophthalmologic assessments included visual acuity measurements and semiquantitative, stereoscopic, seven-field, color, 30° ETDRS fundus photography. The Wisconsin Central Reading Center graded the fundus photographs according to ETDRS criteria. The primary outcome was DR progression (octreotide vs. placebo) as defined by the ETDRS retinopathy severity scale for one or two eyes. Key secondary outcomes included change in overall visual acuity, which was defined as time to loss of ≥15 letters on the ETDRS visual acuity scale between baseline and follow-up visits. Octreotide has shown efficacy as a treatment for refractory cystoid macular edema and therefore macular edema was an end point in the study *(43)*. Thus macular edema (changes between baseline and follow-up visits) was a secondary outcome.

Similar mean age, gender ratios, body mass index (BMI), and blood pressure characteristics were observed in both the 802 and 804 studies but there was a greater proportion of Caucasians in the European study. In both studies, similar proportions (roughly 75%) of patients had Type 2 diabetes, similar percentage of patients had ≥10-year duration of diabetes, and similar number of patients used insulin for glycemic control. Approximately 60% of patients had DR of ≤5-year duration since detection, and almost 10% had nephropathy. Slightly lower proportion of patients in Europe had hypertension (56%) or neuropathy (21%) compared with those in study 804 (69% and 42%, respectively). Similar distribution of retinopathy severity was seen in study 802 vs. 804 as defined by the ETDRS severity scale: 20–25% of patients were already at low-risk PDR at study entry. Similar distribution of ETDRS-rated visual acuity was observed. Most patients scored within or above 70–84 letters (almost 80% overall) and approximately 20% scored within or below 55–69 letters. The primary endpoint was to determine the efficacy of octreotide in delaying time to progression of retinopathy, and this was by ≥3 steps on the ETDRS severity scale or by ≥2 steps on the ETDRS severity scale for individual eyes. The secondary end points were to determine the efficacy of octreotide in delaying time to the development or progression of edema or to the loss of ≥15 letters on the ETDRS visual acuity scale. In study 804, the patients received either octreotide 30 mg intramuscularly every 4 weeks or placebo every 4 weeks. In the 804 study, IGF-1 levels in the serum were significantly reduced, with the percent change from baseline being approximately 20%, which remained consistent for the 160 weeks it was examined.

In the study 804, the time to progression of retinopathy was delayed with a *p*-value = 0.0430 over the 304 weeks of the study. There was no effect of octreotide on the time to development or progression of macular edema ($p = 0.8751$). Loss of ≥15 letters on the ETDRS visual acuity scale was delayed in the octreotide-treated patients but did not reach statistical significance ($p = 0.1054$). In contrast, the result of the study 802 was not as encouraging because the primary end point, being time to progression of retinopathy, was not achieved. Interestingly, however, IGF-1 levels were not suppressed during this study, suggesting that the systemic endocrine effects of octreotide may indeed be important to having this drug achieve the optimal results. In study 802, there was a trend for improvement in visual acuity; however, it did not achieve statistical significance.

From an endocrine perspective, octreotide treatment resulted in a reduction of the blood glucose level in patients treated with insulin and they required lower insulin doses. Typically, insulin doses have to be reduced by 25–50% in patients with octreotide treatment. Close daily monitoring of blood glucose levels is mandatory under octreotide treatment because of the risk of hypoglycemia. The side-effect profile was similar to that observed in other large, long-term studies. Diarrhea and tenesmus are common at the beginning of octreotide treatment but rapidly improve. Nausea and vomiting are less common. Hypothyroidism due to TSH suppression and gallstones are additional side effects.

POTENTIAL REASONS FOR MIXED SUCCESS IN CLINICAL TRIALS

The cumulative results suggest that the clinical therapeutic effect of octreotide in DR may be due to both an endocrine effect and a direct effect on SSTR in ocular target tissues. High doses of octreotide required for clinical efficacy in PDR and ultimately other neovascular ocular diseases are likely because of inadequate penetration of the BRB by this peptide drug after systemic administration. Activation of one or more of the other ocular tissue target SSTRs for which octreotide has much lower potency (such as SSTR3) may be as important as SSTR2 activation. The activation of native SSTR2 receptors on endothelial cells inhibits growth factor-stimulated proliferation by a signaling mechanism that is fundamentally less efficient than in other cell types, resulting in higher concentrations being needed. In these antiproliferative studies, IC50 values are 2–3 orders of magnitude greater than those observed with GH release from pituitary cells, typical target cells of SSTR analogs. Moreover, pharmacokinetic studies have not been conducted to determine the relative distribution of octreotide or other SST peptide analogs in the retina or other ocular tissue compartments after systemic administration.

The expression of SSTRs in diverse ocular cells and in endothelial cell types from various beds may differ, and studies have rarely been performed with rigorous quantitation. To date, these studies have not been performed with human retinal endothelial cells (HRECs). Watson *et al.* reported that SSTR2 receptors were expressed at higher levels in proliferating relative to quiescent human umbilical vascular endothelial cells (HUVEC). However, reverse transcriptase polymerase chain reaction (RT-PCR) studies were conducted only using probes for the SSTR2 subtype. Furthermore, the anti-angiogenic effect has been attributed to SSTR2 activation based on the activity of octreotide as an SSTR2-selective agonist in the endothelial cells and in vitro vascular tissue model systems *(44)*. Octreotide inhibits proliferation of HRECs *(31)*, bovine choriocapillary endothelial cells (BCECs) *(45)*, and HUVECs *(44)*, and has antiangiogenic activity in the chick chorioallantoic membrane (CAM) *(44)* and human placental vein (HVPM) models *(46)*. However, octreotide also has affinity for SSTR5 and SSTR3 with selectivity of 1 and 2 orders of magnitude higher, respectively, in cloned receptor binding studies *(47)*. This is in sharp contrast with the nanomolar potency of octreotide both in SSTR2 binding affinity and in SSTR2-mediated functional assay, such as the antisecretory effect (e.g., on GH release) in neuroendocrine cells both in vitro and in vivo. We have shown, using SSTR-selective agonists in HREC, that SSTR 3- and SSTR 2-selective agonists had dramatic antiproliferative effects *(47)*. Furthermore, this is highly relevant, as human eye specimens showed expression of SSTR2 in CNV lesions *(48)*.

In vivo studies proved that SST analogs are good therapies for proliferative conditions of the eye and are tolerated with little toxicity even when administered by intravitreal injection *(47)*. Octreotide reproducibly inhibited neovascularization in vivo in many different systems *(44, 49–51)*.

We showed using the oxygen-induced retinopathy (OIR) mouse model and the laser rupture of Bruch's membrane CNV model that small non-peptide molecules mimic octreotide's effects. These selective SSTR3 and SSTR2 agonists are less expensive to produce, have efficiencies comparable to octreotide, and are specific for SSTR2 or 3.

This work presents a rationale for further clinical studies of these drugs. Moreover, trials of DR therapies must pay close attention to both the progression and severity of DR, as well as appropriate targeting of stage(s) for intervention, assessment of relevant outcomes, observation over a sufficiently long time period, and adequate sample size.

FUTURE DIRECTION: SST ANALOGS IN COMBINATION THERAPY

There is a continued need to add new pharmacological treatment modalities in order to improve the management of neovascular diseases, both as novel monotherapies and combination therapies. In recent years, there has been a burst in relevant studies. The most interesting examples of new drugs against ocular neovascularization are anti-VEGF therapeutics, bevacizumab (Avastin), ranibizumab (Lucentis) (both from Genentech), and pegaptanib (Macugen) (OSI-Pfizer), for treatment of the wet form of AMD *(52, 53)*. The success of these drugs for AMD may be related to the major role of VEGF in the development of neovascularization in this disorder. Avastin has been also tried for PDR; the most pronounced effect, however, was a decrease of neovascular leakage, again consistent with the role of VEGF *(54, 55)*.

Currently, the major challenge in DR treatment is to be able to stop the progression to vision-threatening PDR; data to this effect on clinical use of octreotide have been discussed above. When PDR still develops, an effective anti-angiogenic therapy substituting or complementing panretinal photocoagulation is badly needed. It should be noted that PDR development could be dependent on more factors than just VEGF

(56–58). It was also shown that retinal endothelial cells respond much more strongly to growth factor combinations than any single factor *(59, 60)*. In a complex, apparently multifactorial, disease as exemplified by DR and PDR, some potentially successful drug monotherapies may rely on targeting master regulators of the angiogenic process, such as HIF-1α or protein kinase CK2 *(29)*.

Another powerful approach is to develop efficient drug combinations. This principle is the mainstream of drug therapy for cancer and AIDS *(61–63)*, but until very recently it was not considered for PDR. In 2004, we pioneered this approach using a mouse OIR model of retinal neovascularization *(57)*. This model is widely used to test anti-angiogenic drugs because diabetic animal models, with very rare exceptions *(64)*, fail to reproduce human PDR with preretinal neovascularization unless genetically manipulated *(65)*. In our experiments, protein kinase CK2 inhibitors, emodin or tetrabromobenzotriazole (TBB), were administered alone or in combination with octreotide. Each compound was able to significantly reduce preretinal neovascularization in mouse pups with systemic administration *(57, 66)*. Combination therapy produced an additive effect. Moreover, using only 1 mg kg^{-1} per day octreotide in combination with a CK2 inhibitor, it was possible to achieve the same degree of inhibition of neovascularization as with 5 mg kg^{-1} per day octreotide alone (Fig. 3). Since emodin is a component of some laxatives and is known to be essentially nontoxic, *(57)* these experiments pave the way to clinical trials using its combination with octreotide for inhibiting DR progression.

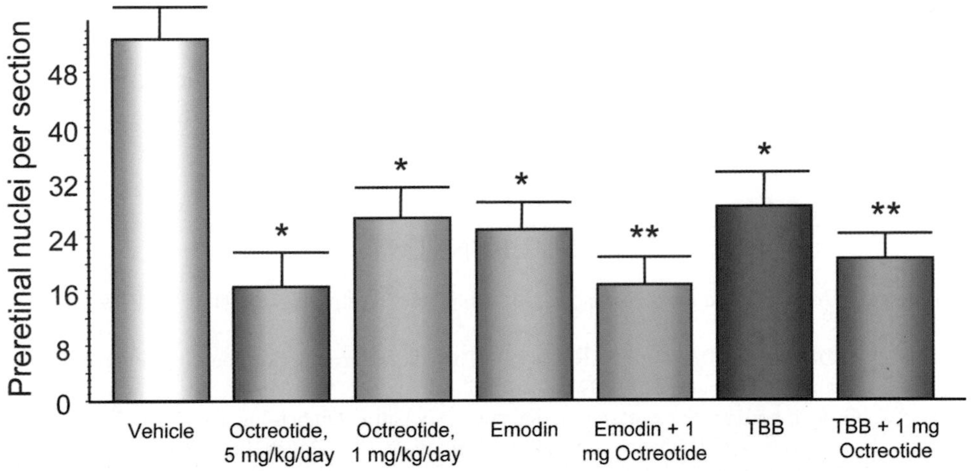

Fig. 3. Combination therapy with octreotide. Counts of preretinal nuclei as a measure of neovascularization in various groups of mice are shown. Intraperitoneal treatment with 30 mg kg^{-1} per day emodin reduced retinal neovascularization by about 57%, and with 30 mg kg^{-1} per day TBB, by 46%. Treatment with 5 mg kg^{-1} per day octreotide yielded about 67% reduction, and with 1 mg kg^{-1} per day octreotide, about 50% reduction. Emodin combined with 1 mg kg^{-1} per day octreotide reduced neovascularization by 69%, and TBB combined with 1 mg kg^{-1} per day octreotide, by 61%. Ten sections per eye from each mouse were counted. Five mice were used per each group in three independent experiments. Vehicle represents emodin solvent since octreotide solvent was just PBS. Bars = mean ± SD. $^{*}p < 0.001$ vs. vehicle; $^{**}p < 0.05$ vs. single drug or vehicle. (Reprinted from *(66)* with permission from the American Society for Investigative Pathology.)

Other recent studies also convincingly showed that a combination of several drugs produced a more potent inhibitory effect on retinal neovascularization than single-drug therapy *(67–69)*. Future treatment of pathologic ocular neovascularization may well rely on combined drug therapy. In this respect, the promising anti-DR agent octreotide may emerge as a key player in such drug combinations.

CONCLUSION

The endogenous peptide SST was isolated from mammalian hypothalamus nearly three decades ago as a potent inhibitory factor of pituitary GH secretion. Now it is appreciated that SST is widely distributed throughout diverse cell types and its actions affect a variety of biological processes such as hormone secretion, neurotransmission, cell proliferation, and angiogenesis. These effects are mediated through five G-protein coupled receptor subtypes, SSTR 1–5. Systemic therapy with the SST peptide analog drug octreotide can result in regression of neovascularization and improve visual acuity in patients with advanced DR. However, the clinical results with octreotide have been variable and have been most favorable for patients receiving high dosage regimens that are well above effective doses required for lowering systemic GH in acromegaly patient. Moreover, the more ischemic the eye, the greater the likelihood of observing a beneficial effect. Therapeutic potential of SST analogs for DR and PDR treatment may be potentially increased if they are used in combination with other anti-angiogenic drugs. The combination therapy may become the mainstream of PDR treatment in the near future.

ACKNOWLEDGEMENTS

A portion of the work described here was supported by the NIH Grant EY015952 to M.B. Grant and G. Shapiro. The authors thank the members of the Grant laboratory for helpful discussion.

REFERENCES

1. Roberts CT, Jr. IGF-1 and prostate cancer. Novartis Found Symp 2004;262:193–9; discussion 9–204, 65–8.
2. Alzaid AA, Dinneen SF, Melton LR, Rizza RA. The role of growth hormone in the development of diabetic retinopathy. Diabetes Care 1994;17(6):531–4.
3. Hyer SL. Growth hormone suppression in diabetic retinopathy. Diabetologia 1987;30(7):534A.
4. Kohner EM, Oakley NW. Diabetic retinopathy. Metabolism 1975;24(9):1085–102.
5. Poulsen J. The Houssay phenomenon in man: recovery from retinopathy in a case of diabetes with Simmonds' disease. Diabetes 1953;2:7–12.
6. Merimee TJ. Metabolic and clinical studies in growth hormone deficient dwarfs: a ten year follow-up. N Engl J Med 1978;298:1217–22.
7. Grant MB, Caballero S, Bush DM, Spoerri PE. Fibronectin fragments modulate human retinal capillary cell proliferation and migration. Diabetes 1998;47(8):1335–40.
8. Grant MB, Caballero S, Tarnuzzer RW, Bass KE, Ljubimov AV, Spoerri PE, Galardy RE. Matrix metalloproteinase expression in human retinal microvascular cells. Diabetes 1998;47(8):1311–7.
9. Grant MB, Schmetz I, Russell B, Harwood HJ, Jr., Silverstein J, Merimee TJ. Changes in insulin-like growth factors I and II and their binding protein after a single intramuscular injection of growth hormone. J Clin Endocrinol Metab 1986;63(4):981–4.

10. Cohen BD, Baker DA, Soderstrom C, Tkalcevic G, Rossi AM, Miller PE, Tengowski MW, Wang F, Gualberto A, Beebe JS, Moyer JD. Combination therapy enhances the inhibition of tumor growth with the fully human anti-type 1 insulin-like growth factor receptor monoclonal antibody CP-751,871. Clin Cancer Res 2005;11(5):2063–73.
11. Sakai K, Busby WH, Jr., Clarke JB, Clemmons DR. Tissue transglutaminase facilitates the polymerization of insulin-like growth factor-binding protein-1 (IGFBP-1) and leads to loss of IGFBP-1's ability to inhibit insulin-like growth factor-I-stimulated protein synthesis. J Biol Chem 2001;276(12):8740–5.
12. Firth SM, Baxter RC. Cellular actions of the insulin-like growth factor binding proteins. Endocr Rev 2002;23(6):824–54.
13. Chang KH, Chan-Ling T, McFarland EL, Afzal A, Pan H, Baxter LC, Shaw LC, Caballero S, Sengupta N, Calzi SL, Sullivan SM, Grant MB. IGF binding protein-3 regulates hematopoietic stem cell and endothelial precursor cell function during vascular development. Proc Natl Acad Sci USA 2007;104(25):10595–600.
14. Lofqvist C, Chen J, Connor KM, Smith AC, Aderman CM, Liu N, Pintar JE, Ludwig T, Hellstrom A, Smith LE. From the Cover: IGFBP3 suppresses retinopathy through suppression of oxygen-induced vessel loss and promotion of vascular regrowth. Proc Natl Acad Sci USA 2007;104(25): 10589–94.
15. Grant MB, King GL. IGF-1 and blood vessels. Diabetes Rev 1995;3(1):113–28.
16. Grant MB, Mames RN, Fitzgerald C, Ellis EA, Aboufriekha M, Guy J. Insulin-like growth factor I acts as an angiogenic agent in rabbit cornea and retina: comparative studies with basic fibroblast growth factor. Diabetologia 1993;36(4):282–91.
17. Grant MB, Caballero S, Millard WJ. Inhibition of IGF-I and b-FGF stimulated growth of human retinal endothelial cells by the somatostatin analogue, octreotide: a potential treatment for ocular neovascularization. Regul Pept 1993;48(1–2):267–78.
18. Merimee TJ, Zapf J, Froesch ER. Insulin-like growth factors: studies in diabetics with and without retinopathy. N Engl J Med 1983;309(9):527–30.
19. Hellstrom A, Engstrom E, Hard AL, Albertsson-Wikland K, Carlsson B, Niklasson A, Lofqvist C, Svensson E, Holm S, Ewald U, Holmstrom G, Smith LE. Postnatal serum insulin-like growth factor I deficiency is associated with retinopathy of prematurity and other complications of premature birth. Pediatrics 2003;112(5):1016–20.
20. Lofqvist C, Andersson E, Sigurdsson J, Engstrom E, Hard AL, Niklasson A, Smith LE, Hellstrom A. Longitudinal postnatal weight and insulin-like growth factor I measurements in the prediction of retinopathy of prematurity. Arch Ophthalmol 2006;124(12):1711–8.
21. Merimee TJ, Zapf J, Froesch ER. Insulin-like growth factors in the fed and fasted states. J Clin Endocrinol Metab 1982;55(5):999–1002.
22. Grant MB. Insulinlike growth factor-I in diabetic vascular complications. Curr Opin Endocrin Diabetes 1996;3(4):335–45.
23. Smith LE, Shen W, Perruzzi C, Soker S, Kinose F, Xu X, Robinson G, Driver S, Bischoff J, Zhang B, Schaeffer JM, Senger DR. Regulation of vascular endothelial growth factor-dependent retinal neovascularization by insulin-like growth factor-1 receptor. Nat Med 1999;5(12):1390–5.
24. Daneman D, Lobes LA, Becker DJ, Drash AL. Diabetic retinopathy in Mauriac's syndrome. Paradoxical deterioration with improved metabolic control. Retina 1981;1(2):84–7.
25. Chantelau E, Eggert H, Seppel T, Schonau E, Althaus C. Elevation of serum IGF-1 precedes proliferative diabetic retinopathy in Mauriac's syndrome. Br J Ophthalmol 1997;81(2):169–70.
26. Hyer SL, Sharp PS, Brooks RA, Burrin JM, Kohner EM. Serum IGF-1 concentration in diabetic retinopathy. Diabet Med 1988;5(4):356–60.
27. The effect of intensive treatment of diabetes on the development and progression of long-term complications in insulin-dependent diabetes mellitus. The Diabetes Control and Complications Trial Research Group. N Engl J Med 1993;329(14):977–86.
28. Spranger J, Mohlig M, Osterhoff M, Buhnen J, Blum WF, Pfeiffer AF. Retinal photocoagulation does not influence intraocular levels of IGF-I, IGF-II and IGF-BP3 in proliferative diabetic retinopathy-evidence for combined treatment of PDR with somatostatin analogues and retinal photocoagulation? Horm Metab Res 2001;33(5):312–6.

29. Afzal A, Shaw LC, Ljubimov AV, Boulton ME, Segal MS, Grant MB. Retinal and choroidal microangiopathies: Therapeutic opportunities. Microvasc Res 2007;74:131–44.
30. Lang GE. Pharmacological treatment of diabetic retinopathy. Ophthalmologica 2007;221(2):112–7.
31. Grant MB, Mames RN, Fitzgerald C, Ellis EA, Caballero S, Chegini N, Guy J. Insulin-like growth factor I as an angiogenic agent. In vivo and in vitro studies. Ann N Y Acad Sci 1993;692:230–42.
32. Boulton M, Dayhaw-Barker P. The role of the retinal pigment epithelium: topographical variation and ageing changes. Eye 2001;15(Pt 3):384–9.
33. Klisovic DD, O'Dorisio MS, Katz SE, Sall JW, Balster D, O'Dorisio TM, Craig E, Lubow M. Somatostatin receptor gene expression in human ocular tissues: RT-PCR and immunohistochemical study. Invest Ophthalmol Vis Sci 2001;42(10):2193–201.
34. Sall JW, Klisovic DD, O'Dorisio MS, Katz SE. Somatostatin inhibits IGF-1 mediated induction of VEGF in human retinal pigment epithelial cells. Exp Eye Res 2004;79(4):465–76.
35. van Hagen PM, Baarsma GS, Mooy CM, Ercoskan EM, ter Averst E, Hofland LJ, Lamberts SW, Kuijpers RW. Somatostatin and somatostatin receptors in retinal diseases. Eur J Endocrinol 2000;143 Suppl 1:S43–51.
36. Vasilaki A, Papadaki T, Notas G, Kolios G, Mastrodimou N, Hoyer D, Tsilimbaris M, Kouroumalis E, Pallikaris I, Thermos K. Effect of somatostatin on nitric oxide production in human retinal pigment epithelium cell cultures. Invest Ophthalmol Vis Sci 2004;45(5):1499–506.
37. Luo Q, Peyman GA, Conway MD, Woltering EA. Effect of a somatostatin analog (octreotide acetate) on the growth of retinal pigment epithelial cells in culture. Curr Eye Res 1996;15(9):909–13.
38. Spraul CW, Kaven CK, Kampmeier JK, Lang GK, Lang GE. Effect of thalidomide, octreotide, and prednisolone on the migration and proliferation of RPE cells in vitro. Curr Eye Res 1999;19(6):483–90.
39. Garlington W, Afzal A, LiCalzi S, Jarajupa Y, Chang K-H, Grant MB, Boulton M, Brooks HL. The effect of a somatostatin analog on the transepithelial transport of ARPE 19 cells. In: ARVO; Fort Lauderdale, FL; 2006.
40. Zamiri P, Masli S, Streilein JW, Taylor AW. Pigment epithelial growth factor suppresses inflammation by modulating macrophage activation. Invest Ophthalmol Vis Sci 2006;47(9):3912–8.
41. Boehm BO, Lang GK, Jehle PM, Feldman B, Lang GE. Octreotide reduces vitreous hemorrhage and loss of visual acuity risk in patients with high-risk proliferative diabetic retinopathy. Horm Metab Res 2001;33(5):300–6.
42. Grant MB, Mames RN, Fitzgerald C, Hazariwala KM, Cooper-DeHoff R, Caballero S, Estes KS. The efficacy of octreotide in the therapy of severe nonproliferative and early proliferative diabetic retinopathy: a randomized controlled study. Diabetes Care 2000;23(4):504–9.
43. Hernaez-Ortega MC, Soto-Pedre E, Martin JJ. Sandostatin LAR for cystoid diabetic macular edema: a 1-year experience. Diabetes Res Clin Pract 2004;64(1):71–2.
44. Watson JC, Balster DA, Gebhardt BM, O'Dorisio TM, O'Dorisio MS, Espenan GD, Drouant GJ, Woltering EA. Growing vascular endothelial cells express somatostatin subtype 2 receptors. Br J Cancer 2001;85(2):266–72.
45. Adams RL, Adams IP, Lindow SW, Zhong W, Atkin SL. Somatostatin receptors 2 and 5 are preferentially expressed in proliferating endothelium. Br J Cancer 2005;92(8):1493–8.
46. Meyers MO, Gagliardi AR, Flattmann GJ, Su JL, Wang YZ, Woltering EA. Suramin analogs inhibit human angiogenesis in vitro. J Surg Res 2000;91(2):130–4.
47. Palii SS, Caballero S, Jr., Shapiro G, Grant MB. Medical treatment of diabetic retinopathy with somatostatin analogues. Expert Opin Investig Drugs 2007;16(1):73–82.
48. Lambooij AC, Kuijpers RW, van Lichtenauer-Kaligis EG, Kliffen M, Baarsma GS, van Hagen PM, Mooy CM. Somatostatin receptor 2A expression in choroidal neovascularization secondary to age-related macular degeneration. Invest Ophthalmol Vis Sci 2000;41(8):2329–35.
49. Danesi R, Del Tacca M. The effects of the somatostatin analog octreotide on angiogenesis in vitro. Metabolism 1996;45(8 Suppl 1):49–50.
50. Demir T, Celiker UO, Kukner A, Mogulkoc R, Celebi S, Celiker H. Effect of Octreotide on experimental corneal neovascularization. Acta Ophthalmol Scand 1999;77(4):386–90.
51. Higgins RD, Yan Y, Schrier BK. Somatostatin analogs inhibit neonatal retinal neovascularization. Exp Eye Res 2002;74(5):553–9.

52. Emerson MV, Lauer AK, Flaxel CJ, Wilson DJ, Francis PJ, Stout JT, Emerson GG, Schlesinger TK, Nolte SK, Klein ML. Intravitreal bevacizumab (Avastin) treatment of neovascular age-related macular degeneration. Retina 2007;27(4):439–44.
53. Takeda AL, Colquitt JL, Clegg AJ, Jones J. Pegaptanib and ranibizumab for neovascular age-related macular degeneration: a systematic review. Br J Ophthalmol 2007;91:1177–82.
54. Avery RL, Pearlman J, Pieramici DJ, Rabena MD, Castellarin AA, Nasir MA, Giust MJ, Wendel R, Patel A. Intravitreal bevacizumab (Avastin) in the treatment of proliferative diabetic retinopathy. Ophthalmology 2006;113(10):1695 e1–15.
55. Jorge R, Costa RA, Calucci D, Cintra LP, Scott IU. Intravitreal bevacizumab (Avastin) for persistent new vessels in diabetic retinopathy (IBEPE study). Retina 2006;26(9):1006–13.
56. Kvanta A. Ocular angiogenesis: the role of growth factors. Acta Ophthalmol Scand 2006;84(3):282–8.
57. Ljubimov AV, Caballero S, Pinna LA, Grant MB. Antiangiogenic effects of protein kinase CK2 inhibitors and octreotide in mouse oxygen-induced retinopathy. In: 5th International Symposium on Ocular Pharmacology and Therapeutics; 2004; Monte Carlo; 2004. p. A45.
58. Zhang SX, Ma JX. Ocular neovascularization: Implication of endogenous angiogenic inhibitors and potential therapy. Prog Retin Eye Res 2007;26(1):1–37.
59. Castellon R, Caballero S, Hamdi HK, Atilano SR, Aoki AM, Tarnuzzer RW, Kenney MC, Grant MB, Ljubimov AV. Effects of tenascin-C on normal and diabetic retinal endothelial cells in culture. Invest Ophthalmol Vis Sci 2002;43(8):2758–66.
60. Ljubimov AV. Growth factor synergy in angiogenesis. In: Retinal and Choroidal Angiogenesis: Kluwer; 2007.
61. Brem H, Gresser I, Grosfeld J, Folkman J. The combination of antiangiogenic agents to inhibit primary tumor growth and metastasis. J Pediatr Surg 1993;28(10):1253–7.
62. Habtemariam T, Yu P, Oryang D, Nganwa D, Ayanwale O, Tameru B, Abdelrahman H, Ahmad A, Robnett V. Modelling viral and CD4 cellular population dynamics in HIV: approaches to evaluate intervention strategies. Cell Mol Biol (Noisy-le-grand) 2001;47(7):1201–8.
63. Haskell CM. ed. Cancer Treatment. 5th ed. Philadelphia: W.B. Saunders Company; 2001.
64. Kador PF, Blessing K, Randazzo J, Makita J, Wyman M. Evaluation of the vascular targeting agent combretastatin a-4 prodrug on retinal neovascularization in the galactose-fed dog. J Ocul Pharmacol Ther 2007;23(2):132–42.
65. Lebherz C, Maguire AM, Auricchio A, Tang W, Aleman TS, Wei Z, Grant R, Cideciyan AV, Jacobson SG, Wilson JM, Bennett J. Nonhuman primate models for diabetic ocular neovascularization using AAV2-mediated overexpression of vascular endothelial growth factor. Diabetes 2005;54(4):1141–9.
66. Kramerov AA, Saghizadeh M, Pan H, Kabosova A, Montenarh M, Ahmed K, Penn JS, Chan CK, Hinton DR, Grant MB, Ljubimov AV. Expression of protein kinase CK2 in astroglial cells of normal and neovascularized retina. Am J Pathol 2006;168(5):1722–36.
67. Bradley J, Ju M, Robinson GS. Combination therapy for the treatment of ocular neovascularization. Angiogenesis 2007;10(2):141–8.
68. Dorrell MI, Aguilar E, Scheppke L, Barnett FH, Friedlander M. Combination angiostatic therapy completely inhibits ocular and tumor angiogenesis. Proc Natl Acad Sci USA 2007;104(3):967–72.
69. Jo N, Mailhos C, Ju M, Cheung E, Bradley J, Nishijima K, Robinson GS, Adamis AP, Shima DT. Inhibition of platelet-derived growth factor B signaling enhances the efficacy of anti-vascular endothelial growth factor therapy in multiple models of ocular neovascularization. Am J Pathol 2006;168(6):2036–53.

21 Diabetic Retinopathy and Systemic Complications

Ning Cheung and Tien Y. Wong

CONTENTS

Key Words: Retinopathy, stroke, heart failure, coronary heart disease, nephropathy, complications, microvascular disease, macrovascular disease, cardiovascular disease prediction, mortality.

INTRODUCTION

Diabetic retinopathy is the most common and specific complication of diabetes *(1)*. Its adverse impact on vision is well known. The clinical significance of retinopathy signs beyond the eyes of diabetic individuals, however, is less clear. The routine ophthalmic examination to detect retinopathy signs presents ophthalmologists and physicians with the unique opportunity to directly visualize and assess actual pathology of diabetic microvascular damage. New studies now show that early signs of retinopathy are associated with a wide range of systemic complications in persons with diabetes, including the development of stroke, coronary heart disease, heart failure, nephropathy, and peripheral vascular disease *(2–8)*. Diabetic retinopathy signs therefore not only reflect microvascular dysfunction in the retina, but also may be markers of more widespread

From: *Diabetic Retinopathy*
Edited by: MD Elia Duh © Humana Press, Totowa, NJ

deleterious effects of abnormal glucose metabolism on the systemic vasculature. This chapter will discuss the relationships of diabetic retinopathy with mortality and various systemic micro- and macrovascular morbidities.

DIABETIC RETINOPATHY AND MORTALITY

It has long been known that in persons with diabetes, the presence of retinopathy is associated with an increased risk of mortality (Table 1). Studies suggest this association is more consistently seen in patients with type 2 as compared to type 1 diabetes, reflecting older age and possibly the higher prevalence of cardiovascular risk factors in type 2 diabetes.

In the Wisconsin Epidemiological Study of Diabetic Retinopathy (WESDR), a large population-based study in the United States, both nonproliferative (NPDR) and proliferative (PDR) diabetic retinopathy were associated with a 34–89% excess risk of death in participants with type 2 diabetes after 16 years of follow-up *(9)*. Importantly, this association was independent of age, sex, diabetes duration, glycemic control, and other survival-related risk factors. Consistent with this finding are data from other studies in Caucasians *(10–14)*, Asians *(15)*, and Mexicans *(16)*.

While retinopathy also predicts poorer survival in persons with type 1 diabetes, some studies suggest that the association is largely explained by coexisting cardiovascular risk factors *(9, 17, 18)*. Not all studies have found this association consistently. In the Early Treatment Diabetic Retinopathy Study, a large clinical trial with a relatively short follow-up, retinopathy was shown to have no association with mortality in type 1 diabetes *(14)*. Some *(19, 20)*, but not all *(13)*, investigators believe that, besides the traditional cardiovascular risk factors, coexisting nephropathy (e.g., end-stage renal disease) is a major determinant for the poorer survival in patients with diabetic retinopathy.

The association of diabetic retinopathy with mortality is largely related to the increased risk of cardiovascular mortality in persons with retinopathy (Table 2). The World Health Organization Multinational Study of Vascular Disease in Diabetes (WHO-MSVDD) consists of a large cohort of type 1 and 2 diabetic persons who were followed up for 12 years for incidence of fatal and nonfatal cardiovascular outcomes *(21)*. In the WHO-MSVDD, the presence of diabetic retinopathy predicted higher risk of cardiovascular disease and mortality *(21)*. This association was seen in persons with type 2, but not type 1, diabetes and was stronger in women than in men, and remained significant even after adjusting for traditional cardiovascular risk factors *(21)*. In addition, some studies show a "dose-dependent" association between diabetic retinopathy and cardiovascular disease risk, with increasing risk in eyes with more severe retinopathy *(11, 12)*. These associations are supported by other studies, such as prospective data from the EURODIAB Study and cross-sectional data from the Cardiovascular Health Study *(10, 13, 18, 22–24)*.

DIABETIC RETINOPATHY AND CEREBROVASCULAR DISEASE

Stroke and other cerebrovascular diseases (e.g., vascular dementia) are major sources of morbidity and mortality in people with diabetes. Over the past decade, despite the significant progress made in stroke prevention and treatment, most advances have been

Table 1
Selected Studies on the Relationship of Diabetic Retinopathy and All-cause Mortality.

Study and population	*Follow-up*	*Retinal status*	*RR/HR (95% CI)*	*Adjusted covariates*
WESDR *(9)* 1,370 T2DM	16-year	Mild NPDR	1.34 (1.14, 1.57)	Age, sex, diabetes duration, HbA1c, hypertension, urine protein, cardiovascular disease history, current smoking, pack-years smoked, diuretic use, history of tactile sensation loss
		Moderate NPDR	1.44 (1.12, 1.84)	
		PDR	1.89 (1.43, 2.50)	
		ME	1.25 (0.98, 1.60)	
ETDRS (14) 2,267 T2DM	5-year	Moderate NPDR	1.27 (0.94, 1.72)	Age, sex, body mass index, HbA1c, total cholesterol, triglycerides, fibrinogen, smoking, insulin use, antihypertensive use, other baseline diabetic complications
		Severe NPDR	1.48 (1.03, 2.15)	
		Mild PDR	1.28 (0.80, 2.06)	
		Moderate/high PDR	2.02 (1.28, 3.19)	
824 Finnish T2DM *(12)*	18-year	NPDR in men	1.34 (0.98, 1.83)	Age, area of residence, HbA1c, smoking, hypertension, cholesterols, diabetes duration, urinary protein
		PDR in men	3.05 (1.70–5.45)	
		NPDR in women	1.61 (1.17–2.22)	
		PDR in women	2.92 (1.41–6.06)	
WESDR *(9)*	16-year	Mild NPDR	1.02 (0.52, 1.99)	Age, sex, diabetes duration, HbA1c, diastolic blood pressure, hypertension, urine protein, cardiovascular disease history, pack-years smoked, units of insulin, history of loss of temperature sensitivity
996 T1DM		Moderate NPDR	1.42 (0.68, 2.98)	
		PDR	1.28 (0.62, 2.62)	
		ME	0.80 (0.50, 1.27)	
ETDRS *(14)*	6-year	Moderate NPDR	0.88 (0.43, 1.80)	Age, sex, body mass index, HbA1c, total cholesterol, triglycerides, fibrinogen, smoking, insulin use, antihypertensive use, other baseline diabetic complications
1,444 T1DM		Severe NPDR	1.33 (0.59, 2.99)	
		Mild PDR	0.54 (0.21, 1.38)	
		Moderate/high PDR	1.21 (0.54, 2.73)	
EURODIAB *(18)* 2,237 T1DM	8-year	NPDR	0.54 (0.19, 1.53)	Age, sex, diabetes duration, HbA1c, hypertension, body mass index, LDL cholesterol, albumin excretion rate, prior cardiovascular disease
		PDR	2.06 (0.63, 6.73)	

WESDR Wisconsin Epidemiological Study of Diabetic Retinopathy, *ETDRS* Early Treatment Diabetic Retinopathy Study, *NPDR* Nonproliferative diabetic retinopathy, *PDR* Proliferative diabetic retinopathy, *CVD* Cardiovascular disease, *T1DM* Type 1 diabetes, *T2DM* Type 2 diabetes, *HR (95% CI)* Hazard rate ratio (95% confidence interval), *HbA1c* Glycosylated hemoglobin

Table 2
Selected Studies on the Relationship of Diabetic Retinopathy with Cardiovascular Disease and Mortality.

Study and population	*Follow-up*	*Retinal status*	*RR/HR (95% CI)*	*Adjusted covariates*
WHO-MSVDD (21)	12-year	DR in T1DM men	1.1 (0.7, 1.9)	Age, diabetes duration, blood pressure, cholesterol, smoking, proteinuria, ECG abnormalities
1,126 T1DM		DR in T1DM women	1.3 (0.7, 2.5)	
3,179 T2DM		DR in T2DM men	1.4 (1.1, 2.0)	
		DR in T2DM women	2.3 (1.6, 3.3)	
824 T2DM (12)	18-year	NPDR in men	1.30 (0.86, 1.96)	Age, area of residence, HbA1c, smoking, hypertension, cholesterols, diabetes duration, urinary protein
		PDR in men	3.32 (1.61–6.78)	
		NPDR in women	1.71 (1.17–2.51)	
		PRD in women	3.17 (1.38–7.30)	
VHS (22)	5-year	NPDR	1.8 (1.2, 2.3)	Age, sex, body mass index, smoking, lipids, HbA1c, diabetes duration and treatment
744 T2DM		PDR	4.1 (2.0, 8.9)	
EURODIAB (18)	8-year	NPDR	1.30 (0.74, 2.29)	Age, sex, diabetes duration, HbA1c, hypertension, body mass index, LDL cholesterol, AER, prior CVD
2,237 T1DM		PDR	1.63 (0.80, 3.33)	
483 T1DM and 2,737 T2DM (11)	3-year	Mild NPDR	2.1 (1.3, 3.2)	Age, sex
		Moderate NPDR	3.2 (1.7, 6.0)	
		Severe NPDR/PDR	4.8 (2.7, 8.6)	

WHO-MSVDD World Health Organization Multinational Study of vascular disease in diabetes, *VHS* Valpolicella Heart Diabetes Study, *NPDR* Nonproliferative diabetic retinopathy, *PDR* Proliferative diabetic retinopathy, *CVD* Cardiovascular disease, *T1DM* Type 1 diabetes, *T2DM* Type 2 diabetes; *RR/HR (95% CI)* Relative risk or hazard rate ratio (95% confidence interval), *HbA1c* Glycosylated hemoglobin confined to the management of strokes that are caused by large vessel disease (e.g., carotid atherosclerosis). However, up to one-third of symptomatic strokes can be attributed to the disease of the small arteries/arterioles in the cerebral circulation *(25)*, especially in people with diabetes *(26–28)*. Little is known about these small vessel pathologies due to the paucity of noninvasive methods to study the cerebral microcirculation.

Because the retinal and cerebral vasculatures share similar embryological origin, anatomical features, and physiological properties *(29, 30)*, pathological lesions seen in eyes with diabetic retinopathy may actually indicate similar pathological disease processes in the cerebral microcirculation. In support of this theory is the strong and consistent evidence that retinopathy signs are associated with both clinical and subclinical stroke, independent of cerebrovascular risk factors.

Since the 1970s, physicians have reported that the presence of retinopathy is associated with stroke, particularly in persons with hypertension *(31–37)*. New population-based studies, using standardized photographic evaluation of retinal images to ascertain retinopathy lesions, have confirmed these early observations (Table 3). In the WESDR, PDR was associated with incident stroke mortality in both type 1 and 2 diabetes, independent of diabetes duration, glycemic control, and other risk factors *(9, 17, 20)*. In type 1 diabetes, retinopathy severity was also associated with higher stroke risk *(20)*. These findings are in keeping with data from the WHO-MSVDD in both men and women with type 2 diabetes *(21)*, although an association was not seen in type 1 diabetes.

More recently, the Atherosclerosis Risk in Communities (ARIC) study, a large prospective cohort study of 1,617 middle-aged white and black Americans with type 2 diabetes, showed that the presence of NPDR, even of the mildest phenotype (presence of microaneurysms and/or retinal hemorrhages only), was associated with a two- to threefold higher risk of ischemic stroke *(38, 39)*. In a substudy of the ARIC cohort in which participants had cranial MRI scans, synergistic interaction between the presence of retinopathy and the presence of MRI-defined cerebral white matter lesions on subsequent risk of clinical stroke development was seen. Participants with both retinopathy and white matter lesions had nearly a 20 times higher stroke risk than those without either findings (relative risk 18.1, 95% confidence intervals, 5.9–55.4) *(40)*. This confirms the theory that subclinical cerebrovascular pathology may be more severe or extensive in persons with both cerebral and retinal markers of microvascular disease. Findings from the ARIC study are further reinforced by cross-sectional data from the Cardiovascular Health Study of an older population *(41)* and other studies *(37, 42)*. Finally, there is new evidence that retinopathy signs are associated with stroke risk even in persons without clinically defined diabetes *(43)* and in persons with impaired glucose tolerance *(44)*.

Apart from stroke events, diabetic retinopathy signs have also been linked with other cerebrovascular disorders. For example, among the ARIC study participants without clinical stroke, retinopathy lesions were related to cognitive decline *(45)* and MRI-detected cerebral atrophy *(46)*. In the CHS and other studies, retinopathy was also modestly associated with cognitive dysfunction and dementia *(47, 48)*.

The importance of the reported associations of retinopathy signs with stroke, white matter lesions, cerebral atrophy, and cognitive impairment is that it directly supports a

Table 3
Selected Studies on the Relationship of Diabetic Retinopathy and Stroke.

Study and population	*Follow-up*	*Retinal status*	*RR/HR (95% CI)*	*Adjusted covariates*
WESDR (17)	4-year	PDR in T1DM	2.9 (1.2, 6.8)	Age and sex
996 T1DM and 1,370 T2DM		PDR in T2DM	6.0 (1.1, 32.6)	
WESDR (9)	16-year	Mild NPDR	1.30 (0.92, 1.85)	Age, sex, diabetes duration, HbA1c, hypertension, urinary protein, CVD history, current smoking, pack-years smoked, diuretic use, history of tactile sensation loss
1,370 T2DM		Moderate NPDR	0.96 (0.51, 1.82)	
		PDR	1.88 (1.03, 3.43)	
		ME	1.17 (0.65, 2.10)	
WESDR (20)	20-year	DR severity	1.6 (1.1, 2.3)	Age, sex, hypertension, neuropathy, smoking, HbA1c, aspirin use, pulse pressure
996 T1DM				
ARIC (38)	8-year	Any DR	2.34 (1.13, 4.86)	Age, sex, race, study center, blood pressure, anti-hypertensive medications, fasting glucose, insulin use, diabetes duration, HDL and LDL cholesterols, smoking
1,617 T2DM		Mild DR	2.52 (1.16, 5.48)	
		MA	2.25 (1.03, 4.90)	
ARIC (40)	5-year	DR with WML	2.5 (1.5, 4.0)	Age, sex, race, blood pressure, smoking and vascular risk factors
1,684 with and without DM		DR with stroke	4.9 (2.0, 11.9)	
		DR and WML with stroke	18.1 (5.9, 55.4)	
WHO-MSVDD (21)	12-year	DR in T1DM men	1.5 (0.8, 3.0)	Age
1,126 T1DM		DR in T1DM women	1.3 (0.6, 2.8)	
			2.1 (1.4, 3.2)	
3,179 T2DM		DR in T2DM men	2.4 (1.6, 3.4)	
		DR in T2DM women		

WESDR Wisconsin Epidemiological Study of diabetic retinopathy, *ARIC* Atherosclerosis Risk in Communities Study, *WHO-MSVDD* World Health Organization Multinational Study of vascular disease in diabetes, *NPDR* Nonproliferative diabetic retinopathy, *PDR* Proliferative diabetic retinopathy, *CVD* Cardiovascular disease, *HbA1c* Glycosylated hemoglobin, *T1DM* Type 1 diabetes, *T2DM* Type 2 diabetes, *RR/HR (95% CI)* Relative risk or hazard rate ratio (95% confidence interval) contribution of small vessel disease (evident in the retina) in the pathogenesis of a wide spectrum of cerebrovascular conditions in persons with diabetes. In addition, because diabetic retinopathy is usually the end result of a disruption in the blood–retinal barrier, it is possible to infer that these cerebral conditions may also be related to breakdown of the blood–brain barrier *(49)*.

DIABETIC RETINOPATHY AND HEART DISEASE

Microvascular dysfunction is now recognized as an important pathogenic factor in the development of heart disease in persons with diabetes. However, similar to cerebral circulation, there are no simple and noninvasive techniques for the assessment of coronary microcirculation *(50)*, and studies that have traditionally evaluated the role of coronary microvascular dysfunction in diabetic heart disease have been limited by small clinic-based samples using highly specialized methods *(51–55)*.

More than two decades ago, the Framingham Heart and Eye Study proposed that retinopathy signs may reflect a generalized microangiopathic process that affects organs elsewhere in the body, such as the heart, in people with diabetes *(56)*. This hypothesis is consistent with earlier clinical studies based on ophthalmoscopic examinations linking retinopathy signs with ischemic T-wave changes on electrocardiogram *(57, 58)*, severity of coronary artery stenosis on angiography *(59)*, and more recently, with incident clinical coronary heart disease vents *(60)*.

Recent population-based studies using standardized photographic grading of retinopathy have produced stronger evidence in support of these previous observations. It is now clear that diabetic retinopathy signs are associated with risk of coronary heart disease and congestive heart failure (Table 4). In the ARIC study, the presence of retinopathy was associated with twofold higher risk of incident coronary heart disease, threefold higher risk of fatal coronary heart disease, and fourfold higher risk of congestive heart failure, independent of diabetes duration, glycemic control, smoking, lipid profile, and other risk factors *(61, 62)*. The population-attributable risk of retinopathy to congestive heart failure has been estimated to be 30.5% *(62)*. In addition, there is a graded, dose-dependent association of increasing diabetic retinopathy severity with increasing coronary heart disease risk *(61)*. These findings are consistent with data from the WHO-MSVDD *(21)* and other studies showing associations of not only NPDR but also PDR with coronary heart disease *(12, 63, 64)*.

As for associations with cardiovascular mortality and stroke, the association of retinopathy with coronary heart disease risk is not consistently present in younger persons with type 1 diabetes. In the WESDR type 1 diabetes cohort, while NPDR, PDR, and retinopathy severity were all associated with an excess risk of deaths from ischemic heart disease, ascertained from death certificates, these associations were not significant after adjusting for cardiovascular risk factors, including nephropathy *(9, 17, 20)*. The authors have suggested that misclassification of cause of death could have limited their study *(9)*. In the EURODIAB study of type 1 diabetes, retinopathy was also not significantly associated with incident CHD after multivariate analysis *(65)*.

Apart from epidemiological studies, there are clinical studies that suggest the presence of retinopathy can be used as an indicator of silent myocardial ischemia and help guide investigative approaches in diabetic patients with suspected heart disease *(66–71)*.

Table 4
Selected Studies on the Relationship of Diabetic Retinopathy and Heart Disease.

Study and population	*Follow-up*	*Retinal status*	*RR/HR (95% CI)*	*Adjusted covariates*
ARIC (61)	8-year	DR with any	2.07 (1.38, 3.11)	Age, sex, race, study center, fasting glucose, HbA1c,
1,524 T2DM		CHD event	3.35 (1.40, 8.01)	diabetes duration, blood pressure, antihypertensive,
		DR with fatal CHD	1.88 (1.06, 3.32)	smoking, BMI, lipid profile, nephropathy, carotid
		DR with MI	1.93 (1.17, 3.19)	intima-media thickness
		DR with cardiac revascularization		
ARIC (62) 627 T2DM	7-year	DR	4.32 (2.13, 8.76)	Age, sex, race, study center, education, blood pressure, antihypertensive, glucose, LDL, smoking, BMI
WHO-MSVDD (21)	12-year	DR in T1DM men	2.2 (1.2, 3.9)	Age
1,126 T1DM		DR in T1DM women	1.8 (1.0, 3.2)	
3,179 T2DM		DR in T2DM men	1.6 (1.2, 2.2)	
		DR in T2DM women	1.7 (1.2, 2.4)	
824 Finnish	18-year	NPDR	1.18 (0.74, 1.89)	Age, area of residence, HbA1c, smoking, hypertension,
T2DM (12)		PDR in men	2.54 (1.07–6.04)	cholesterol, HDL, diabetes duration, urinary protein
		NPDR in women	1.79 (1.13–2.85)	
		PDR in women	4.98 (2.06–12.06)	
1,040 Finnish	7-year	NPDR	1.38 (0.95, 2.00)	Age, area, sex, triglycerides, HbA1c, smoking, hyperten-
T2DM (63)		PDR	2.12 (1.02, 4.39)	sion, cholesterol, HDL, urinary protein
WESDR (9)	16-year	Mild NPDR	1.30 (0.92, 1.85)	Age, sex, diabetes duration, HbA1c, hypertension, urinary
1,370 T2DM		Moderate NPDR	1.26 (0.88, 1.80)	protein, CVD history, current smoking, pack-years
		PDR	1.43 (0.94, 2.17)	smoked, diuretic use, history of tactile sensation loss
		ME	1.10 (0.76, 1.58)	

WESDR (9) 996 T1DM	16-year	Mild NPDR	1.97 (0.44, 8.80)	Age, sex, diabetes duration, HbA1c, diastolic blood pressure, hypertension, urinary protein, CVD history, pack-years smoked, units of insulin, history of loss of temperature sensitivity
		Moderate NPDR	3.06 (0.65, 14.35)	
		PDR	3.00 (0.66, 13.61)	
		ME	0.84 (0.43, 1.66)	
WESDR (20) 996 T1DM	20-year	DR severity with angina	1.2 (1.0, 1.5)	Age, sex, hypertension, neuropathy, smoking, HbA1c, aspirin use, pulse pressure, (confounded by nephropathy)
		DR severity with MI	1.2 (1.0, 1.5)	
		DR severity with IHD	1.3 (1.1, 1.5)	

WESDR Wisconsin Epidemiological Study of diabetic retinopathy, *ARIC* Atherosclerosis Risk in Communities Study, *WHO-MSVDD* World Health Organization Multinational Study of vascular disease in diabetes, *NPDR* Nonproliferative diabetic retinopathy, *PDR* Proliferative diabetic retinopathy, *CVD* Cardiovascular disease, *T1DM* Type 1 diabetes, *T2DM* Type 2 diabetes, *RR/HR (95% CI)* Relative risk or hazard rate ratio (95% confidence interval), *BMI* Body mass index, *HbA1c* glycosylated hemoglobin

Furthermore, retinopathy may also be a valuable prognostic predictor for diabetic patients undergoing cardiac revascularization procedures. For instance, studies show that compared with patients without diabetic retinopathy, patients with retinopathy are more likely to sustain major adverse cardiac events or complications (e.g., death, myocardial infarction, heart failure, in-stent restenosis) after percutaneous coronary intervention or coronary artery bypass surgery, even after factoring effects of age, gender, diabetes duration, insulin use, and other factors that may affect prognosis after these procedures *(72–75)*. Thus, it may be useful to assess retinopathy status when making clinical decision regarding the need for revascularization in diabetic patients with established coronary heart disease *(76)*.

The associations of retinopathy with cardiac morbidity and mortality are consistent with other observations that diabetic retinopathy is associated with subclinical coronary micro- and macrovascular pathology. Studies showed that persons with retinopathy are more likely to have myocardial arteriolar abnormalities *(51)*, coronary perfusion defects *(71, 77, 78)*, poorer coronary flow reserve *(79)*, and lower coronary collateral score *(80)*, than those without retinopathy. The presence of retinopathy signs has also been associated with higher degrees of coronary artery calcification (unpublished data from the Multi-Ethnic Study of Atherosclerosis, Wong TY 2007) *(81)* and more diffuse/severe coronary artery stenosis on angiograms *(70)*, two robust measures of coronary atherosclerotic burden. Nevertheless, the fundamental question of whether the association of retinopathy with heart disease is driven by micro- or macrovascular disease remains unclear but it is likely that a mixture of micro- and macrovascular disease processes, mediated by common pathogenic pathways, contributes to the observed associations.

DIABETIC RETINOPATHY, NEPHROPATHY, AND NEUROPATHY

Nephropathy is another well-known microvascular complication of diabetes. Experimental studies show a high correlation of pathological changes in the retinal vasculature with those that occur in the renal vasculature *(82, 83)*. This is in keeping with epidemiological studies consistently demonstrating an association between diabetic retinopathy and nephropathy, independent of shared risk factors (Table 5). Studies of individuals with hypertension show that retinopathy signs are strongly related to microalbuminuria, a preclinical marker of renal dysfunction *(84)*. More recent studies of clinical kidney disease support this observation. In the WESDR, more severe diabetic retinopathy was associated with an increased 4-year risk of nephropathy in persons with type 1 diabetes *(17, 85)*. Moreover, the presence of specific retinopathy signs, such as retinal hemorrhages, microaneurysms, and cotton wool spots, was associated with higher risk of renal dysfunction, even in persons without clinical diabetes *(86)*. Similarly, in the Cardiovascular Health Study, the presence of retinopathy was independently associated with prevalent gross protenuria *(23)* and an increased risk of progression of renal impairment *(87)*. These findings suggest that retinopathy and nephropathy share pathogenic pathways (e.g., inflammation, endothelial dysfunction) and highlight the need to monitor renal function in diabetic persons with retinopathy.

There is also evidence that retinopathy may be related to risk of neuropathy in people with diabetes *(88, 89)* or abnormal glucose metabolism *(90)*. In a longitudinal study of

Table 5
Diabetic Retinopathy and Other Diabetic Microvascular Complications.

Study and population	*Design*	*Summary of results*
WESDR (85)	Prospective	DR was associated with declining renal function (reduced creatinine clearance) (RR 1.77–2.31 for NPDR and RR 3.18 for PDR)
765 T1DM	10-year follow-up	DR was associated with incident renal insufficiency (RR 9.54 for moderate NPDR and 24.73 for PDR)
ARIC (86) 1,338 T2DM	Cross-sectional	DR was associated with retinal dysfunction (OR 2.6; 95% CI: 1.6, 4.3), adjusted for age, sex, race, center, glucose, antihypertensive, blood pressure, BMI, smoking, alcohol, HDL, triglyceride
CHS (87) 1,394 with and without DM	Cross-sectional	DR was associated with progression of retinal impairment (4-year changes in creatinine and eGFR) (OR 3.20; 95% CI: 1.58, 6.50 for increased creatinine and OR 2.84; 95% CI: 1.56, 5.16 for reduced eGFR), adjusted for age, sex, race, weight, diabetes, hypertension, ACEi, proteinuria
CHS (23) 296 T2DM	Cross-sectional	DR was associated with gross proteinuria (OR 4.76; 95% CI: 1.53, 14.86), adjusted for age, sex, glucose, diabetes duration
AusDiab (90) 1,154 with IFG/IGT	Cross-sectional	DR was associated with neuropathy (OR 4.0; 95% CI: 1.8, 9.0), adjusted for age, sex, hypertension, cholesterol, lipid-lowering medication, micro/macroalbuminuria

WESDR Wisconsin Epidemiological Study of diabetic retinopathy, *ARIC* Atherosclerosis Risk in Communities Study, *CHS* Cardiovascular Health Study, *AusDiab* Australian Diabetes Obesity and Lifestyle Study, *IFG* impaired fasting glucose, *IGT* impaired glucose tolerance, *OR* Odds ratio, *RR* Relative risk, *CI* Confidence interval, *DR* Diabetic retinopathy

264 diabetic individuals, the presence of more severe microvascular diseases, including retinopathy, was associated with more severe diabetic polyneuropathy. Recently, the Australian Diabetes Obesity and Lifestyle Study, a population-based study of Australian adults aged 25 years or more, reported a strong association between retinopathy and neuropathy in persons without clinical diabetes but with abnormal glucose metabolism *(90)*. Furthermore, in the WESDR, participants with PDR had a higher risk of incident lower leg amputation, a complication of diabetic peripheral neuropathy, as compared to those with no or minimal retinopathy at baseline *(17)*.

PATHOGENIC BASIS BETWEEN DIABETIC RETINOPATHY AND SYSTEMIC DISEASE

Although epidemiological and clinical studies have now clearly demonstrated associations of diabetic retinopathy with a range of systemic complications, the exact underlying pathophysiological mechanisms remain unclear. In part, this is due to several unresolved issues regarding the basic pathogenesis of diabetic retinopathy *(1)*.

Nonetheless, several mechanisms have been hypothesized. First, the excess risk of systemic complications in persons with diabetic retinopathy has been suggested to be due to the more adverse cardiovascular profile in diabetic individuals. However, most studies have accounted in statistical analyses for the potential confounding effects of cardiovascular risk factors.

Second, it is important to note that diabetic retinopathy is related not only to microvascular complications (e.g., nephropathy), but also macrovascular diseases. For example, retinopathy has been associated with several direct measures of atherosclerosis, including carotid artery intima-media thickness or carotid plaque, arterial stiffness (a measure of early atherosclerosis), coronary artery calcification, as well as atherosclerotic lesions detected on angiograms *(23, 41, 70, 81, 91)*. This later observation raises the possibility that common pathophysiological processes may underlie the development of both micro- and macrovascular disease in diabetes. These common pathways may include inflammation, endothelial dysfunction, and advanced glycation end products *(10, 61, 92)*.

Third, it has been suggested, based on the Steno hypothesis, that retinopathy may reflect generalized vascular dysfunction caused by endothelial dysfunction *(93)* and genetically determined alterations in the basement membrane metabolism *(94)* associated with hyperglycemia. These diabetic vascular insults increase arterial/arteriolar wall permeability and leakage. In small arteriolar/capillary beds, retinopathy and nephropathy develop as a result. In large arterial wall, increased permeability facilitates entry and accumulation of lipids, thus promoting the pathogenic cascade of atherosclerosis formation. Such hypothesis, though attractive, remains to be further validated.

CLINICAL SIGNIFICANCE OF RETINOPATHY IN SYSTEMIC DISEASE SCREENING

The relationships of diabetic retinopathy with systemic vascular diseases are clinically important to ophthalmologists and other healthcare providers who treat and counsel patients with diabetes. Current cardiovascular risk prediction for diabetic populations is inaccurate *(95–97)*. As a recent systematic review of data from more than 70,000 participants shows, the Framingham risk scores significantly underestimate the absolute risk of cardiovascular disease in diabetic populations *(95)*. Clearly, there is need to search for more specific predictor for cardiovascular disease risk in people with diabetes. There is now good evidence that retinopathy, reliably detectable from retinal photographs, is an early marker of subclinical vascular disease and a strong independent predictor of clinical cardiovascular events. Thus, incorporating retinopathy into the currently available risk prediction tools *(98, 99)* may refine cardiovascular disease prediction in asymptomatic persons with diabetes. Retinopathy has already been proposed to be used in clinical settings to guide preoperative assessment and counseling of diabetic patients planning for elective cardiac revascularization procedures *(72–76)*.

Apart from people with diabetes, there is emerging evidence that classical signs of early "diabetic" retinopathy (e.g., microaneurysms, retinal hemorrhages, and cotton wool spots) are relatively common even in people without clinically diagnosed diabetes *(100, 101)*. Studies have reported high prevalence (up to 14%) and incidence (6–10%) rates of these retinopathy lesions in nondiabetic general populations *(102, 103)*. Retinopathy signs in people without diabetes have also been associated with an increased risk of stroke *(39, 43, 104)*, ischemic heart disease *(105)*, congestive heart failure *(62)*, and impaired renal function *(86, 87)*; and may also indicate a greater risk of hypertension and an excess risk of future diabetes *(106)*, particularly if there is a family history of diabetes *(107, 108)*. These "nondiabetic" retinopathy signs may therefore reflect masked abnormalities in glucose metabolism, blood pressure regulation, and other processes. Additional research is needed to delineate further the pathogenic basis and clinical significance of retinopathy signs in nondiabetic individuals.

CONCLUSION

Diabetic retinopathy is a common microvascular complication in the eyes of diabetic individuals *(109)*. Besides its serious threat to vision, the presence of retinopathy also signifies an excess risk of morbidity and mortality attributable to systemic micro- and macrovascular disease. It is increasingly clear that retinopathy may reflect diabetic vascular injury not only in the eyes but also in the other organs such as the brain (stroke), heart (coronary heart disease, heart failure), and kidneys (renal dysfunction). Studying these retinopathy lesions provides a unique channel to further our understanding of the pathogenesis of various systemic diseases in diabetes, and early detection of retinopathy may also offer a means to implement therapeutic measures that can prevent the development or halt the progression of these systemic complications. For ophthalmologists and other eye care providers, it is therefore important not to overlook the broader clinical implications of retinopathy beyond the eyes of their diabetic patients.

REFERENCES

1. Frank RN. Diabetic retinopathy. *N Engl J Med* 2004;**350**(1):48–58
2. Wong TY, Klein R, Klein BE, Tielsch JM, Hubbard L, Nieto FJ. Retinal microvascular abnormalities and their relationship with hypertension, cardiovascular disease, and mortality. *Surv Ophthalmol* 2001;**46**(1):59–80
3. Wong TY, Mitchell P. Hypertensive retinopathy. *N Engl J Med* 2004;**351**(22):2310–7

4. Wong TY, McIntosh R. Hypertensive retinopathy signs as risk indicators of cardiovascular morbidity and mortality. *Br Med Bull* 2005;**73–74**:57–70
5. Wong TY, McIntosh R. Systemic associations of retinal microvascular signs: A review of recent population-based studies. *Ophthalmic Physiol Opt* 2005;**25**(3):195–204
6. St Clair L, Ballantyne CM. Biological surrogates for enhancing cardiovascular risk prediction in type 2 diabetes mellitus. *Am J Cardiol* 2007;**99**(4A):80B–88B
7. Nguyen TT, Wong TY. Retinal vascular manifestations of metabolic disorders. *Trends Endocrinol Metab* 2006;**17**(7):262–8
8. Cheung N, Wong TY. Retinal vascular changes as biomarkers of systemic cardiovascular diseases. In: Jelinek Hand Cree M (eds). Automated image detection of retinal pathology (In press)
9. Klein R, Klein BE, Moss SE, Cruickshanks KJ. Association of ocular disease and mortality in a diabetic population. *Arch Ophthalmol* 1999;**117**(11):1487–95
10. Van Hecke MV, Dekker JM, Nijpels G, et al. Retinopathy is associated with cardiovascular and all-cause mortality in both diabetic and nondiabetic subjects: The hoorn study. *Diabetes Care* 2003;**26**(10):2958
11. Henricsson M, Nilsson A, Heijl A, Janzon L, Groop L. Mortality in diabetic patients participating in an ophthalmological control and screening programme. *Diabet Med* 1997;**14**(7):576–83
12. Juutilainen A, Lehto S, Ronnemaa T, Pyorala K, Laakso M. Retinopathy predicts cardiovascular mortality in type 2 diabetic men and women. *Diabetes Care* 2007;**30**(2):292–9
13. Rajala U, Pajunpaa H, Koskela P, Keinanen-Kiukaanniemi S. High cardiovascular disease mortality in subjects with visual impairment caused by diabetic retinopathy. *Diabetes Care* 2000;**23**(7):957–61
14. Cusick M, Meleth AD, Agron E, et al. Associations of mortality and diabetes complications in patients with type 1 and type 2 diabetes: Early treatment diabetic retinopathy study report no. 27. *Diabetes Care* 2005;**28**(3):617–25
15. Sasaki A, Uehara M, Horiuchi N, Hasegawa K, Shimizu T. A 15-year follow-up study of patients with non-insulin-dependent diabetes mellitus (NIDDM) in Osaka, Japan. Factors predictive of the prognosis of diabetic patients. *Diabetes Res Clin Pract* 1997;**36**(1):41–7
16. Hanis CL, Chu HH, Lawson K, et al. Mortality of Mexican Americans with NIDDM. Retinopathy and other predictors in Starr County, Texas. *Diabetes Care* 1993;**16**(1):82–9
17. Klein R, Klein BE, Moss SE. Epidemiology of proliferative diabetic retinopathy. *Diabetes Care* 1992;**15**(12):1875–91
18. van Hecke MV, Dekker JM, Stehouwer CD, et al. Diabetic retinopathy is associated with mortality and cardiovascular disease incidence: The EURODIAB prospective complications study. *Diabetes Care* 2005;**28**(6):1383–9
19. Torffvit O, Lovestam-Adrian M, Agardh E, Agardh CD. Nephropathy, but not retinopathy, is associated with the development of heart disease in Type 1 diabetes: A 12-year observation study of 462 patients. *Diabet Med* 2005;**22**(6):723–9
20. Klein BE, Klein R, McBride PE, et al. Cardiovascular disease, mortality, and retinal microvascular characteristics in type 1 diabetes: Wisconsin epidemiologic study of diabetic retinopathy. *Arch Intern Med* 2004;**164**(17):1917–24
21. Fuller JH, Stevens LK, Wang SL. Risk factors for cardiovascular mortality and morbidity: The WHO Multinational Study of Vascular Disease in Diabetes. *Diabetologia* 2001;**44**(Suppl 2):S54–64
22. Targher G, Bertolini L, Tessari R, Zenari L, Arcaro G. Retinopathy predicts future cardiovascular events among type 2 diabetic patients: The Valpolicella Heart Diabetes Study. *Diabetes Care* 2006;**29**(5):1178
23. Klein R, Marino EK, Kuller LH, et al. The relation of atherosclerotic cardiovascular disease to retinopathy in people with diabetes in the Cardiovascular Health Study. *Br J Ophthalmol* 2002;**86**(1):84–90
24. Jager A, van Hinsbergh VW, Kostense PJ, et al. Prognostic implications of retinopathy and a high plasma von Willebrand factor concentration in type 2 diabetic subjects with microalbuminuria. *Nephrol Dial Transplant* 2001;**16**(3):529–36
25. Greenberg SM. Small vessels, big problems. *N Engl J Med* 2006;**354**(14):1451–3
26. Alex M, Baron EK, Goldenberg S, Blumenthal HT. An autopsy study of cerebrovascular accident in diabetes mellitus. *Circulation* 1962;**25**:663–73

27. Aronson SM. Intracranial vascular lesions in patients with diabetes mellitus. *J Neuropathol Exp Neurol* 1973;**32**(2):183–96
28. Bell DS. Stroke in the diabetic patient. *Diabetes Care* 1994;**17**(3):213–9
29. Wong TY. Is retinal photography useful in the measurement of stroke risk? *Lancet Neurol* 2004;**3**(3):179–83
30. Patton N, Aslam T, Macgillivray T, Pattie A, Deary IJ, Dhillon B. Retinal vascular image analysis as a potential screening tool for cerebrovascular disease: A rationale based on homology between cerebral and retinal microvasculatures. *J Anat* 2005;**206**(4):319–48
31. Okada H, Horibe H, Yoshiyuki O, Hayakawa N, Aoki N. A prospective study of cerebrovascular disease in Japanese rural communities, Akabane and Asahi. Part 1: Evaluation of risk factors in the occurrence of cerebral hemorrhage and thrombosis. *Stroke* 1976;**7**(6):599–607
32. Tanaka H, Hayashi M, Date C, et al. Epidemiologic studies of stroke in Shibata, a Japanese provincial city: Preliminary report on risk factors for cerebral infarction. *Stroke* 1985;**16**(5):773–80
33. Svardsudd K, Wedel H, Aurell E, Tibblin G. Hypertensive eye ground changes. Prevalence, relation to blood pressure and prognostic importance. The study of men born in 1913. *Acta Med Scand* 1978;**204**(3):159–67
34. Nakayama T, Date C, Yokoyama T, Yoshiike N, Yamaguchi M, Tanaka H. A 15.5-year follow-up study of stroke in a Japanese provincial city. The Shibata Study. *Stroke* 1997;**28**(1):45–52
35. Goto I, Katsuki S, Ikui H, Kimoto K, Mimatsu T. Pathological studies on the intracerebral and retinal arteries in cerebrovascular and noncerebrovascular diseases. *Stroke* 1975;**6**(3):263–9
36. Schneider R, Rademacher M, Wolf S. Lacunar infarcts and white matter attenuation. Ophthalmologic and microcirculatory aspects of the pathophysiology. *Stroke* 1993;**24**(12):1874–9
37. Petitti DB, Bhatt H. Retinopathy as a risk factor for nonembolic stroke in diabetic subjects. *Stroke* 1995;**26**(4):593–6
38. Cheung N, Rogers S, Couper DJ, Klein R, Sharrett AR, Wong TY. Is diabetic retinopathy an independent risk factor for ischemic stroke? *Stroke* 2006;**38**(2):398–401
39. Wong TY, Klein R, Couper DJ, et al. Retinal microvascular abnormalities and incident stroke: The Atherosclerosis Risk in Communities Study. *Lancet* 2001;**358**(9288):1134–40
40. Wong TY, Klein R, Sharrett AR, et al. Cerebral white matter lesions, retinopathy, and incident clinical stroke. *J Am Med Assoc* 2002;**288**(1):67–74
41. Wong TY, Klein R, Sharrett AR, et al. The prevalence and risk factors of retinal microvascular abnormalities in older persons: The Cardiovascular Health Study. *Ophthalmology* 2003;**110**(4):658–66
42. Wong TY, Klein R, Nieto FJ, et al. Retinal microvascular abnormalities and 10-year cardiovascular mortality: A population-based case–control study. *Ophthalmology* 2003;**110**(5):933–40
43. Mitchell P, Wang JJ, Wong TY, Smith W, Klein R, Leeder SR. Retinal microvascular signs and risk of stroke and stroke mortality. *Neurology* 2005;**65**(7):1005–9
44. Wong TY, Barr EL, Tapp RJ, et al. Retinopathy in persons with impaired glucose metabolism: The Australian Diabetes Obesity and Lifestyle (AusDiab) study. *Am J Ophthalmol* 2005;**140**(6):1157–9
45. Wong TY, Klein R, Sharrett AR, et al. Retinal microvascular abnormalities and cognitive impairment in middle-aged persons: The Atherosclerosis Risk in Communities Study. *Stroke* 2002;**33**(6):1487–92
46. Wong TY, Mosley TH, Jr., Klein R, et al. Retinal microvascular changes and MRI signs of cerebral atrophy in healthy, middle-aged people. *Neurology* 2003;**61**(6):806–11
47. Tekin O, Cukur S, Uraldi C, et al. Relationship between retinopathy and cognitive impairment among hypertensive subjects. A case–control study in the ankara-pursaklar region. *Eur Neurol* 2004;**52**(3):156–61
48. Baker ML, Larsen EK, Kuller LH, et al. Retinal microvascular signs, cognitive function, and dementia in older persons. The Cardiovascular Health Study. *Stroke* 2007;**38**:2041
49. Wardlaw JM, Sandercock PA, Dennis MS, Starr J. Is breakdown of the blood–brain barrier responsible for lacunar stroke, leukoaraiosis, and dementia? *Stroke* 2003;**34**(3):806–12
50. Duran JR, 3rd, Taffet G. Coronary microvascular dysfunction. *N Engl J Med* 2007;**356**(22):2324–5; author reply 2325
51. Factor SM, Okun EM, Minase T. Capillary microaneurysms in the human diabetic heart. *N Engl J Med* 1980;**302**(7):384–8
52. Di Carli MF, Janisse J, Grunberger G, Ager J. Role of chronic hyperglycemia in the pathogenesis of coronary microvascular dysfunction in diabetes. *J Am Coll Cardiol* 2003;**41**(8):1387–93

53. Miura H, Wachtel RE, Loberiza FR, Jr., et al. Diabetes mellitus impairs vasodilation to hypoxia in human coronary arterioles: Reduced activity of ATP-sensitive potassium channels. *Circ Res* 2003;**92**(2):151–8
54. Li Q, Wang J, Sun Y, et al. Efficacy of postoperative transarterial chemoembolization and portal vein chemotherapy for patients with hepatocellular carcinoma complicated by portal vein tumor thrombosis – a randomized study. *World J Surg* 2006;**30**(11):2004–11; discussion 2012–3
55. Pitkanen OP, Nuutila P, Raitakari OT, et al. Coronary flow reserve is reduced in young men with IDDM. *Diabetes* 1998;**47**(2):248–54
56. Hiller R, Sperduto RD, Podgor MJ, Ferris FL, 3rd, Wilson PW. Diabetic retinopathy and cardiovascular disease in type II diabetics. The Framingham Heart Study and the Framingham Eye Study. *Am J Epidemiol* 1988;**128**(2):402–9
57. Breslin DJ, Gifford RW, Jr., Fairbairn JF, 2nd, Kearns TP. Prognostic importance of ophthalmoscopic findings in essential hypertension. *J Am Med Assoc* 1966;**195**(5):335–8
58. Breslin DJ, Gifford RW, Jr., Fairbairn JF, 2nd. Essential hypertension. A twenty-year follow-up study. *Circulation* 1966;**33**(1):87–97
59. Michelson EL, Morganroth J, Nichols CW, MacVaugh H, 3rd. Retinal arteriolar changes as an indicator of coronary artery disease. *Arch Intern Med* 1979;**139**(10):1139–41
60. Duncan BB, Wong TY, Tyroler HA, Davis CE, Fuchs FD. Hypertensive retinopathy and incident coronary heart disease in high risk men. *Br J Ophthalmol* 2002;**86**(9):1002–6
61. Cheung N, Wang JJ, Klein R, Couper DJ, Richey Sharrett AR, Wong TY. diabetic retinopathy and the risk of coronary heart disease: The Atherosclerosis risk in communities study. *Diabetes Care* 2007;**30**:1742–6
62. Wong TY, Rosamond W, Chang PP, et al. Retinopathy and risk of congestive heart failure. *J Am Med Assoc* 2005;**293**(1):63–9
63. Miettinen H, Haffner SM, Lehto S, Ronnemaa T, Pyorala K, Laakso M. Retinopathy predicts coronary heart disease events in NIDDM patients. *Diabetes Care* 1996;**19**(12):1445–8
64. Faglia E, Favales F, Calia P, et al. Cardiac events in 735 type 2 diabetic patients who underwent screening for unknown asymptomatic coronary heart disease: 5-year follow-up report from the Milan Study on Atherosclerosis and Diabetes (MiSAD). *Diabetes Care* 2002;**25**(11):2032–6
65. Soedamah-Muthu SS, Chaturvedi N, Toeller M, et al. Risk factors for coronary heart disease in type 1 diabetic patients in Europe: The EURODIAB Prospective Complications Study. *Diabetes Care* 2004;**27**(2):530–7
66. Araz M, Celen Z, Akdemir I, Okan V. Frequency of silent myocardial ischemia in type 2 diabetic patients and the relation with poor glycemic control. *Acta Diabetol* 2004;**41**(2):38–43
67. Gokcel A, Aydin M, Yalcin F, et al. Silent coronary artery disease in patients with type 2 diabetes mellitus. *Acta Diabetol* 2003;**40**(4):176–80
68. Janand-Delenne B, Savin B, Habib G, Bory M, Vague P, Lassmann-Vague V. Silent myocardial ischemia in patients with diabetes: Who to screen. *Diabetes Care* 1999;**22**(9):1396–400
69. Naka M, Hiramatsu K, Aizawa T, et al. Silent myocardial ischemia in patients with non-insulin-dependent diabetes mellitus as judged by treadmill exercise testing and coronary angiography. *Am Heart J* 1992;**123**(1):46–53
70. Norgaz T, Hobikoglu G, Aksu H, et al. Retinopathy is related to the angiographically detected severity and extent of coronary artery disease in patients with type 2 diabetes mellitus. *Int Heart J* 2005;**46**(4):639–46
71. Yoon JK, Lee KH, Park JM, et al. Usefulness of diabetic retinopathy as a marker of risk for thallium myocardial perfusion defects in non-insulin-dependent diabetes mellitus. *Am J Cardiol* 2001;**87**(4):456–9, A6
72. Briguori C, Condorelli G, Airoldi F, et al. Impact of microvascular complications on outcome after coronary stent implantations in patients with diabetes. *J Am Coll Cardiol* 2005;**45**(3):464–6
73. Kim YH, Hong MK, Song JM, et al. Diabetic retinopathy as a predictor of late clinical events following percutaneous coronary intervention. *J Invasive Cardiol* 2002;**14**(10):599–602
74. Ono T, Kobayashi J, Sasako Y, et al. The impact of diabetic retinopathy on long-term outcome following coronary artery bypass graft surgery. *J Am Coll Cardiol* 2002;**40**(3):428–36
75. Ono T, Ohashi T, Asakura T, et al. Impact of diabetic retinopathy on cardiac outcome after coronary artery bypass graft surgery: Prospective observational study. *Ann Thorac Surg* 2006;**81**(2):608–12
76. Ohno T, Ando J, Ono M, et al. The beneficial effect of coronary-artery-bypass surgery on survival in patients with diabetic retinopathy. *Eur J Cardiothorac Surg* 2006;**30**(6):881–6

77. Giugliano D, Acampora R, De Rosa N, et al. Coronary artery disease in type-2 diabetes mellitus: A scintigraphic study. *Diabete Metab* 1993;**19**(5):463–6
78. Ioannidis G, Peppa M, Rontogianni P, et al. The concurrence of microalbuminuria and retinopathy with cardiovascular risk factors; reliable predictors of asymptomatic coronary artery disease in type 2 diabetes. *Hormones (Athens)* 2004;**3**(3):198–203
79. Akasaka T, Yoshida K, Hozumi T, et al. Retinopathy identifies marked restriction of coronary flow reserve in patients with diabetes mellitus. *J Am Coll Cardiol* 1997;**30**(4):935–41
80. Celik T, Berdan ME, Iyisoy A, et al. Impaired coronary collateral vessel development in patients with proliferative diabetic retinopathy. *Clin Cardiol* 2005;**28**(8):384–8
81. Yoshida M, Takamatsu J, Yoshida S, et al. Scores of coronary calcification determined by electron beam computed tomography are closely related to the extent of diabetes-specific complications. *Horm Metab Res* 1999;**31**(10):558–63
82. Nag S, Robertson DM, Dinsdale HB. Morphological changes in spontaneously hypertensive rats. *Acta Neuropathol (Berl)* 1980;**52**(1):27–34
83. Chavers BM, Mauer SM, Ramsay RC, Steffes MW. Relationship between retinal and glomerular lesions in IDDM patients. *Diabetes* 1994;**43**(3):441–6
84. Pontremoli R, Cheli V, Sofia A, et al. Prevalence of micro- and macroalbuminuria and their relationship with other cardiovascular risk factors in essential hypertension. *Nephrol Dial Transplant* 1995;**10**(Suppl 6):6–9
85. Klein R, Klein BE, Moss SE, Cruickshanks KJ, Brazy PC. The 10-year incidence of renal insufficiency in people with type 1 diabetes. *Diabetes Care* 1999;**22**(5):743–51
86. Wong TY, Coresh J, Klein R, et al. Retinal microvascular abnormalities and renal dysfunction: The atherosclerosis risk in communities study. *J Am Soc Nephrol* 2004;**15**(9):2469–76
87. Edwards MS, Wilson DB, Craven TE, et al. Associations between retinal microvascular abnormalities and declining renal function in the elderly population: The Cardiovascular Health Study. *Am J Kidney Dis* 2005;**46**(2):214–24
88. Dyck PJ, Davies JL, Wilson DM, Service FJ, Melton LJ, 3rd, O'Brien PC. Risk factors for severity of diabetic polyneuropathy: Intensive longitudinal assessment of the Rochester Diabetic Neuropathy Study cohort. *Diabetes Care* 1999;**22**(9):1479–86
89. Savage S, Estacio RO, Jeffers B, Schrier RW. Urinary albumin excretion as a predictor of diabetic retinopathy, neuropathy, and cardiovascular disease in NIDDM. *Diabetes Care* 1996;**19**(11):1243–8
90. Barr EL, Wong TY, Tapp RJ, et al. Is peripheral neuropathy associated with retinopathy and albuminuria in individuals with impaired glucose metabolism? The 1999–2000 AusDiab. *Diabetes Care* 2006;**29**(5):1114–6
91. Rema M, Mohan V, Deepa R, Ravikumar R. Association of carotid intima-media thickness and arterial stiffness with diabetic retinopathy: The Chennai Urban Rural Epidemiology Study (CURES-2). *Diabetes Care* 2004;**27**(8):1962–7
92. Goldin A, Beckman JA, Schmidt AM, Creager MA. Advanced glycation end products: Sparking the development of diabetic vascular injury. *Circulation* 2006;**114**(6):597–605
93. Parving HH, Nielsen FS, Bang LE, et al. Macro-microangiopathy and endothelial dysfunction in NIDDM patients with and without diabetic nephropathy. *Diabetologia* 1996;**39**(12):1590–7
94. Deckert T, Feldt-Rasmussen B, Borch-Johnsen K, Jensen T, Kofoed-Enevoldsen A. Albuminuria reflects widespread vascular damage. The Steno hypothesis. *Diabetologia* 1989;**32**(4):219–26
95. Brindle P, May M, Gill P, et al. Primary prevention of cardiovascular disease: A web-based risk score for seven British black and minority ethnic groups. *Heart* 2006;**92**(11):1595–602
96. Stephens JW, Ambler G, Vallance P, Betteridge DJ, Humphries SE, Hurel SJ. Cardiovascular risk and diabetes. Are the methods of risk prediction satisfactory? *Eur J Cardiovasc Prev Rehabil* 2004;**11**(6):521–8
97. Guzder RN, Gatling W, Mullee MA, Mehta RL, Byrne CD. Prognostic value of the Framingham cardiovascular risk equation and the UKPDS risk engine for coronary heart disease in newly diagnosed Type 2 diabetes: Results from a United Kingdom study. *Diabet Med* 2005;**22**(5):554–62
98. Lee ET, Howard BV, Wang W, et al. Prediction of coronary heart disease in a population with high prevalence of diabetes and albuminuria: The Strong Heart Study. *Circulation* 2006;**113**(25):2897–905
99. Donnan PT, Donnelly L, New JP, Morris AD. Derivation and validation of a prediction score for major coronary heart disease events in a U.K. Type 2 diabetic population. *Diabetes Care* 2006;**29**(6):1231–6

100. Wong TY, Klein R, Klein BEK. The epidemiology of diabetic retinopathy. In: Scott I, Harry Flynn H, Smiddy W (eds). Diabetic Retinopathy. Oxford University Press (In press)
101. Wong TY, Klein R. The epidemiology of eye diseases in diabetes. In: Ekoe JM, Zimmet P, Williams R, Rewers M (eds). The Epidemiology of Diabetes Mellitus. John Wiley and Sons (In press)
102. Cugati S, Cikamatana L, Wang JJ, Kifley A, Liew G, Mitchell P. Five-year incidence and progression of vascular retinopathy in persons without diabetes: The Blue Mountains Eye Study. *Eye* 2006;**20**(11):1239–45
103. Klein R, Klein BE, Moss SE. The relation of systemic hypertension to changes in the retinal vasculature: The Beaver Dam Eye Study. *Trans Am Ophthalmol Soc* 1997;**95**:329–48; discussion 348–50
104. Cooper LS, Wong TY, Klein R, et al. Retinal microvascular abnormalities and MRI-defined subclinical cerebral infarction: The Atherosclerosis Risk in Communities Study. *Stroke* 2006;**37**(1):82–6
105. Hirai FE, Moss SE, Knudtson MD, Klein BE, Klein R. Retinopathy and survival in a population without diabetes: The Beaver Dam Eye Study. *Am J Epidemiol* 2007;**166**(6):724–30
106. Klein R, Klein BE, Moss SE, Wong TY. The relationship of retinopathy in persons without diabetes to the 15-year incidence of diabetes and hypertension: Beaver Dam Eye Study. *Trans Am Ophthalmol Soc* 2006;**104**:98–107
107. Wong TY, Mohamed Q, Klein R, Couper DJ. Do retinopathy signs in non-diabetic individuals predict the subsequent risk of diabetes? *Br J Ophthalmol* 2006;**90**(3):301–3
108. Cugati S, Mitchell P, Wang JJ. Do retinopathy signs in non-diabetic individuals predict the subsequent risk of diabetes? *Br J Ophthalmol* 2006;**90**(7):928–9
109. Hubbard LD, Brothers RJ, King WN, et al. Methods for evaluation of retinal microvascular abnormalities associated with hypertension/sclerosis in the Atherosclerosis Risk in Communities Study. *Ophthalmology* 1999;**106**(12):2269–80

Subject Index

W

X

Z